Atlas of Diagnostic and Therapeutic Gastrointestinal Endoscopy

-ASGE AudioVisual Award Winner & Recipient (2006-2010)-

Joo Young Cho, M.D. Ph D.

Institute for Digestive Research, Digestive Disease Center,
Soonchunhyang University, College of Medicine,
Seoul, Republic of Korea

This textbook is dedicated to our family

Therapeutic endoscopy ; ASGE audiovisual awards(2006~2010)

First published 2011 by Sohn poong sam the President of Soonchunhyang University

Soonchunhyang University Publication Department

646 Sinchang-myeon, Asan-si, Chungcheongnam-do, SEOUL 336-745 KOREA)

tel : 82-41-530-1115
fax : 82-41-530-1719
www.sch.ac.kr

ISBN : 978-89-964627-9-7-93510
Price : ₩ 30,000

Contributors

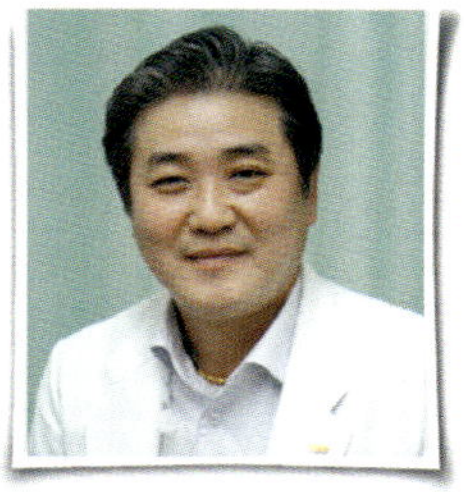

Joo Young Cho, M.D. Ph D.

Institute for Digestive Research, Digestive Disease Center, Soonchunhyang University, College of Medicine, Seoul, Republic of Korea

Specialty: Upper gastrointestinal tract (ESD and NOTES)

E-mail: schcjy@schmc.ac.kr

2006 ASGE Audiovisual Award Recipient

2007 ASGE Audiovisual Award Recipient

2008 ASGE Audiovisual Award Recipient

2009 ASGE Audiovisual Award Winner

2010 ASGE Audiovisual Award Winner

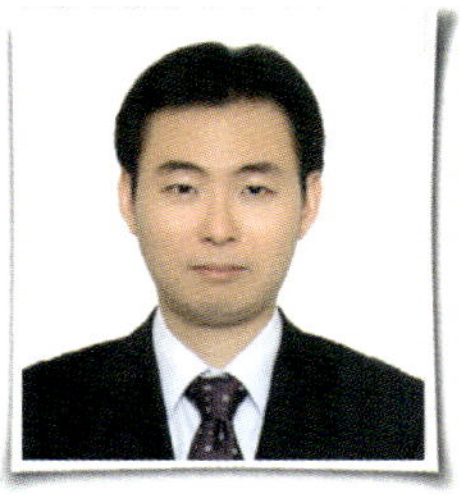

Tae Hee Lee, M.D.

Institute for Digestive Research, Digestive Disease Center, Soonchunhyang University, College of Medicine, Seoul, Republic of Korea

Specialty: Functional gastrointestinal disorders and EUS

E-mail: iman0825@ schmc.ac.kr

2008 ASGE Audiovisual Award Recipient

2010 ASGE Audiovisual Award Winner

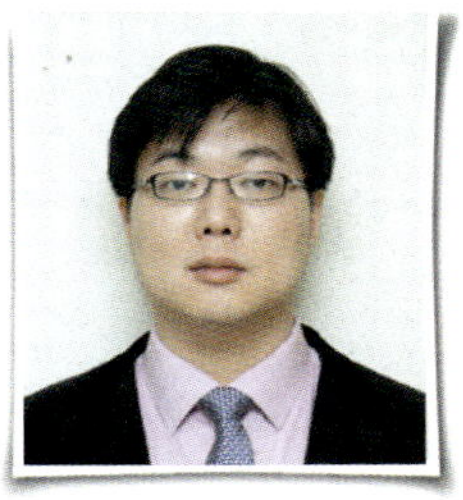

Won Young Cho, M.D. Ph D.

Institute for Digestive Research, Digestive Disease Center, Soonchunhyang University, College of Medicine, Seoul, Republic of Korea

Specialty: Upper gastrointestinal tract (ESD and NOTES)

E-mail: wychomd@ schmc.ac.kr

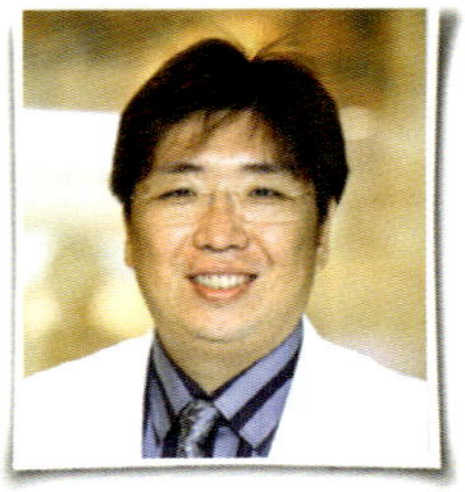

Jae Young Jang, M.D. Ph D.

Institute for Digestive Research, Digestive Disease Center, Soonchunhyang University, College of Medicine, Seoul, Republic of Korea

Specialty: Liver

E-mail: jyjang@schmc.ac.kr

2009 ASGE Audiovisual Award Winner

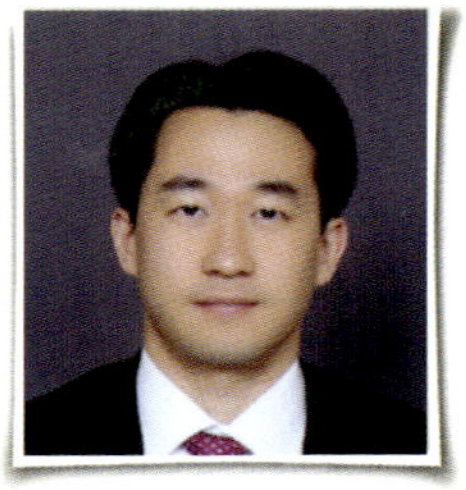

Soung Won Jeong, M.D. Ph D.

Institute for Digestive Research, Digestive Disease Center, Soonchunhyang University, College of Medicine, Seoul, Republic of Korea

Specialty: Liver

E-mail: jeongsw@schmc.ac.kr

2009 ASGE Audiovisual Award Winner

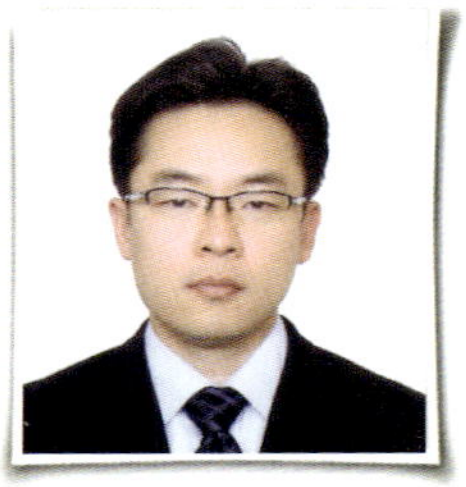

Hyun Gun Kim, M.D. Ph D.

Institute for Digestive Research, Digestive Disease Center, Soonchunhyang University, College of Medicine, Seoul, Republic of Korea

Specialty: colon

E-mail: medgun@schmc.ac.kr

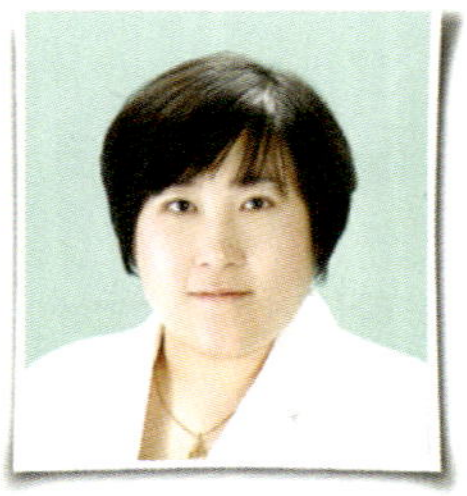

Youn Sun Park, M.D. Ph D.

Institute for Digestive Research, Digestive Disease Center, Soonchunhyang University, College of Medicine, Seoul, Republic of Korea

Specialty: Upper gastrointestinal tract

E-mail: younsun@schmc.ac.kr

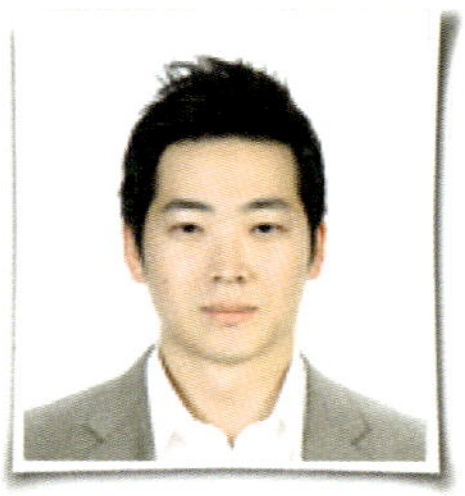

Gene Hyun Bok, M.D.

Institute for Digestive Research, Digestive Disease Center, Soonchunhyang University, College of Medicine, Seoul, Republic of Korea

E-mail: genehyun@hanmail.net

Preface

It is a great pleasure for me and my colleagues to present this colored atlas of the American society of gastroenterology (ASGE) 'Audio Visual Awards' that were presented to our department. The Annual ASGE Audiovisual Award is given to outstanding educational video productions relating to GI endoscopy techniques. From 2006 to 2010 our department has won 5 consecutive awards including 2 winners in 2009 and 2010. These programs consist of comprehensive reviews and practical suggestions for the endoscopic treatment of GI disorders ranging from benign diseases such as GI bleeding to early cancer of the GI tract.

Endoscopy is a dynamic area where new methods are introduced continuously. It is my hope that this material will enable future endoscopists to gain a new perspective and continue to challenge the boundaries of the field.

I would also like to acknowledge professor Tae Hee Lee, Won Young Cho, Jae Young Jang, Gene Hyun Bok, Soung Won Jeong, Hyun Gun Kim, Youn Sun Park, ASGE, and PENTAX KOREA. Without their dedication and inspiration, this atlas and the awards would not be possible.

Joo Yonug Cho
2011. 3. 30

Foreword

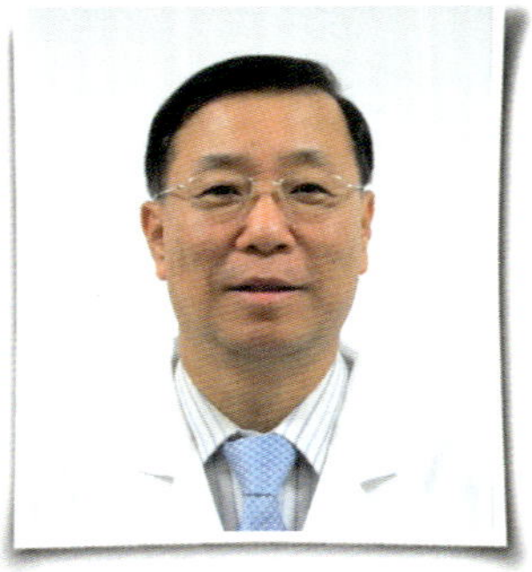

Endoscopic procedure, both therapeutic and diagnostic, is one of the fastest developing fields in medicine today. With new techniques and cutting edge technology being introduced continuously, it is difficult to keep up with all the information, and even more difficult to acquire the procedural skills needed to perform endoscopic procedures. This colored atlas presents a comprehensive review of advanced endoscopic techniques as well as indications and useful tips for beginners and expert endoscopists alike.

Dr. Cho and his team of expert endoscopists have gained international acknowledgement for their educational endoscopy guideline presentations. This atlas will not only inform the readers of current endoscopic trends, but will also provide insightful information on endoscopic techniques easily overlooked, and commonly encountered problems during endoscopic procedures.

Prof. Young Woon Chang
Department of Internal Medicine,
Kyung Hee University Hospital

ASGE AudioVisual Award

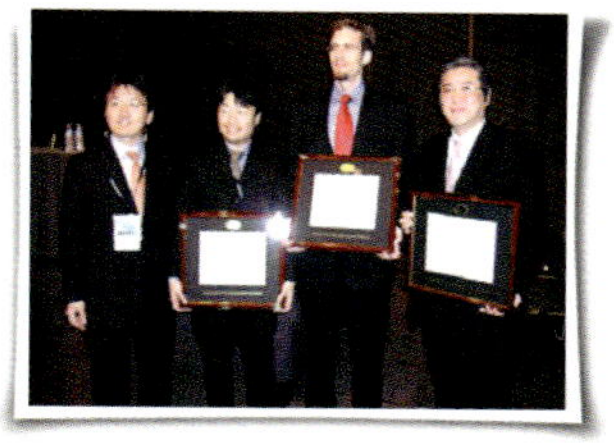

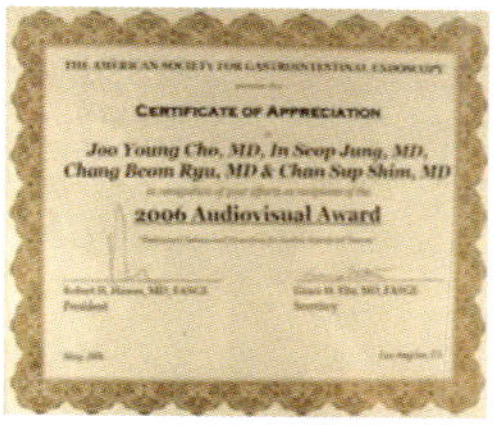

THE AMERICAN SOCIETY FOR GASTROINTESTINAL ENDOSCOPY

CERTIFICATE OF APPRECIATION

Joo Young Cho, MD, In Seop Jung, MD, Chang Beom Ryu, MD & Chan Sup Shim, MD

2006 Audiovisual Award

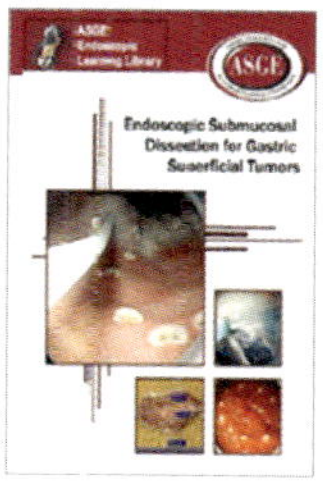

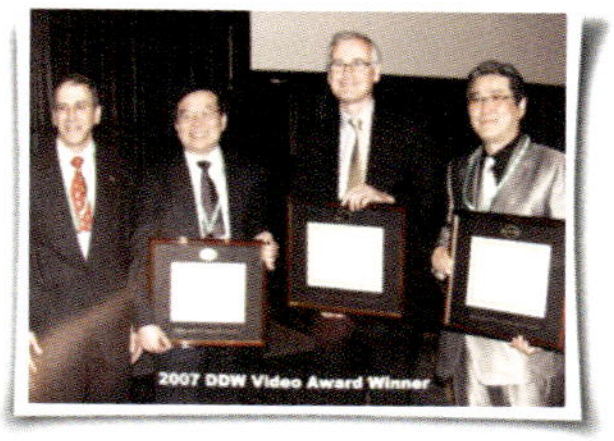

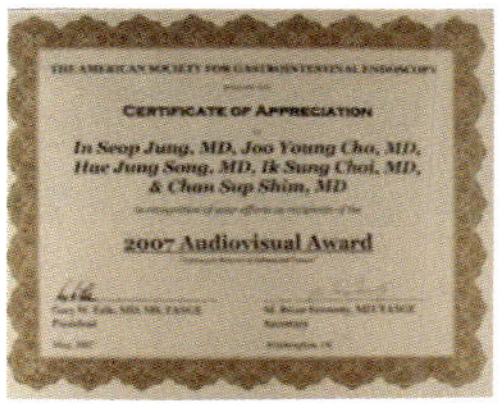

THE AMERICAN SOCIETY FOR GASTROINTESTINAL ENDOSCOPY

CERTIFICATE OF APPRECIATION

In Seop Jung, MD, Joo Young Cho, MD, Hae Jung Song, MD, Ik Sung Choi, MD, & Chan Sup Shim, MD

2007 Audiovisual Award

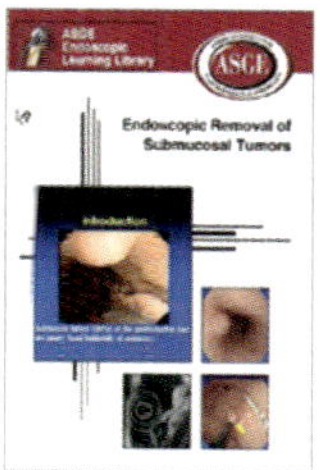

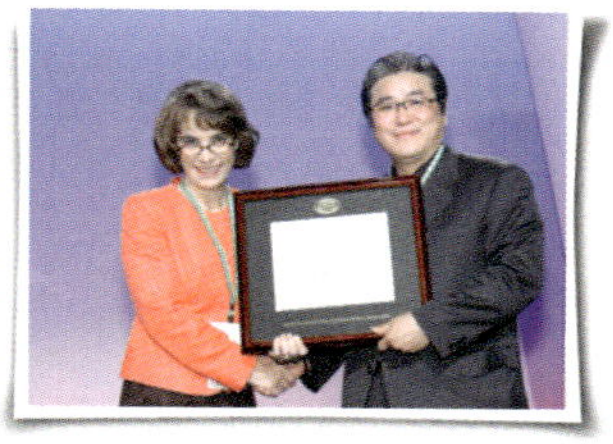

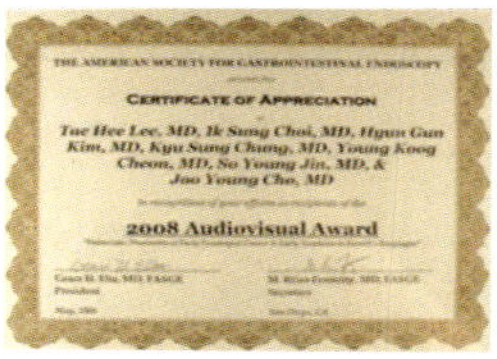

THE AMERICAN SOCIETY FOR GASTROINTESTINAL ENDOSCOPY

CERTIFICATE OF APPRECIATION

Tae Hee Lee, MD, Ik Sung Choi, MD, Hyun Gun Kim, MD, Kyu Sung Chung, MD, Young Koog Cheon, MD, So Young Jin, MD, & Joo Young Cho, MD

2008 Audiovisual Award

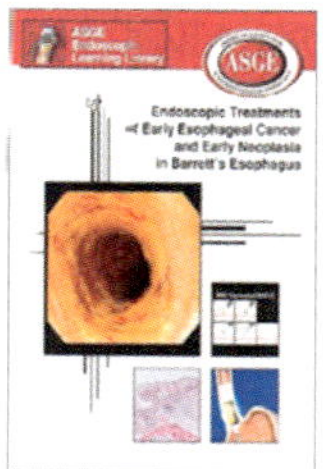

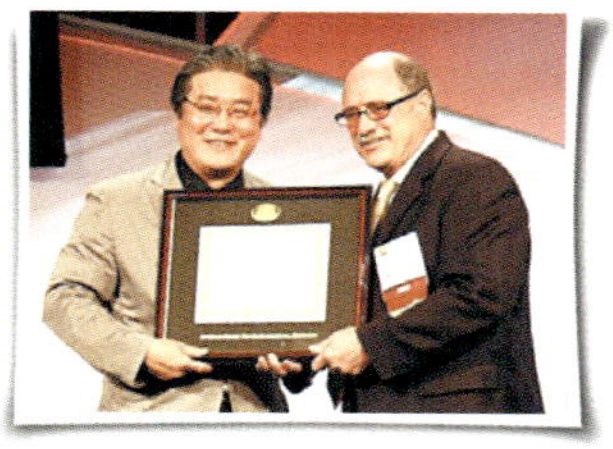

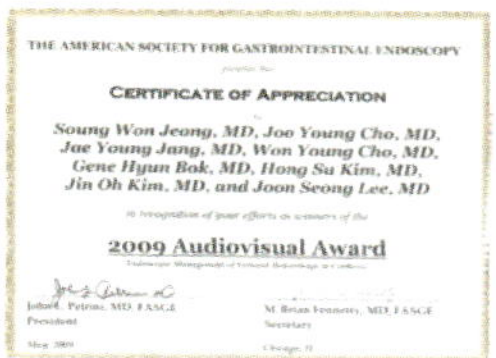

THE AMERICAN SOCIETY FOR GASTROINTESTINAL ENDOSCOPY

CERTIFICATE OF APPRECIATION

Soung Won Jeong, MD, Joo Young Cho, MD, Jae Young Jang, MD, Won Young Cho, MD, Gene Hyun Bok, MD, Hong Su Kim, MD, Jin Oh Kim, MD, and Joon Seong Lee, MD

in recognition of your efforts as winners of the

2009 Audiovisual Award

John... Petrini, MD, FASGE
President

M. Brian Fennerty, MD, FASGE
Secretary

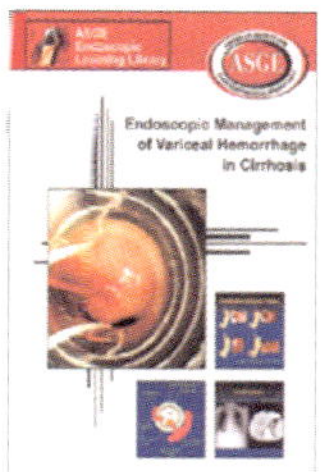

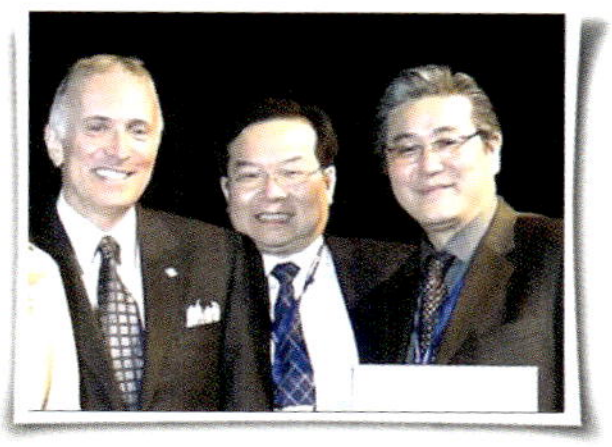

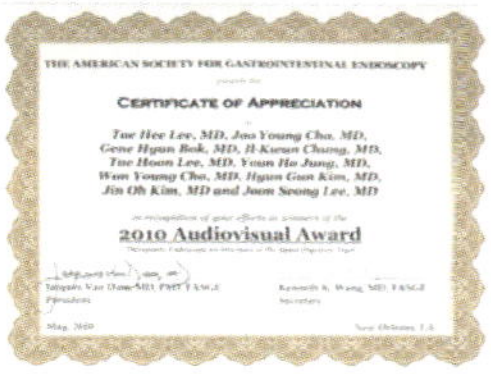

THE AMERICAN SOCIETY FOR GASTROINTESTINAL ENDOSCOPY

CERTIFICATE OF APPRECIATION

Tae Hee Lee, MD, Joo Young Cho, MD, Gene Hyun Bok, MD, Il-Kwun Chung, MD, Tae Hoon Lee, MD, Youn Ho Jung, MD, Won Young Cho, MD, Hyun Gun Kim, MD, Jin Oh Kim, MD and Joon Seong Lee, MD

2010 Audiovisual Award

Kenneth K. Wang, MD, FASGE
Secretary

May, 2010

New Orleans, LA

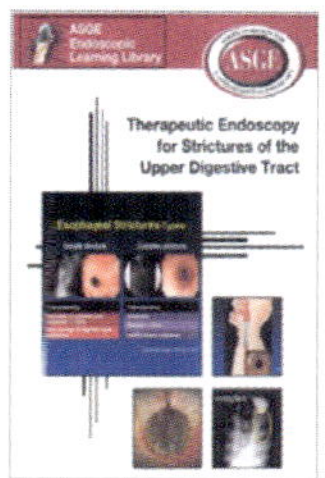

Contents

Chapter 1

Endoscopic Submucosal Dissection for Gastric Superficial Tumors

2006 ASGE Audiovisual Award Recipient
Joo Young Cho, M.D. Ph D.

Chapter 1 Endoscopic Submucosal Dissection for Gastric Superficial Tumors

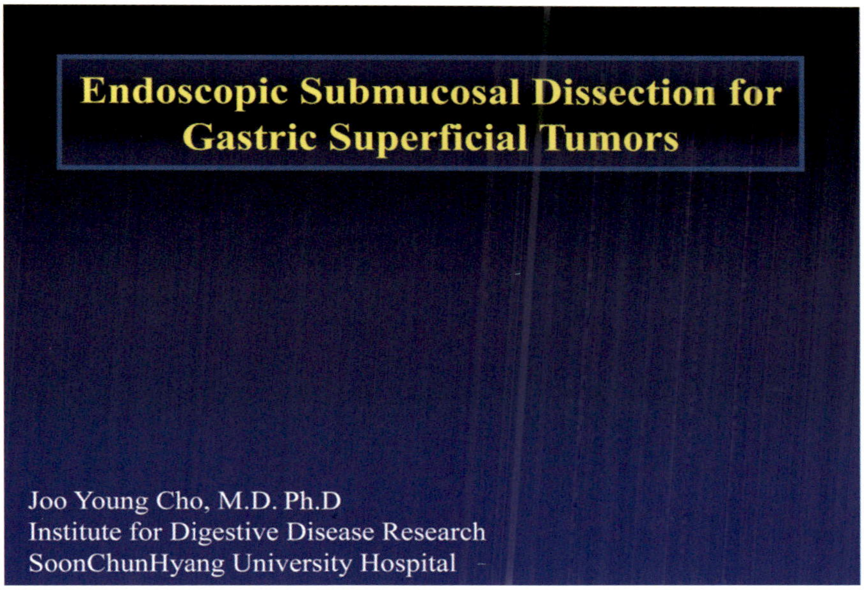

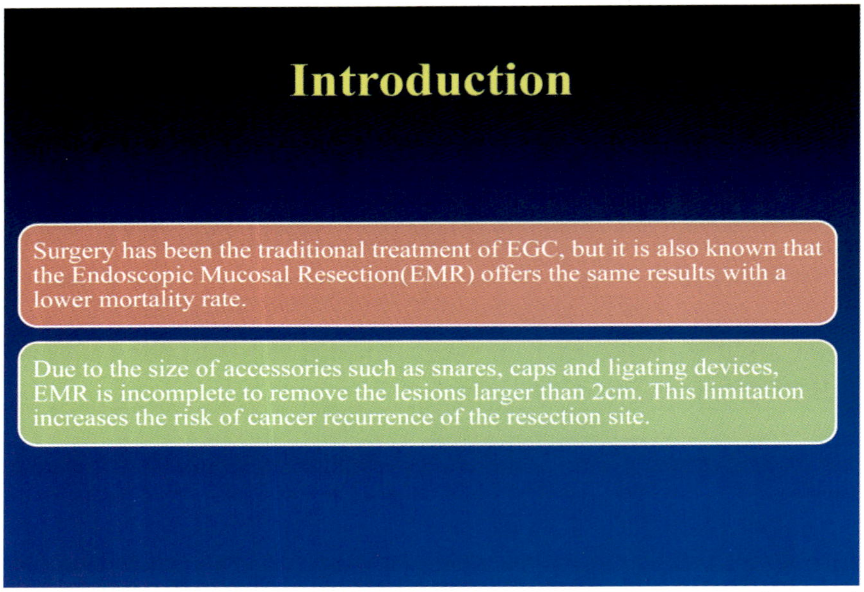

Surgery has been the traditional treatment of EGC, but it is also known that endoscopic mucosal resection (EMR) offers the same results with a lower mortality rate.
Due to the size of accessories such as snares, caps and ligating divices, EMR is incomplete to remove lesions larger than 2cm. This limitation increases the risk of cancer recurrence at the resection site.

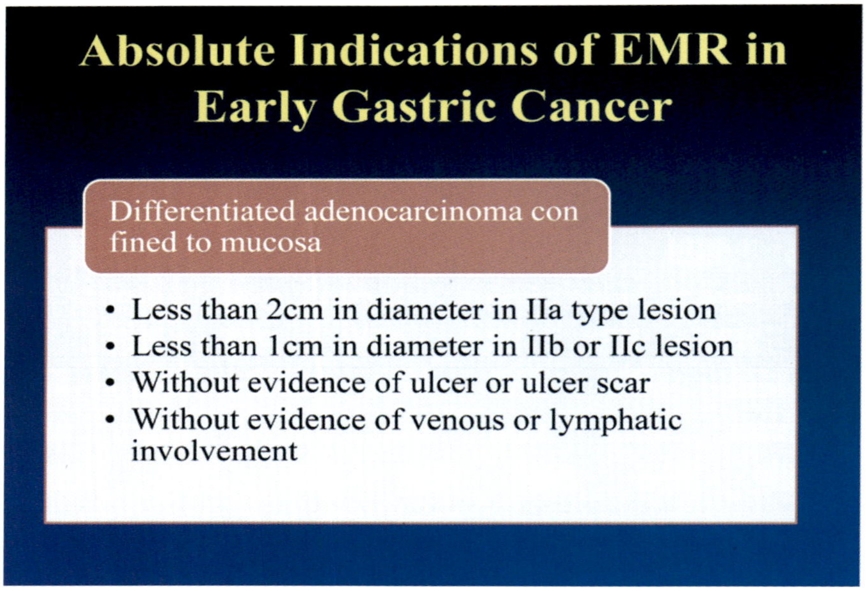

The absolute indications for treatment of early gastric cancer includes histopathologies of well or moderately differentiated adenocarcinoma or papillary carcinoma. Such lesions must be confined to the mucosa. And they must be smaller than 2cm for superficially elevated type lesions, and smaller than 1cm for the flat and depressed type lesions. They must be without ulceration or ulcer scars and there must be no evidence of venous or lymphatic involvement.

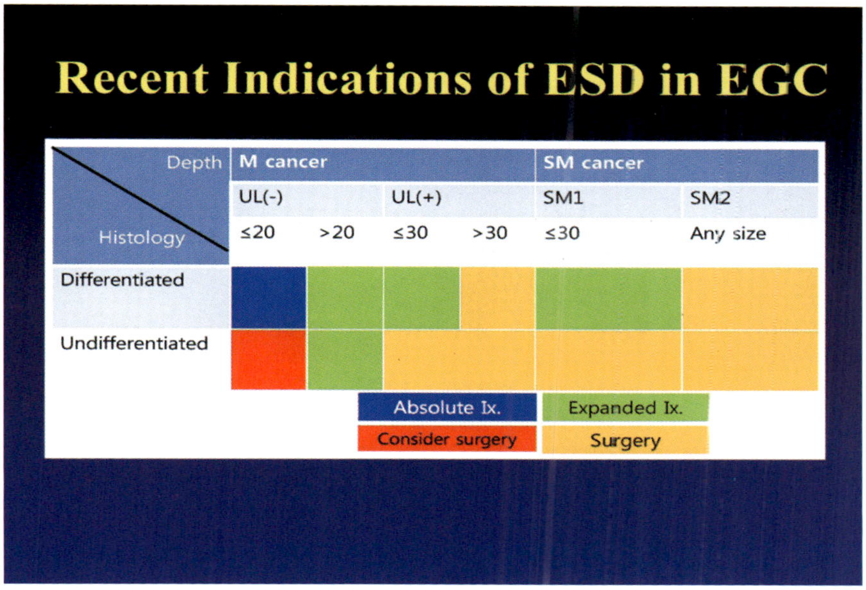

Recent indications of ESD in early gastric cancer are depicted in this table. The blue box indicates the absolute indications of EMR in early gastric cancer. The green boxes show expanded indications of ESD. The expanded indications allow ESD in early gastric cancer with well or moderately differentiated adenocarcinoma of any size if there is no ulceration, and in well or moderately differentiated adenocarcinoma less than 3cm with an ulcerated type confined to the mucosa or the submucosa 1 layer. The red box represents poorly differentiated adenocarcinoma less than 2cm confined to the mucosa. Surgery must be considered regardless of ulceration in this case. The orange color boxes represents definite surgery.

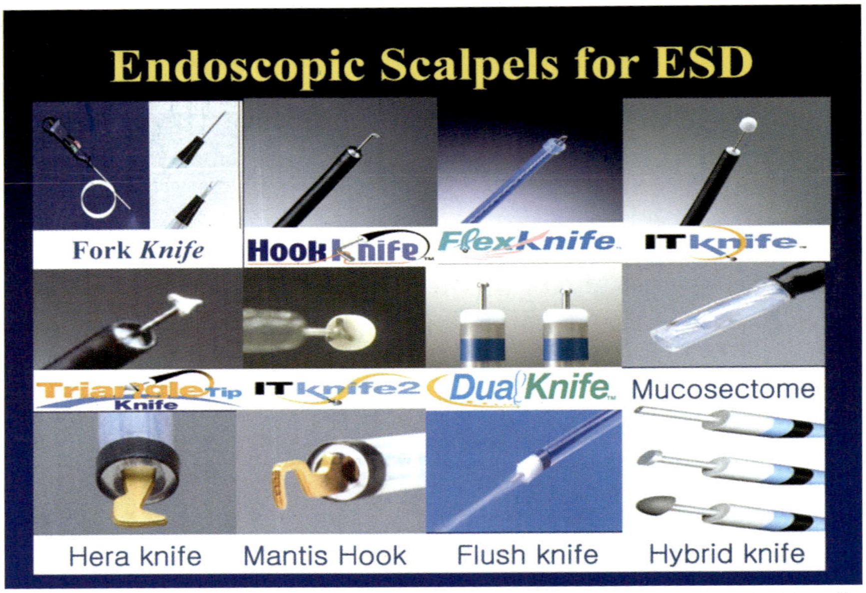

These are some of the scalpels used in ESD. These scalpels are known as the fixed flexible knife and Fork knife they were developed and produced in Korea. The IT Knife or insulated tip knife, the HookKnife and FlexKnife were developed and produced in Japan.

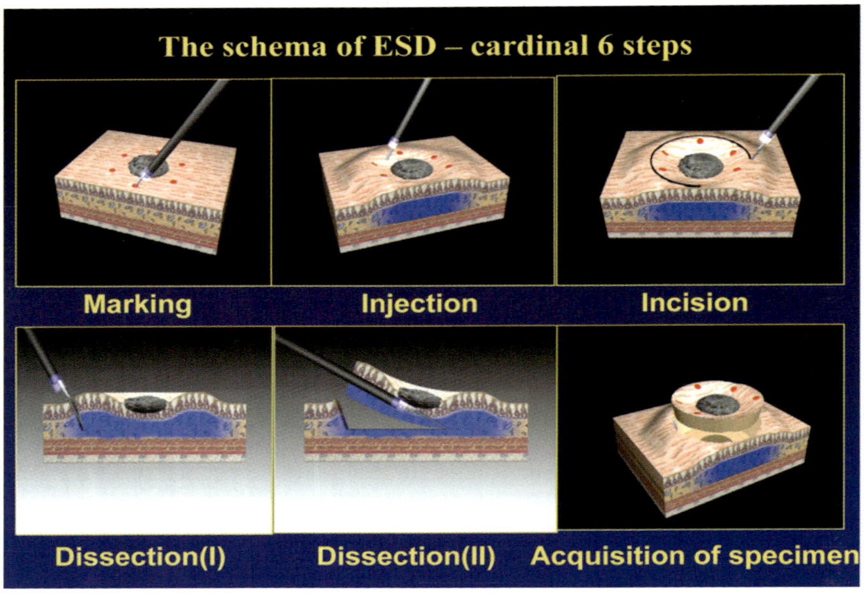

These are the six procedural steps of ESD. The first step is confirmation of the lateral margin, followed by marking around the lateral margin, injection into the submucosal layer, incision, dissection and acquisition of the specimen.

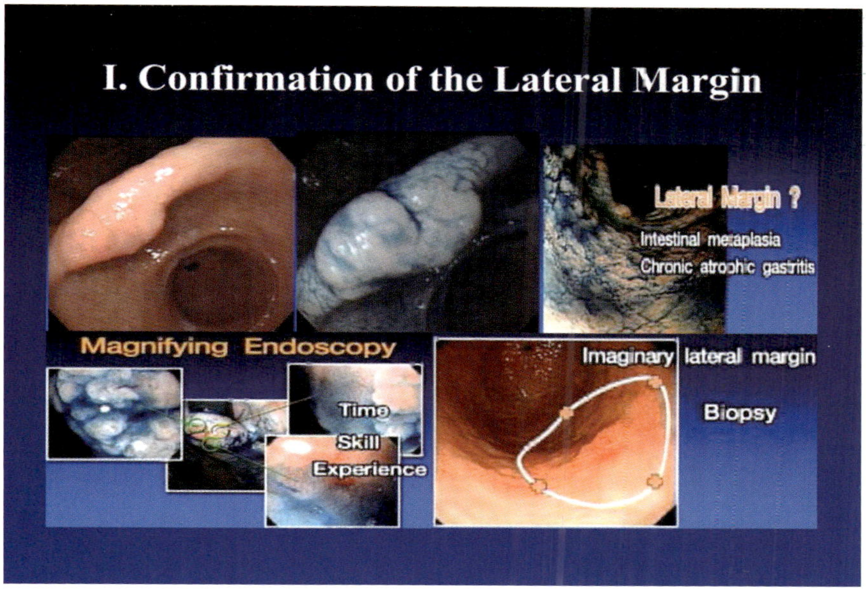

For complete resection of a given lesion confirmation of the lateral margin of the tumor is most important. Unfortunately in many cases, it is difficult to identify this margin solely with routine endoscopy. In these situations chromoendoscopy using Indigocarmine is helpful to demarcate the lateral margins. However, using indigocarmine is ineffective in patients with intestinal metaplasia or severe chronic atrophic gastritis. Magnifying endoscopy can be useful in such cases. But this procedure requires time and an experienced endoscopist. An alternative approach is to draw imaginary lateral margins around the lesion and perform biopsies on all four corner points to eliminate the possibility of tumor margin inclusion. These biopsy sites can also later be used as markers for ESD.

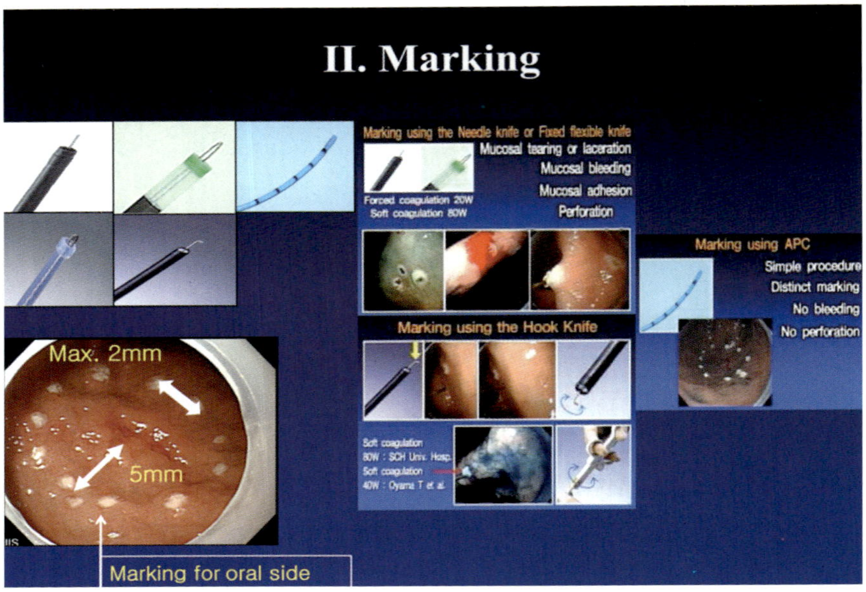

Markings can be performed using almost any knife including the needle knife, fixed flexible knife, flex knife, hook knife and argon plasma coagulation (APC). A minimum of approximately 5mm distal spacing centered around the tumor margin is required to prevent damaging the tumor area. This is because the markings themselves take up 2mm of space. Also a marking to represent the oral side of the lesion is important for the acquisition of a specimen. Forced coagulation of 20W of soft coagulation of 80W is applied for marking using the needle knife or fixed flexible knife. The disadvantages of this procedure are the occurrence of tears or frequent bleeding of the mucosa, adhesion of tissue on the knife and perforation. When using the hook knife 40 of 80W of soft coagulation should be applied to the reverse tip for marking. However constant flipping to maintain the reverse tip and visual blocking of the tip by tissue adherence makes this procedure difficult. Argon plasma coagulation is a simple method to perform marking without the risk of bleeding, perforation and burns to the mucosa. One important thing to remember for APC, is to bring the probe as close as possible in order to make the markings small and clear.

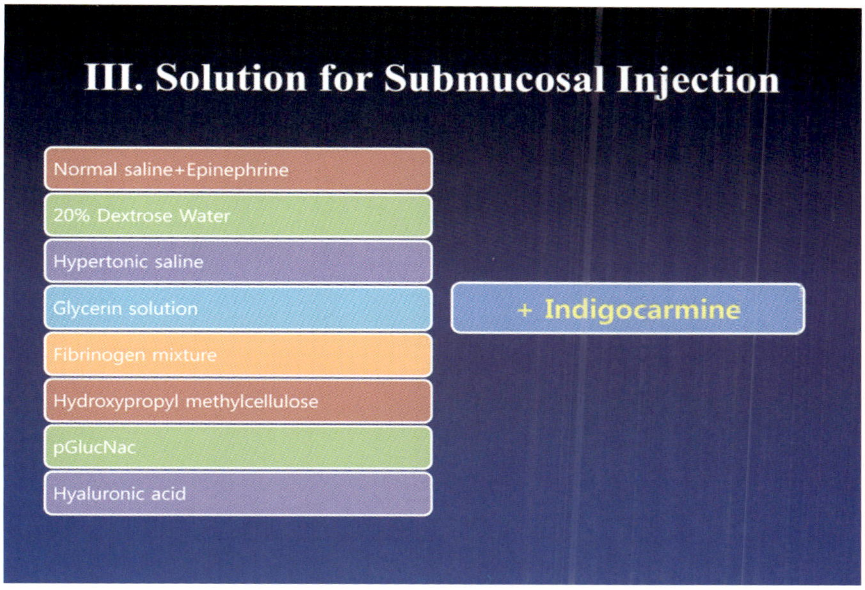

For submucosal injection, solutions such as normal saline and epinephrine mixture, 20% dextrose water, hypertonic saline, glycerin solution, fibrinogen mixture solution, hydroxypropyl methyl cellulose, pGlucNac and sodium hyaluronate solution are being used. These injections are mixed with indigocarmine to stain the submucosa blue in order to distinguish it from the proper muscle layer.

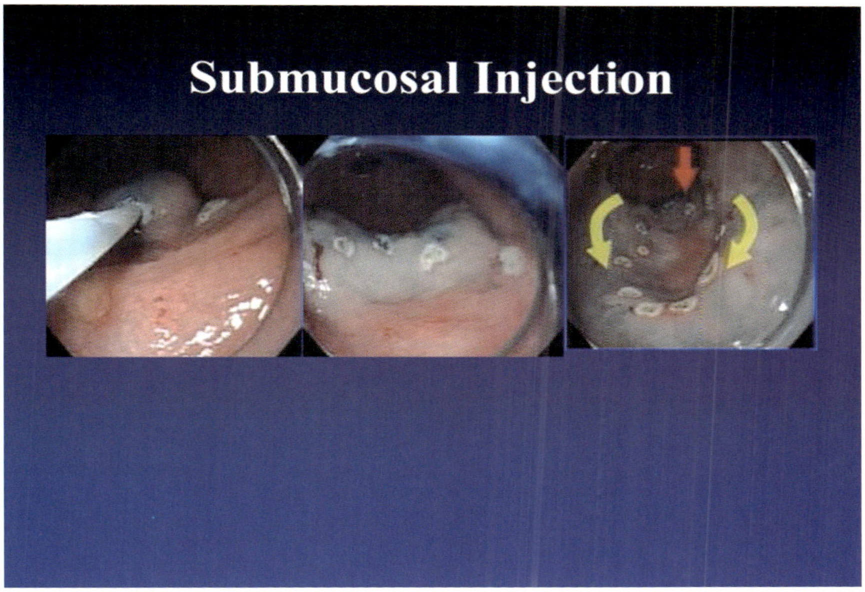

Submucosal injection starts from the distal point of the endoscopic field down to the proximal area. This method eliminates distal point injection interruptions by elevating the proximal injected area.

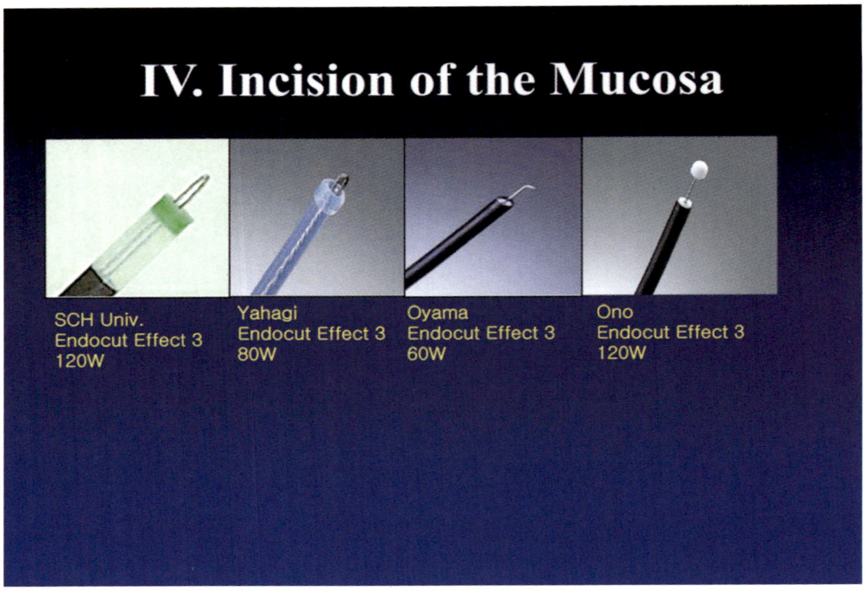

The selection of the knife and the mode of the electrosurgical unit for incision are slightly different according to the preference of the endoscopist.

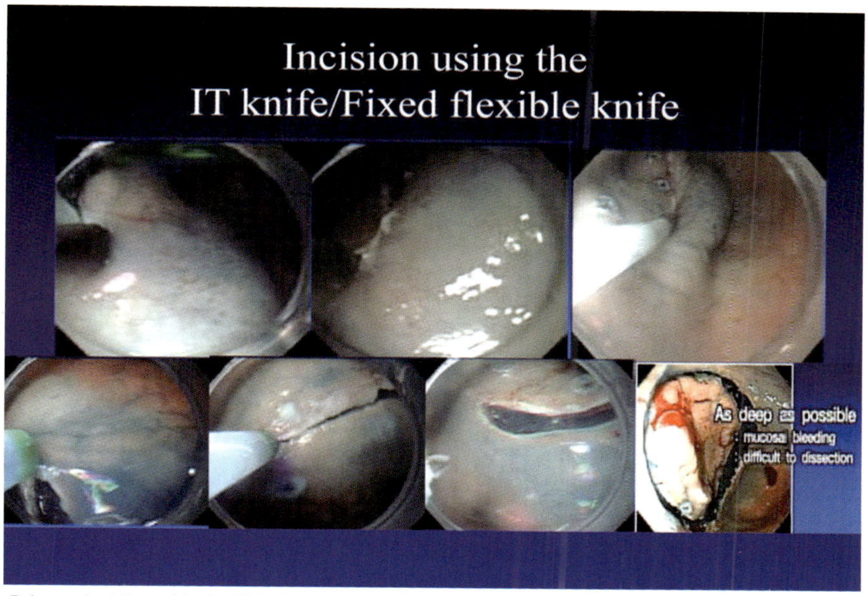

Prior to incision with the IT knife, a precutting incision or hole is made in the mucosa with the needle knife or fixed flexible knife. The tip of the IT knife is then inserted for incison. Incision with the IT knife is performed from the distal point of the endoscopic field and proceeded along both lateral sides of the lesion. During the incision of the antral greater curvature with the IT knife, often only the folded layers of the mucosa are coagulated. In this case a submucosal injection or pressing the layer with the cap of the endoscope to make the incision is recommended.

The tip of the fixed flexible knife is exposed approximately 2mm from its sheath. Incision using the fixed flexible knife is the same as the IT knife, starting from the distal to the proximal side. The main difference is there is no limitation in the initial incision point. The initial incision point can be anywhere according to the margins of the tumor and the positioning of the endoscope. Caution is required when a proper angle cannot be acquired for the endoscope. Over extension of the knife can result in incision of layers in uneven depth and perforation. In such cases approximation of the endoscope to the mucosa as close as possible, with a minimal deployment of the knife after confirmation of the incision boundary is strongly recommended, in order to ensure an even incision and safe removal of the mucosa. A thin layer of incision often causes more bleeding, and we suggest the deepest incision possible.

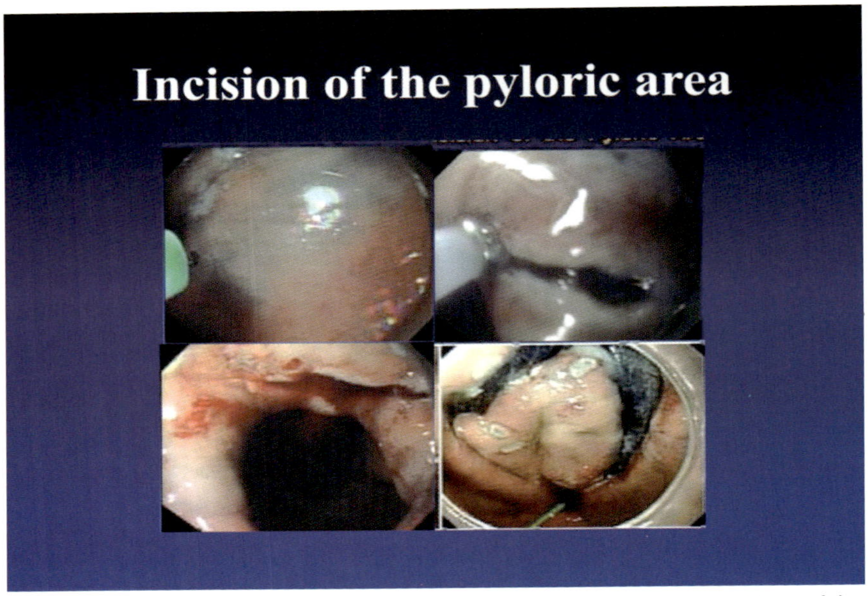

Incision around tumors located near the pylorus may be difficult due to the folded layer of the pyloric area resulting from prior injections of the surrounding mucosa. Subsequently initiating an incision after injecting only the pyloric area is recommended, rather than injecting other areas if the tumor margin is located near the pylorus. Bleeding control is often required during incision in the pyloric area due to the abundant vasculature.

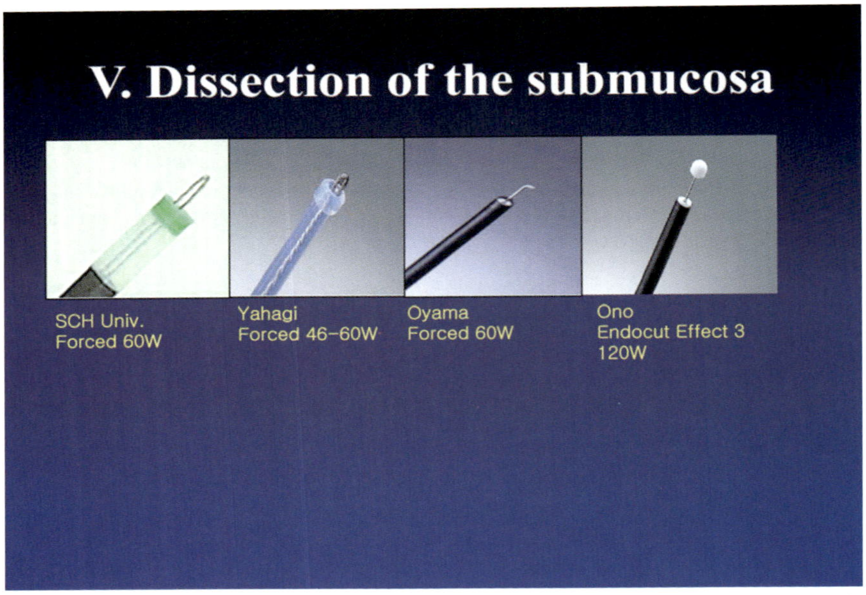

Different knife can be used for submucosal dissection, and the mode of the electrosurgical unit depends of the preference of the endoscopist.

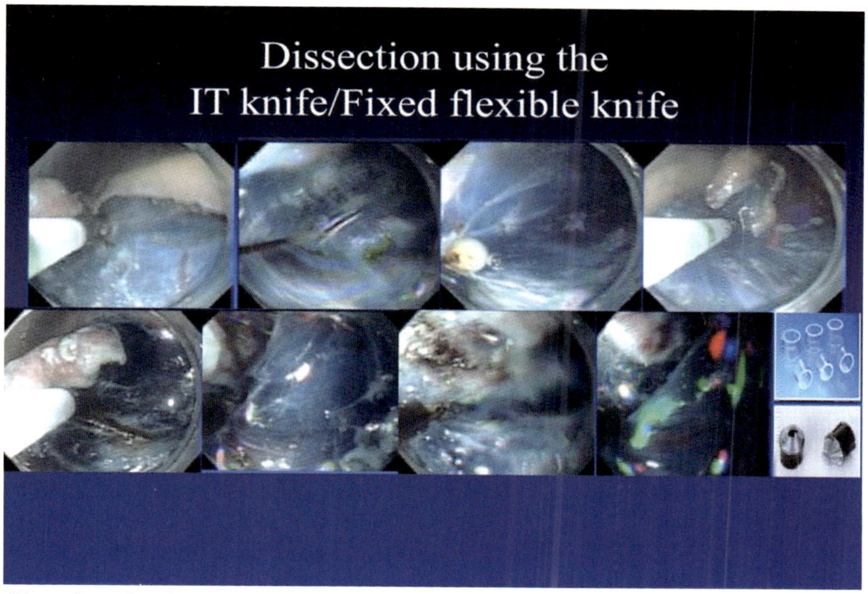

Dissection using the IT knife. Submucosal dissection with an IT knife requires elevation of the submucosal layer with an injection to dissect it laterally from the proper muscle. When doing this, it is easier to hook the ceramic ball tip of the IT knife under the layer of the dissected submucosa to pull it inward from the distal field towards the endoscope.

Both the fixed flexible knife and the fork knife should be approximated close to the tumor margins with careful monitoring of the submucosal layer through the endoscope. Incision should proceed from the tumor margins close to the proper muscle area towards the distal location viewed from the endoscopic field. The fork can save time because it can be used simultaneously to perform injection and saline irrigation during bleeding without changing accessories. The saw-toothed blade of the fork can promote dissection while the cap of the endoscope holds down the layer for a better view.

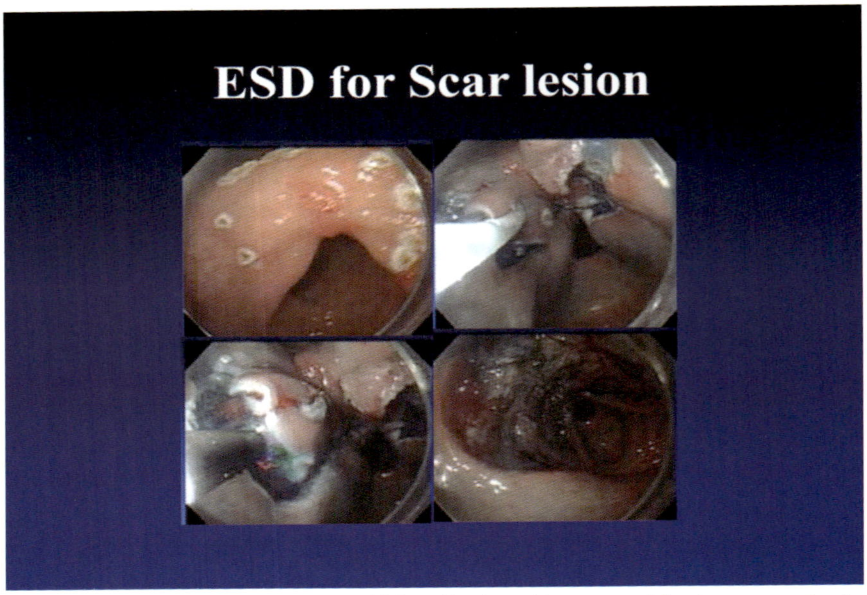

To perform re-ESD on scar lesions, sufficient distal markings around the tumor margins is suggested. After the incision elevate the submucosal layer by injecting around the non-fibrotic band area. Then, the removal of the fibrotic band begins with either the fixed flexible knife or fork knife by pressing the dissected layer with the cap of the endoscope at a straight angle. For this procedure, the IT knife is too flexible to dissect the hardened band.

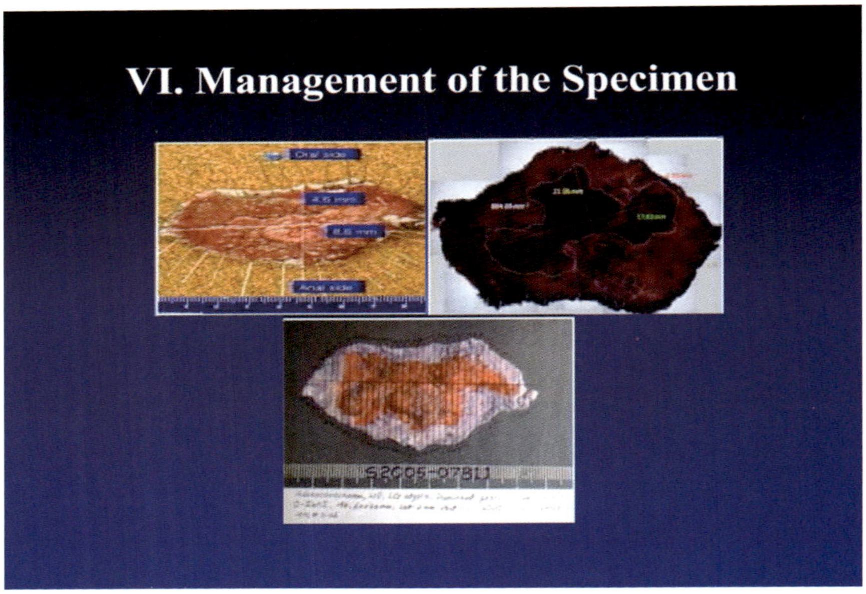

It is important to fix, spread and pin down the tumor on styrofoam or rubber panels. This will prevent the edges from rolling up. After fixation it is important to confirm complete tumor margin inclusion through a stereoscope. The closest margin spot from the tumor to the proper muscle should be marked for the pathologist to examine and section the specimen properly.

Results(1)

Duration	Feb 2003-Feb 2005
Male/Female(n)	109/55
Median age(yrs)	61.1(29-85)
Number of lesion	
1	151(92.0%)
2	11(6.7%)
3	2(1.3%)
Total	164(100%)

Size	No(%)
≤ 10	18(10.0)
11-20	83(46.3)
21-30	50(30)
≥ 31	28(13.7)
Total	179
Morphology	No(%)
Elevated	114(63.7)
Flat or depressed	65(38.3)

The total number of patients who underwent ESD form Feb of 2003 to Feb of 2005 at our department was 164. The male to female ratio was 2:1. Median age was 61.1 years. 8% of the patients had multiple tumors. 56.3% of the gastric tumors were under the size of 2 cm. 30% were between 2-3 cm, and 15.6% were over 3 cm.

Results(2)

The Distribution of location		
Antrum(%)	Mid to lower Body (%)	Upper body to cardia(%)
106 (59.2)	64(35.8)	9(5)

Anterior wall	47(26.2)
Lesser curvature	28(15.7)
Posterior wall	63(35.2)
Greater curvature	41(22.9)

Histologic Findings of Specimen	
Pathology	Number of lesions(%)
Adenocardinoma	126(70.3)
Well	73(58.0)
Moderate	41(32.5)
Poorly	12(9.5)
Tubular Adenoma	42(23.4)
Low grade	28(66.7)
High grade	14(33.3)
Others	11(6.0)
Total	179

63.7% of tumors were elevated and 36.3% were flat or depressed. 59.2% of the tumors were located in the antrum, and 35.1% were located on the posterior wall. Of the 179 cases 70.3% were adenocarcinoma and 23.4% were tubular adenoma. 9.5% of adenocarcinoma was poorly differentiated.

Results(3)

Depth of invasion	No. of lesion (%)	Vertical margin(+)
M1	1(0.9)	0
M2	46(38.3)	0
M3	57(47.5)	0
Sm1	14(11.7)	3/14(21.1)
sm2	2(1.6)	2/2(100)
Total	120	5

Size(mm)	No. of lesion(%)	En bloc resection (%)	Piecemeal resection (%)
≤ 10	18	18(100)	0
11-20	81	80(98.8)	1(1.2)
21-30	49	45(91.8)	4(8.2)
≥ 31	28	26(92.9)	2(7.1)
Total	176	169(96.0)	7(4.0)

87% of adenocarcinoma was confined to the mucosa. 11.7% invaded up to the sm1 layer. Of the patients with sm1 layer invasion, 3 had vertical margin involvement of the tumor. 2 patients were confirmed to have invasion into the sm2 layer. In both cases, vertical margins were positive for tumor involvement. En-bloc resection rate in ESD was 100% for tumors with a size less than 1cm. Overall the total en-bloc resection rate was 96%.

Results(4)

Size(mm)	Lesions	Complete resection (%)
≤ 10	18	18 (100)
11-20	81	71(87.7)
21-30	49	38(77.5)
≥31	28	23(82.1)
Total	176	150(85.2)

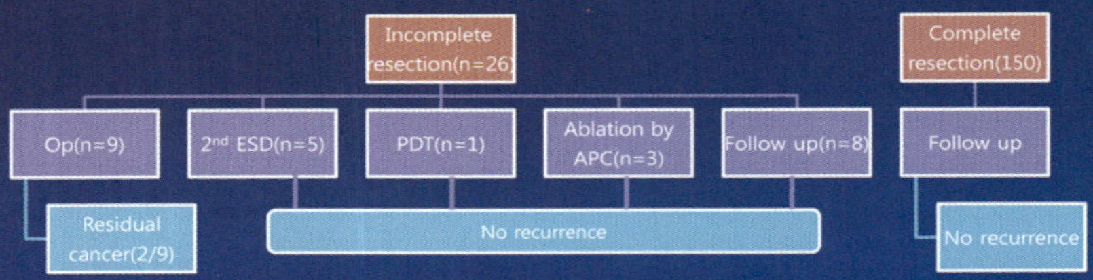

The complete resection rate for ESD was 100% for tumors less than 1cm. The complete resection rate for 176 tumors was 85.2%. Out of 26 incomplete resection cases, 5 underwent 2nd ESD, 4 received APC or other ablation therapy such as photodynamic therapy, and 9 received a gastrectomy. Out of the 9 patients who had surgery, 6 were found to have no remnant lesions.

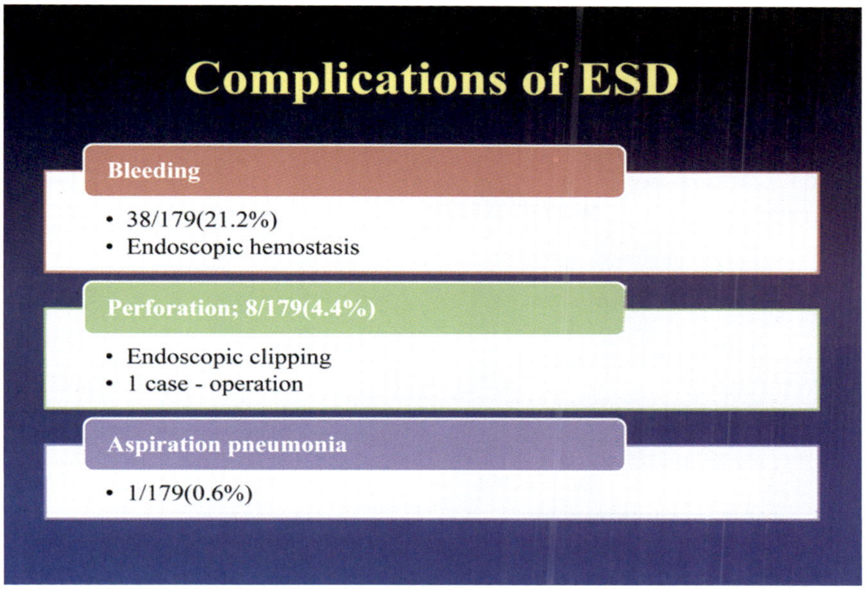

There are several complications for ESD. Bleeding occurred in 21.2%. Endoscopic hemostasis was sufficient for controlling the bleeding. Perforation occurred in 4.4% of patients and aspiration pneumonia in 0.6% of patients. Endoscopic clipping was performed on 7 of the 8 patients who developed perforation.

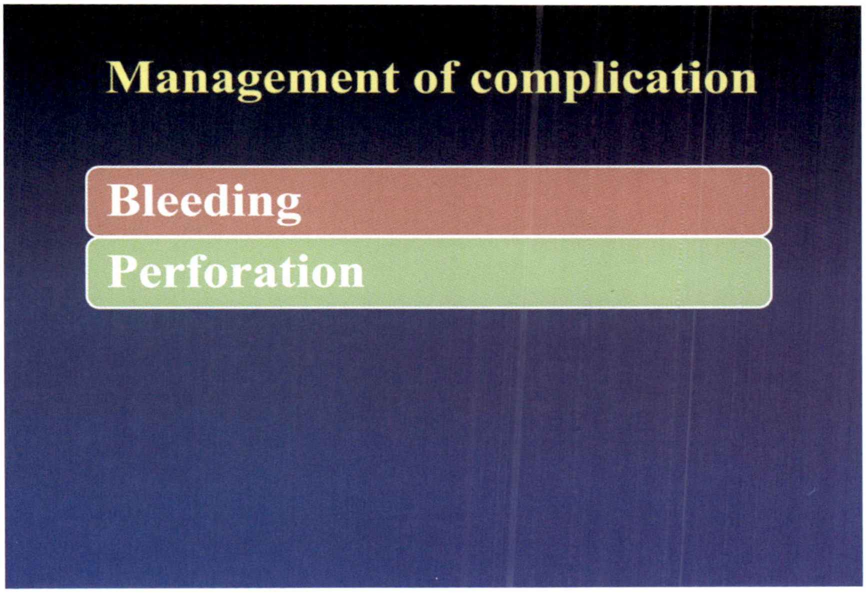

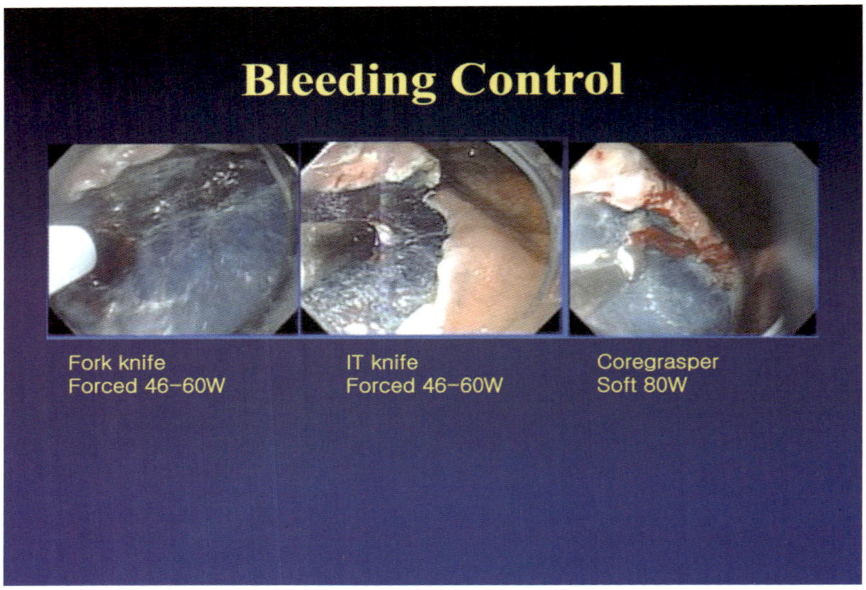

To control the bleeding from a 1mm blood vessel using the fork knife, forced coagulation of 50W is used (left). To control the bleeding from a 1mm blood vessel using an IT knife, allow the contact of the IT knife to generate 50W of current (middle). However, for bleeding control of blood vessels 2-3mm in size usually in the center of the submucosa, soft coagulation of 80W with hemostatic forceps is required (right).

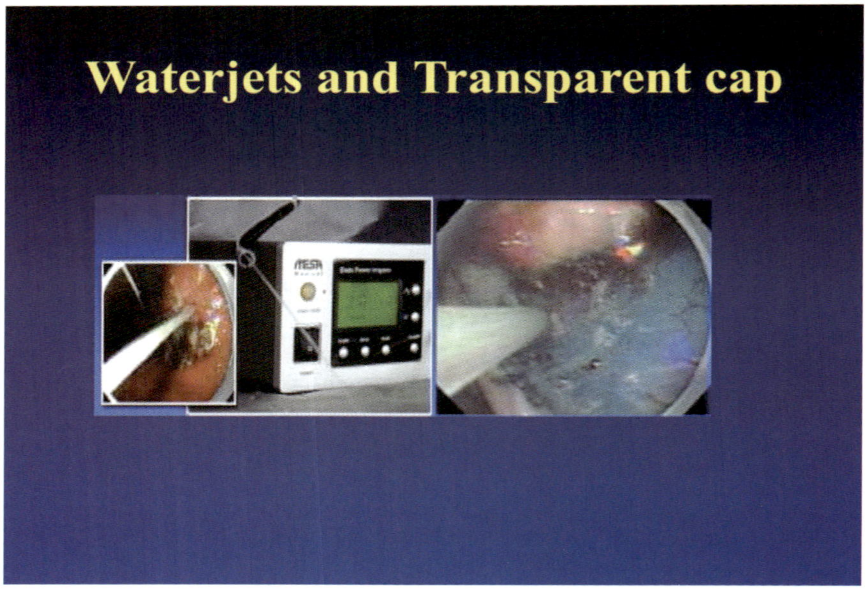

A high pressure water jet pump with a transparent cap is useful during severe bleeding or when blood clots obscure the dissection area.. A high pressure water jet pump can be used to clear the view and locate the origin of bleeding during dissection.

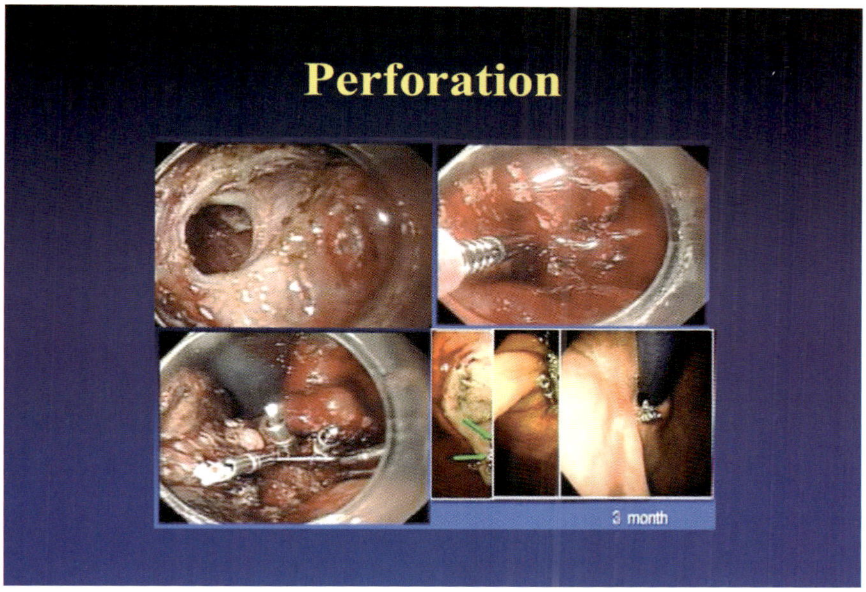

During dissection, perforation develops at the cardia. When perforation occurs it is necessary to deflate and close the involved area with hemoclips. Water irrigation should be avoided.

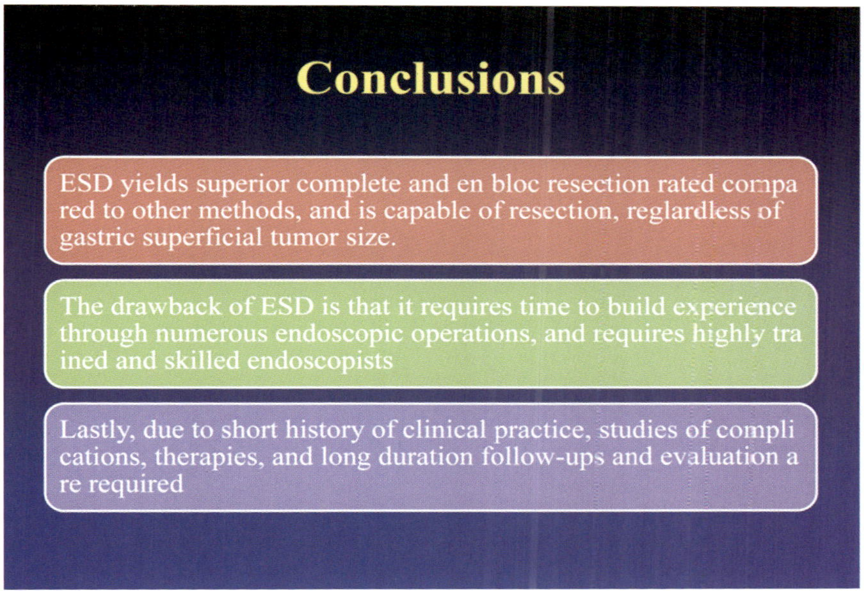

ESD yields superior complete and en-bloc resection rates compared to other methods, and is capable of resection, regardless of gastric tumor size. The drawback of ESD is that it requires time to build experience through numerous endoscopic operations, and requires highly trained and skilled endscopists. Lastly, due to its short history of clinical practice, further studies of complications, therapies, and long term duration follow-ups and evaluation are required.

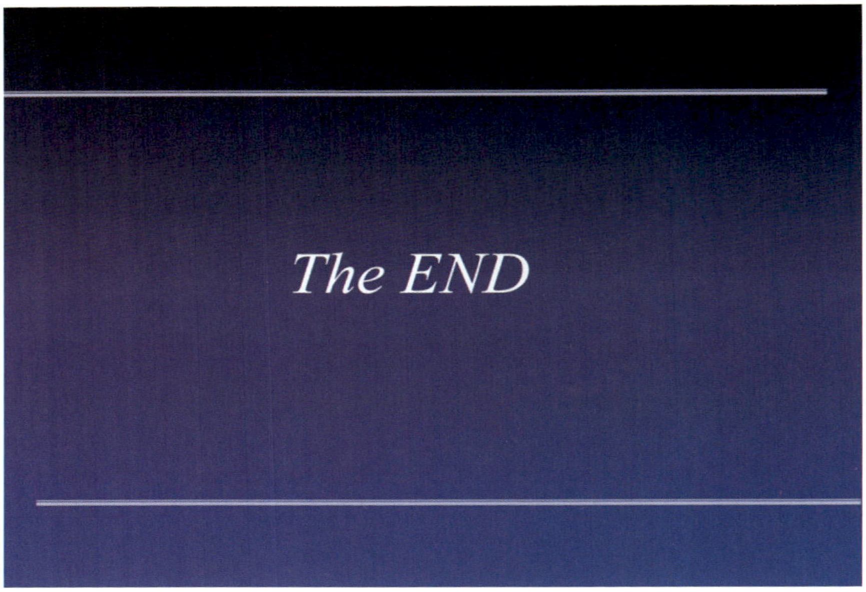
The END

Chapter 2

Endoscopic Removal of Submucosal Tumors

2007 ASGE Audiovisual Award Recipient

Joo Young Cho, M.D. Ph D.
Won Young Cho, M.D. Ph D.

Chapter 2 Endoscopic Removal of Submucosal Tumors

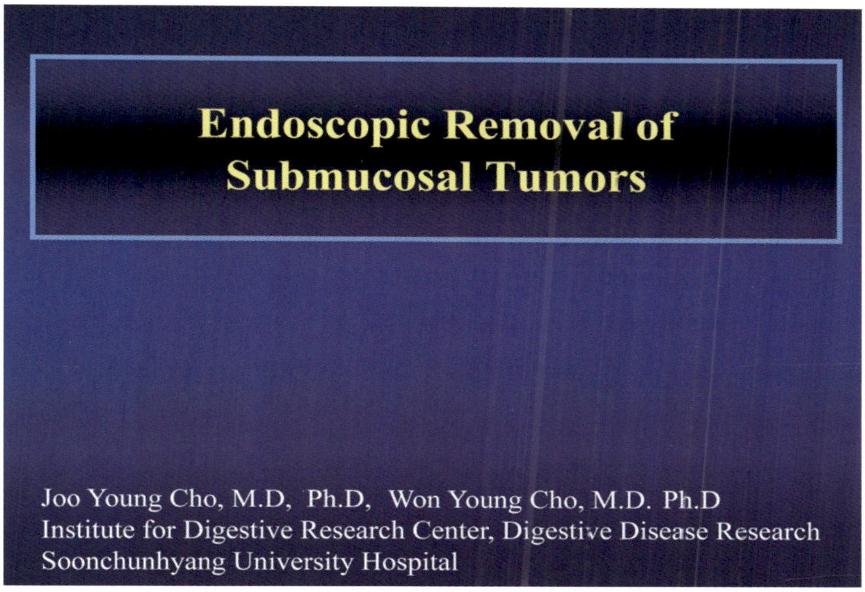

Submucosal tumors of the gastrointestinal tract are uncommon and are usually found incidentally during endoscopic examination. The use of EUS for diagnosis of SMTs is now established as the most sensitive diagnostic procedure for detection of SMTs.

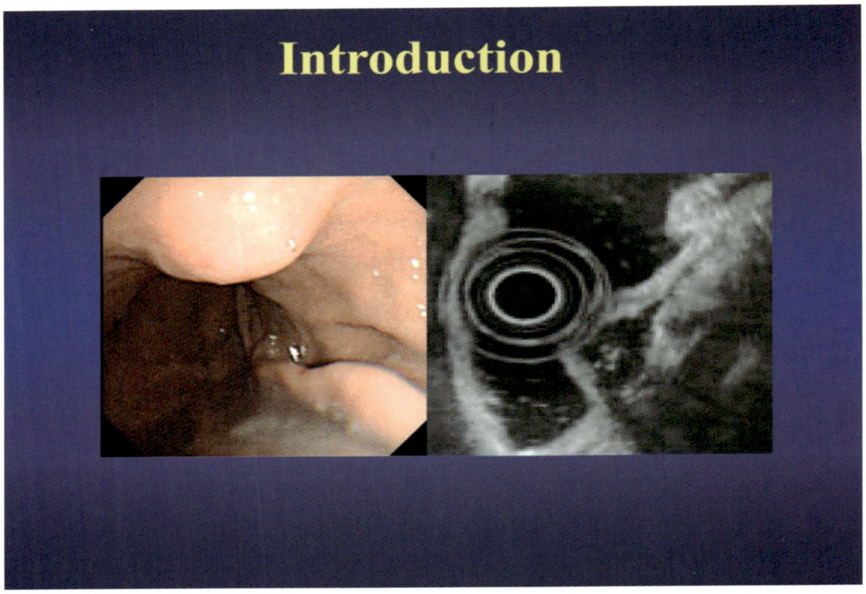

Until recently, management of SMT' s is consisted of two relatively unsatisfactory options; observation without a definitive tissue diagnosis, or surgical resection. As endoscopic techniques continuously develop, less invasive techniques such as endoscopic resection are becoming the preferred method of treating SMT' s.

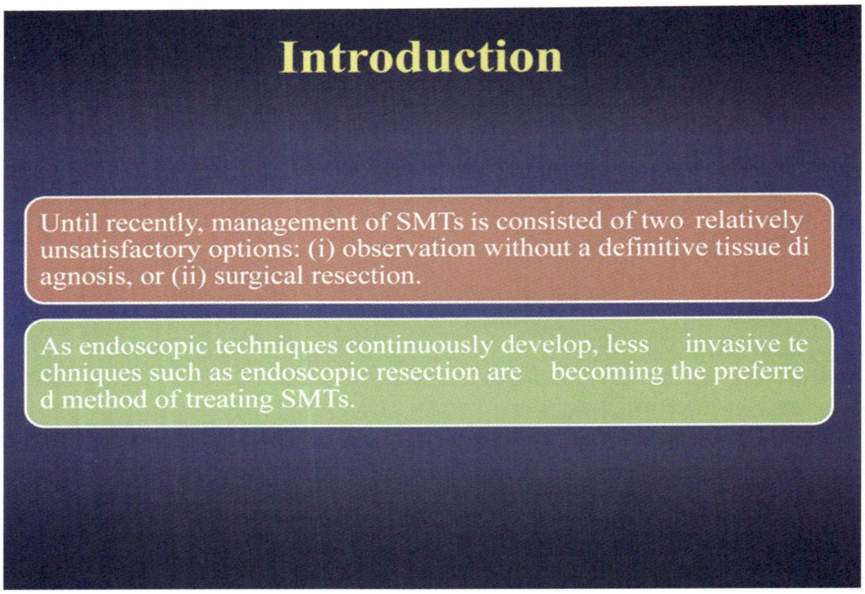

Therapeutic options of SMT' s are as follows, Standard snare polypectomy, strip biopsy using physiologic saline and a snare device, endoscopic submucosal resection with a ligating device(ESMR-L), Endoscopic submucosal tumor resection with a transparent cap(ESMR-C), Unroofing technique, and Endoscopic submucosal dissection (ESD).

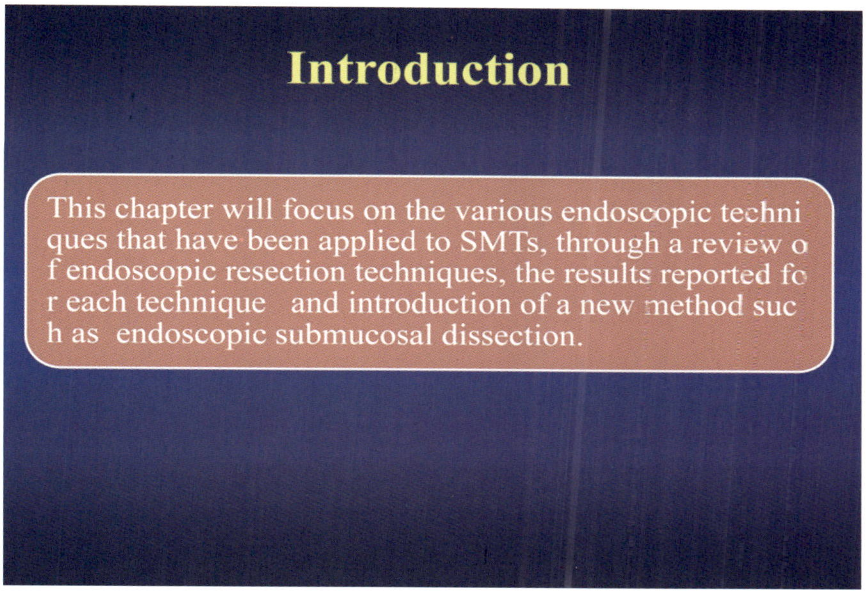
Introduction
This chapter will focus on the various endoscopic techni
ques that have been applied to SMTs, through a review o
f endoscopic resection techniques, the results reported fo
r each technique and introduction of a new method suc
h as endoscopic submucosal dissection.

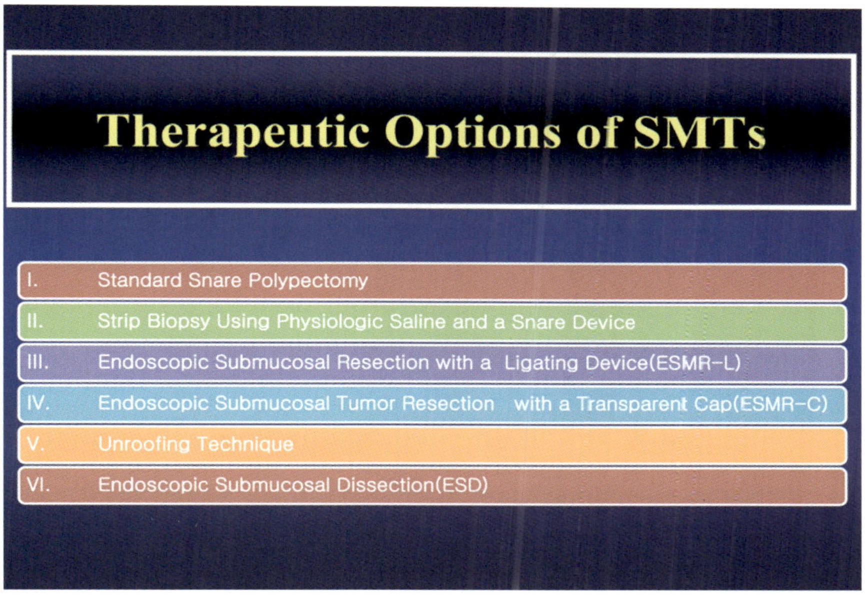
Therapeutic Options of SMTs
I. Standard Snare Polypectomy
II. Strip Biopsy Using Physiologic Saline and a Snare Device
III. Endoscopic Submucosal Resection with a Ligating Device(ESMR-L)
IV. Endoscopic Submucosal Tumor Resection with a Transparent Cap(ESMR-C)
V. Unroofing Technique
VI. Endoscopic Submucosal Dissection(ESD)

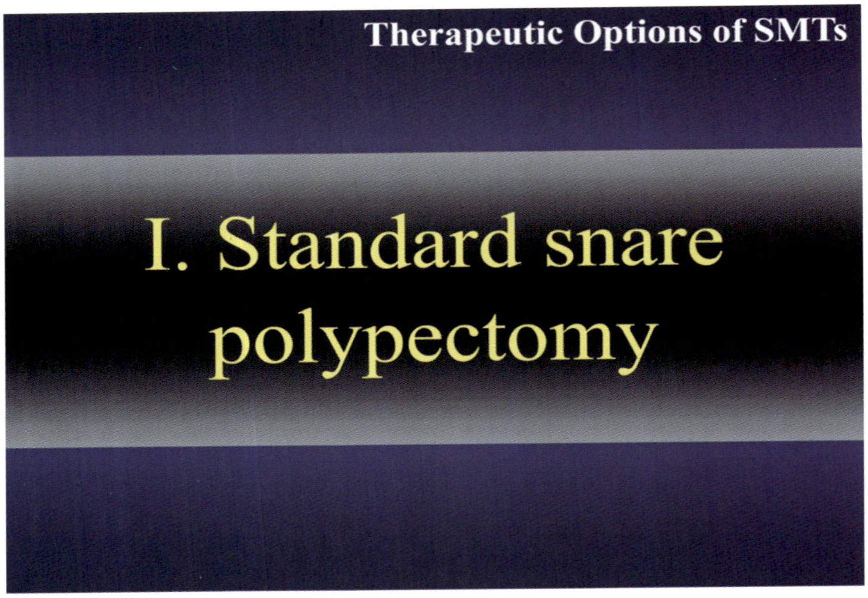

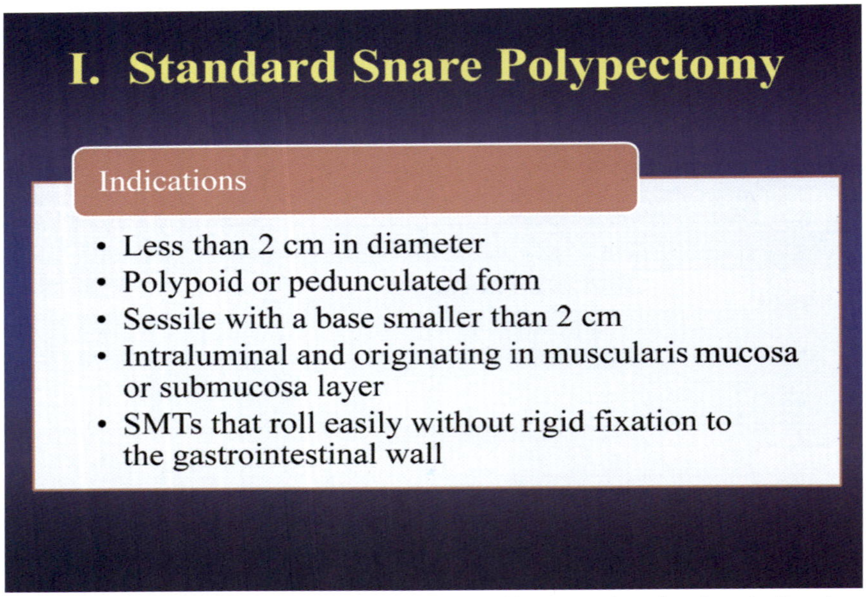

Standard snare polypectomy is indicated for patients with a tumor less than 2 cm in diameter, tumors that are polypoid or pedunculated in form, sessile tumors with a base smaller than 2 cm, and intraluminal tumors originating in the muscularis mucosa or submucosa. This method may also be applied to SMT' s that roll easily without rigid fixation to the gastrointestinal wall when pushed by forceps during the endoscopic examination.

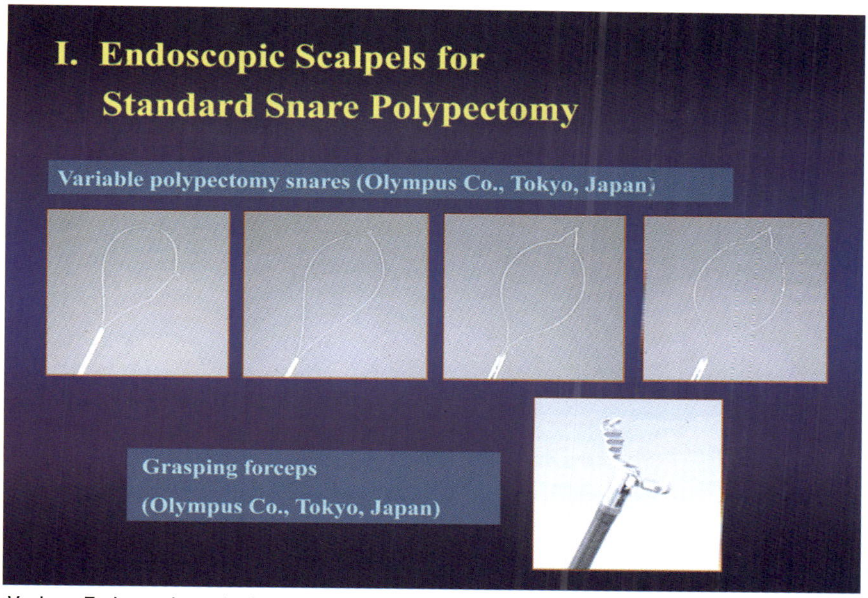

Various Endoscopic scalpels can be used for standard snare polypectomy. Crescent shaped, hexagonal shaped and oval shaped snares as well as grasping forceps are used.

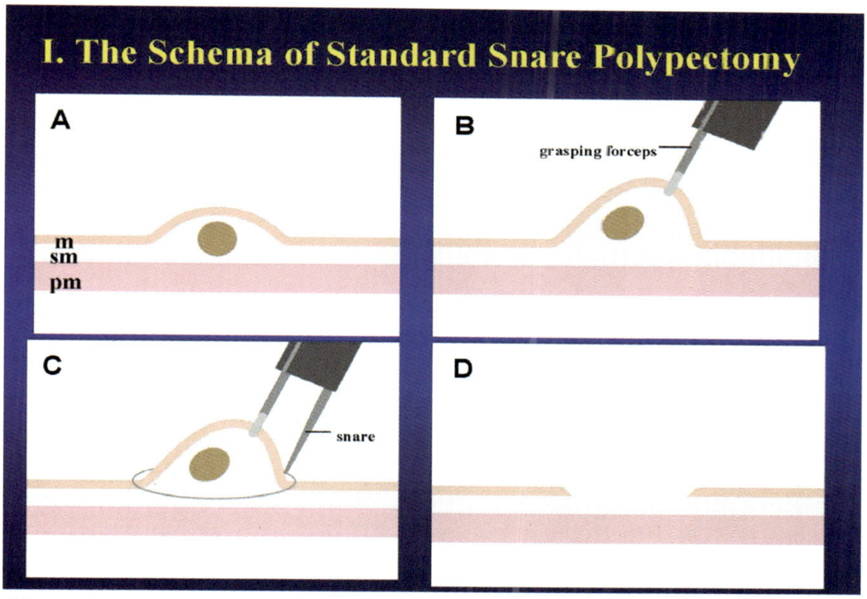

When using the snare polypectomy method for resection of SMT' s, grasping forceps and a diathermic snare are inserted through the two instrument channels into the gastrointestinal lumen. The grasping forceps are passed through the loop of the snare and used to firmly grasp the oral aspect of the tumor and pull it as far as possible to the center of the lumen. The snare is then placed around the center of the tumor and tightened to excise the tumor by electrocoagulation with a blended current.

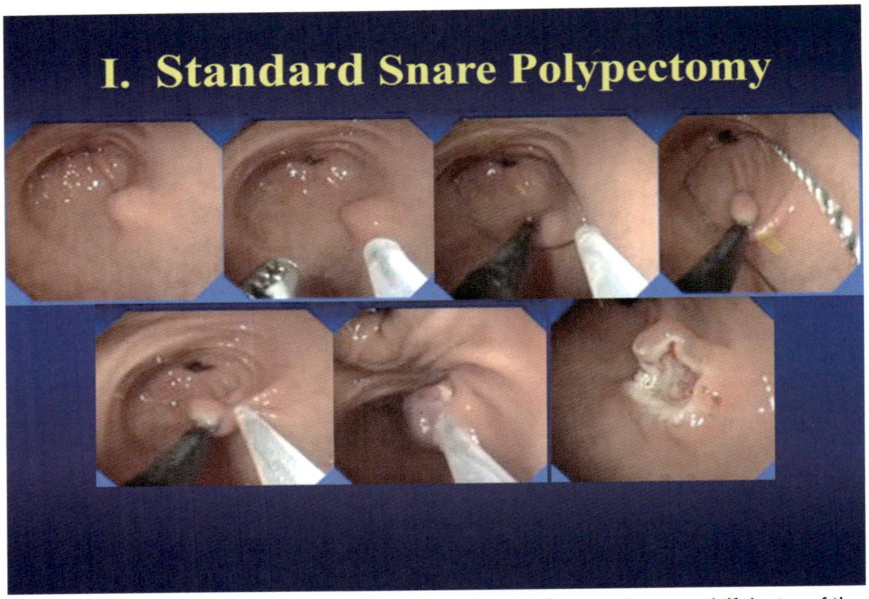

The critical element of this method is the location at which the tumor is grasped. If the top of the tumor is grasped and pulled by grasping forceps, it is very likely that only the upper part of the mucosa of the SMT will be resected. Therefore the mucosa covering the oral side of the tumor should be strongly grasped and pulled toward the center of the lumen before placing the snare.

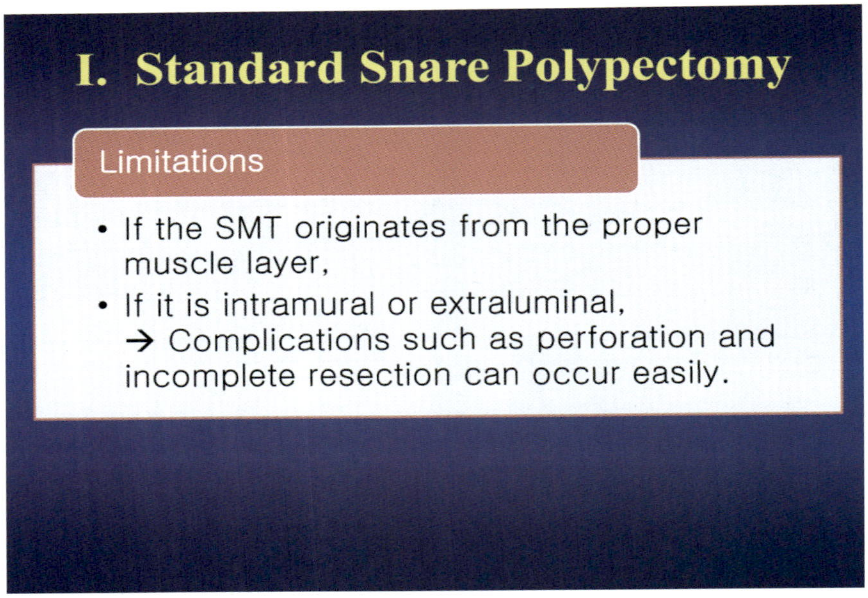

There are several limitations to this method. If the SMT originates from the proper muscle layer or if it is an intramural or extraluminal tumor, complication such as perforation or incomplete resection can occur easily.

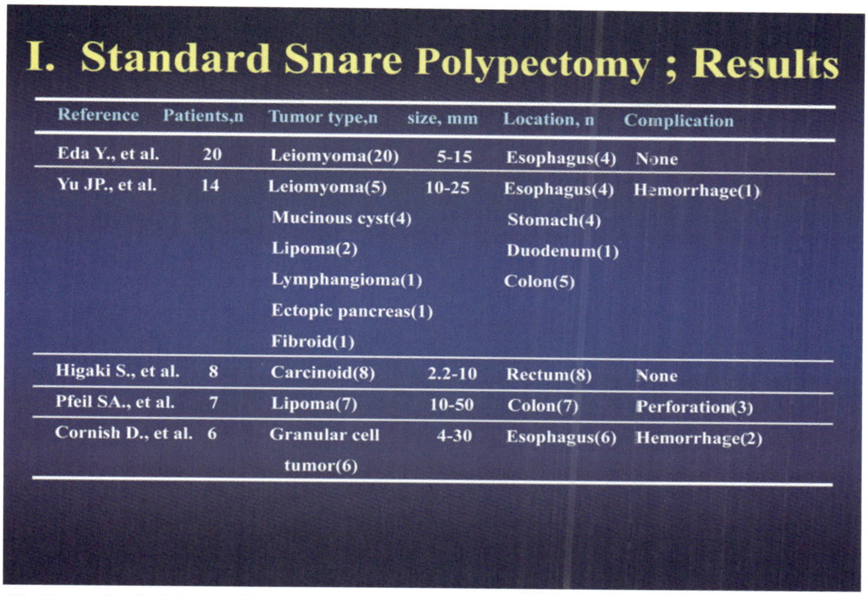

I. Standard Snare Polypectomy ; Results

Reference	Patients,n	Tumor type,n	size, mm	Location, n	Complication
Eda Y., et al.	20	Leiomyoma(20)	5-15	Esophagus(4)	None
Yu JP., et al.	14	Leiomyoma(5) Mucinous cyst(4) Lipoma(2) Lymphangioma(1) Ectopic pancreas(1) Fibroid(1)	10-25	Esophagus(4) Stomach(4) Duodenum(1) Colon(5)	Hemorrhage(1)
Higaki S., et al.	8	Carcinoid(8)	2.2-10	Rectum(8)	None
Pfeil SA., et al.	7	Lipoma(7)	10-50	Colon(7)	Perforation(3)
Cornish D., et al.	6	Granular cell tumor(6)	4-30	Esophagus(6)	Hemorrhage(2)

Most reports of clinical applications of the snare polypectomy method showed a high success rate with acceptably few complications. Importantly no serious complications were reported in association with the snare polypectomy method in cases chosen according to the indications previously described.

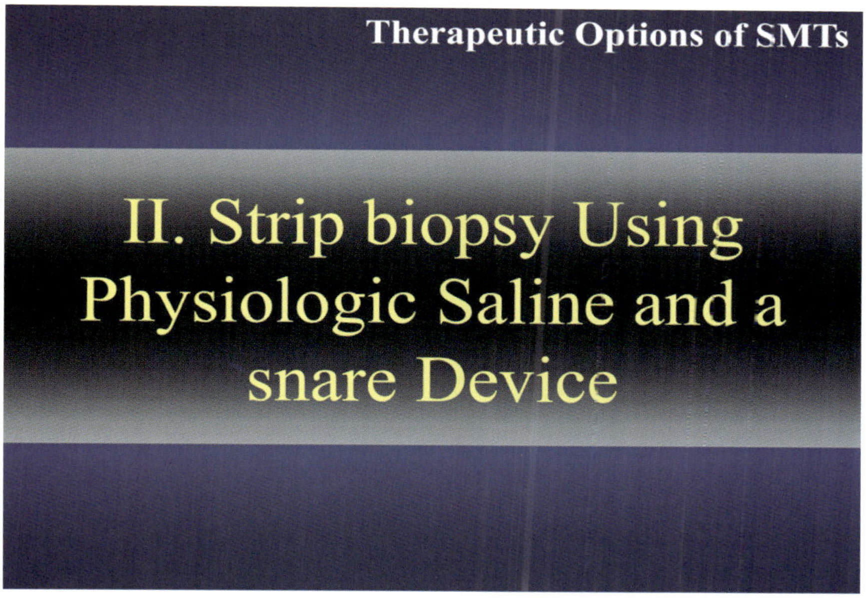

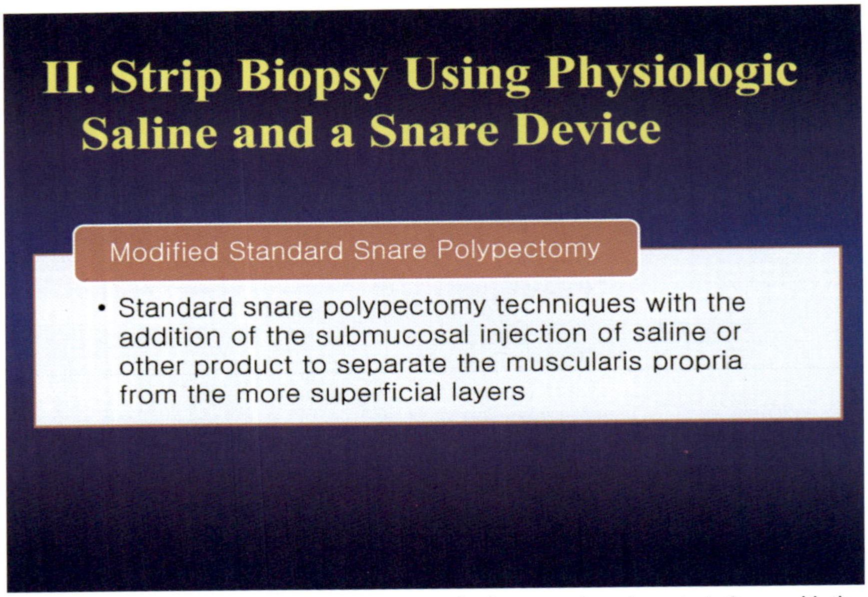

The strip biopsy method is based upon the standard snare polypectomy techniques with the addition of the submucosal injection of saline or other products to separate the muscularis propria from the more superficial layers.

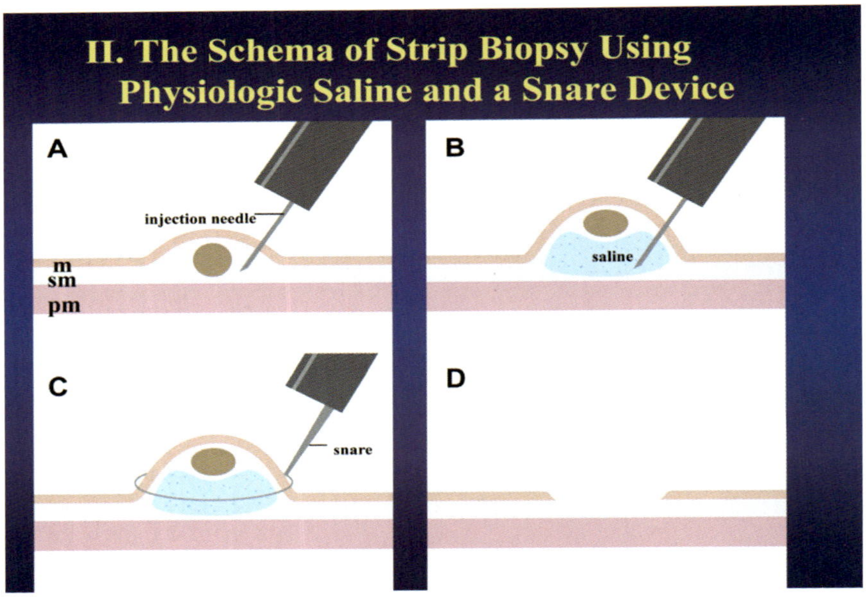

At first, the injection needle is placed at the base of the SMT. Saline solution is injected beneath the SMT to elevate it from the muscularis propria. The snare is placed around the base of the tumor and tightened in order to excise the tumor with electrocoagulation.

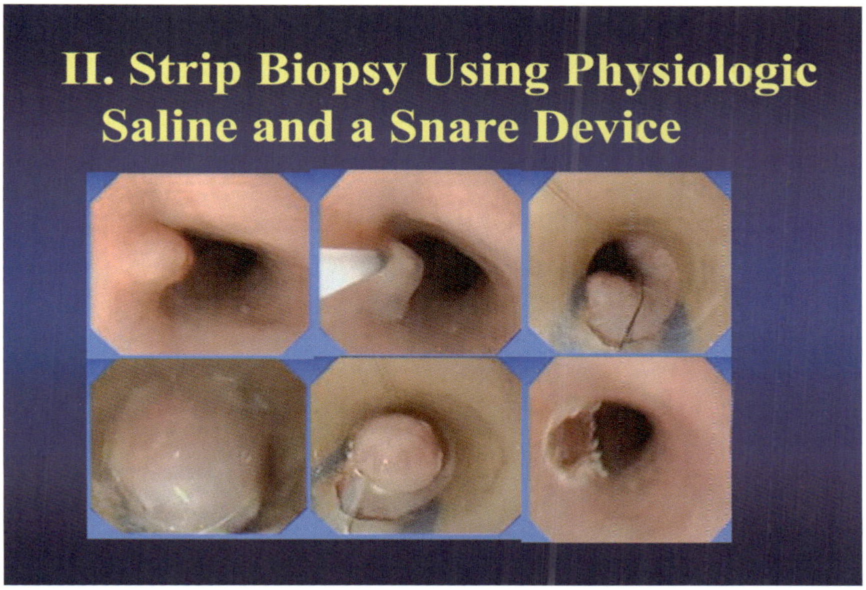

In this case, a submucosal tumor is observed on endsoscopy at the mid esophagus. Saline solution was injection beneath the SMT to elevated it from the muscularis propria. The snare is placed around the base of the tumor and tightened for successful excision.

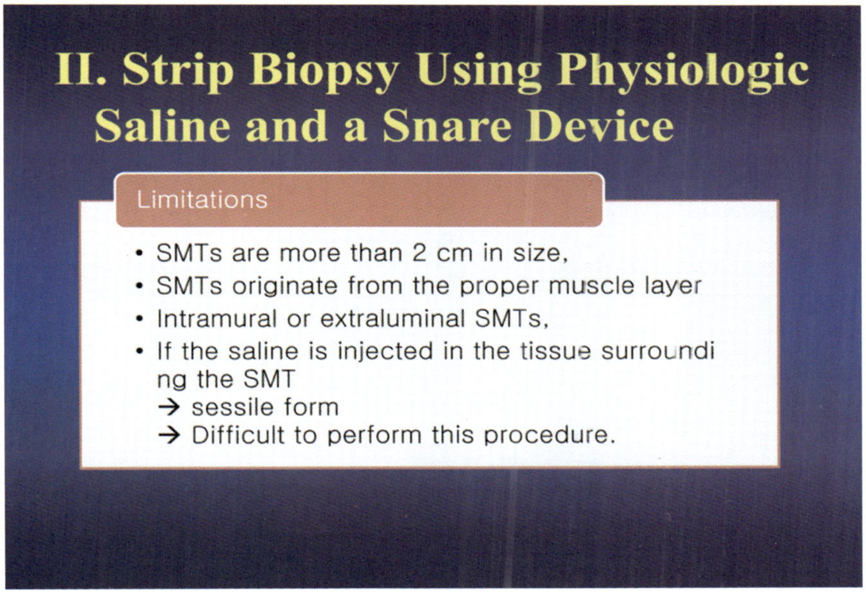

There are several limitations to the strip biopsy technique. The strip biopsy technique is difficult to perform if the SMT is more than 2 cm size, if the SMT originated from the proper muscle layer, or if the SMT is intramural or extraluminal. Additionally if the saline is injected in the tissue surrounding the SMT, and not directly beneath the tumor, the SMT may become sessile in form which in turn makes it difficult to grasp with forceps.

II. Strip Biopsy Using Physiologic Saline and a Snare Device ; Results

Reference	Patients,n	Tumor type,n	size, mm	Location, n	Complication
Kawamoto K., et al.	45	Lipoma (9) Leiomyoma (3) Hemangioma (3) Granular cell tumor (1) Lymphangioma (6) Carcinoid (6)	6-25	Esophagus (5) Stomach (1) Duodenum (16) Colon (23)	Hemorrhage (5)
Sun S., et al.	16	Leiomyoma (10) Ectopic pancreas (2) Lipoma (1) Others (2)	8-35	Esophagus (3) Stomach (13)	Hemorrhage (2)
Kojima T., et al.	17	Leiomyoma (12) Granular cell tumor (5)	5-14	Esophagus (17)	Hemorrhage (1)
Songur Y., et al.	2	Leiomyoma (2)	15-20	Esophagus (2)	None

Like the snare polypectomy method, the strip biopsy technique shows a high success rate for tumor less than 2cm in diameter, and for SMT located in the muscularis mucosa and submucosal layers. No serious complications have been reported for this procedure.

Therapeutic Options of SMTs

III. Endoscopic Submucosal Resection with a Ligating Device (ESMR-L)

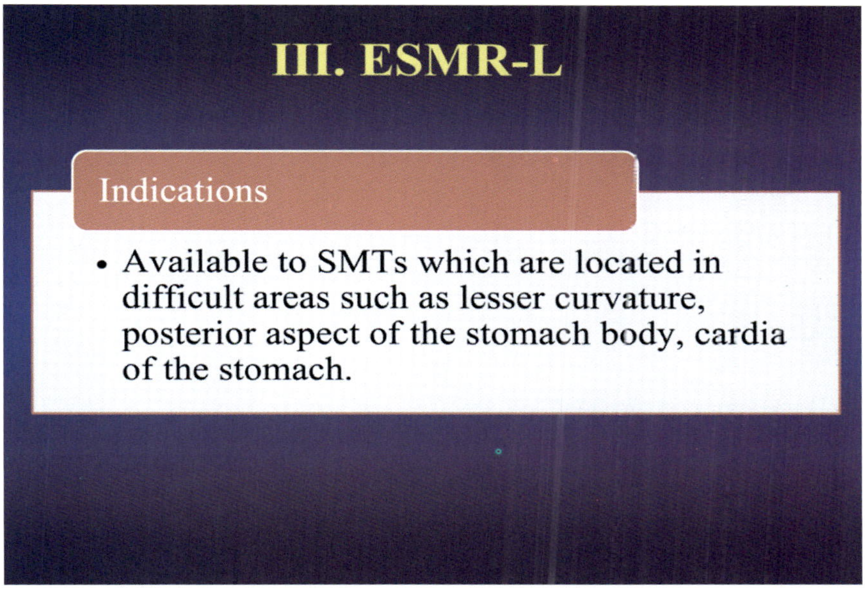

Endoscopic submucosal resction with a ligating device (ESMR-L) is available for removal of difficult SMT' s located on the lesser curvature, the posteror aspect of the body and the cardia of the stomach.

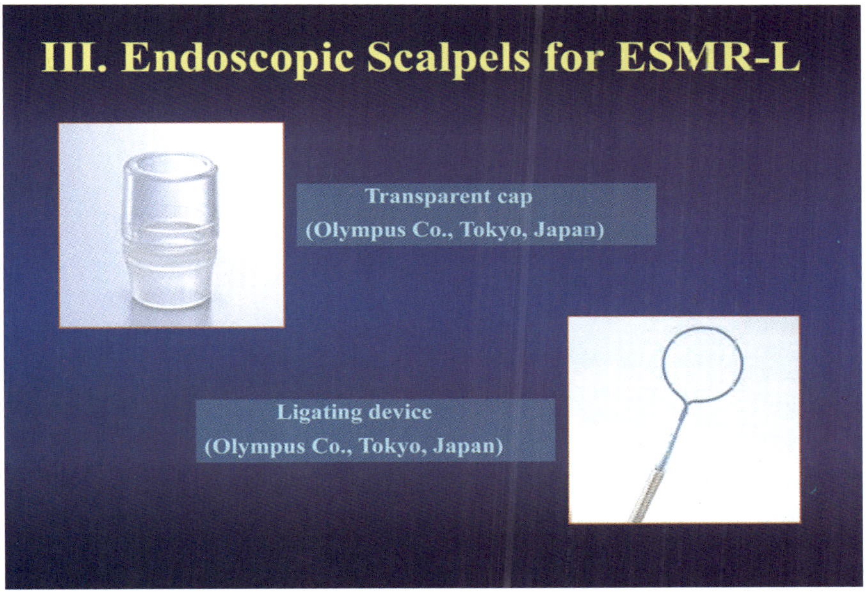

For this method, a transparent cap and ligating device are used.

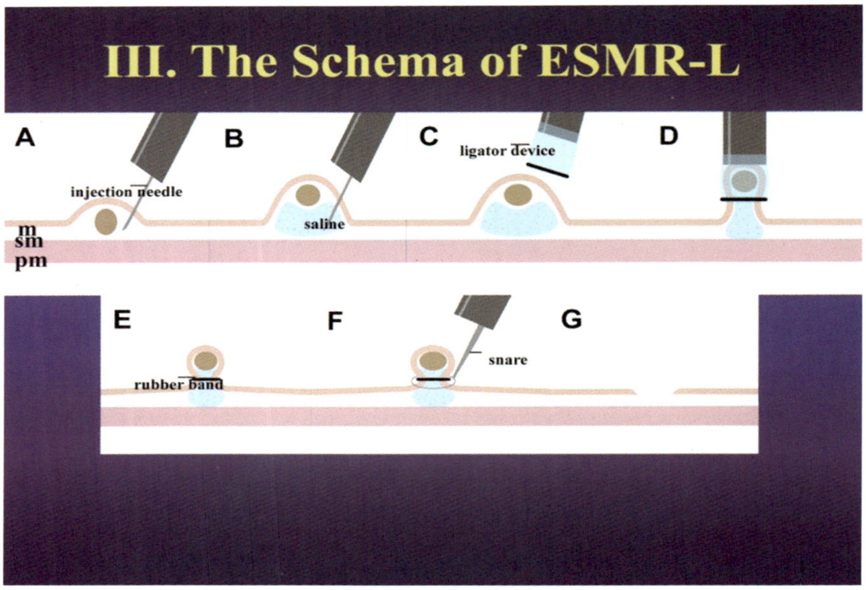

At first, saline solution is injected beneath the SMT to elevate it from the muscularis mucosa. The endoscope with the attached ligating device is brought near to the tumor. The tumor is aspirated into the ligating device and a rubber band is deployed. Then a snare is placed below the band for removal of tumor by electrocoagulation.

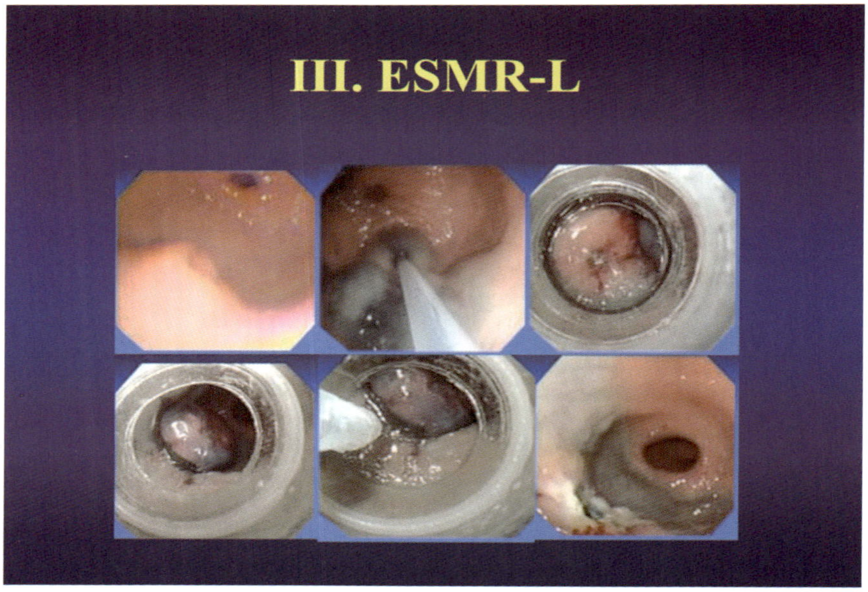

In this case, a submucosal tumor with central umblication is seen on the greater curvature of the gastric antrum. After saline injection removal was attempted using a snare and grasping forceps. However, the tumor was difficult to grasp and removal using ESMR-L was performed.

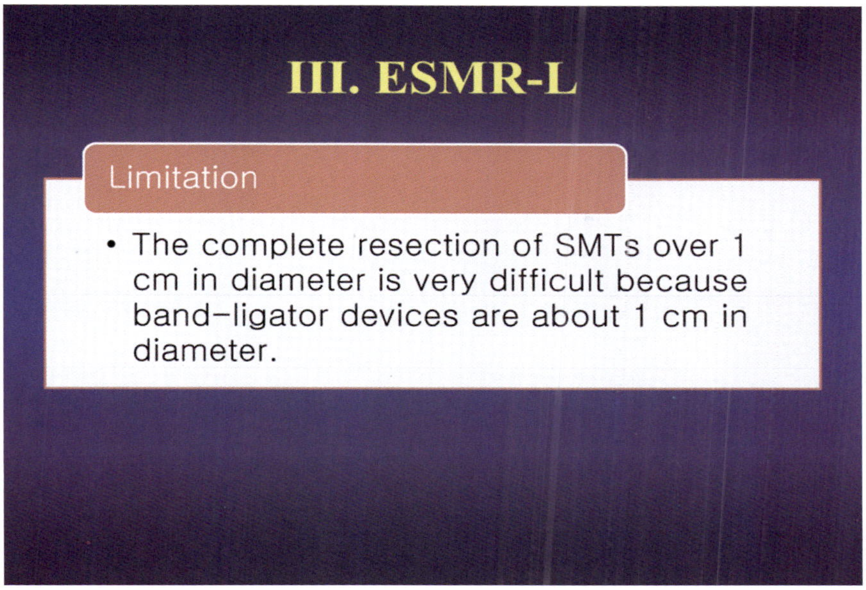

The limitation of this method is that the complete resection of SMT' s over 1 cm in diameter is very difficult due to the limited size of band-ligator devices.

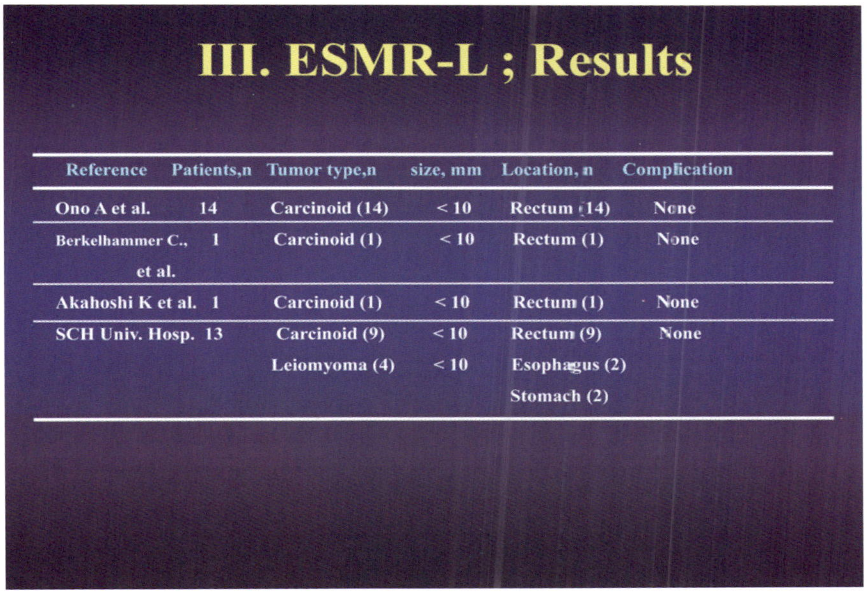

Reference	Patients,n	Tumor type,n	size, mm	Location, n	Complication
Ono A et al.	14	Carcinoid (14)	< 10	Rectum (14)	None
Berkelhammer C., et al.	1	Carcinoid (1)	< 10	Rectum (1)	None
Akahoshi K et al.	1	Carcinoid (1)	< 10	Rectum (1)	None
SCH Univ. Hosp.	13	Carcinoid (9)	< 10	Rectum (9)	None
		Leiomyoma (4)	< 10	Esophagus (2)	
				Stomach (2)	

ESMR-L has been used mainly for the removal of rectal carcinoid tumors. Several authors reported high success rates without any complications for the removal of rectal carcinoid tumors less than 1 cm in diameter. Our group has had success with leiomyomas less than 1 cm originating the esophagus and stomach.

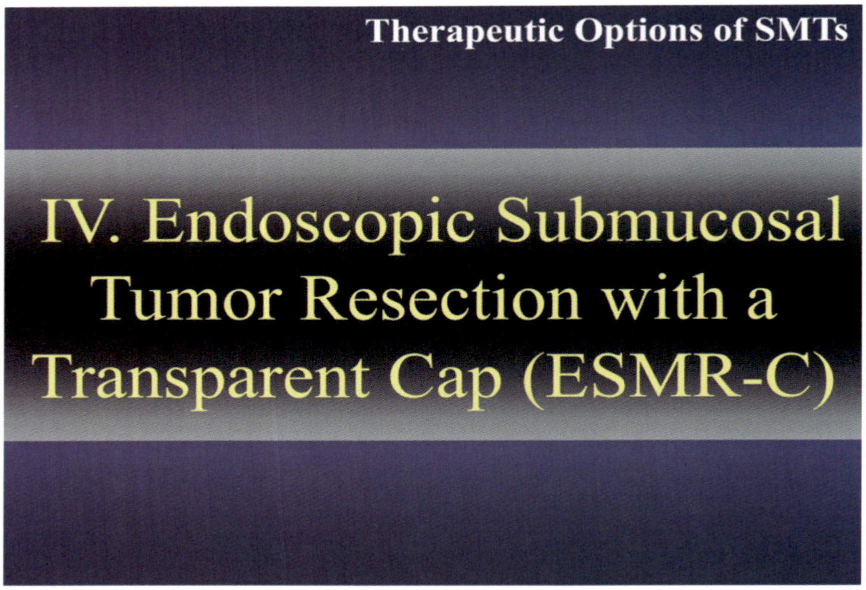

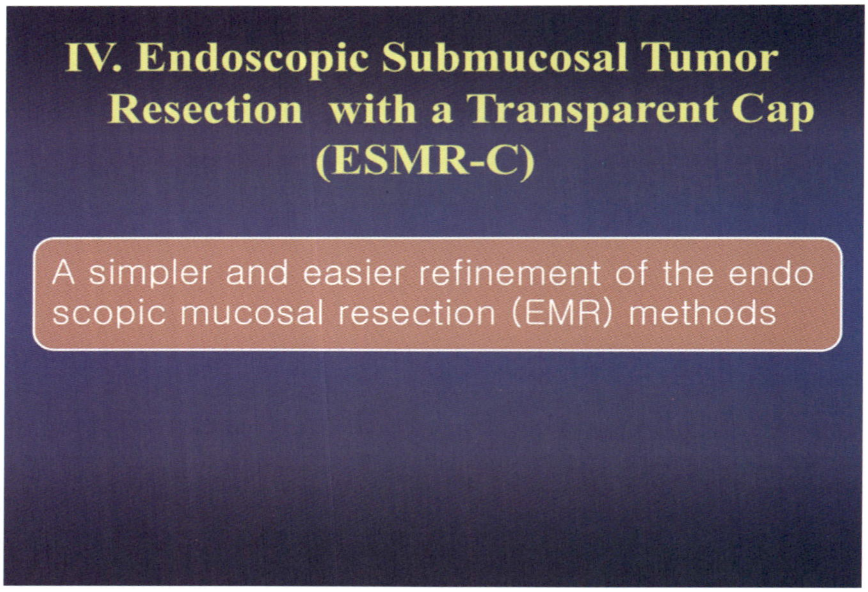

Endoscopic submucosal tumor resection with a transparent cap (ESMR-C) is a simpler and easier refinement of the endoscopic mucosal resection method (EMR).

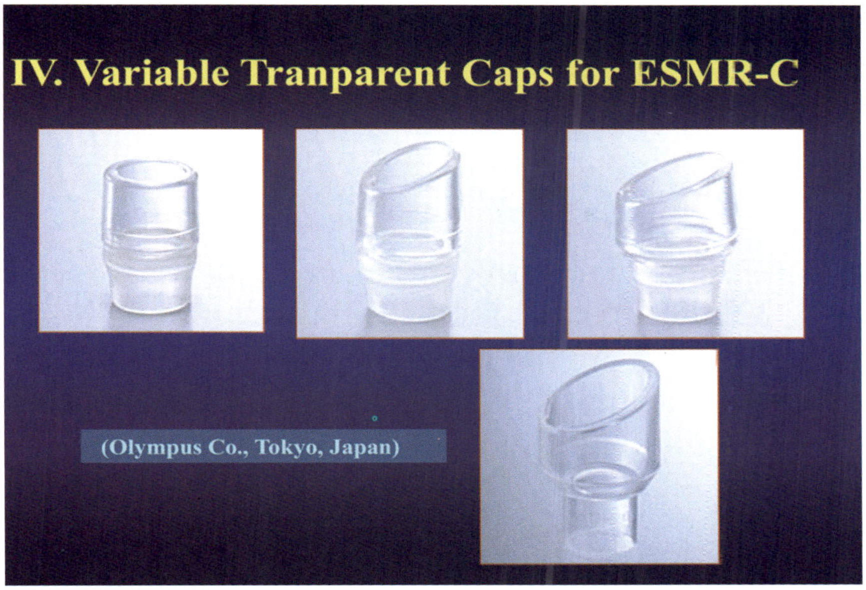

This technique requires a specialized transparent plastic cap, that is fitted on the tip of a standard diagnostic or therapeutic endoscope. Various caps have been developed in sized ranging from 12 to 18 mm for the use in variable endoscopes.

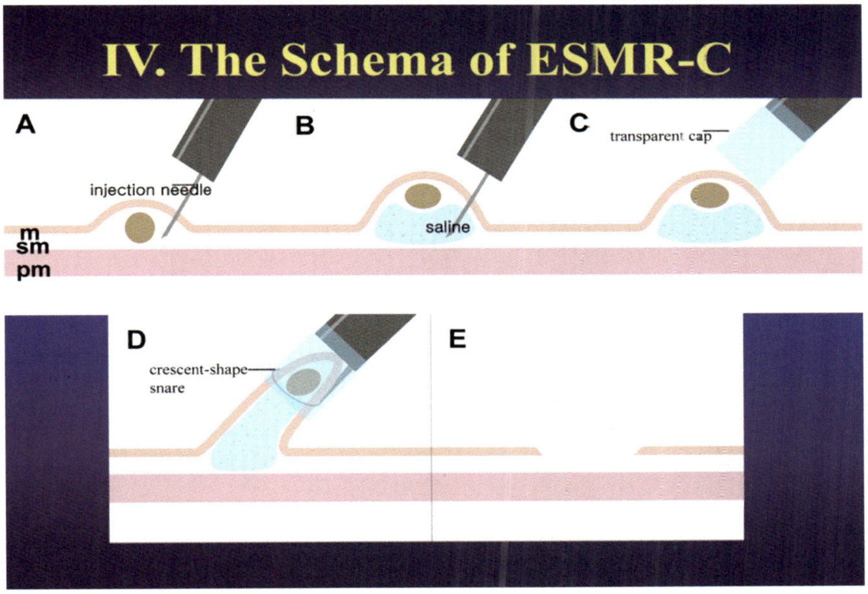

Saline solution is injected beneath the SMT to elevated from the muscularis propria. A transparent cap is fitted at the tip of the endoscope. The snare is then pre-looped into the groove of the rim of the cap. The tumor is aspirated into the transparent cap and electosurgically excised using the snare.

III. ESMR-C

Limitation

- SMTs more than 2 cm in diameter (Pl astic cap size : 12-18 mm)
- SMTs are located in the proper muscle→ Difficult to resect.

In clinical practice, SMT' s more than 2 cm in diameter are difficult to remove due to limitation of cap size. SMT' s located in the proper muscle layer are also difficult to resect.

IV. ESMR-C ; Results

Reference	Patients,n	Tumor type,n	size, mm	Location, n	Complication
Kajiyama T., et al.	38	Leiomyoma(13) Hemangioma (3) Granular cell tumor (2) Ectopic pancreas (5) Submucosal glandular cysts (2) Lipoma (2) Carcinoid (9)	4-20	Esophagus (16) Stomach (12) Colon (8)	Hemorrhage (1)
Imada-Shirakata Y., et al.	8	Carcinoid (8)	3.5-10	Rectum (8)	None
Kajiyama T., et al.	9	Leiomyoma (9)	13-26	Esophagus (9)	None

Kajiyana et al. reported the results of ESMR-C for 38 cases of SMT' s. They reported a 100% resection rate and occurrence of minor hemorrhage in 3% of patients. Other studies have also reported high success rates for this method.

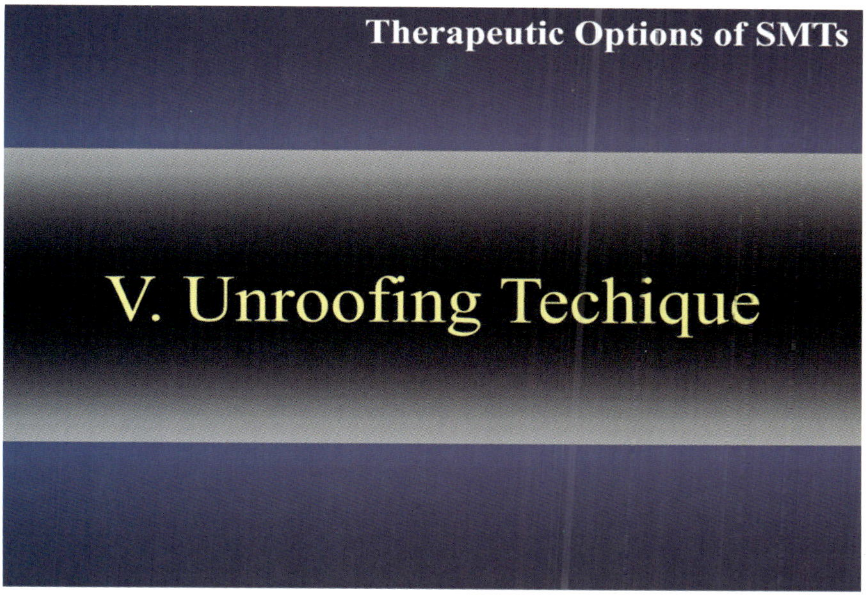

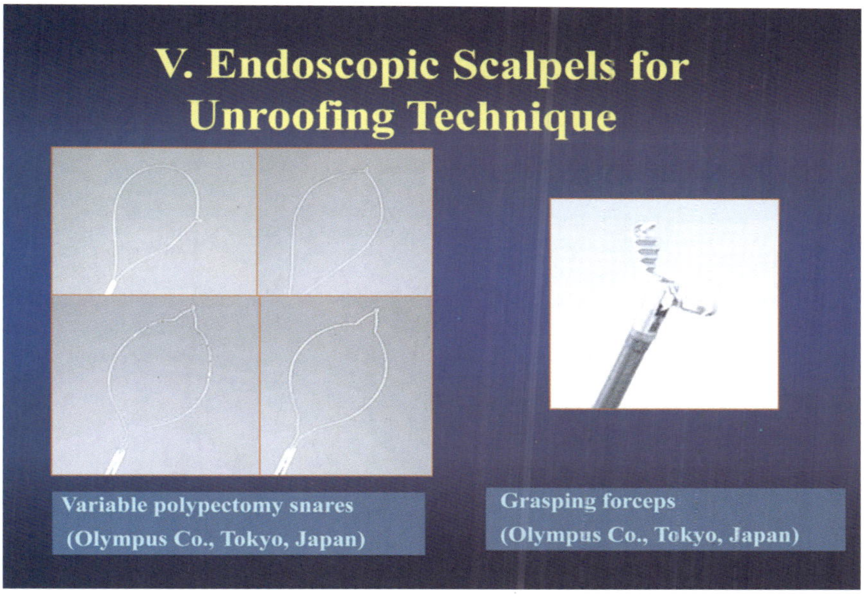

For the unroofing method, various polypectomy snares and grasping forceps are used.

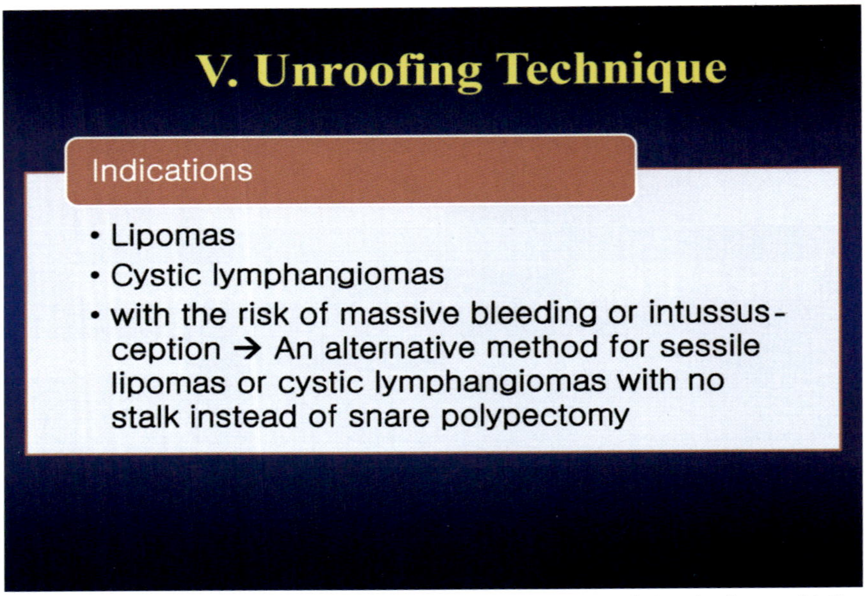

The unroofing technique is applicable, only in cases of lipoma, and cystic lymphagiomas with the risk of massive bleeding or intussusceptions. Use of the snare polypectomy method in these cases may also carry a higher risk of perforation, especially for sessile lipomas or cystic lymphagiomas with no stalk.

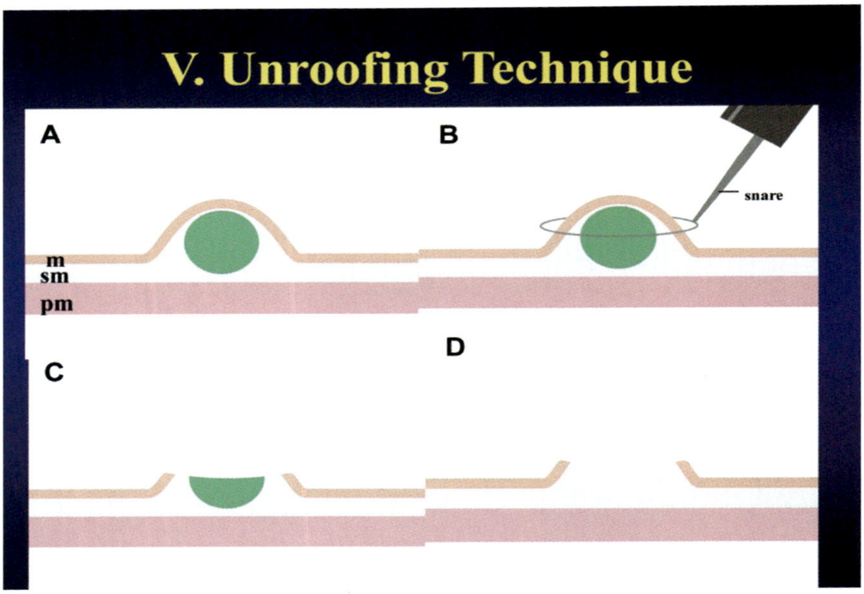

The unroofing method utilizes a snare over the middle of the SMT, creating an opening in the overlying mucosa. In most cases, the remnant lipoma or lymphangioma resolves spontaneously.

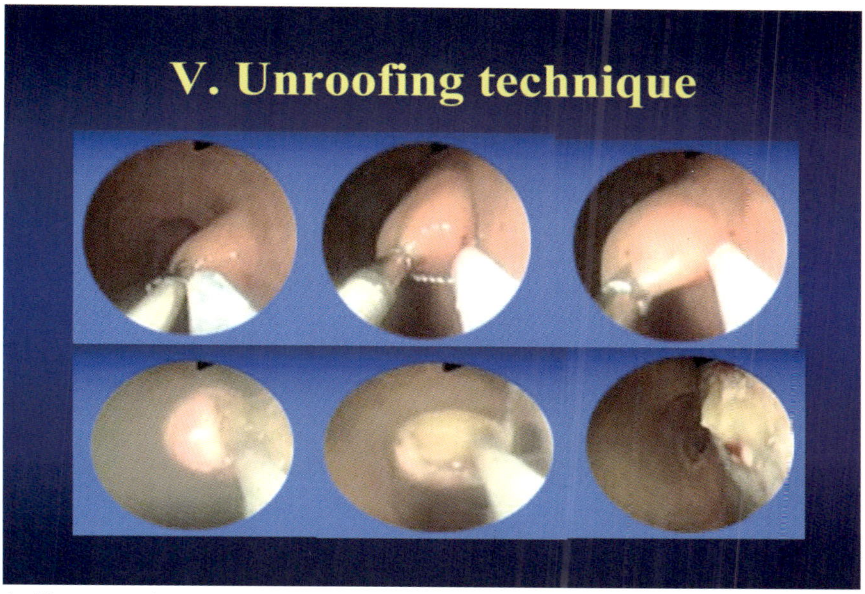

In this case, a submucosal lesion is seen on the posterior wall of the duodenal bulb. The middle of the SMT is snared, creating an opening in the underlying mucosa. The remnant lipoma can be seen following resection.

V. Unroofing Technique ; Results

Reference	Patients, n	Tumor type, n	size, mm	Location, n	Complication
Mimura T., et al.	8	Lymphangioma(8)	8-40	Colorectum	None
Hizawa K., et al.	1	Lipoma (1)	20x30	Duodenum	None
Fukuda S., et al.	1	Lipoma (1)	50x30	Stomach	None
Hizawa K., et al.	9	Simple cystic tumor(4) Multicystic tumor(4) Solid cystic tumor (1)	n.a.	n.a.	None
SCH Univ, Hosp.	6	Lipoma (6)	16-50	Small intestine(1) Colon (5)	Hemorrhage(1)

n.a.: data not available owing to lack of certainty in the literature

Several authors reported successful treatment of lipomas and cystic tumors using this method.

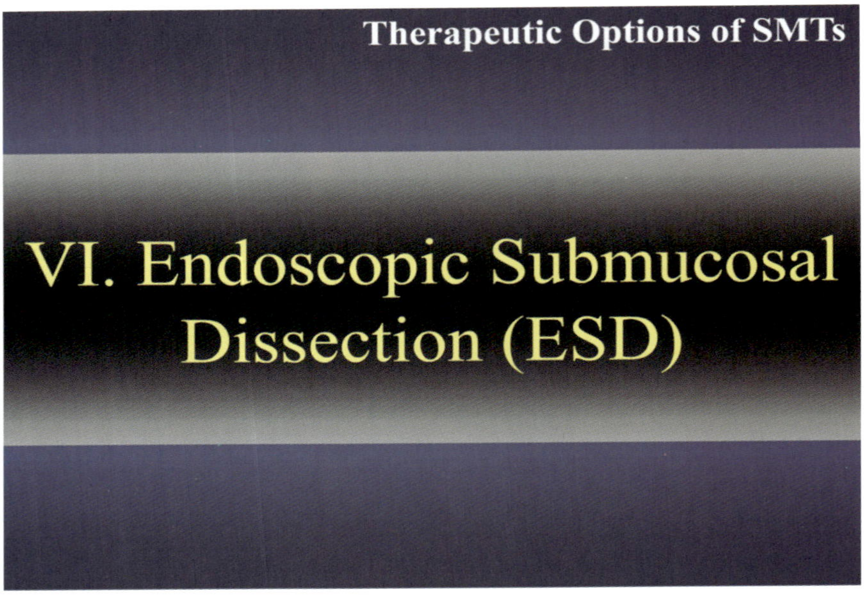

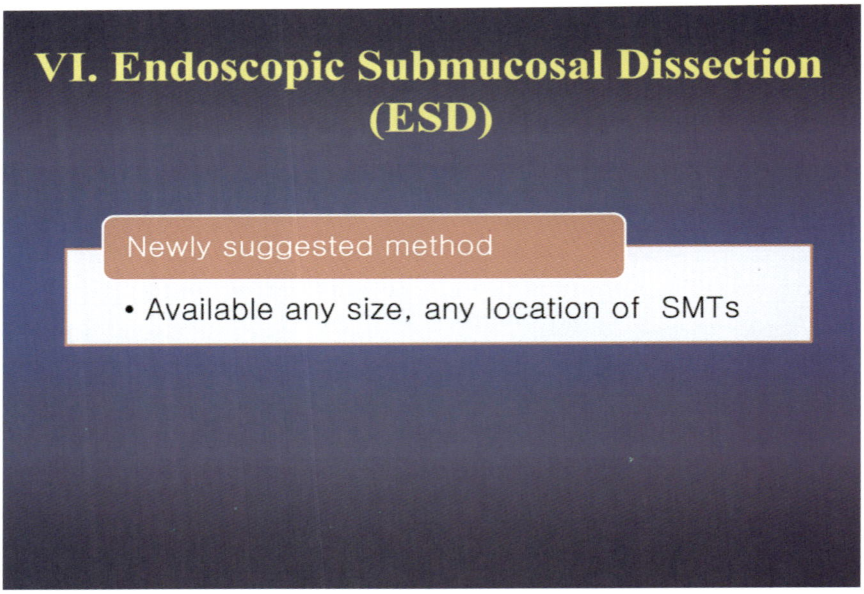

ESD is a newly suggested method for removal of SMT' s. It is available to SMT of any size of location.

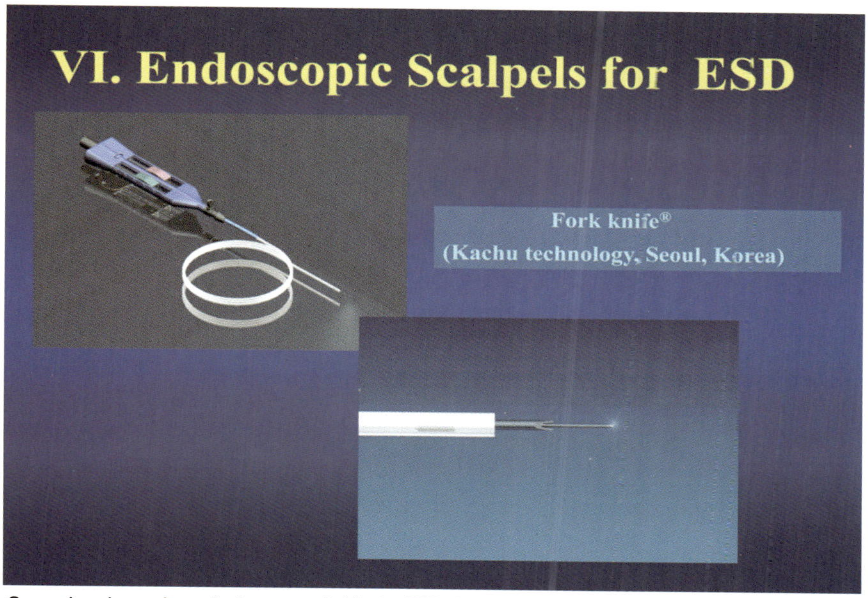

Several endoscopic scalpels are available for ESD. These include the IT knife, the Hook knife, the Flex knife and the Fork knife.

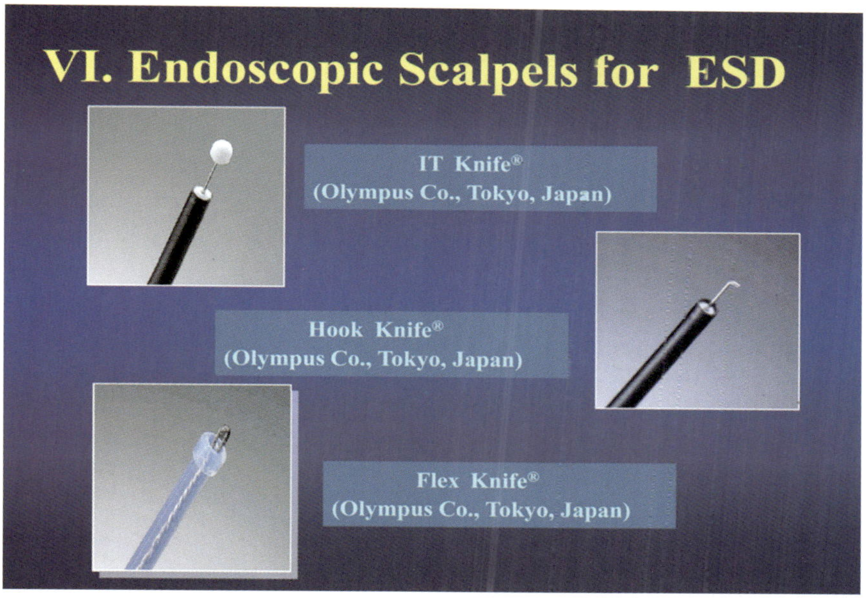

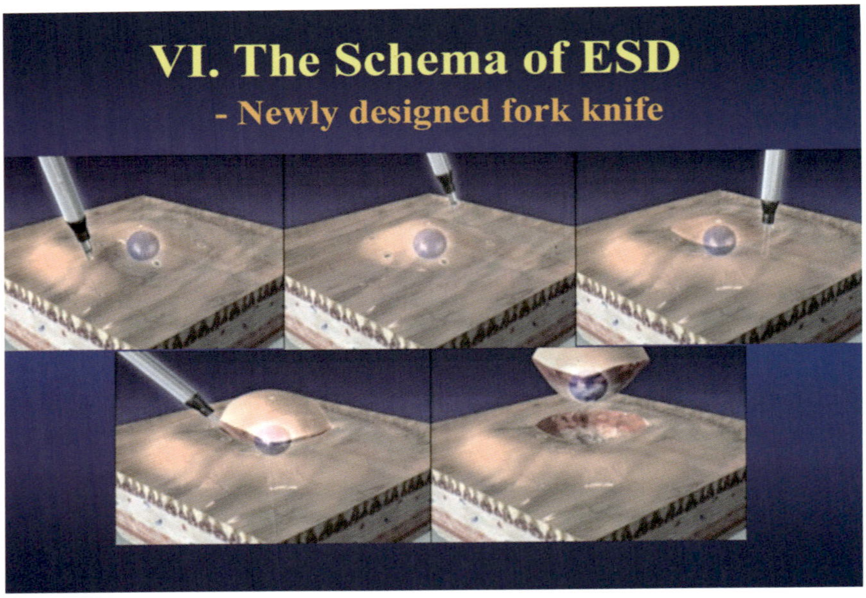

ESD is a five step procedure. First marking dots are made circumferentially around the lesion. Next, submucosal injection is performed and the lesion is elevated. Incision is then performed using an appropriate knife to separate the tumor from the surrounding non-neoplastic mucosa. The submucosal layer is then gradually dissected from the muscle layer and the resected specimen is removed.

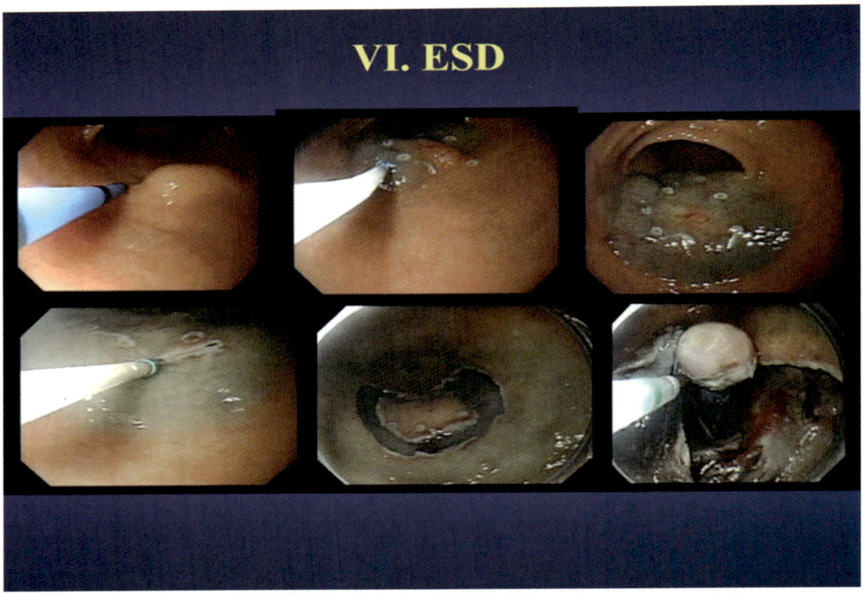

In clinical practice, first marking dots with argon plasma coagulation are made circumferentially around the lesion. Next, submucosal injection is performed and the lesion is elevated. Incision is then performed using an appropriate knife to separate the tumor from the surrounding non-neoplastic mucosa. The submucosal layer is then gradually dissected from the muscle layer and the resected specimen is completely removed.

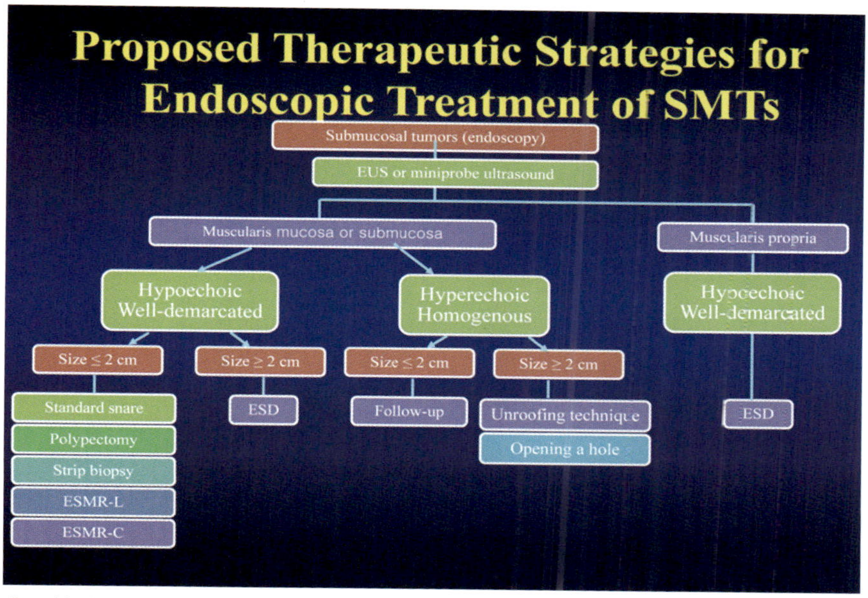

Considering the results of previous investigations of the endoscopic treatment of SMT' s, the following therapeutic strategies can be proposed. Based on the observed endoscopic and endosonographic characteristics of the tumors, well demarcated hypoechoic lesions up to 2 cm in diameter without umblication that are suggestive of ectopic pancreas on endoscopic examination and limited to the muscularis mucosa or submucosa on EUS examination can be removed using the standard snare polypectomy, strip biopsy, ESMR-L, or ESMR-C methods. Hyperechoic homogeneous lesions with or without a clearly evident cystic component can be monitored conservatively. Because these appearences are highly suggestive of benign lesions, such as lipomas , lymphagiomas or ectopic pancreas, based on experience with conventional and miniprobe EUS. However larger submucosal tumors with benign endosonographic characteristics, can be removed using the unroofing technique and ESD. Sessile SMT' s that extend into the proper muscle layer, and large SMT' s which are hyperechoic and well demarcated on EUS can be removed by ESD.

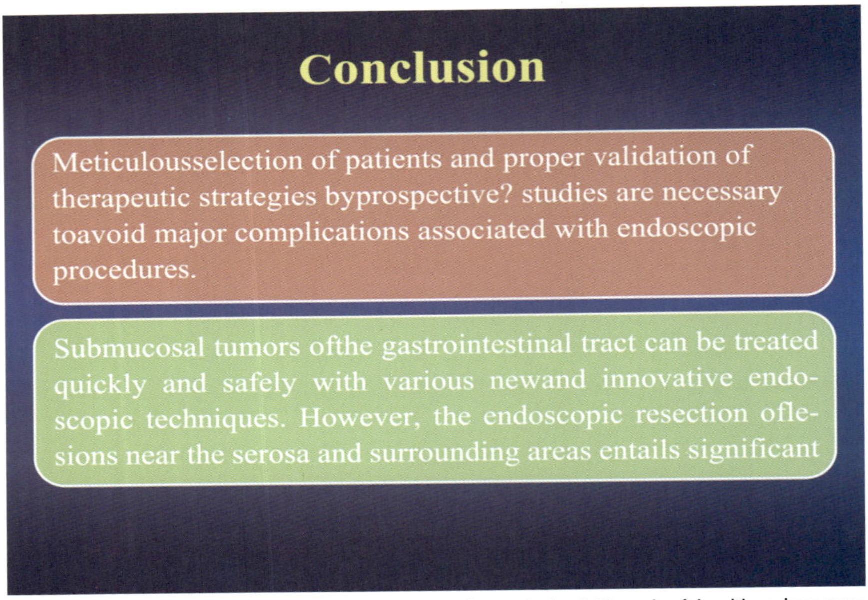

Submucosal tumors of the gastrointestinal tract can be treated quickly and safely with various new and innovative endoscopic techniques. However, the endoscopic resection of lesions near the serosa and surrounding areas entails significant risk such as perforation and hemorrhage. Meticulous selection of patients and proper validation of therapeutic strategies by prospective studies are necessary to avoid major complications associated with endoscopic procedures.

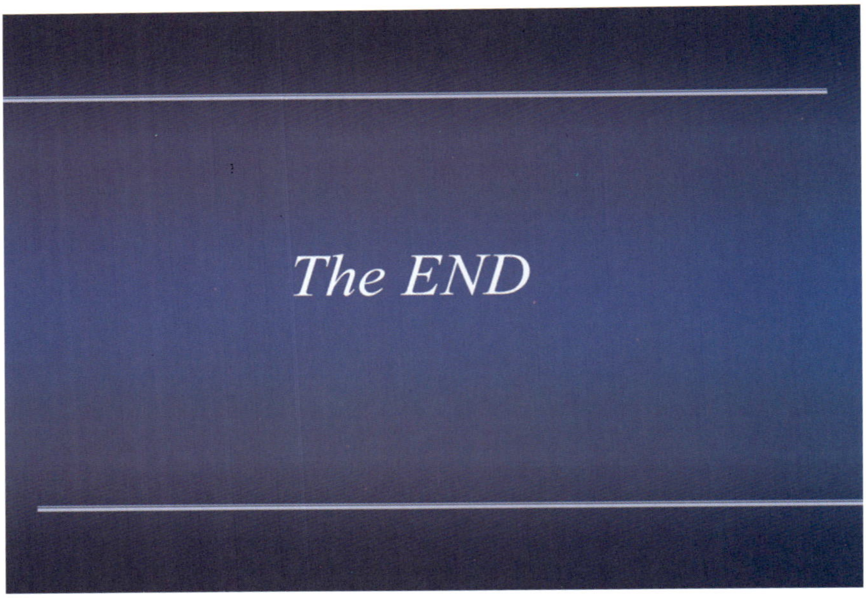

Chapter 3

Endoscopic Treatments of Early Esophageal Cancer & Early Neoplasia in Barrett's Esophagus

2008 ASGE Audiovisual Award Recipient
Tae Hee Lee, M.D.
Joo Young Cho, M.D. Ph D.

Chapter 3 Endoscopic Treatments of Early Esophageal Cancer & Early Neoplasia in Barrett's Esophagus

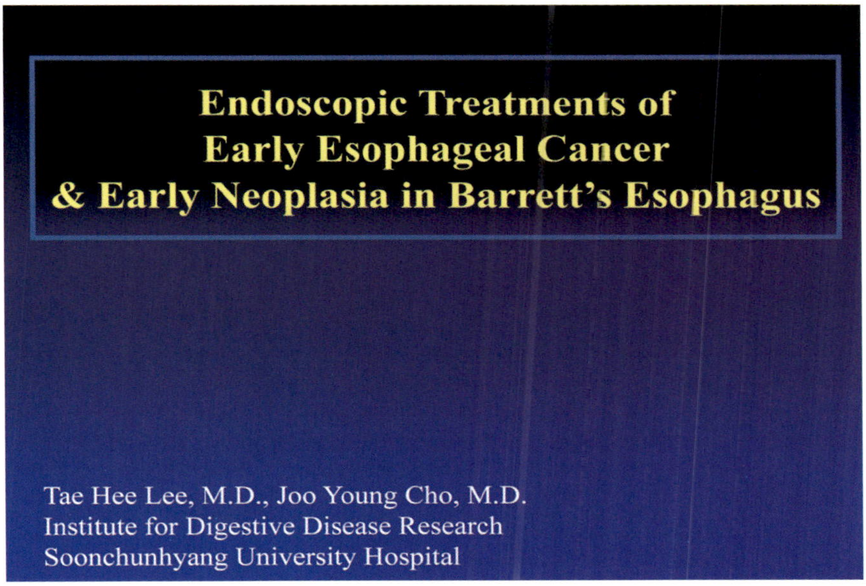

With technologic advances in endoscopy, detection and endoscopic treatment of early esophageal cancer is increasing. This chapter will focus on the various endoscopic treatments that have been applied to early esophageal cancer including early neoplasia in barrett' s esophagus.

Endoscopic Treatments of Early Esophageal Cancer & Early Neoplasia in Barrett's Esophagus

Early Esophageal Cancer

Endoscopic Resection

- EMR (endoscopic Mucosal Resection)
- ESD (endoscopic Submucosal dissection)

Endoscopic Ablation

- PDT(photodynamic therapy)
- Radiofrequency Ablation
- Laser and APC
- Cryoablation
- Endoscopic resection therapy
- Endoscopic ablation therapy

TOPIC (I)

Early esophageal cancer

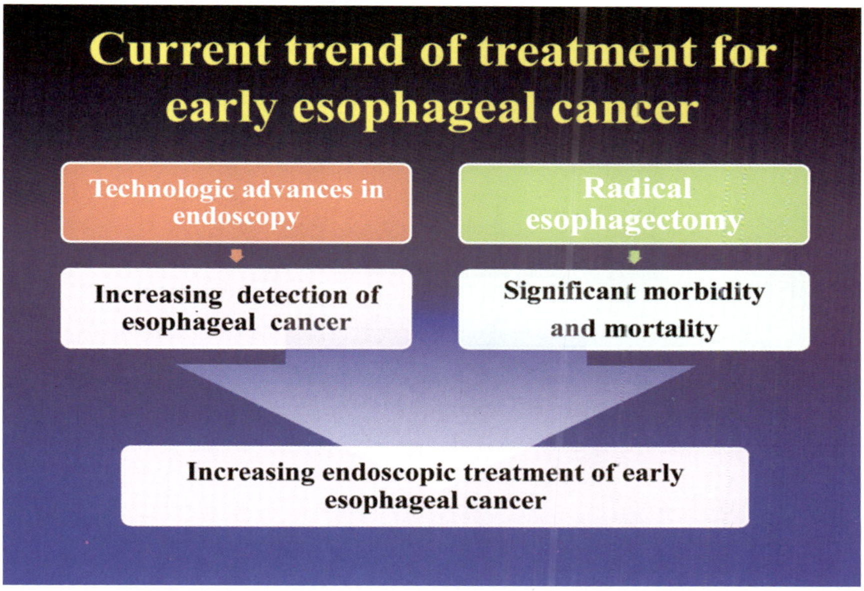

The recent developments in endoscopic technology have enabled the clinician to diagnose early esophageal cancer with increasing frequency. Considering the significant morbidity and mortality related to radical esophagectomy, the option of early treatment of esophageal cancer is increasingly being considered.

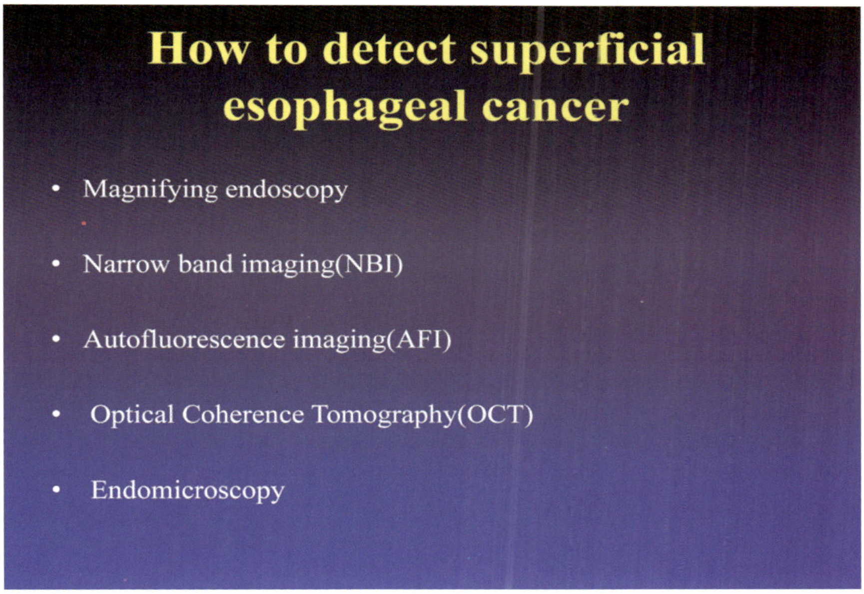

The advances in diagnostic endoscopy that allow us to accurately detect early esophageal cancer include Magnifying endoscopy, Narrow band imaging(NBI), Autofluorescence imaging(AFI), OCT, and Endomicroscopy.

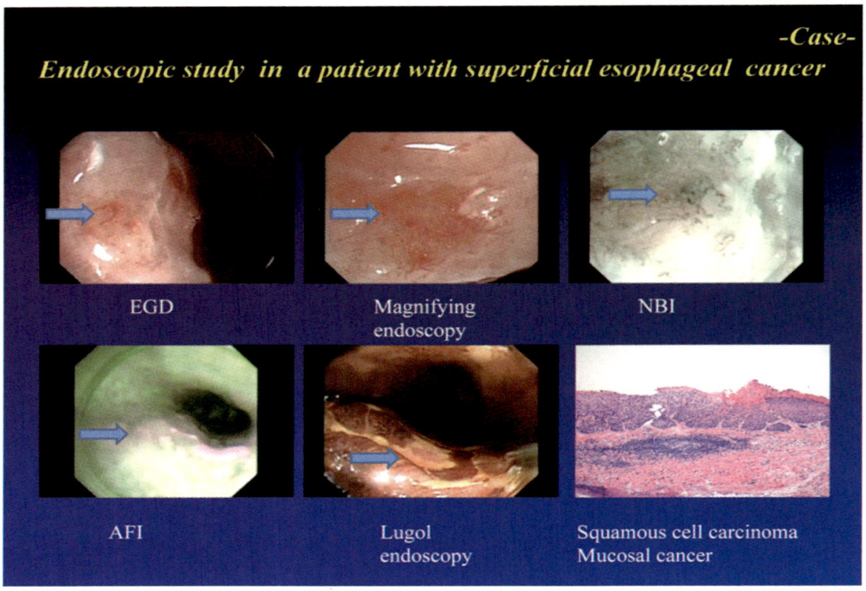

Various diagnostic endoscopy modalities used for detection of superficial esophageal cancer. Magnifying endoscopy can magnify the mucosa up to 100 fold. It shows an intricate image of the IPCL pattern. When NBI is used the mucosal capillaries appear brown while the submucosal veins appear blue. This image shows a relatively spared IPCL pattern adjacent to an abnormal lesion. AFI clearly shows the normal mucosa in green in contrast the abnormal mucosa appears pink. Chromoendoscopy using Lugol' s solution highlights an unstained area of abnormal mucosa.

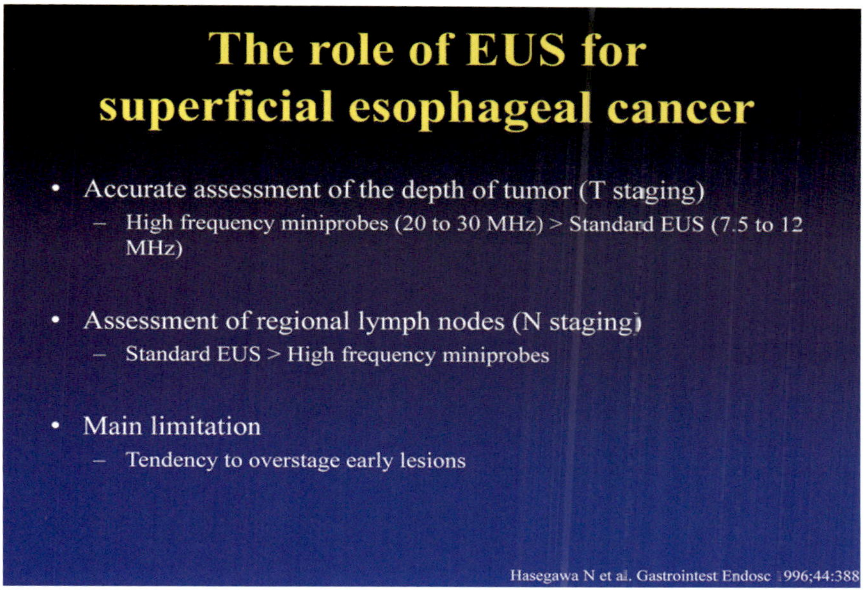

EUS is known to be an extremely useful tool for local and regional staging of esophageal cancer. High frequency EUS using a miniprobe is more accurate for distinguishing tumor invasion into the muscularis mucosa. However the limited depth of penetration precludes the adequate assessment of nodal stage. High frequency miniprobe also has a tendency to overstage early lesions when there is underlying inflammation of the tissue.

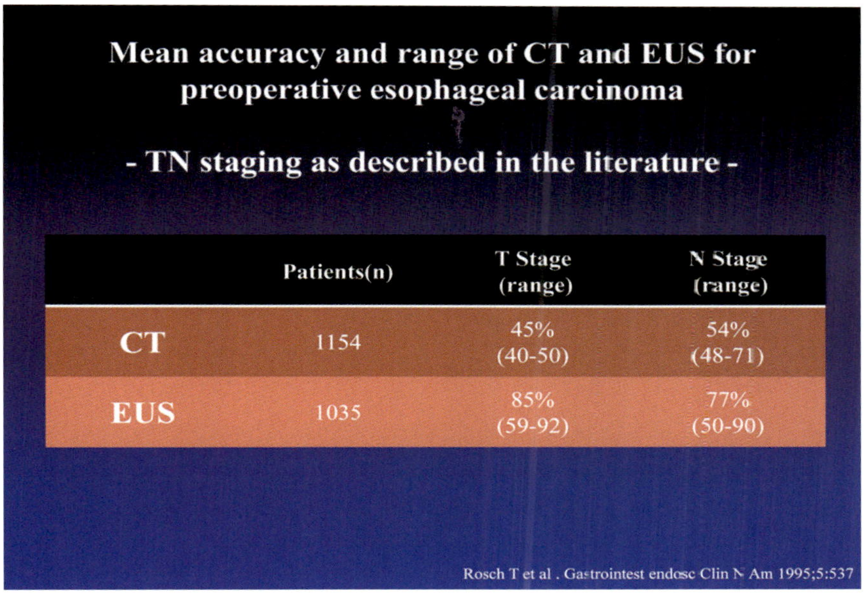

	Patients(n)	T Stage (range)	N Stage (range)
CT	1154	45% (40-50)	54% (48-71)
EUS	1035	85% (59-92)	77% (50-90)

In experienced hands, EUS has been shown to be superior to CT for T and N staging of esophageal cancer.

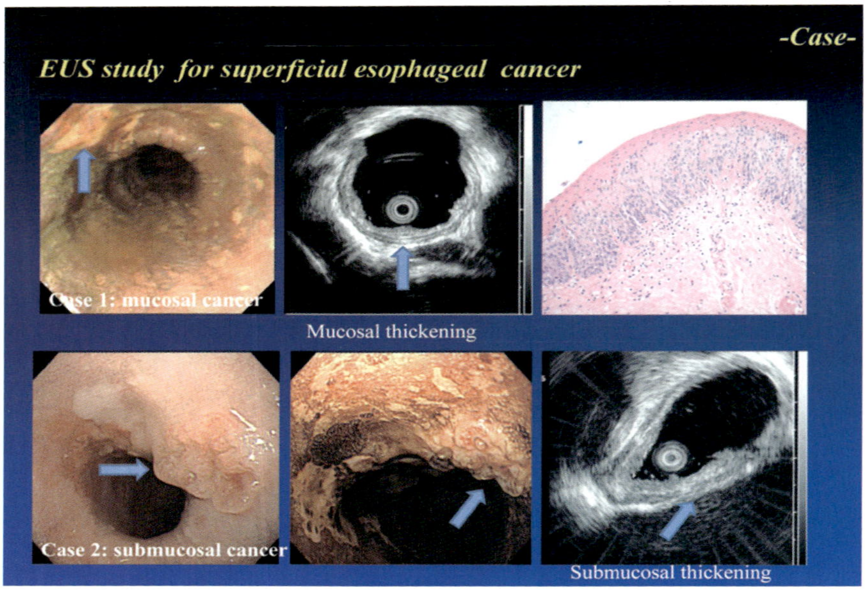

In the case 1, lugol chromoscopy has identified unstained mucosal lesion and EUS indicated its mucosal thickening, which was turned to squamous cell carcinoma, moderate differentiated, confined to the lamina propria. In the case 2, On conventional endoscopy, an ulceroinfiltrative lesion from 30cm upper incisor was suspicious for malignancy. Again, Lugol chromoscopy has made a very clear lesion of iodine unstained that already penetrated up to muscle layer on EUS.

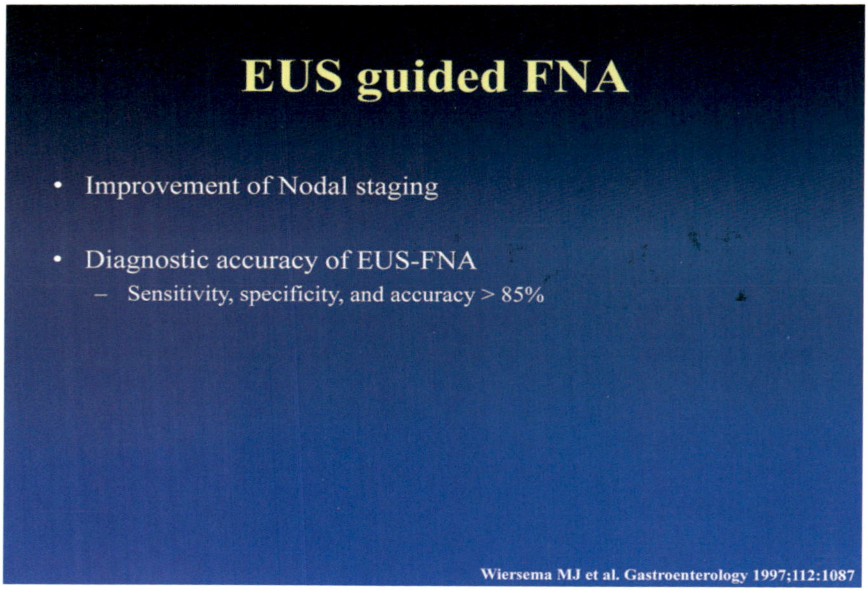

EUS guided fine needle aspiration may improve the accuracy of N staging. The overall accuracy of EUS guided fine needle aspiration for locoregional lymph nodes was more than 85% in one report.

EUS criteria for assessments of lymph nodes

	Benign	Malignant
Size	<10mm	>10mm
Shape	Elongated	Round
Border	Irregular	Smooth
Echogenicity	Hyperechoic	Hypoechoic

Catalano et al. Gastrointest endosc 1994;40:442

Endosonographic criteria that are suggestive of malignant involvement of visible lymph nodes include a width greater than 10 mm, round shape, smooth border, and echo-poor pattern.

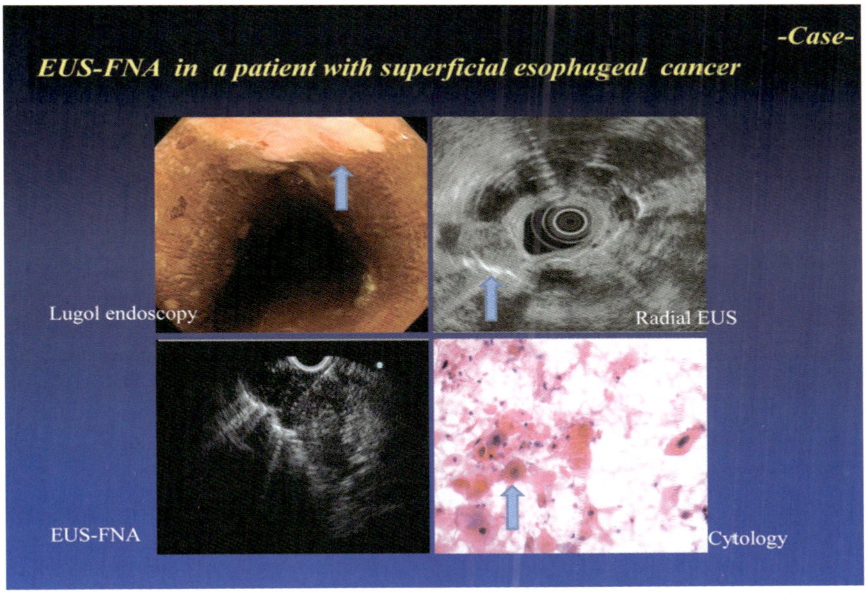

This patient was diagnosed with esophageal cancer. A nonstained lesion is seen on the mid-esophagus. EUS demonstrated multiple enlarged lymph nodes. EUS fine needle aspiration was performed and the results were suggestive of squamous cell carcinoma.

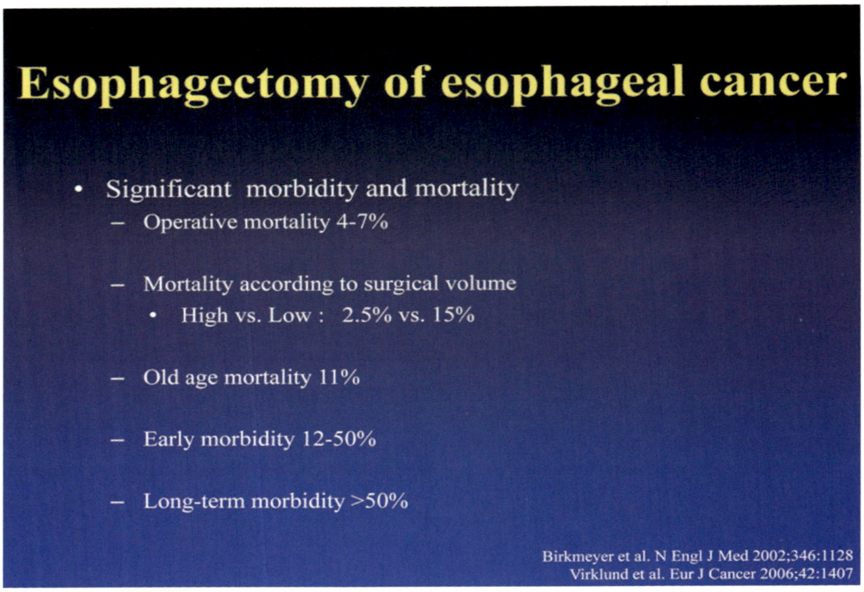

Esophagectomy is associated with significant procedure related mortality and long term morbidity. Mortality rates ranging from 4 to 7% have been reported. The mortality rate differed significantly with the number of procedures the center had performed. In particular, elderly patients had a higher mortality rate. 12 to 50% of patients developed serious postoperative complications. Such as pneumonia, anastomotic leaks and myocardial infarction. Long term morbidity rates of more than 50% have been reported.

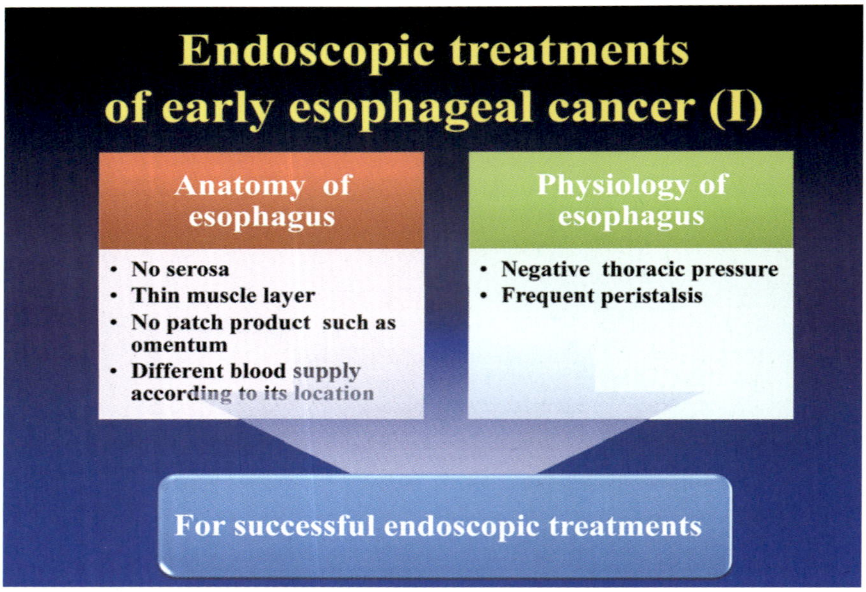

For successful endoscopic treatment the endoscopist must have a complete understanding of the anatomy and physiology of the esophagus. Unlike most of the GI tract, the esophagus is devoid of a serosal layer and the muscular layer is very thin. The endoscopist must have knowledge of the blood supply of the esophagus. And the consequences that negative thoracic pressure and frequent peristalsis may have on the procedure.

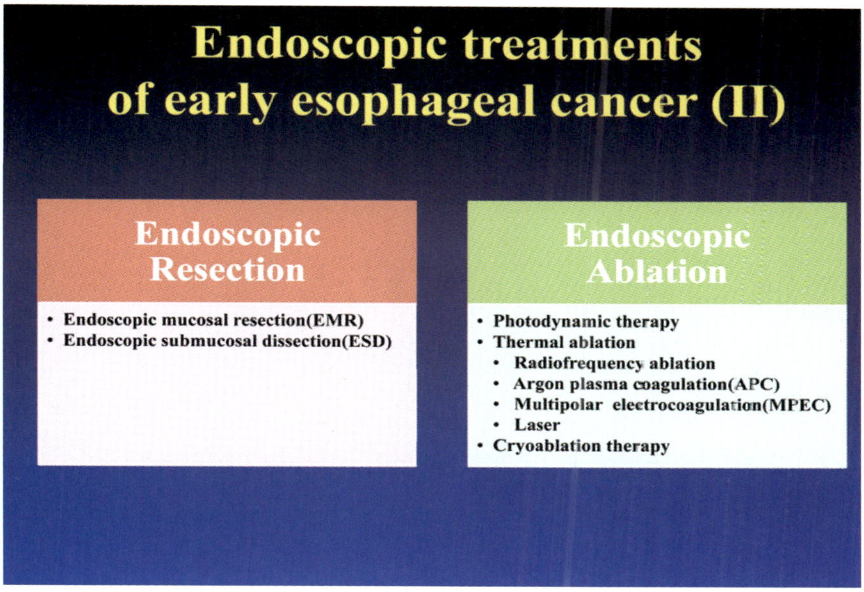

Endoscopic treatment of the esophagus can generally be divided into endoscopic resection and endoscopic ablation. Endoscopic resection can be done with either EMR of ESD. Endoscopic ablation therapies include photodynamic therapy, radiofrequency ablation, APC, MPEC, laser and cyro spray ablation.

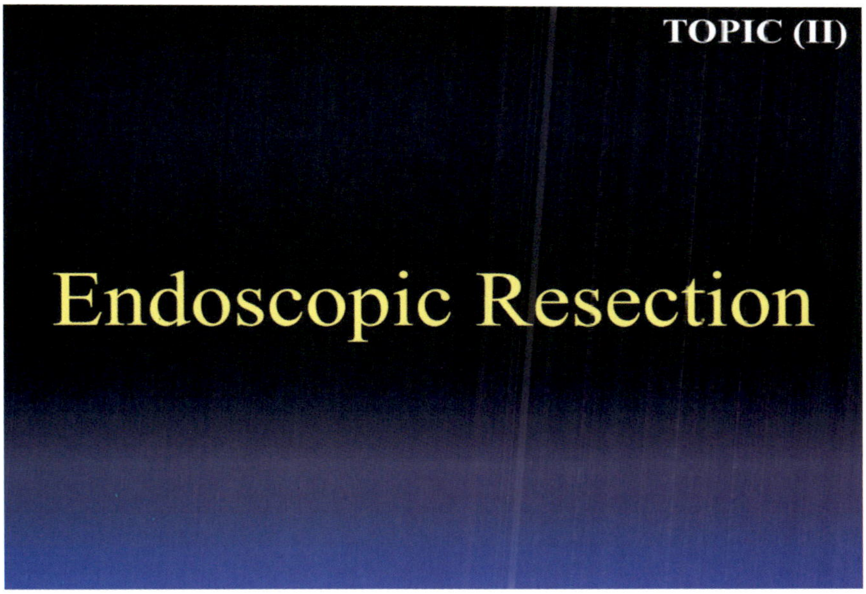

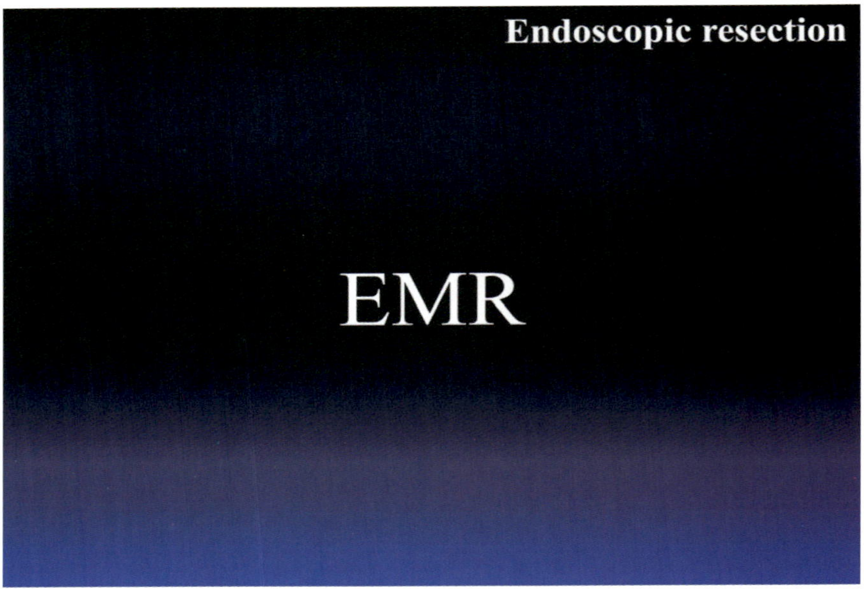

EMR for esophageal cancer was firth developed by Makuuchi in 1988. in the following years, squamous cell dysplasia and early carcinoma were considered as indications for EMR.

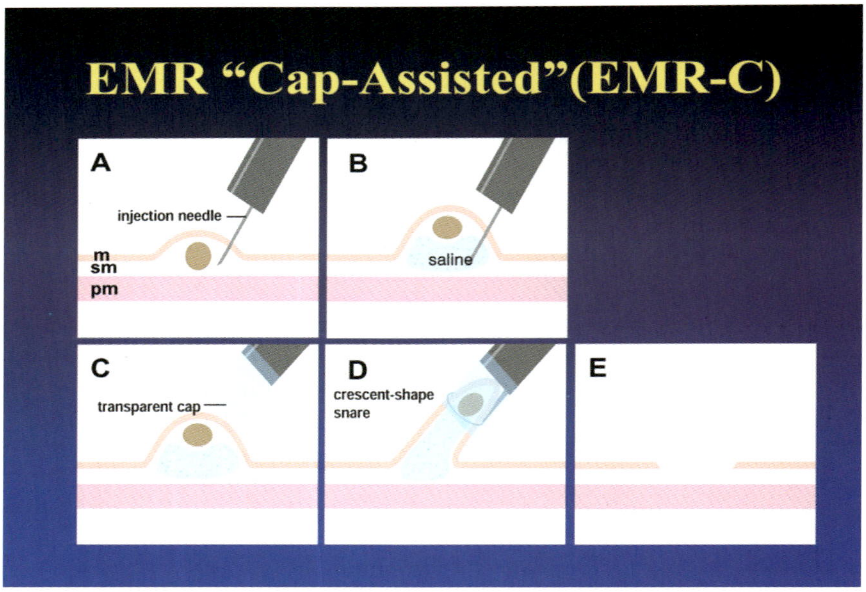

In EMR-C an injection needle is inserted in the margin of the target lesion. The lesion is lifted by a submucosal injection, usually diluted epinephrine. A transparent cap is attached to the distal end of the endoscope. And a snare is positioned at the distal end of the inner cap. Using negative pressure the lesion is suctioned into the cap and is immediately captured by closing the prepositioned snare. The lesion is then removed using electrocoagulaton.

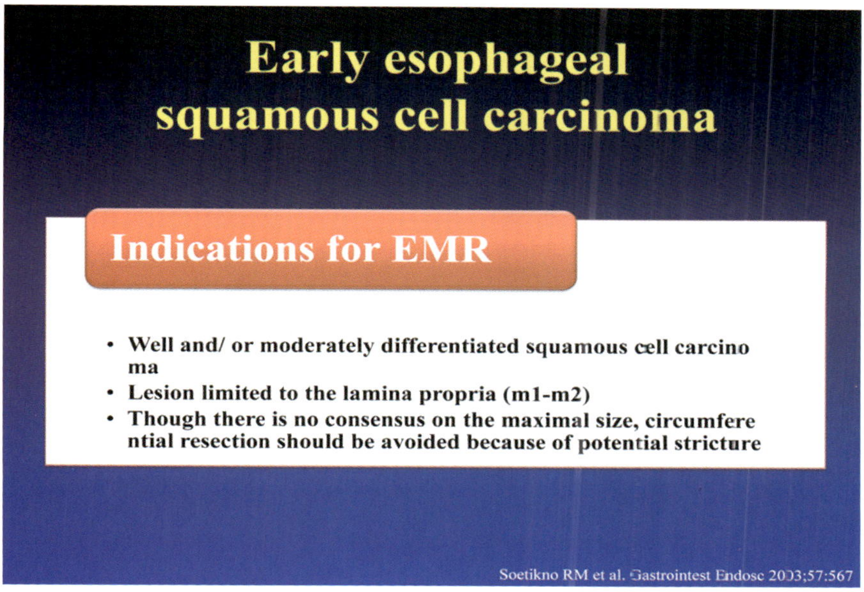

EMR should be only considered if the lesion is well of moderately differentiated and limited to the lamina propria. Although there is no consensus on the maximal size, circumferential lesions should be avoided because of the potential of stricture formation.

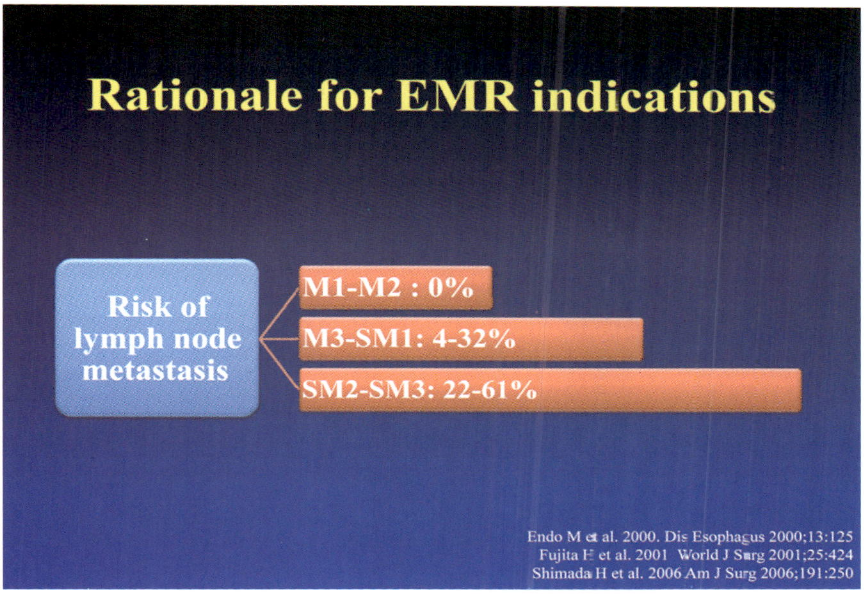

The depth of invasion is an important indicator of the risk for nodal metastasis in patients with superficial esophageal cancer. There have been no reports of nodal metastasis with MI and M2 tumors, making these the most suitable for endoscopic treatment M3 and deeper lesions have a substantial risk for nodal metastasis. Esophagectomy with lymphnode dissection is recommended.

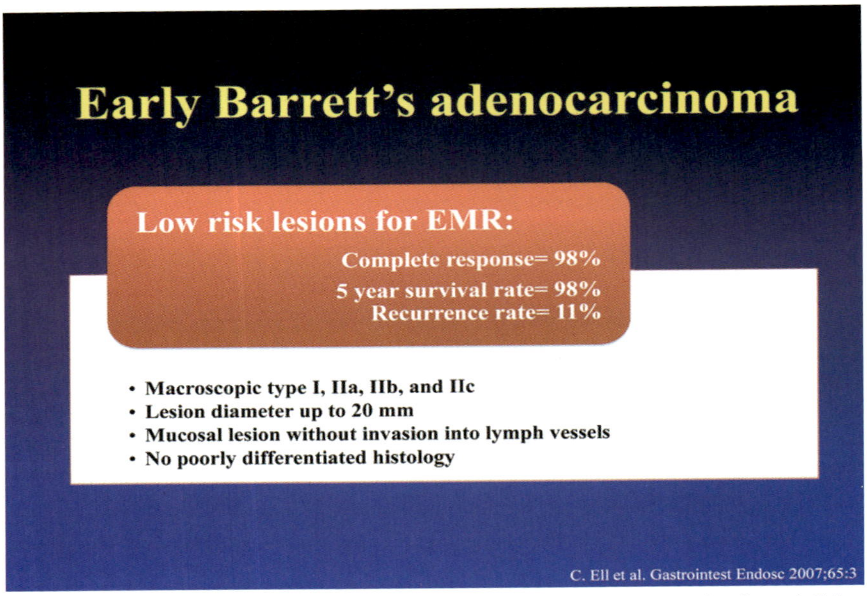

EMR is an alternative treatment for early Barrett' s adenocarcinoma, allowing for a definite histologic diagnosis while also potentially being curative. In a recent report EMR showed excellent results in carefully selected patients with early Barrett' s adenocarcinoma. A 98% complete response, no major complicatons, an 11% recurrence rate and a 98% overall 5 year survival was reported.

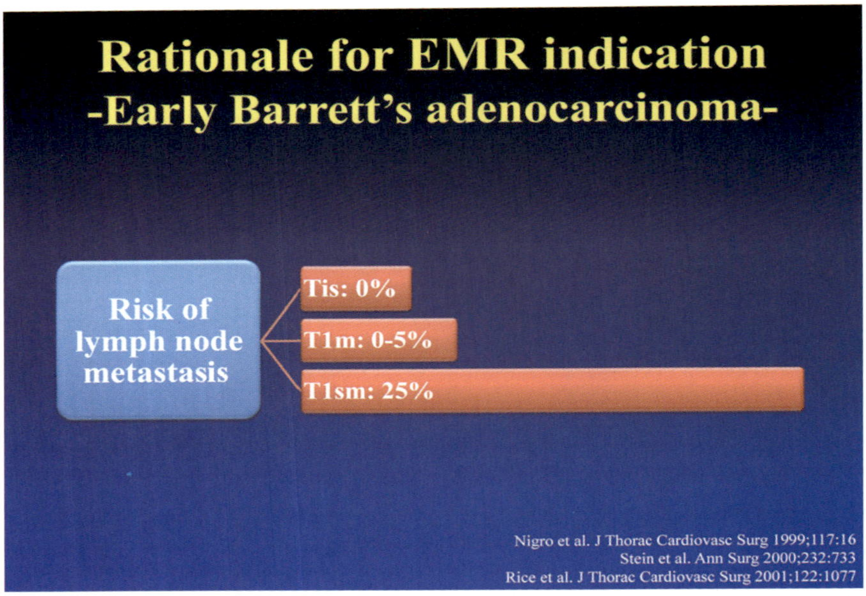

Carcinoma in-situ is not associated with lymph node metastasis. The risk of nodal metastasis is less than 5% for cancer limited to the mucosal layer. When there is submucosal involvement nodal metastasis averages 25%.

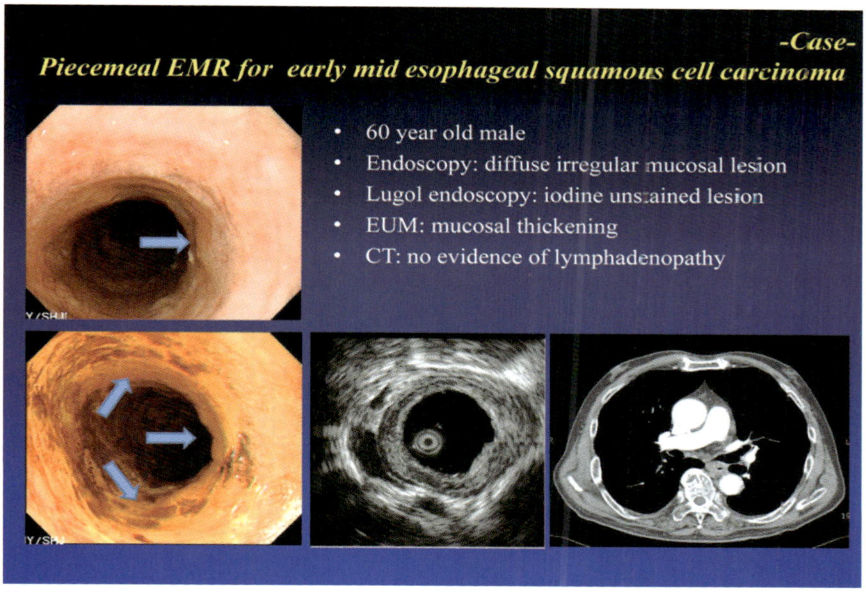

This is a 60 year old male patient. Endoscopy showed an irregular mucosal lesion 30cm from the upper incisors. Chromoendoscopy using Lugol' s solution revealed a segment with 75% circumferential involvement by an unstained lesion. High frequency miniprobe EUS showed mucosal thickening. Chest CT scans showed mild and circumferential wall thickening in the mid-esophagus about 2cm below the carina without evidence of lymph node enlargement.

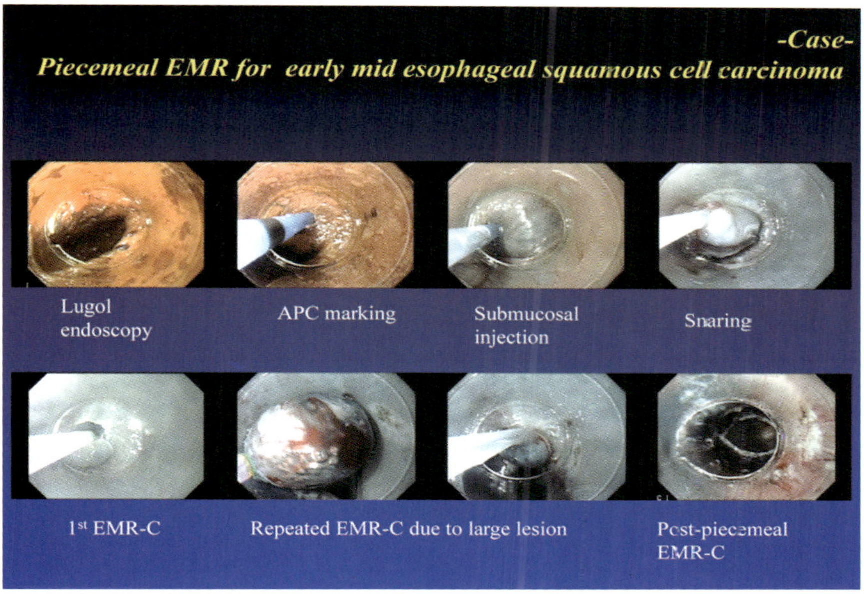

After spraying the esophagus with lugol' s solution marking was done with electorcoagulation dots on the normal tissue surrounding the lesion. A margin of 2mm was obtained. The lesion was then lifted by injection of a saline solution first at the distal and then at the proximal ends. A transparent cap with a snare was position around the lesion and EMR was performed. Due to the large size of the lesion, repeated EMR sessions were required.

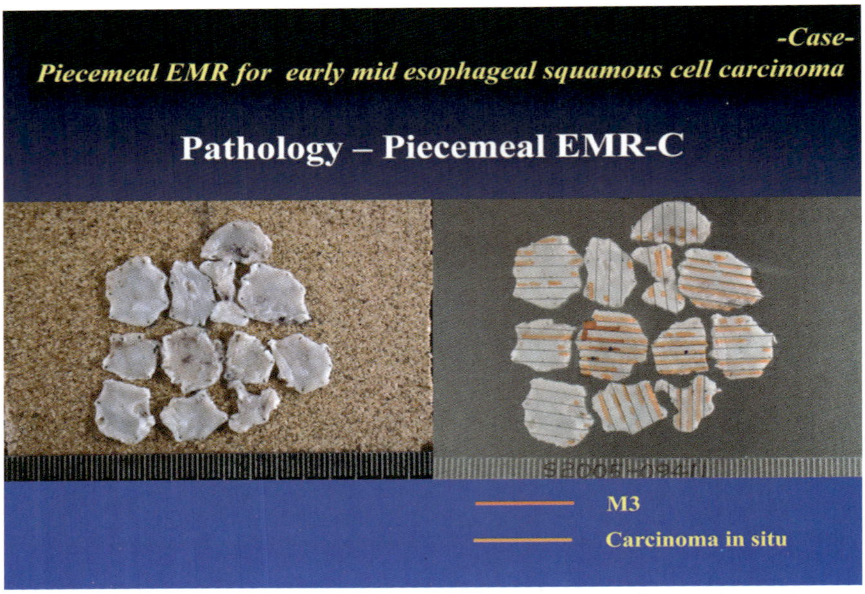

Because of the multiple resection pieces, we were unable to reconstruct the resection specimen or confirm whether the lateral margin was involved.

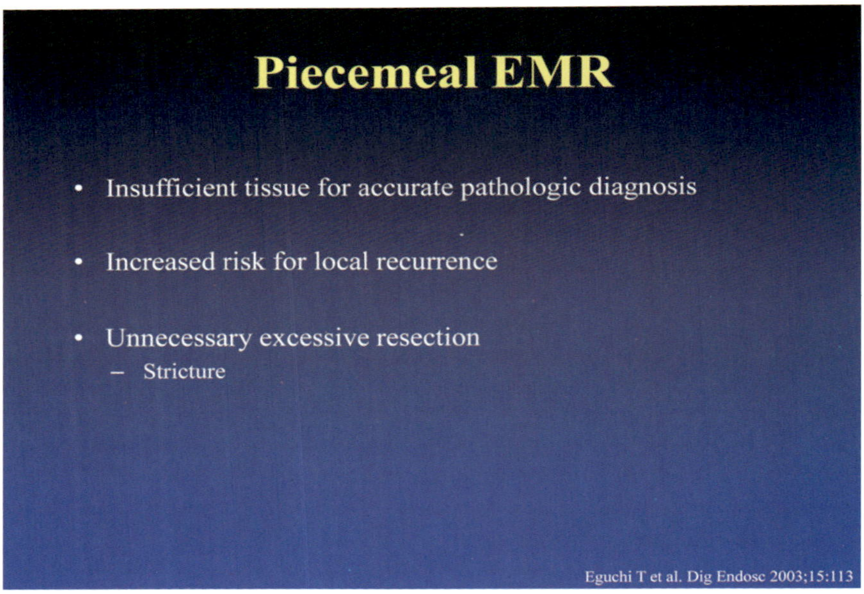

Piecemeal EMR provides insufficient tissue for accurate pathologic diagnosis and increases the risk for local recurrence. Furthermore, the resected area cannot be controlled by the operators. Therefore normal mucosa may be excessively resected. This may cause deformity and strictures of the narrowed esophageal lumen. En-bloc resection with ESD can overcome these limitations.

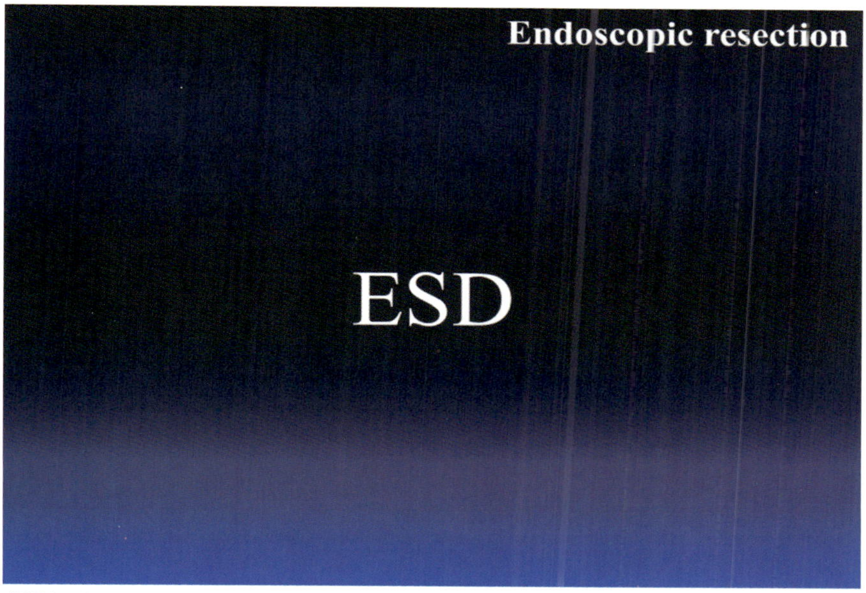

ESD has been introduced to overcome limitations of EMR.

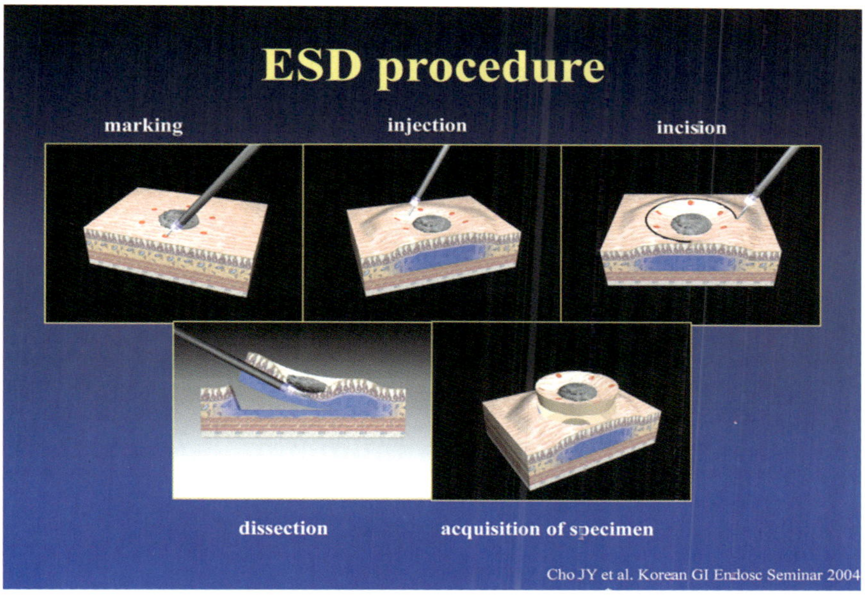

ESD is a five step procedure. First marking dots are made circumferentially around the lesion. Next, submucosal injection is performed and the lesion is elevated. Incision is then performed using an appropriate knife to separate the lesion from the surrounding non-neoplastic mucosa. The submucosal layer is then gradually dissected from the muscle layer and the resected specimen is removed.

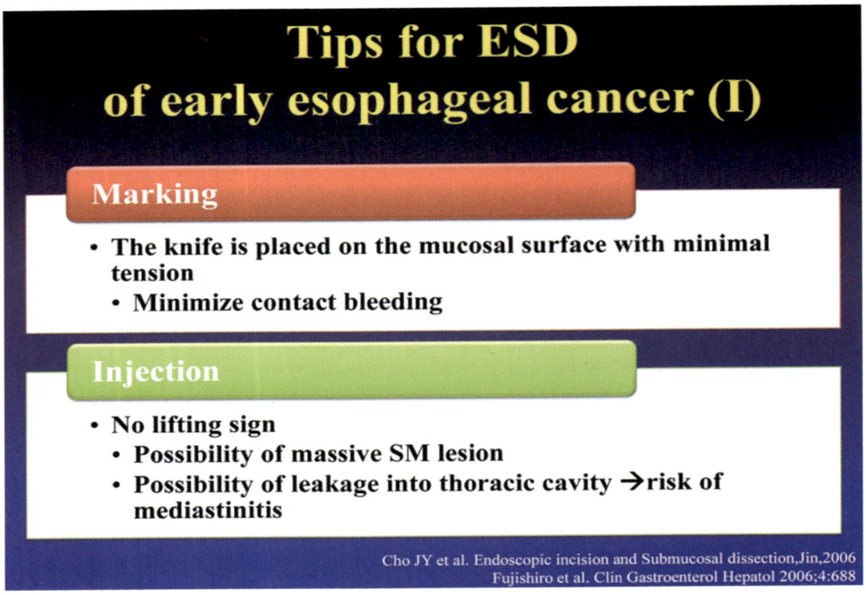

When performing ESD the knife should be placed on the mucosal surface with little tension to minimize contact bleeding. If the mucosa in not elevated after submucosal injection the endoscopist should consider the possibility of massive submucosal lesions or leakage of the injection material into the thoracic cavity.

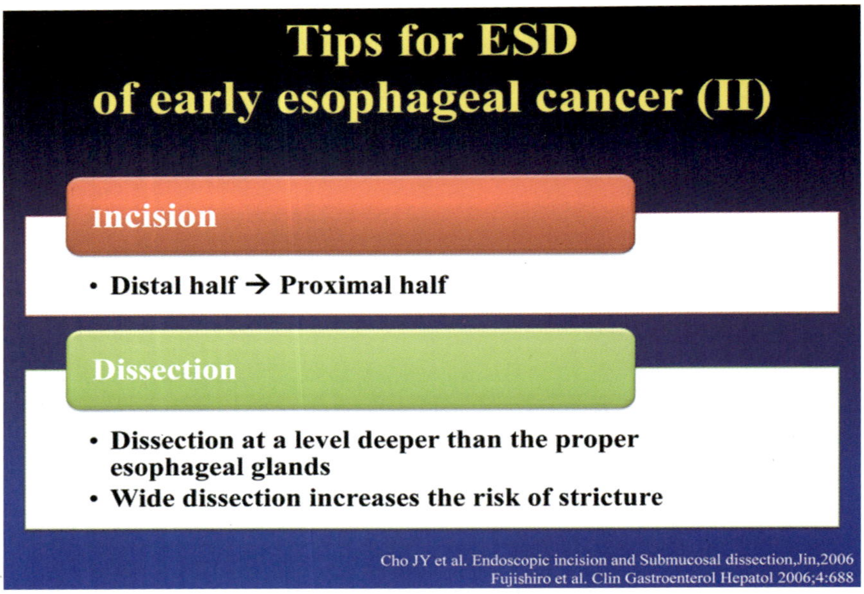

When performing incision the direction should be from the distal half to the proximal half. Dissection should be at a level deeper than the proper esophageal glands. If wide dissection is performed the risk of strictures is increased.

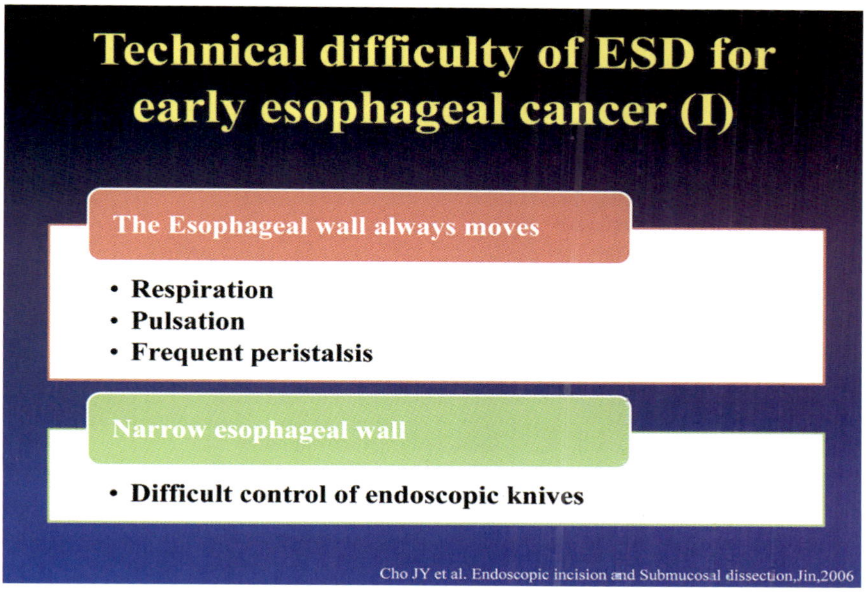

The technical difficulty is substantially greater than EMR, This is because of the frequency movement of the esophagus associated with respiration, pulsation and frequent peristalsis. The narrow lumen of the esophagus also contributes to the difficulty.

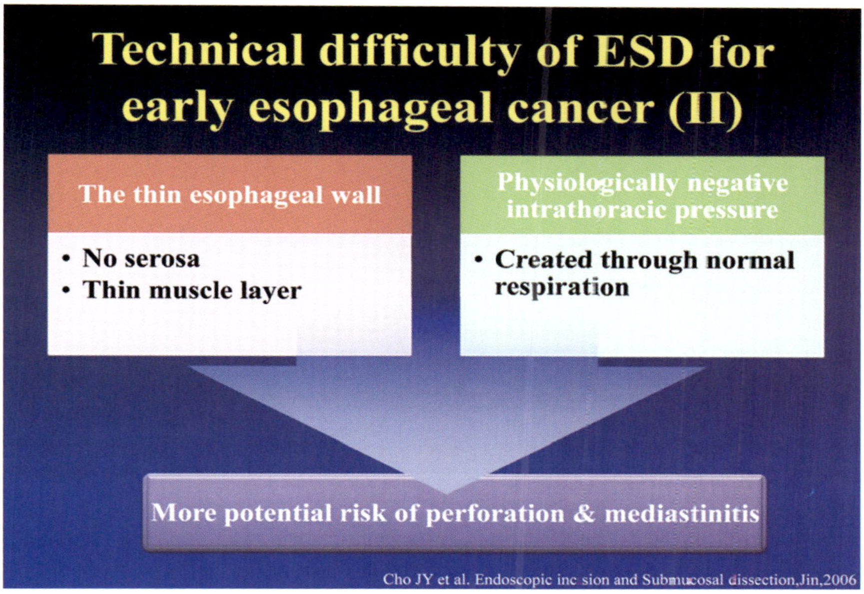

The esophagus does not have a serosal layer and the muscle layer is extremely thin. Moreover, given the negative intrathoracic pressure, esophageal ESD is prone to perforation compared to ESD in the stomach. Perforation in the esophagus is directly related to mediastinitis.

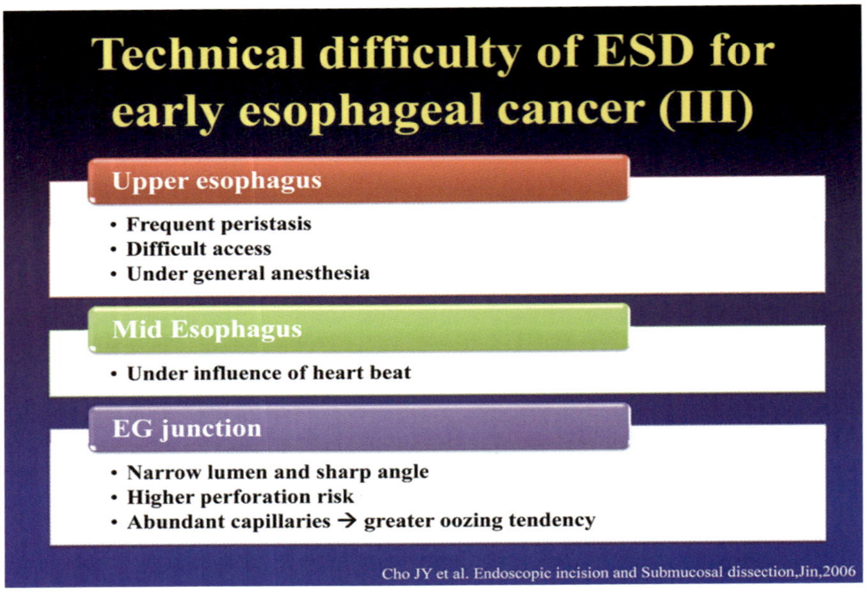

The location of the lesion has direct impact on the difficulty of ESD. Endoscopic assessability is extremely difficult in cervical or high esophageal lesions. The frequency of peristalsis also contributes to the difficulty. Therefore ESD is generally performed under general anesthesia in the operating room. Frequent pulsations can cause difficulty in mid-esophageal cancer. When the lesion is located in the lower esophagus or EG junction as in Barrett' s adenocarcinoma the narrow lumen and sharp angle contribute to the difficulty of resection. Furthermore the mucosa in this area is supplied by abundant capillaries which increases the risk of bleeding.

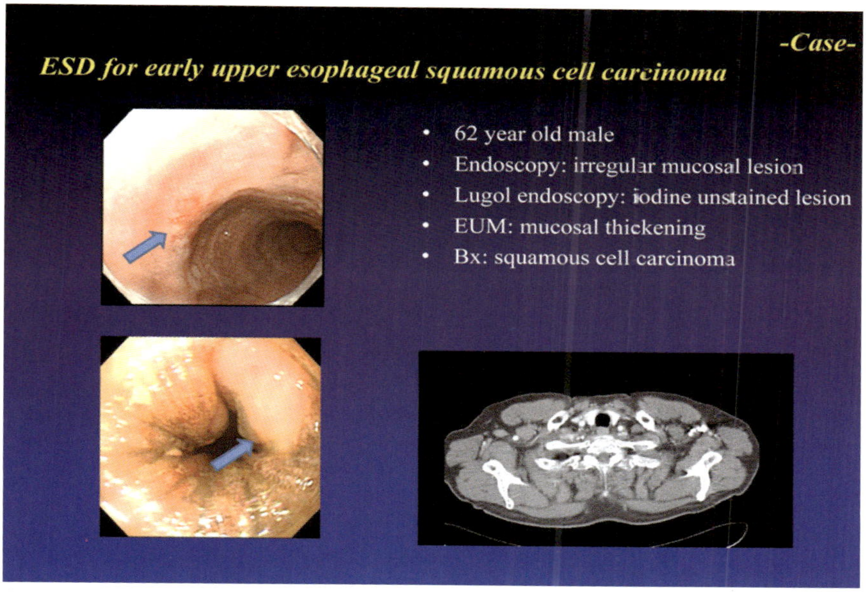

In this patient a non-stained flat lesion was seen just below the cricopharyngeal muscle. EUS showed subtle mucosal thickening and CT scans were normal.

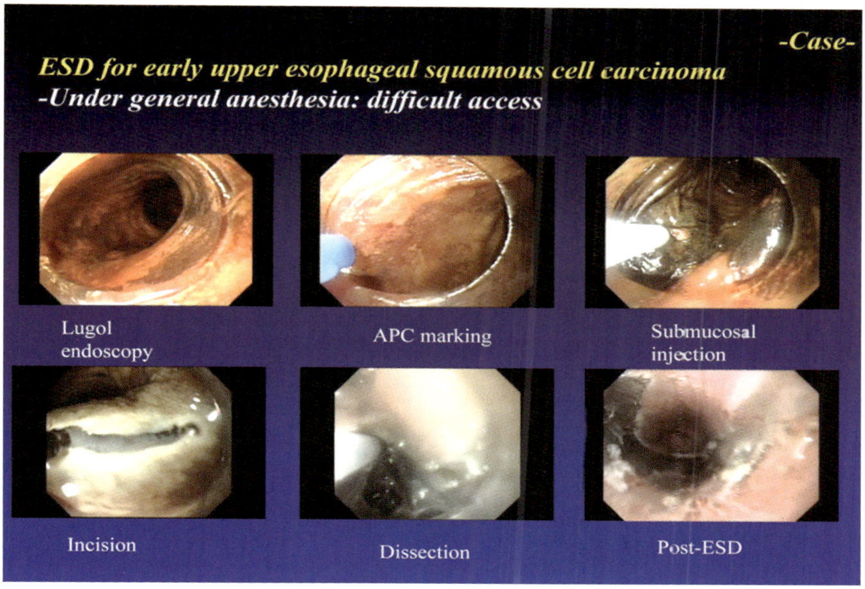

Under general anesthesia marking around the lesion and injection of a mixture of sodium alginate, indigocarmine and epinephrine was performed. The incision was performed with the fixed flexible knife. Dissection was performed with both the IT knife and the fixed flexible knife. En-bloc resection of the specimen was successfully completed.

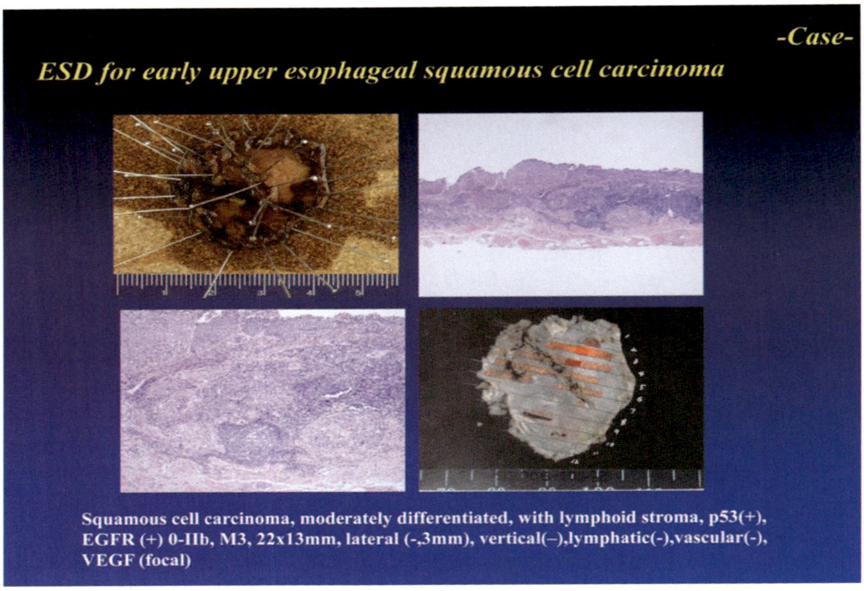

The resected specimen measured 3x3cm. An area unstained by Lugol' s solution is seen on the upper half of the resected specimen. The pathologic report showed squamous cell carcinoma limited to the lamina propria. All margins were free from tumor involvement.

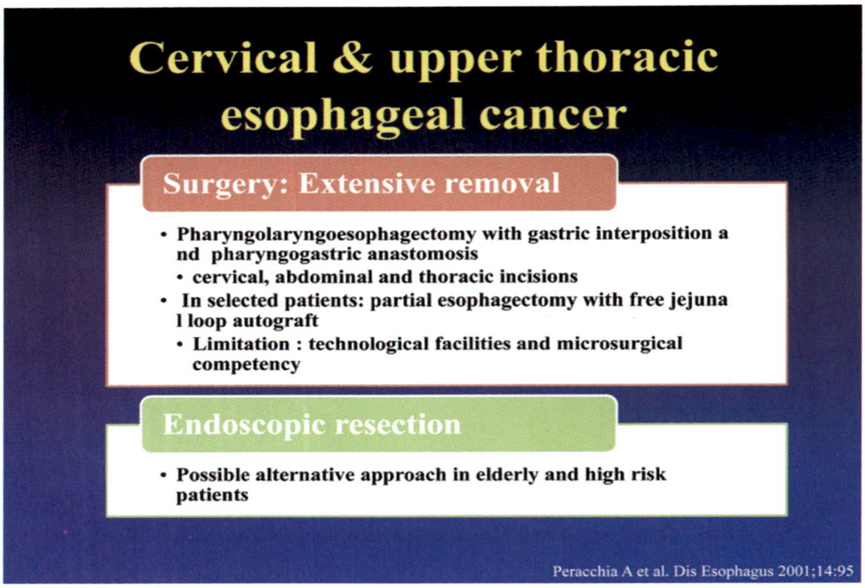

Currently extensive surgery is the only recommended treatment for upper thoracic esophageal cancer. Considering the high risk of operation minimally invasive endoscopic resection may be an acceptable alternative for elderly and high risk patients.

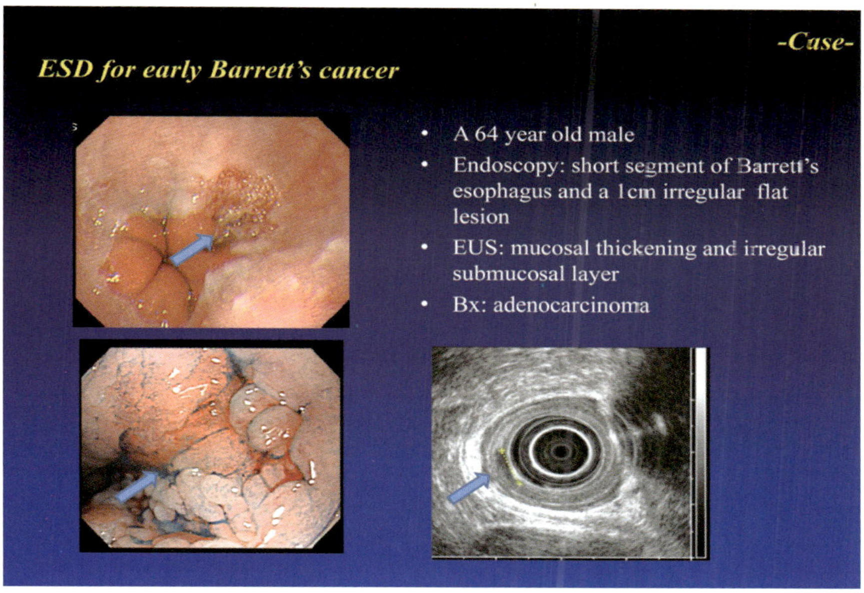

This a 64 year old male who was referred for management of Barrett' s adenocarcinoma. Conventional endoscopy demonstrated a short segment of Barrett' s esophagus and a 1 cm irregular flat lesion on the distal esophagus. EUS showed mucosal thickening and an irregular submucosal layer. Although surgery was initially recommended, he refuses operation and we decided to perform ESD.

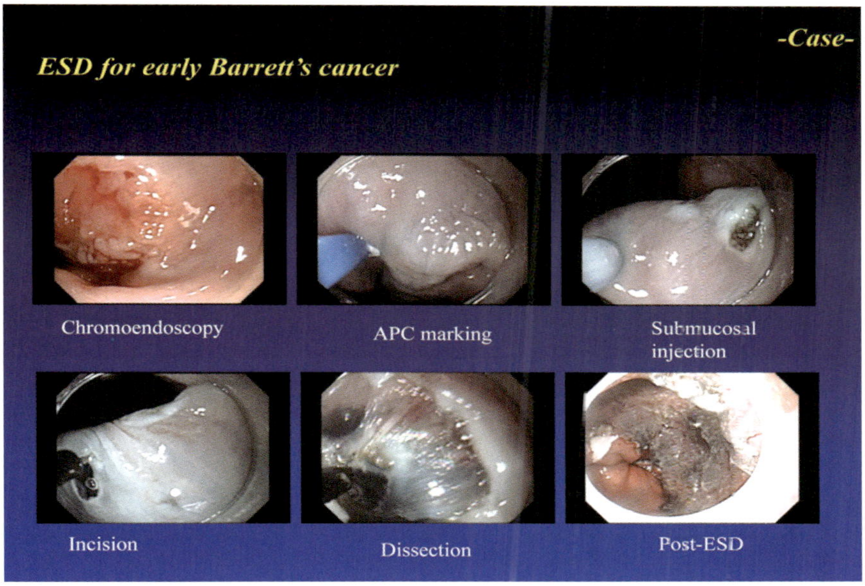

Endoscopy and chromoendoscopy showed an ulcerative lesion with a destructive mucosal and irregular vascular pattern. After marking and injection around the target area, incision was performed with the fixed flexible knife. Dissection of the submucosa was performed with Fork knife and the IT knife. En-bloc resection was successful, without any complications.

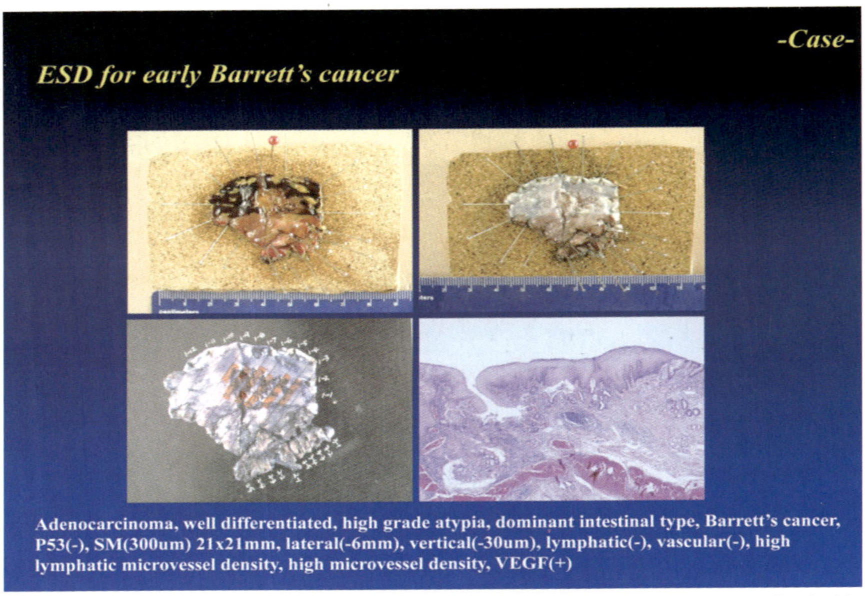

An ulcerative lesion is seen in the center of the resected specimen. The lesion is not stained with Lugol' s solution. The lateral margins were free from tumor involvement and the orange area was identified as well differentiated adenocarcinoma. The depth of invasion was 300um and limited to the submucosal layer. There was no evidence of lymphvascular invasion.

ESD for early esophageal cancer

En bloc resection

- Conventional EMR is limited by the blindness of the resection and the size of the specimen(<2cm)

Advantages over EMR

- Accurate pathologic diagnosis
- Reduced risk of local recurrence
- Circumferential lesion

Disadvantages over EMR

- The higher complication risk
- Highly operator dependent ; Difficult procedure
- The longer procedure time

Fujishiro et al. Clin Gastroenterol Hepatol 2006;4;688

EMR is unable to resect large or laterally spreading lesions in one piece. However ESD can provide en-bloc resection is these lesions, providing an accurate pathologic diagnosis, a reduced risk of local recurrence, and adequate resection of circumferential lesions. The disadvantages of ESD are the higher complication rate, technical experience of part of the operator, and a longer procedure time.

The outcomes of endoscopic resection in early esophageal cancer

Reference; Year	Patients (n)	Histology	Methods	CR	Mortality	Survival (5YSR)	Recur/ Meta	F/U (mo)	Cx
Fujishiro et al; 2006	58	SCC	ESD	78%	0%	NR	4.5%	17	Perforation (6.9%) Stricture (16%)
Oyama et al; 2006	130	SCC	ESD	93.8%	0%	NR	0%	28	0%
Pech et al;2007	65	SCC	EMR	92%	3%	77% (7YSR)	26%**	39	23%*
Ciocirlan et al; 2007	51***	SCC	EMR	91%	0%	95%	26%	NR	6%*
Cho JY et al ; 2007	20****	SCC *****	EMR ESD	80%	0%	NR	19%	15	15%

CR; Complete resection (free lateral & vertical margins), Cx; complication, Meta;metachronous, NR; not reported, SCC;squamous cell carcinoma Adeno;adenocarcinoma
* No major complication such as perforation and severe bleeding
** 1) independent risk factor for recurrence : multifocal carcinoma 2) these patient all achieved another CR after further ER
*** Including patients with T1sm (16 lesions)
**** Including PDT in 9 cases
***** Including adenocarcinoma in 2 cases

In various studies the overall complete resection rate after endoscopic resection varied from 78 to more than 90% and the 5 year survival rate was reported to be as high as 95% in one study. Although these studies showed promising results for endoscopic resection of early esophageal cancer, larger randomized trials with comparison of EMR and ESD are needed.

The outcomes of endoscopic resection in early Barrett's cancer

Reference; Year	Patients (n)	Histology	Methods	CR
May A et al; 2002	115	HGD(19) AC(96)	EMR*	98%
Ell C et al;2007	100	AC	EMR	99%

Reference ;Year	Mortality	Survival (5YSR)	Recur/ Meta	F/U(mo)	Cx
May A et al; 2002	0%	88% (3YSR)	30%	34	9.5%**
Ell C et al;2007	0%	98%	11 %	36	8%**

CR; Complete resection (free lateral & vertical margins), Cx; complication, Meta; metachronous, AC: adenocarcinoma
* PDT in 32 cases
** No major complication such as perforation and severe bleeding

2 recent studies of endoscopic resection in early Barrett' s cancer showed excellent complete resection rates, no procedure related mortality, and an overall complication rate of 9%. However, after a mean follow up period of 35 months the rates of recurrence was 11 to 30%. The authors attributed the high recurrence rate to the existence of multifocal premalignant and malignant areas in Barrett' s esophagus as well as metachronous developments of foci of new dysplasia.

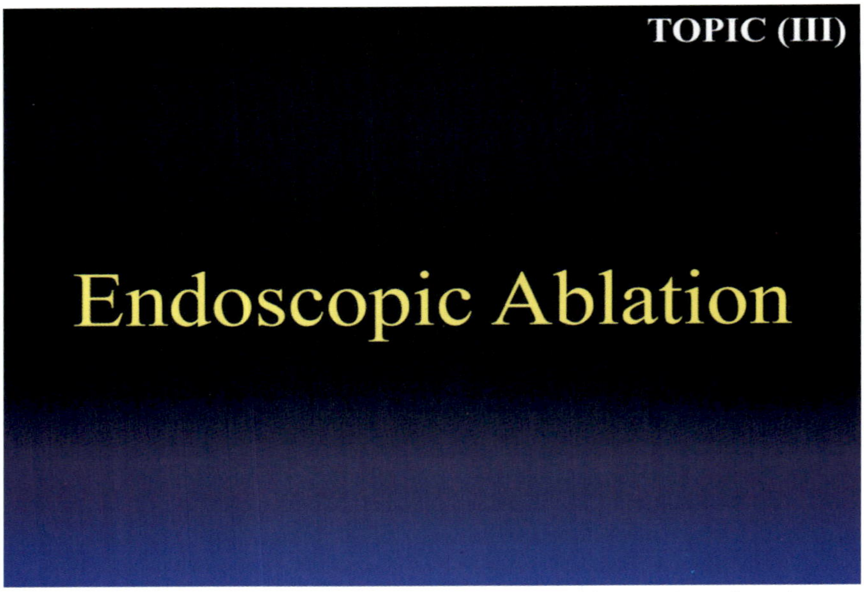

This topic will focus on the endoscopic ablations that have been applied to early esophageal cancer including early neoplasia in Barrett' s esophagus.

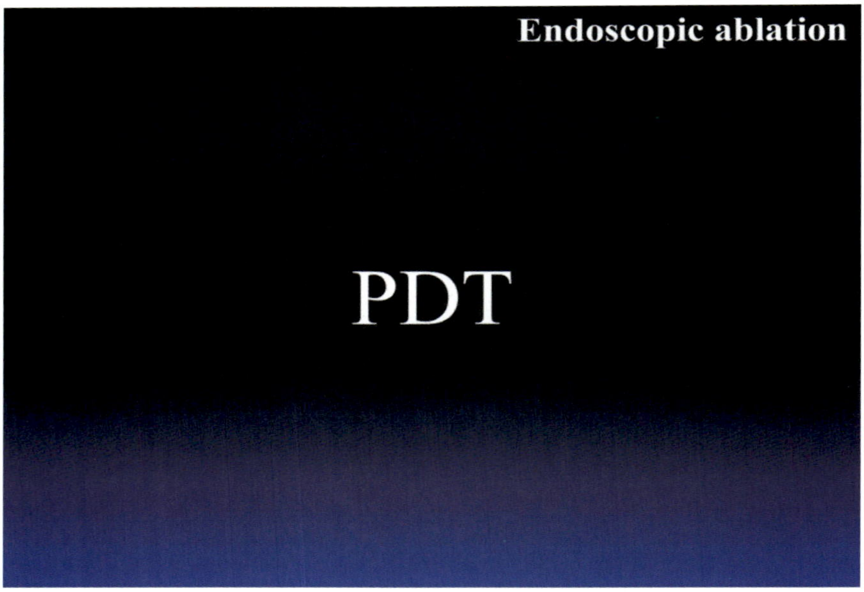

Photodynamic therapy is an endoscopic treatment of early cancers based on the photosensitization of neoplasms following the administration of a photosensitizer prior to lase light-induced tissue destruction.

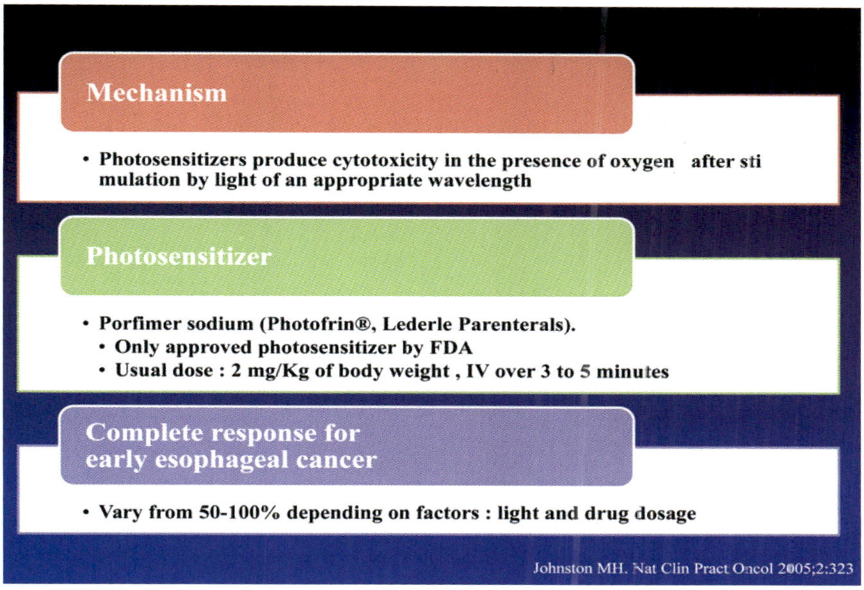

The mechanism of PDT utilizes photosensitizers that are cytotoxic in the presence of oxygen after stimulation with light of an appropriate wavelength. Photophrin is the only photosensitizer approved by the FDA. The complete response rate of PDT for early esophageal cancer varies from 50 to 100%. The response rate is dependent on factors such as the length of light exposure and drug dosage.

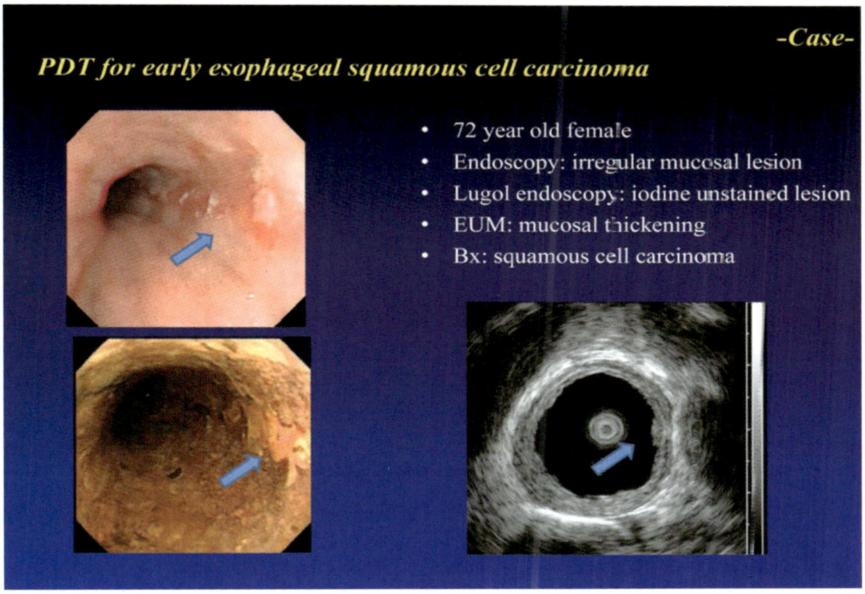

In this patient chromoendoscopy showed unstained mucosal irregularities on the distal esophagus. Mucosal thickening was noted on EUS.

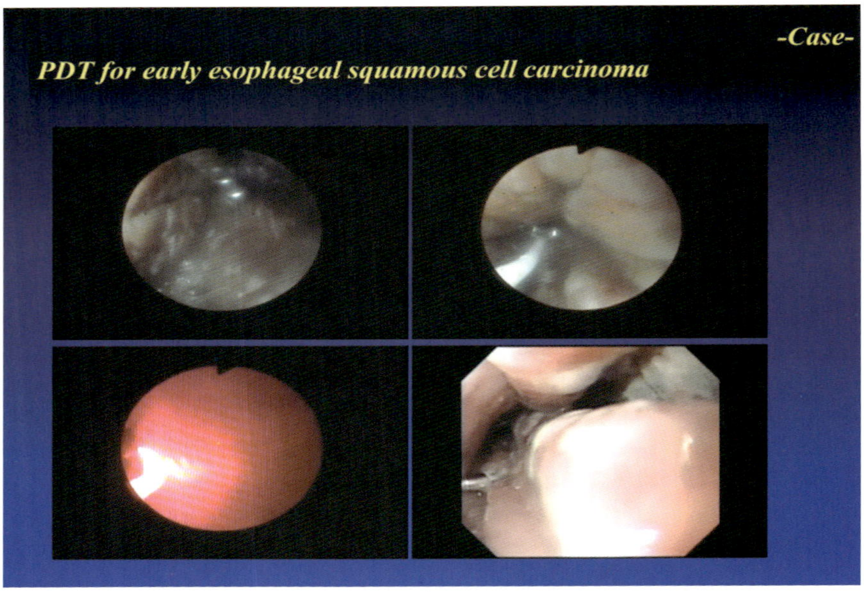

For a proper light illumination, a catheter is applied to the lesion. A hemoclip marks the margin of the lesion. PDT was performed at 180 J/square cm. 2 days later, a post PDT ulceration can be seen.

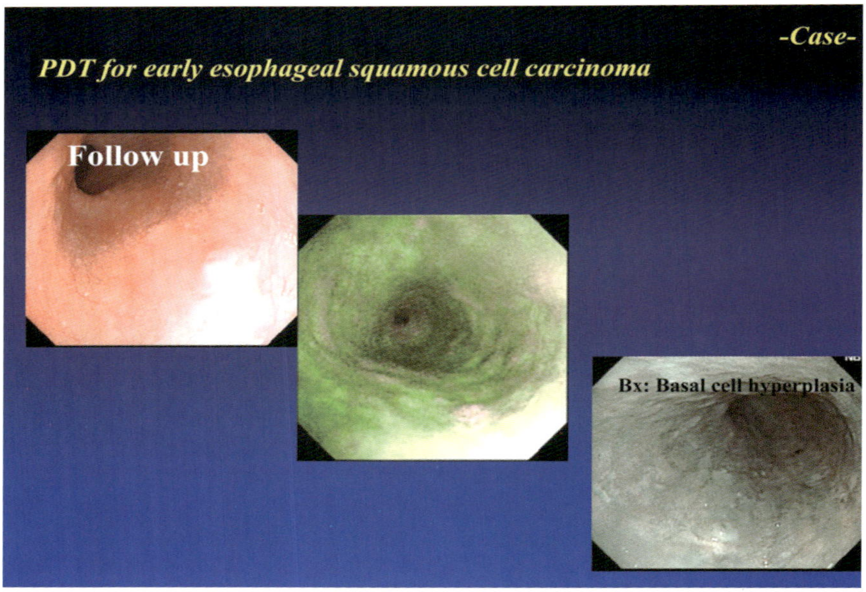

3 months after treatment follow up endoscopy with NBI and AFI showed a scarred area. Biopsy from this area showed basal cell hyperplasia without any evidence of tumor recurrence.

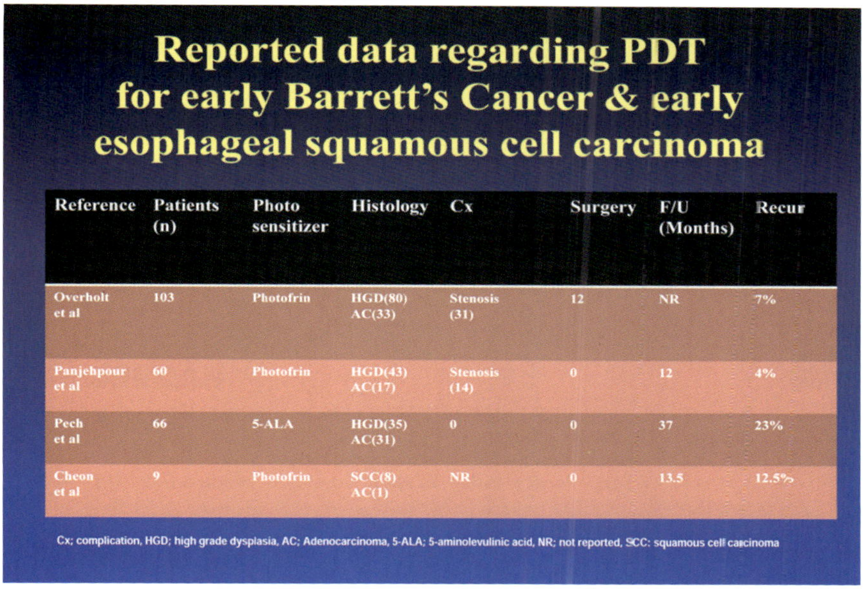
Reported data regarding PDT for early Barrett's Cancer & early esophageal squamous cell carcinoma

Reference	Patients (n)	Photo sensitizer	Histology	Cx	Surgery	F/U (Months)	Recur
Overholt et al	103	Photofrin	HGD(80) AC(33)	Stenosis (31)	12	NR	7%
Panjehpour et al	60	Photofrin	HGD(43) AC(17)	Stenosis (14)	0	12	4%
Pech et al	66	5-ALA	HGD(35) AC(31)	0	0	37	23%
Cheon et al	9	Photofrin	SCC(8) AC(1)	NR	0	13.5	12.5%

Cx; complication, HGD; high grade dysplasia, AC; Adenocarcinoma, 5-ALA; 5-aminolevulinic acid, NR; not reported, SCC: squamous cell carcinoma

The recurrence of esophageal cancer treated with PDT ranged from 4 to 23%. PDT was associated with a relatively high rate of esophageal stenosis. However, in one study, that used 5-aminolevulenic acid as a photosensitizer, there were no reports of post PDT stenosis.

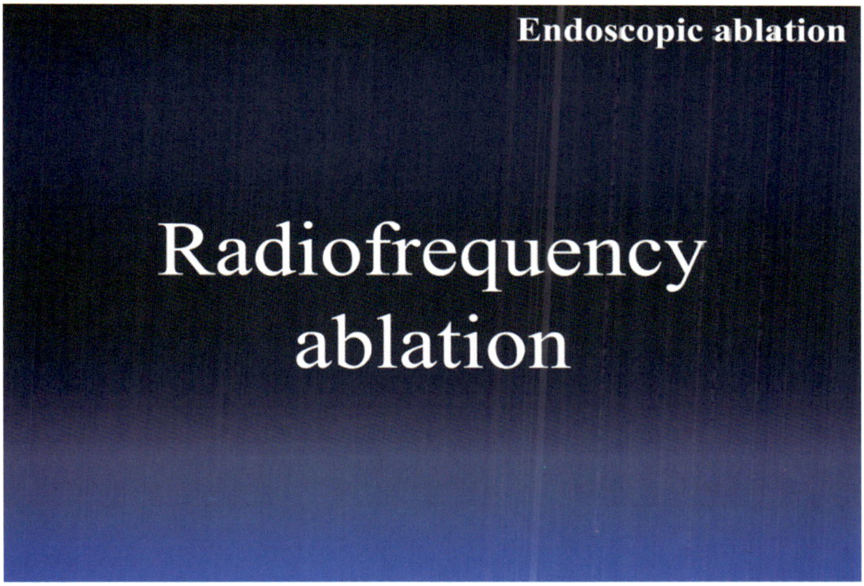

Radiofrequency ablation is also a kind of thermal modality for treating early neoplasia in Barrett' s esophagus.

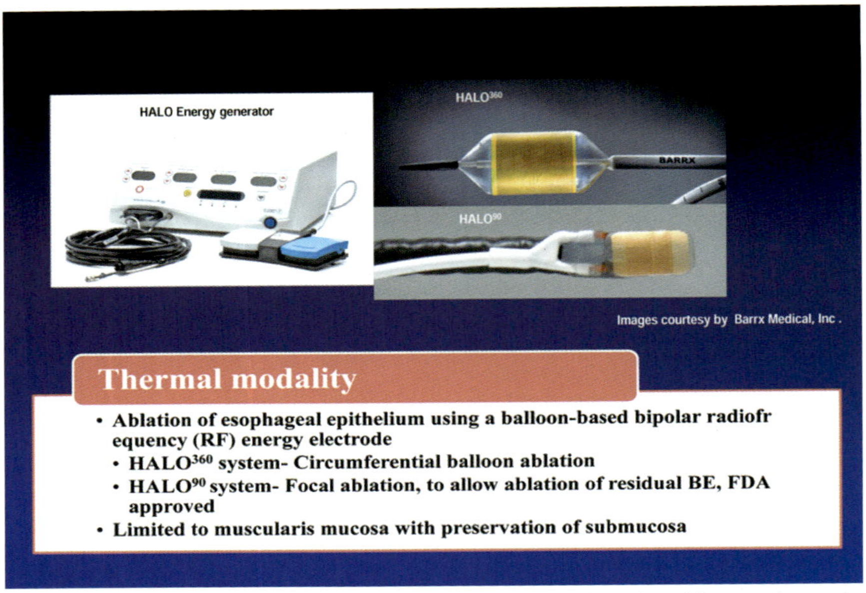

Recently radiofrequency ablation using the Halo system was introduced for treating early neoplasia in Barrett' s esophagus. The Halo 360 system uses a circumferential balloon ablation technique whereas the Halo 90 system can be used for focal ablation and treatment of residual Barrett' s esophagus. The therapeutic depth is limited to the muscularis mucosa with preservation of the submucosa.

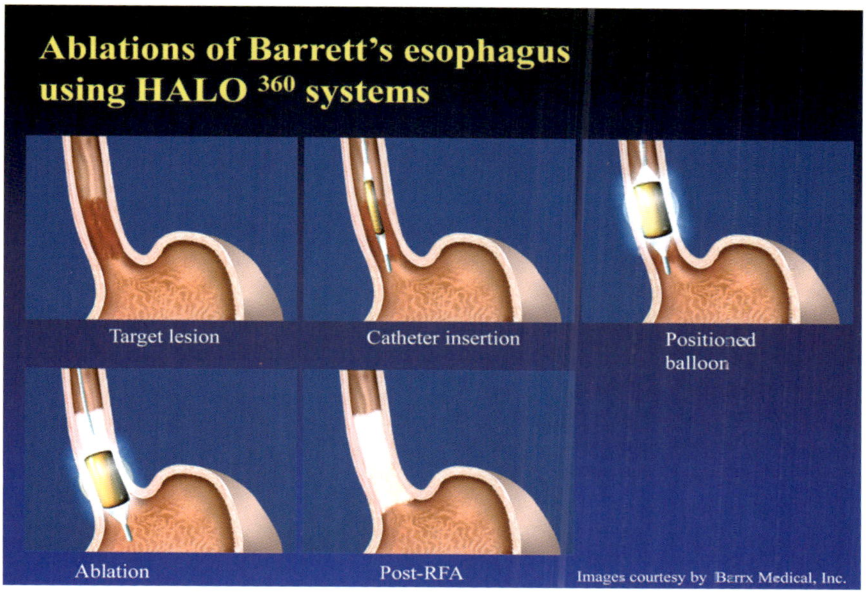

A catheter is inserted into the esophagus alongside the endoscope. At the tip of the catheter there is a small balloon that is inflated once inside the esophagus near the treatment area. The balloon and the HALO360 Energy Generator together measure the diameter of the esophagus. This information is used by the physician to select the appropriate treatment catheter. The sizing balloon is then removed and the treatment or HALO360+ Ablation Catheter is introduced. The HALO360+ Ablation Catheter also has a balloon at the tip, but this balloon is covered by a band of radiofrequency electrodes. Once the electrodes of the balloon are positioned on the desired treatment area the balloon is inflated. The HALO360 Energy Generator and the ablation catheter then work together to deliver a short burst of energy that is circumferential: 360 degrees.

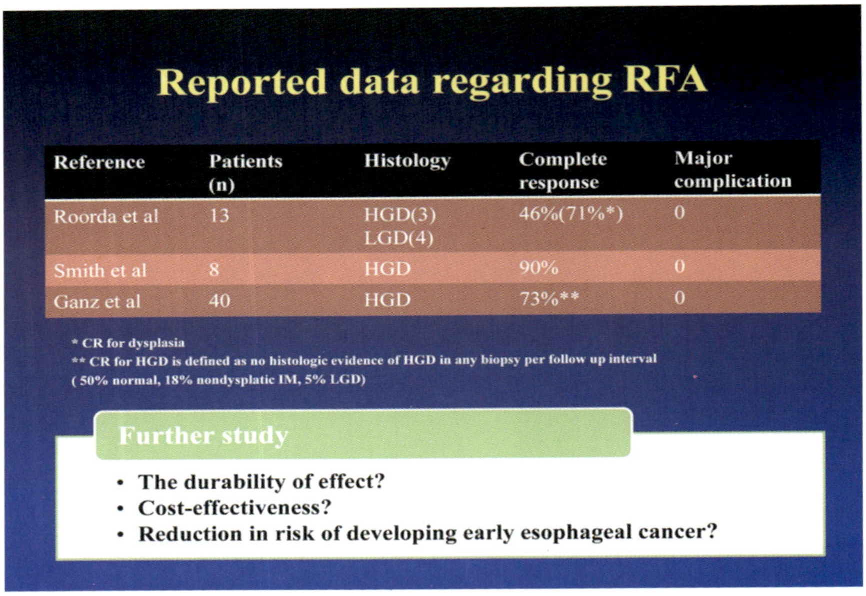

The reported data regarding radiofrequency ablation is limited at the present. Complete response after RFA varies from 46 to 90% in small studies. No major complication was reported. Prospective studies regarding the durability of effect, cost effectiveness and reduction in risk of developing early esophageal cancer are needed.

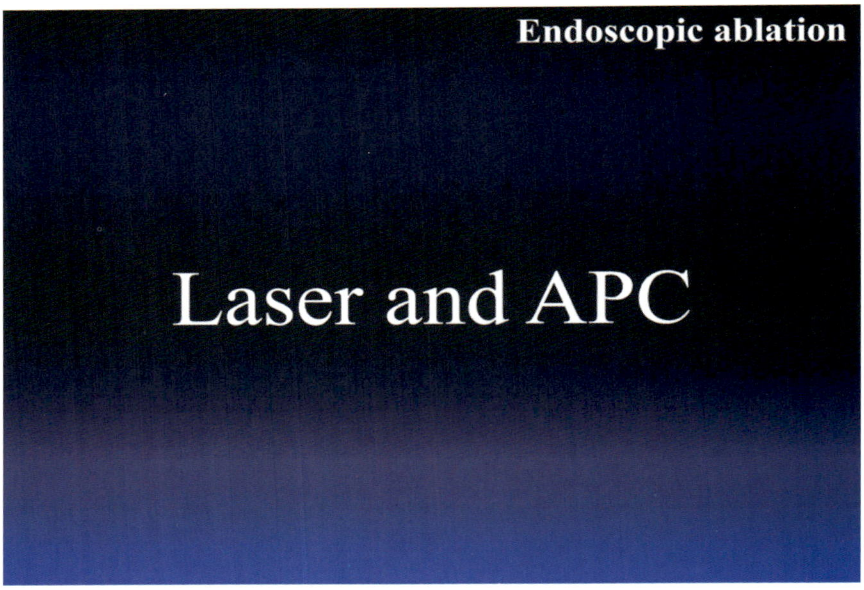

Laser and APC are also thermal modalities for treating early neoplasia in Barrett' s esophagus.

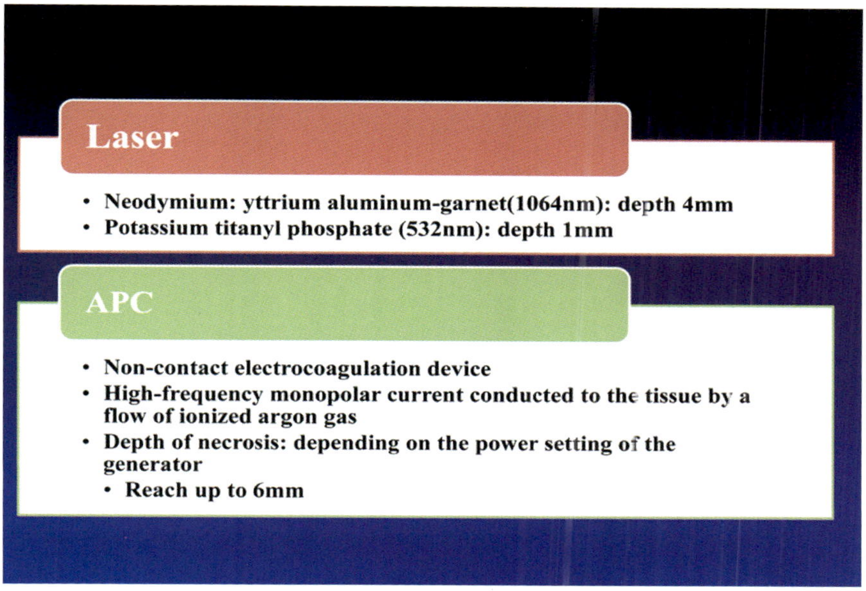

Various lasers and APC can be used for endoscopic ablation. The ND-YAG and penetrate up to 4mm whereas the KTP laser has a penetration depth of 1mm. APC is a non contact electrocoagulation device which used high frequency monopolar current conducted to the tissue by a flow of ionized argon gas. The maximal penetration depth is 6mm.

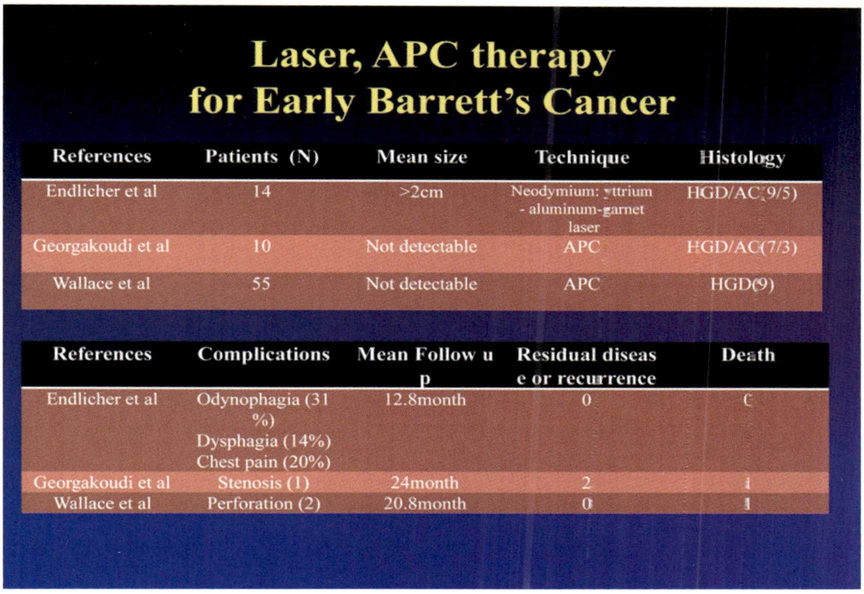

References	Patients (N)	Mean size	Technique	Histology
Endlicher et al	14	>2cm	Neodymium: yttrium - aluminum-garnet laser	HGD/AC(9/5)
Georgakoudi et al	10	Not detectable	APC	HGD/AC(7/3)
Wallace et al	55	Not detectable	APC	HGD(9)

References	Complications	Mean Follow up	Residual disease or recurrence	Death
Endlicher et al	Odynophagia (31%) Dysphagia (14%) Chest pain (20%)	12.8month	0	0
Georgakoudi et al	Stenosis (1)	24month	2	1
Wallace et al	Perforation (2)	20.8month	0	1

Like RFA, only a few small studies have evaluated the efficacy of laser and APC for superficial caner in patients with Barrett' s esophagus. The place of APC and laser ablation in the treatment of superficial esophageal cancer is uncertain. Further experience with this approach is needed.

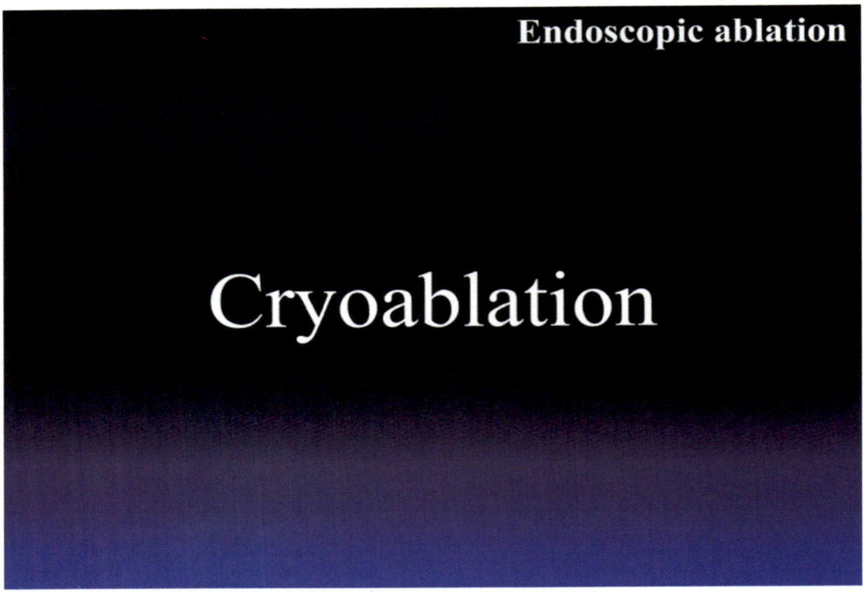

Cryotherapy is routinely utilized for various skin lesions. Recently endoscopic cryotherapy with high pressure spray is used for early Barrett' s neoplasia.

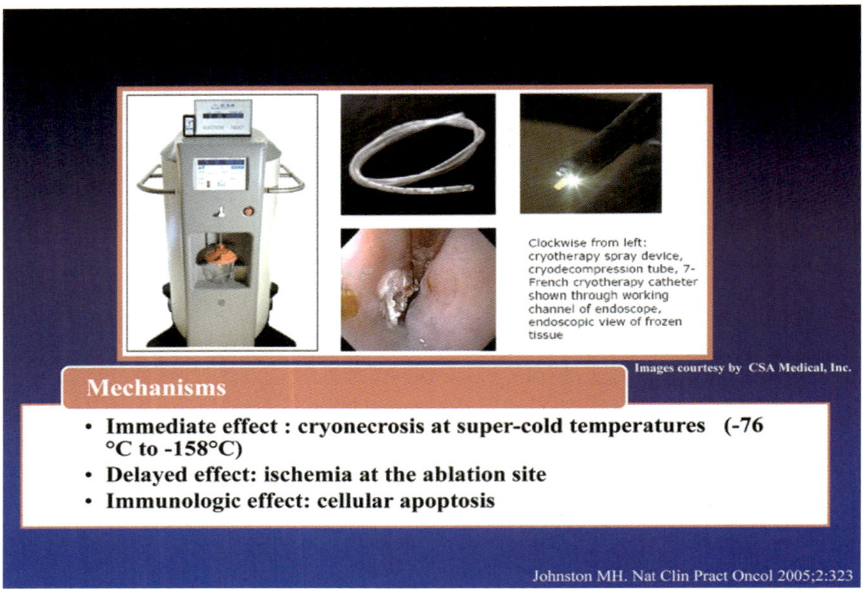

Cryoablation therapy has 3 effects on tissue. Cryonecrosis occurs immediately after the tissue is exposed to supercold temperature. Following cryonecrosis delayed ischemia of the ablation site and an immunologic effect characterized by cellular apoptosis is observed.

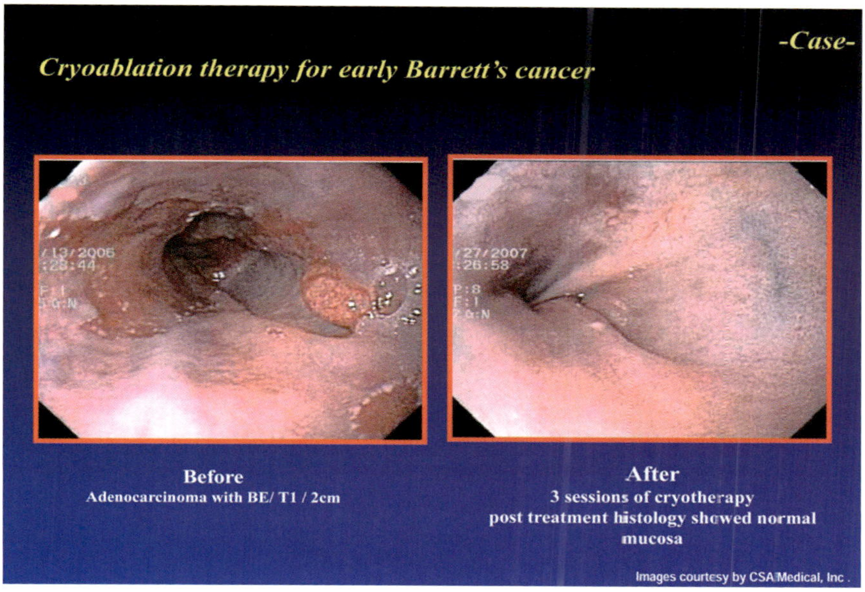

In this patient with Barrett' s esophagus, a cancerous lesion can be seen in the 3 o' clock area. After 3 sessions of cryotherapy, endoscopic and pathologic findings showed a normal mucosa.

Reported data regarding Cryoablation therapy

Reference	Patients (n)	Histology	CR	Cx	Subsquamous SIM
Johnston et al	11	LGD5, HGD1	78%	0	0
Cleveland clinic pilot study *	37	HGD26, IMCA6, SCHGD1	88%**	Perforation(1) ***	NR

CR; Complete response, Cx; Major complication, SIM; Specialized intestinal metaplasia,IMCA;Intramucosal cancer, SCHGD;Squamous cell HGD, NR; Not reported

* A prospective multi-center, longitudinal cohort study

** Eradication of LGD and HGD within BE at 24 months after the final treatment

*** Gastric perforation occurred in one patient with Marfan's syndrome due to overinflation of the stomach
Three patients developed mild stricture easily relieved with dilatation

Further study

- **The durability of effect?**
- **Cost-effectiveness?**
- **Reduction in risk of developing early esophageal cancer?**

Preliminary results of cryoablation therapy showed that complete histologic eradication of Barrett' s esophagus was achieved in 78% of patients with no complications. Likewise further study is required.

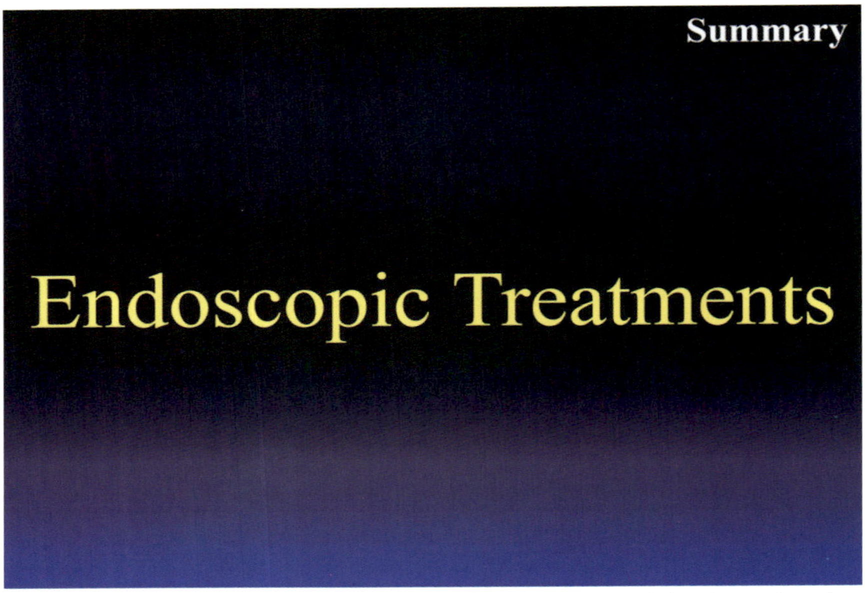

In summary, increasing numbers of early eosphageal neoplasias are being detected, so that endoscopic treatments with a curative intent play an increasing role.

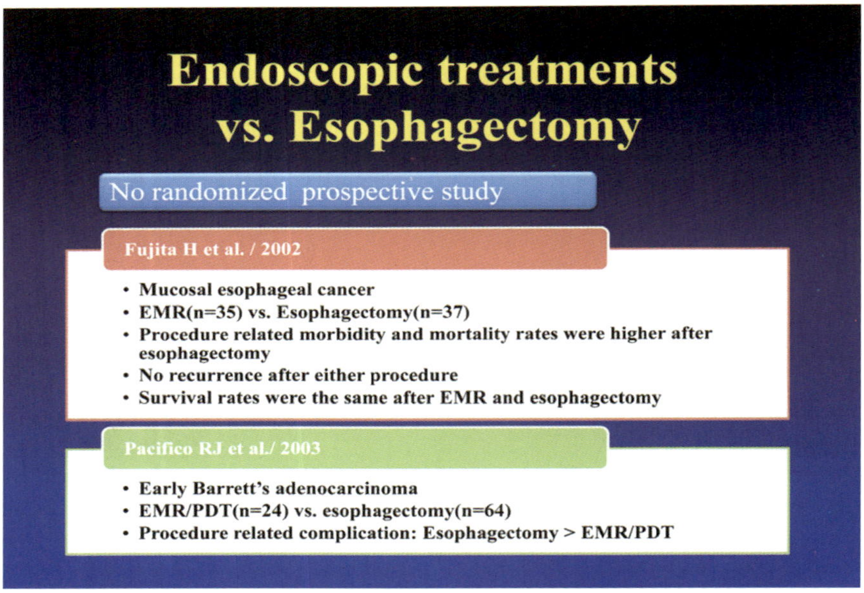

Currently there are no randomized prospective studies that compare endoscopic treatment and esophagectomy. According to Fujita' s report for treating mucosal esophageal cancer EMR was superior to esophagectomy in procedure related morbidity and mortality. Yet, the overall survival and recurrence rates were not significantly different. In another study, the results of EMR with PDT to esophagectomy were compared in early Barrett' s esophagus. The overall results were similar to that of Fujita' s.

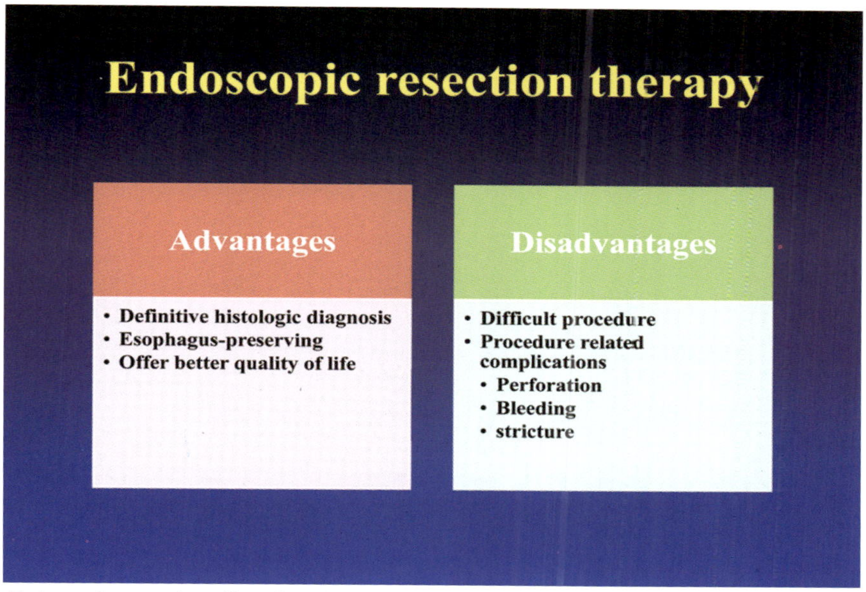

Endoscopic resection offers the advantage of histopathologic diagnosis with preservation of esophageal integrity and quality of life. However it requires substantial technical experience and in associated with severe complications.

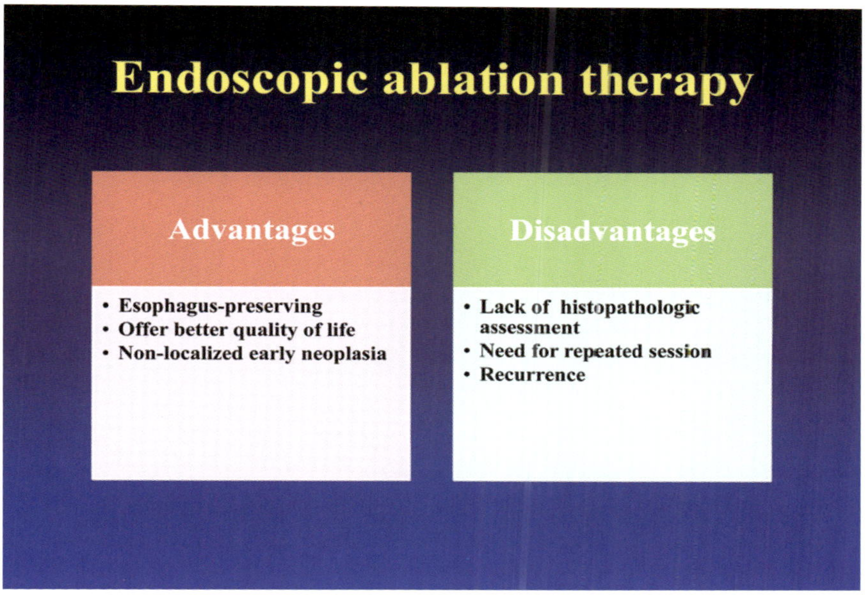

Ablation therapy is also a minimally invasive option that preserves the esophagus. It could be applies for the treatment of non localized early neoplasia. However, histopathologic assessment is not possible. Therefore the need for repeated intervention and tumor recurrence may be a risk.

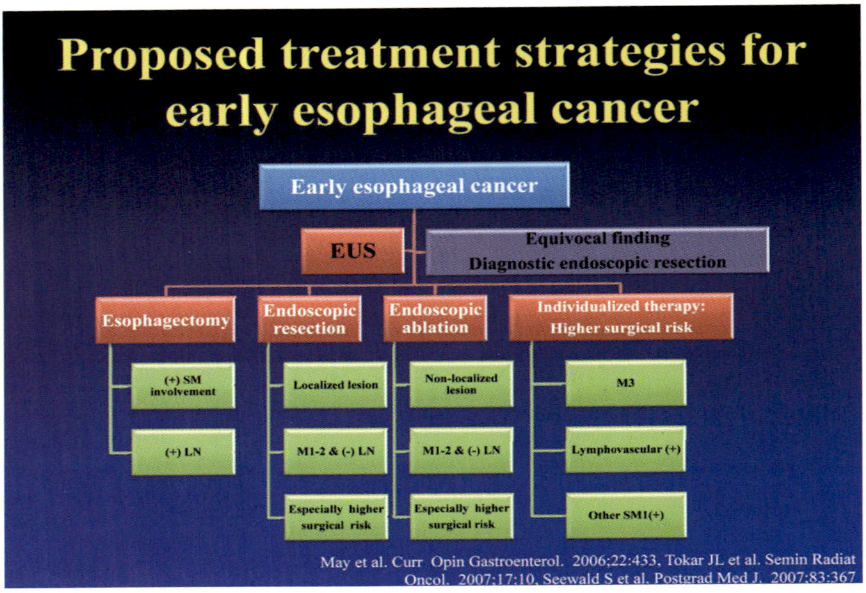

This flowchart illustrates a possible strategy for early esophageal cancer. Careful selection of patients with EUS is imperative for successful endoscopic therapy. If there is involvement of the submucosal layer or regional lymph nodes esophagectomy should be performed. In patients with equivocal findings on EUS, a trial of endoscopic resction may be required for proper diagnostic workup. For high risk patients with lesions confined to the lamina propria endoscopic treatment is expected. Resection is suitable for localized lesions while ablation can be performed on non-localized lesions. Although there is no consensus for high risk patients with M3 or submucosal cancer or cancer with lymphvascular invasion, individualized therapy with endoscopic resection may be a feasible option.

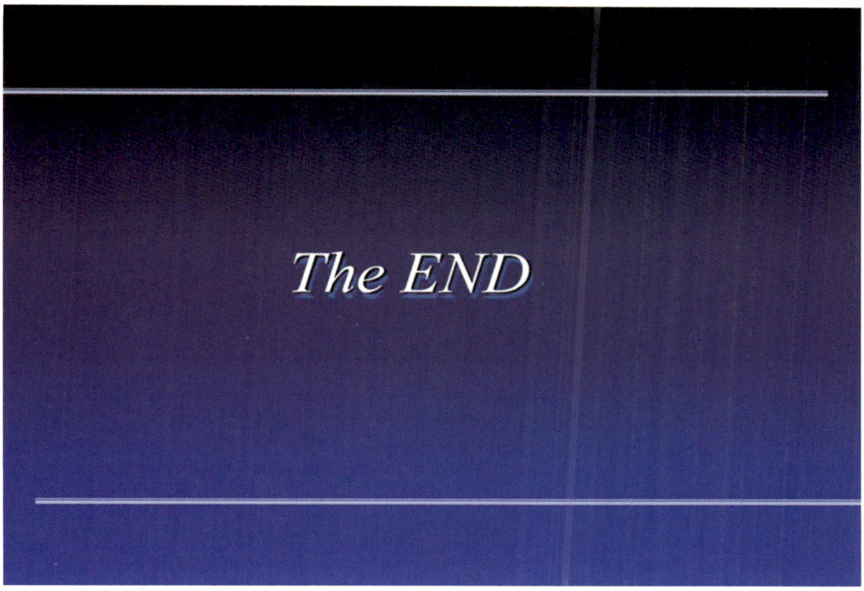

Endoscopic treatments for early esophageal cancer maybe a reasonable alternative to surgery in selected patients. Recent studies show excellent outcomes with endoscopic resection and ablation. As therapeutic endoscopy continues to expand further studies are needed to clarify the exact role of endoscopic treatment for early esophageal cancer.

Chapter 4

Novel Imaging Endoscopy on Upper Digestive Tract

Educational Video Nominated for a 2008 ASGE Audiovisual Award

Hyun Gun Kim, M.D. Ph D.
Joo Young Cho, M.D. Ph D.

Chapter 4 Novel Imaging Endoscopy on Upper Digestive Tract

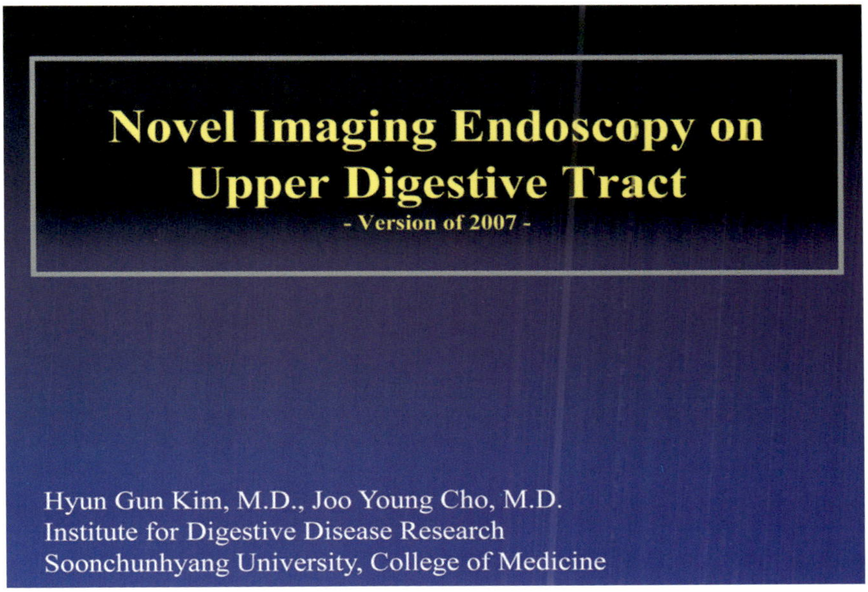

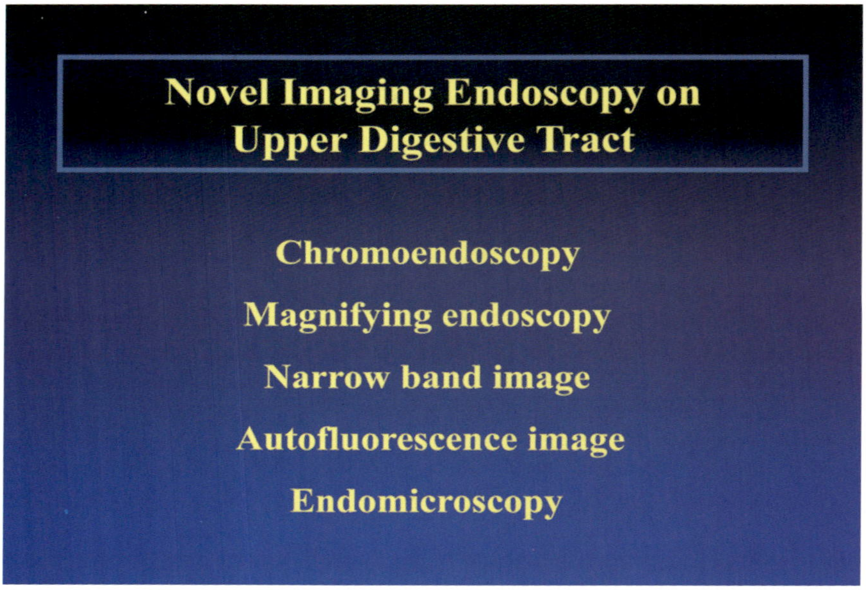

This chapter introduces and focuses on the basic application of advanced endoscopic imaging such as, chromoendoscopy, magnifying endoscopy, narrow band image, auto-fluorescence image and endomicroscopy

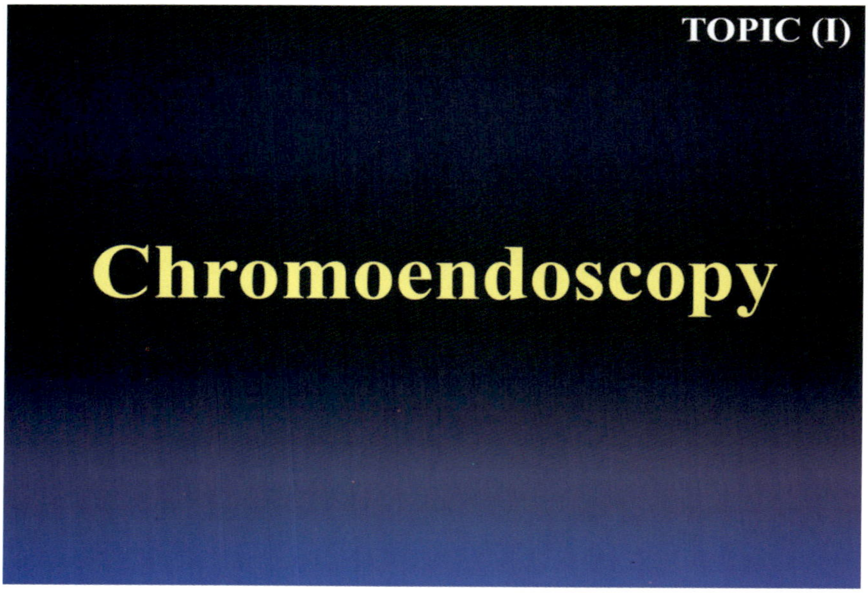

Chromoendoscopy –variable methods-

Stain	Organ	Mechanism	Positive stain	Aim
Lugol	Esophagus	Stains glycogen in normal squamous mucosa	Dark brown	Early esophageal cancer
Toludine blue	Esophagus	Stains nuclear material of malignant epithelial lesions	Blue	Squamous cell cancer
Methylene blue	Esophagus	Actively absorbing epithelium and metaplastic tissue	Blue	Barrett's esophagus, Intestinal metaplasia
Indigo carmine	Stomach	Contrast topography	blue	Screening of early cancer
1.5% Acetic acid + indigo carmine	Stomach	Unknown	blue	Gastric neoplasm

Endoscopy 1999;31:487-96

The table shows the variable stain material used in clinical practice for the upper gastrointestinal(GI) lesion. Chromoendoscopy utilizes the tissue reaction to various chemicals. Frequent stains used in chromoendoscopy of the GI tract are lugol' s solution for early esophageal cancer, methylene blue for Barrett' s esophagus, and indigo carmine for early gastric cancer. Recently the application of a mixture of 1.5% acetic acid indigo carmine has been used for the diagnosis of gastric neoplasms including adenomas.

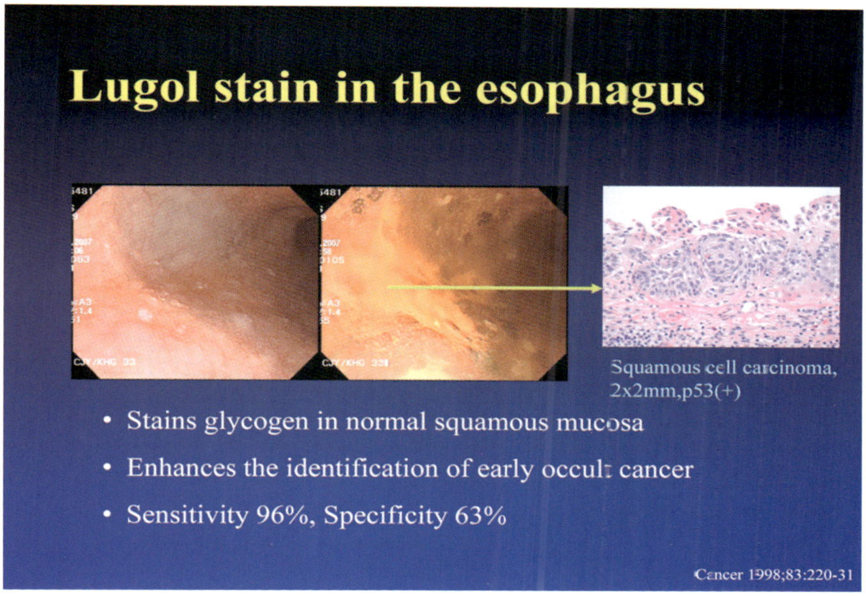

Lugol' s solution facilitates the diagnosis of early esophageal cancer This agent has enhanced the identification of early stage occult cancer in screening programs for high-risk patients such as heavy smokers, alcoholics. In one study, the sensitivity and specificity of lugol' s solution for detect the early esophageal cancer or dysplasia was reported as 98% and 63%.

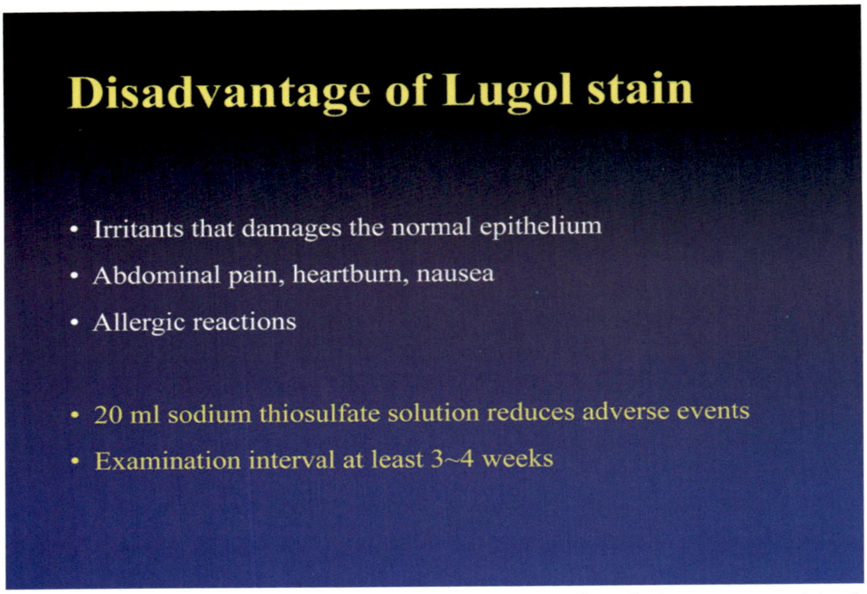

Lugol' s solution is an irritant that damages the normal epithelium. Patients may complain of abdominal pain, heartburn, and nausea. In addition, allergic reactions to iodine, including shock, have rarely been reported. Administration of 20ml of a sodium thiosulfate solution, which substantially reduces these adverse events, is therefore recommended after lugol chromoendoscopy. A subsequent examination with lugol' s solution should be carried out no lesser than 3~4 weeks, to prevent epithelial damage.

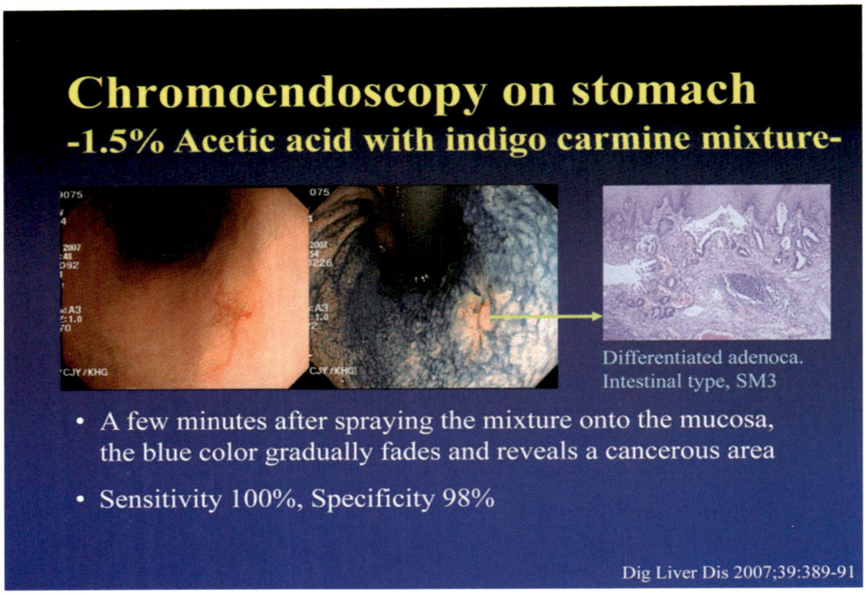

1.5% acetic acid and indigo carmine is a relatively new method for detecting gastric neoplasms. A few minutes after spraying the mixture onto the mucosa, the blue color gradually fades and reveals an unstained abnormal lesion. A sensitivity of 100% and specificity of 98% has been reported.

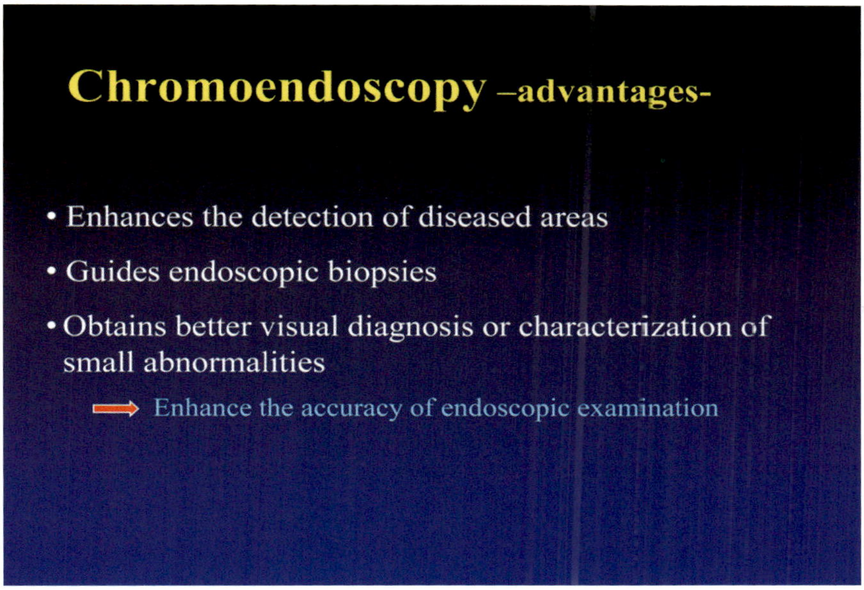

Chromoendoscopy enhances the detection of diseased areas, guide endoscopic biopsies, and obtains better visual diagnosis or characterization of small abnormalities. In all, chromoendoscopy enhances the accuracy of endoscopic examination

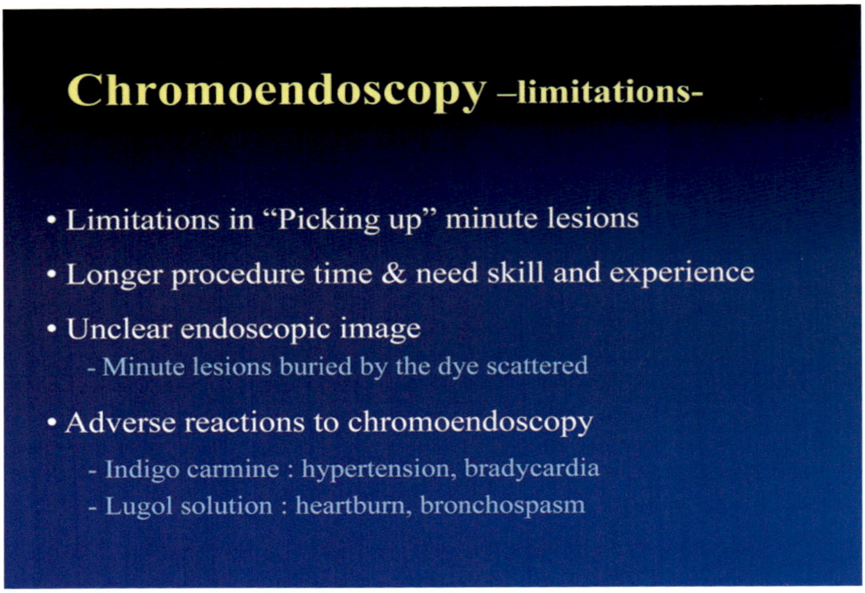

Although chromoendoscopy can enhance the accuracy of endoscopy, there are some limitations of chromoendoscopy. 'Picking up' by conventional endoscopic examination is a necessary precondition for the diagnosis of minute lesions by chromoscopy. But lesions cannot be "picked up" for eventual diagnosis when the color tone and irregularities on their surfaces cannot be distinguished from those of the surroundings. <Chromoendoscopy also requires a longer procedure time and the scattered dye may contribute to unclear endoscopic images.> Additionally, there are a number of adverse reactions related to specific dyes.

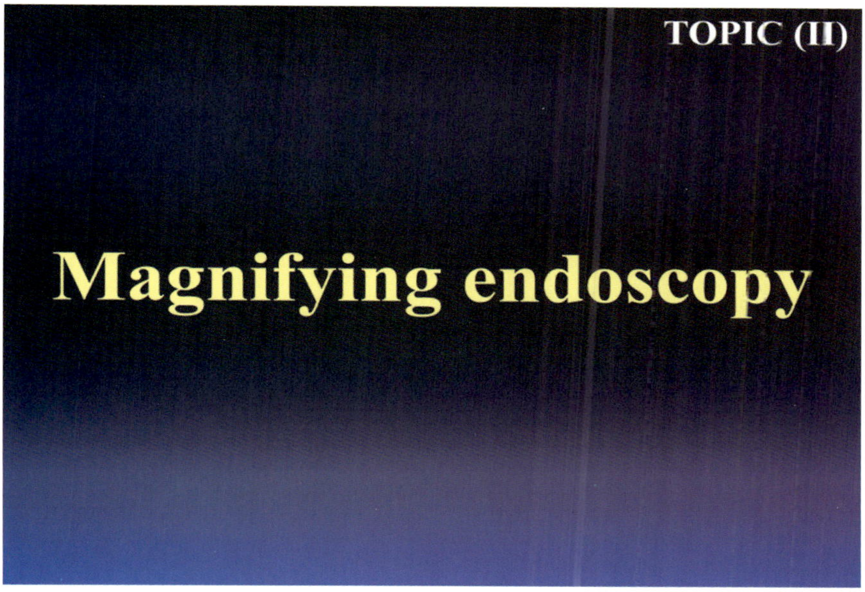

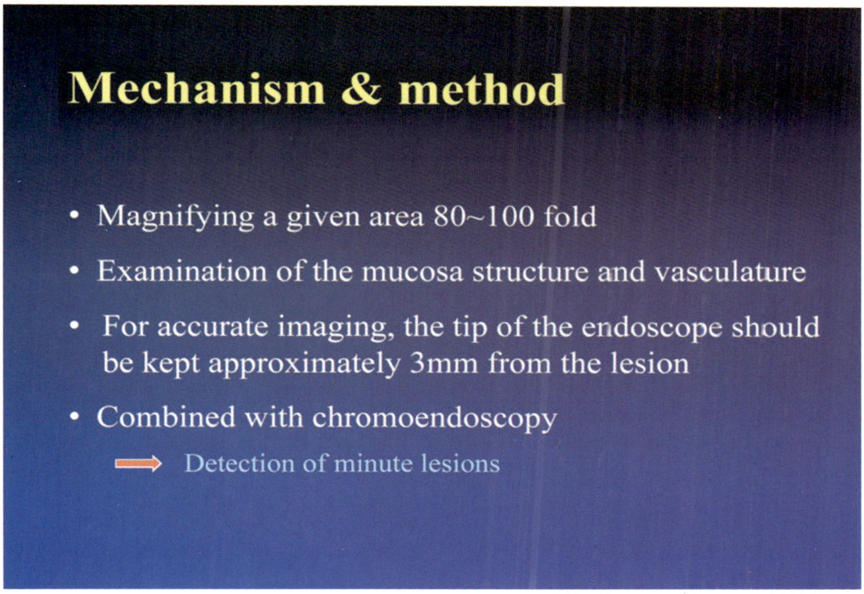

Magnifying endoscopy can magnify a given area 80 to 100 fold, enabling the detailed examination mucosal pit and vascular pattern. The tip of the endoscope should be kept approximately 3 mm from the surface. Magnifying endoscopy can be combined with chromoendoscopy for a more detailed examination.

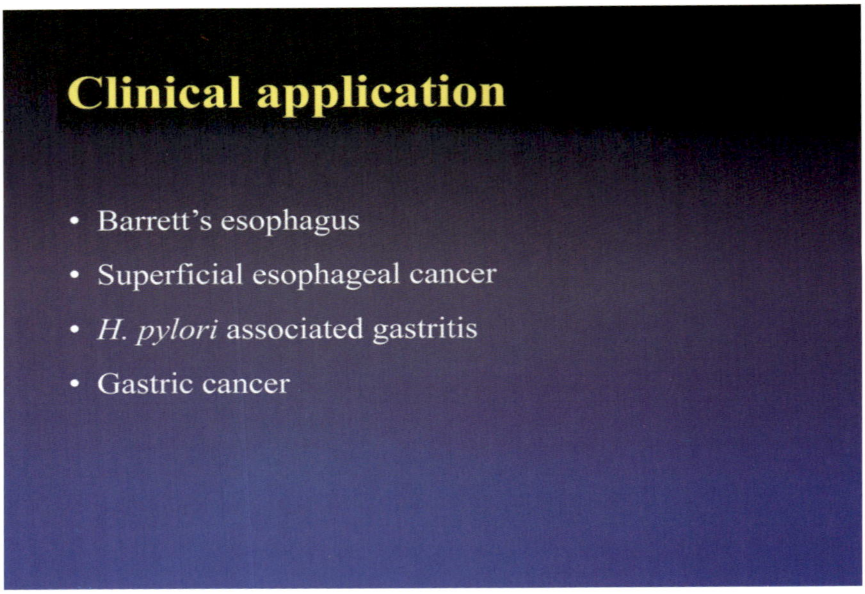

Clinically magnifying endoscopy is used for examination of Barrett' s esophagus, early esophageal cancer, H. pylori associated gastritis, gastric adenomas and early gastric cancer.

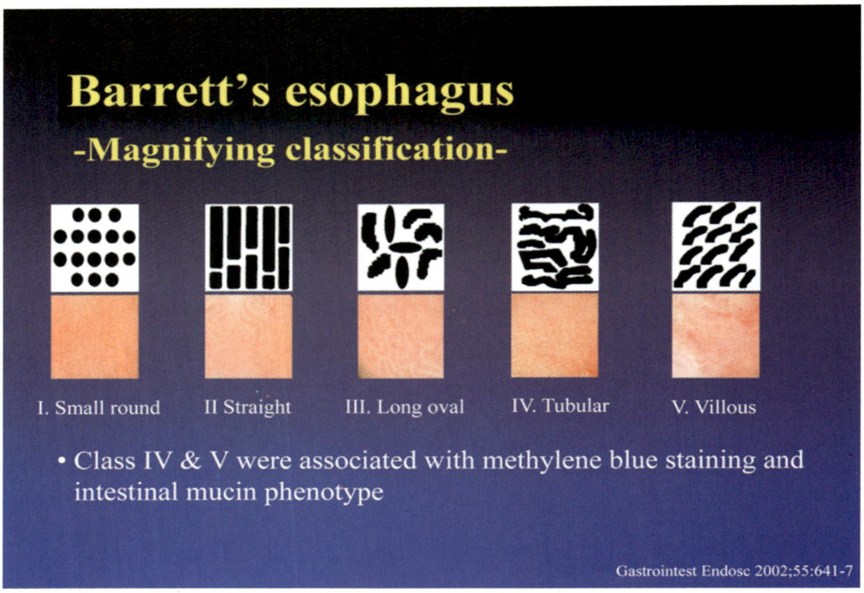

In 2002, Dr. Endo classified Barrett' s esophagus into 5 types according to the magnification image of the mucosa. A tubular or villous mucosal pattern (Type IV, V) was strongly associated with methylene blue staining and intestinal mucin phenotype.

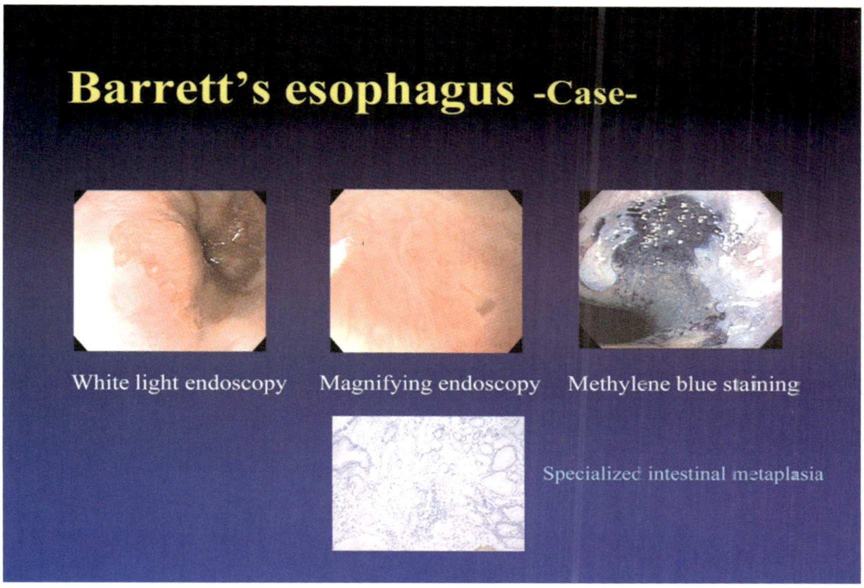

This case shows magnifying endoscopy and methylene blue staining of Barrett's esophagus. White light endoscopy shows short segment Barrett's esophagus proximal to the gastroesophageal junction. Magnifying endoscopy shows a tubular mucosal pit pattern. After magnifying examination, methylene blue staining was performed and biopsies were taken from the stained areas.

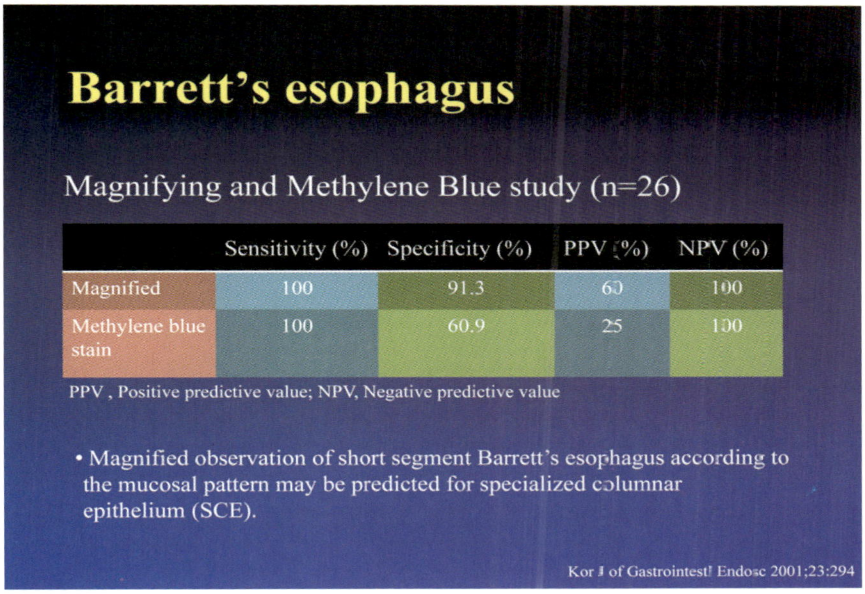

In one study, the sensitivity rate and negative predictive value of both the magnifying endoscopy and methylene blue was 100%. But specificity and positive predictive value of the magnifying endoscopy was higher than methylene blue staining. Magnified observation of short segment Barrett's esophagus according to the mucosal pattern may be predicted for specialized columnar epithelium.

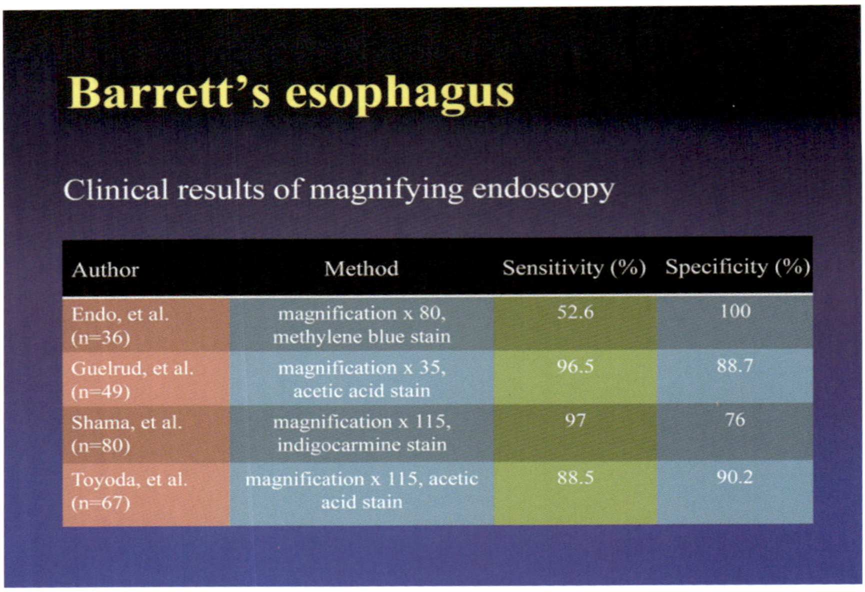

Barrett's esophagus

Clinical results of magnifying endoscopy

Author	Method	Sensitivity (%)	Specificity (%)
Endo, et al. (n=36)	magnification x 80, methylene blue stain	52.6	100
Guelrud, et al. (n=49)	magnification x 35, acetic acid stain	96.5	88.7
Shama, et al. (n=80)	magnification x 115, indigocarmine stain	97	76
Toyoda, et al. (n=67)	magnification x 115, acetic acid stain	88.5	90.2

Several studies have focused upon detection of Barrett' s esophagus and magnifying endoscopy. Magnifying endoscopy was combined with chromoendoscopy and the sensitivity ranges from 52-97% and specificity 76-100%.

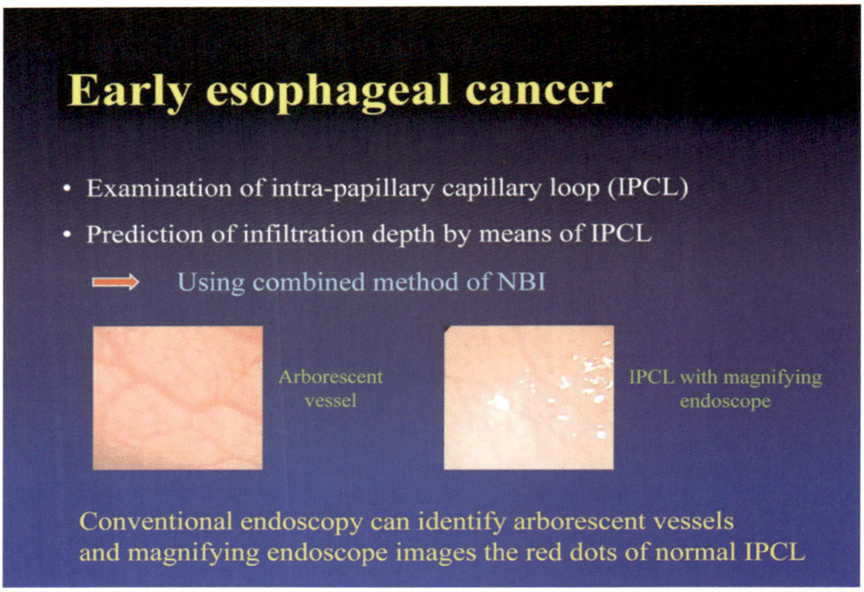

Examination of the intrapapillary capillary loop pattern with magnifying endoscopy helps distinguish early esophageal cancer. The IPCL pattern has also been reported to be related to infiltration depth. Recently Narrow band imaging combined with magnifying endoscopy has been reported to enhance these findings.

Esophageal IPCL

Type	Structure	Morphology	State
Type I	Normal epithelial pattern	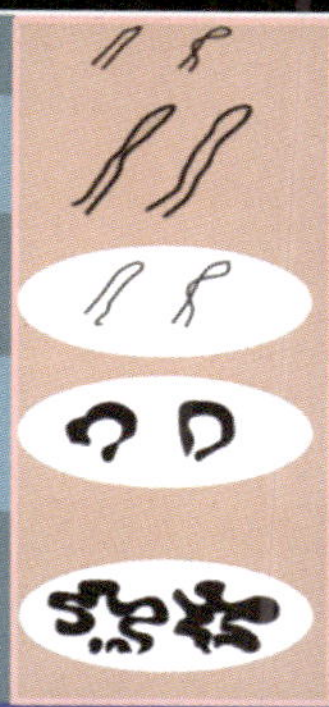	Normal
Type II	Elongation and/or dilatation		Esophagitis
Type III	No change or minimal changes of IPCL		Mild dysplasia
Type IV	IPCL includes three out of four characteristic changes of Type V		Severe dysplasia
Type V	Dilatation, tortuous running, caliber changes, and Irregular shape on each IPCL		Cancer

Digestive endoscopy 2001;13(S1):S40-S41.

IPCL patterns can be classified into 5 groups by magnifying endoscopy. The characteristic changes seen in carcinoma include weaving, dilatation, irregular caliber and varying shapes of individual IPCLs. Lesions with minimal change can be distinguished by iodine staining and lesions with all 4 characteristics are considered to be cancerous.

Esophageal IPCL of early cancer

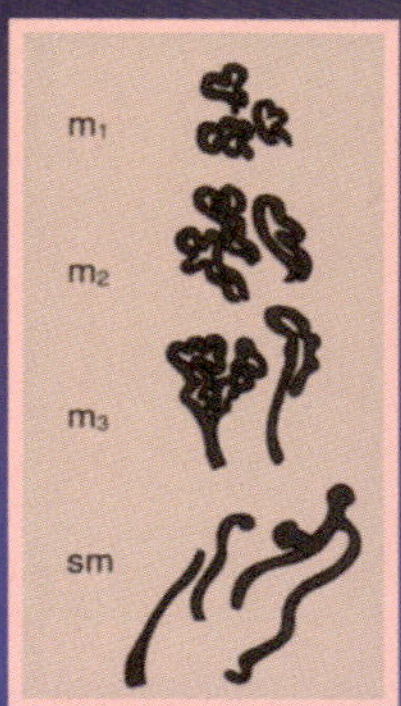

Changes of IPCL with the infiltration of T1 esophageal cancer

More prominent and elongated

↓

Change over the total length

↓

Totally destroyed

Digestive endoscopy 2001;13(S1):S40-S41.

The IPCL pattern may also predict the infiltration depth of the cancerous lesions. n submuiosal cancer, almost complete IPCL destructed and novel tumor vessels are often seen.

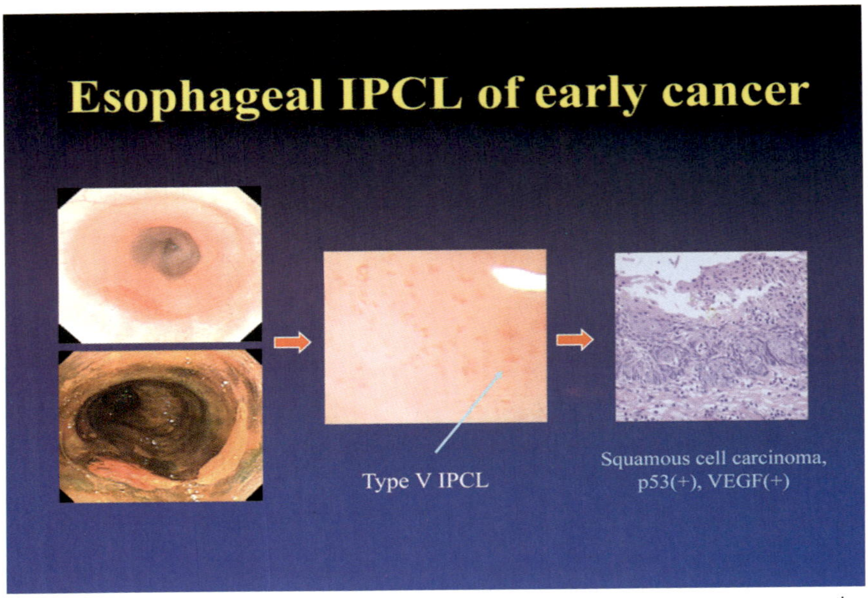

This is a patient with early esophageal cancer. The lesion does not stain after application of lugol' s solution and magnifying endoscopy shows a type 5 dilated tortuous IPCL pattern. Biopsy is consistent with squamous cell cancer.

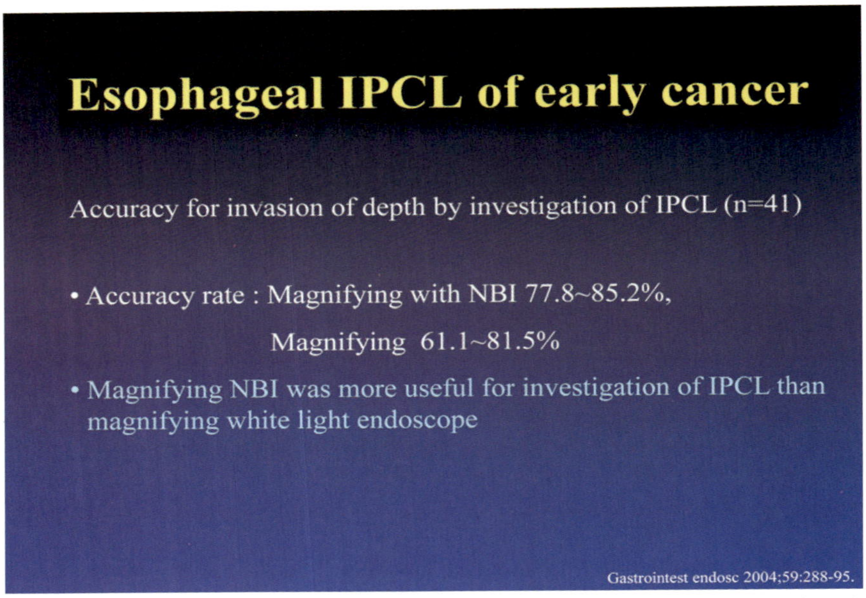

Recently, NBI has been used with magnifying endoscopy to examine the IPCL pattern in esophageal cancer. In this study the accuracy of NBI with magnifying endoscopy was significantly greater than magnifying endoscopy alone.

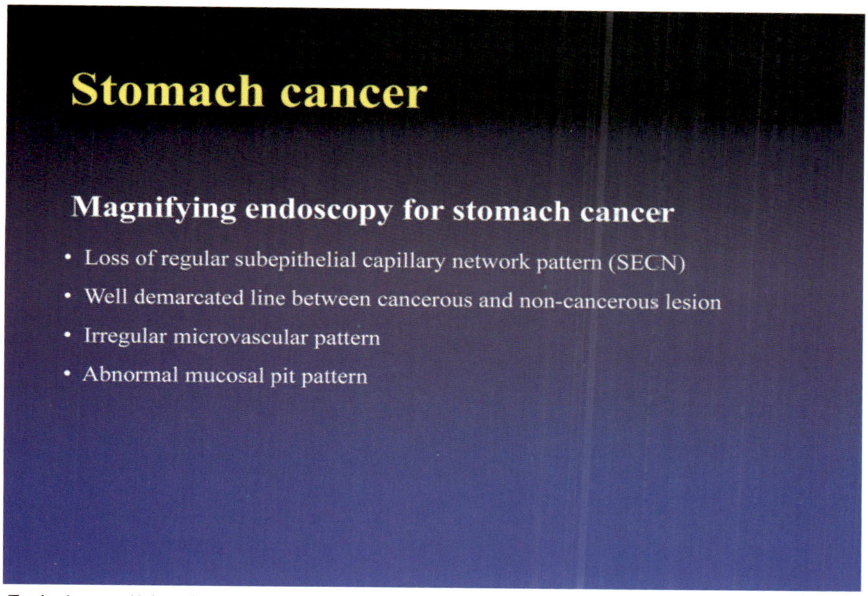

Typical magnifying findings of stomach cancer are loss of the regular subepithelial capillary network pattern, A enhanced demarcated line between cancerous and non-cancerous lesions, an irregular microvascular pattern and abnormal mucosal pit pattern.

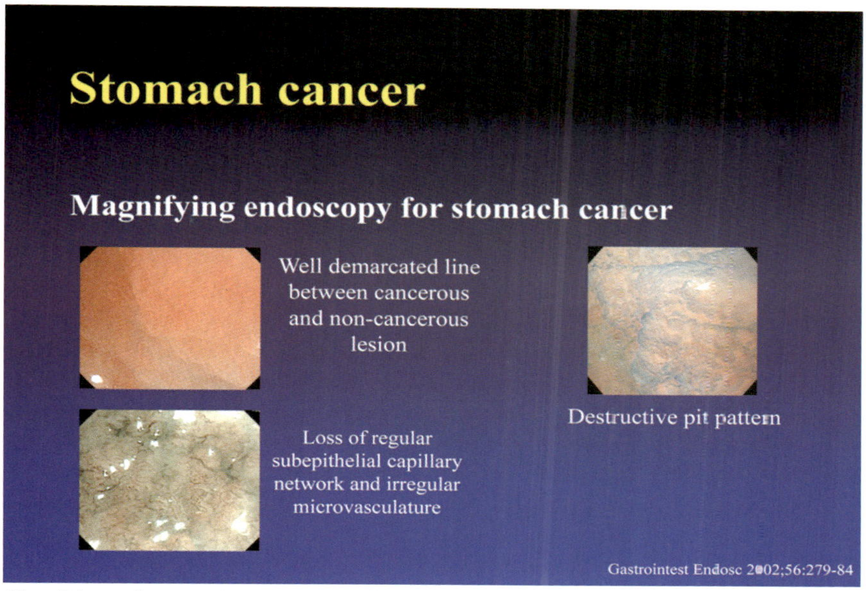

Magnifying endoscopy of stomach cancer. The upper left hand image shows a clear demarcated line between cancerous and non-cancerous regions. The image below shows loss of the regular subepithelial capillary network and irregular microvasculature. The upper right hand image shows a destructive pit pattern.

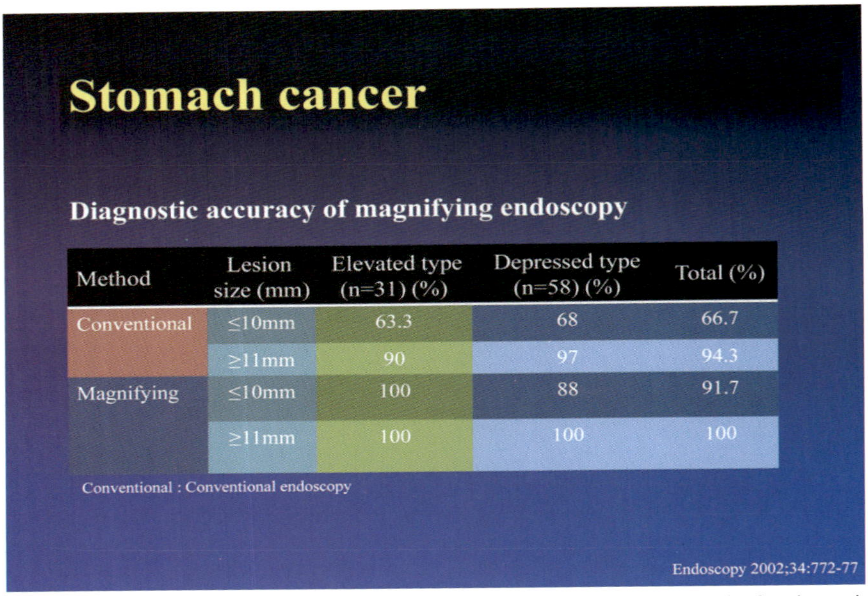

Method	Lesion size (mm)	Elevated type (n=31) (%)	Depressed type (n=58) (%)	Total (%)
Conventional	≤10mm	63.3	68	66.7
	≥11mm	90	97	94.3
Magnifying	≤10mm	100	88	91.7
	≥11mm	100	100	100

The diagnostic accuracy magnifying endoscopy for early gastric cancer was superior for elevated and depressed lesion compared to conventional endoscopy regardless of the size of the lesion.

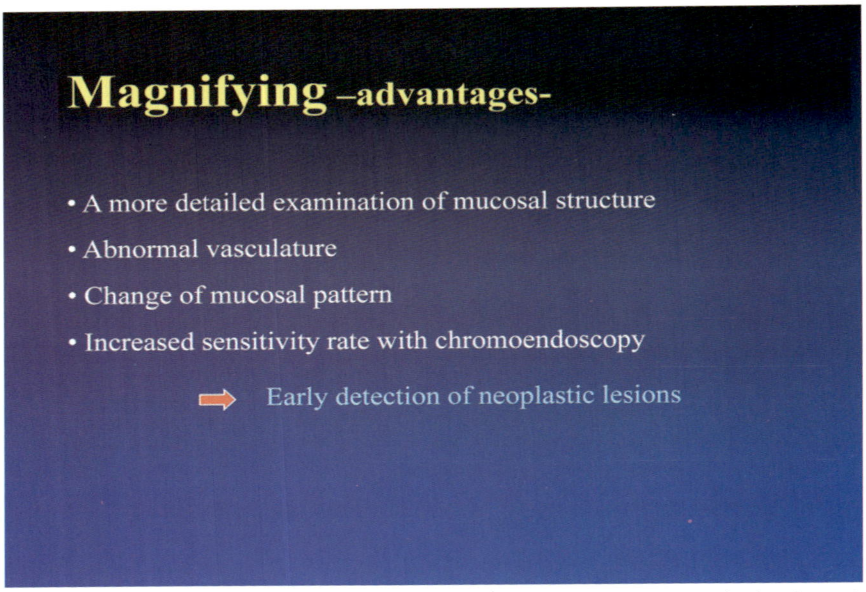

The diagnostic accuracy magnifying endoscopy for early gastric cancer was superior for elevated and depressed lesion compared to conventional endoscopy regardless of the size of the lesion.

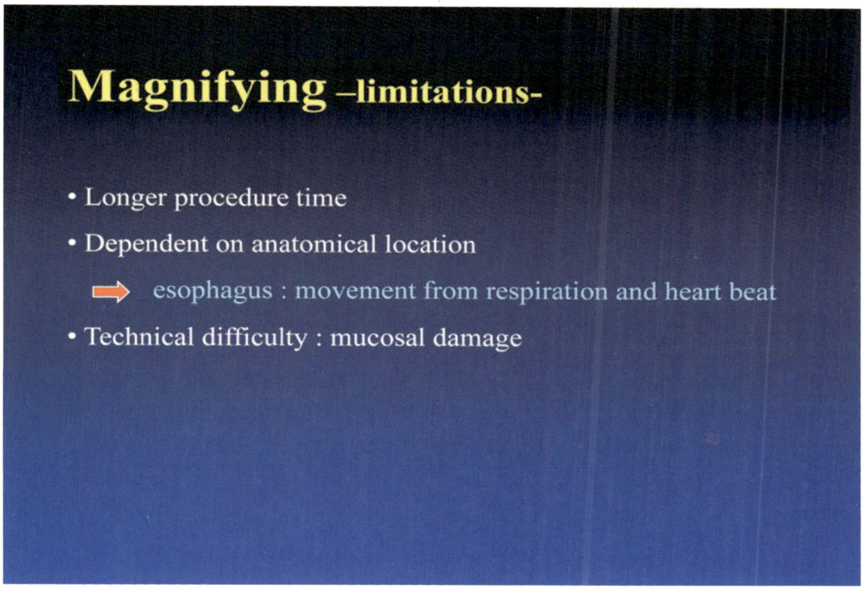

There are limitations of magnifying endoscopy. Mostly procedure related. These include a longer procedure time, factors related to the anatomical location and technical difficulty. When examining the esophagus frequent movement associated with the patients respiration and heart beat may cause difficulty. When examining the mucosa close approximation of the scope may cause unintended injury to the mucosa, which in turn may make the examination even more difficult.

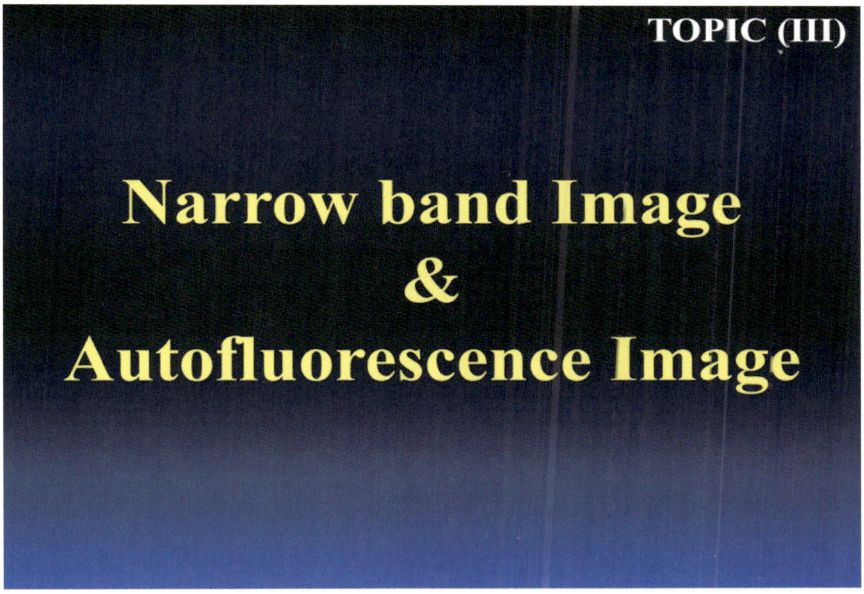

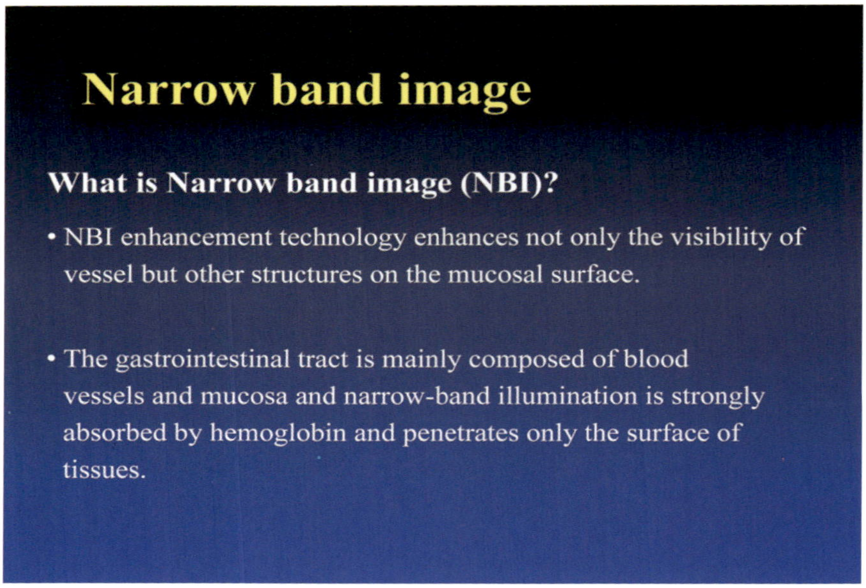

NBI enhancement technology enhances not only the visibility of vessel but other structures on the mucosal surface. The gastrointestinal tract is mainly composed of blood vessels and mucosa and narrow-band illumination is strongly absorbed by hemoglobin and penetrates only the surface of tissues.

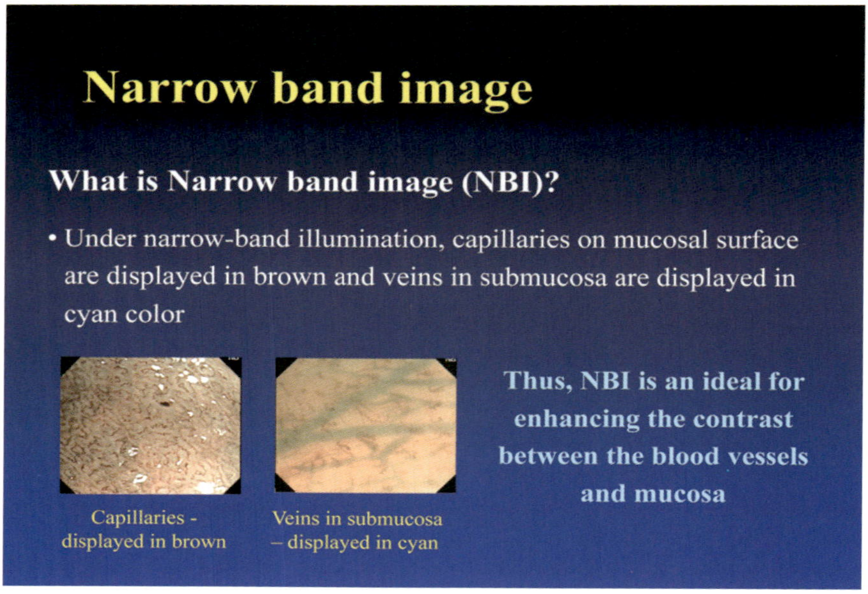

Under narrow-band illumination, capillaries on mucosal surface are displayed in brown and veins in submucosa are displayed in blue. Thus, NBI is ideal for enhancing the contrast between the blood vessels and mucosa.

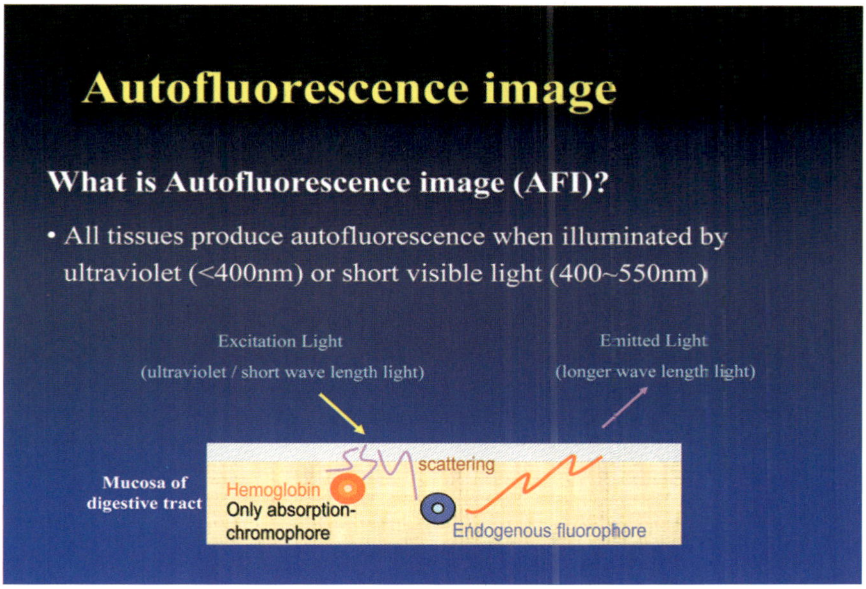

All tissues produce autofluorescence when illuminated by ultraviolet or short visible light. When mucosa is illuminated, excitation light is scattered throughout the tissue, chromophores, mainly hemoglobin of red blood cells absorbs the light without emission. A portion of the light is emitted as a longer wave length by endogenous fluorophores.

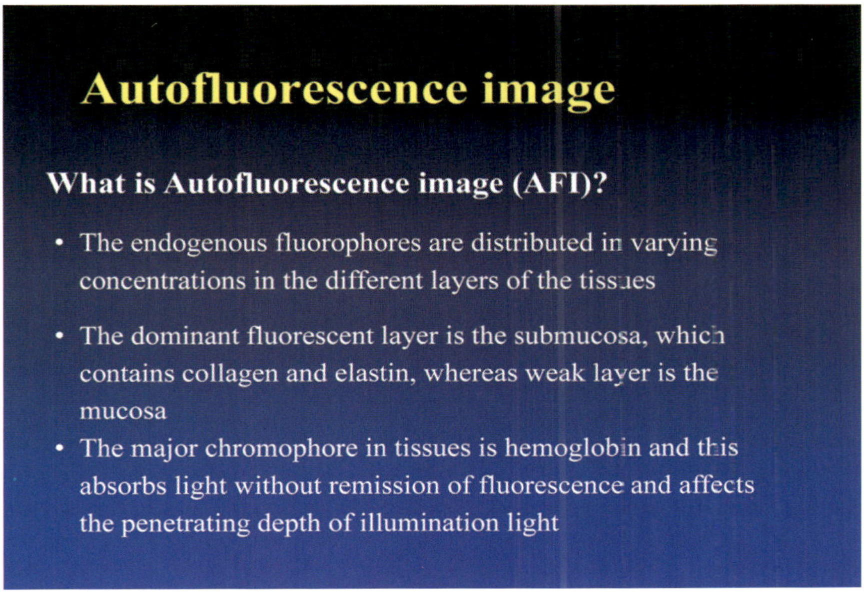

The endogenous fluorophores are distributed in varying concentrations in the different layers of the tissues. The dominant fluorescent layer is the submucosa, which contains collagen and elastin, whereas the weak layer is the mucosa. The Major chromophore in tissues is hemoglobin and this absorbs light without remission of fluorescence and affects the penetrating depth of illumination light.

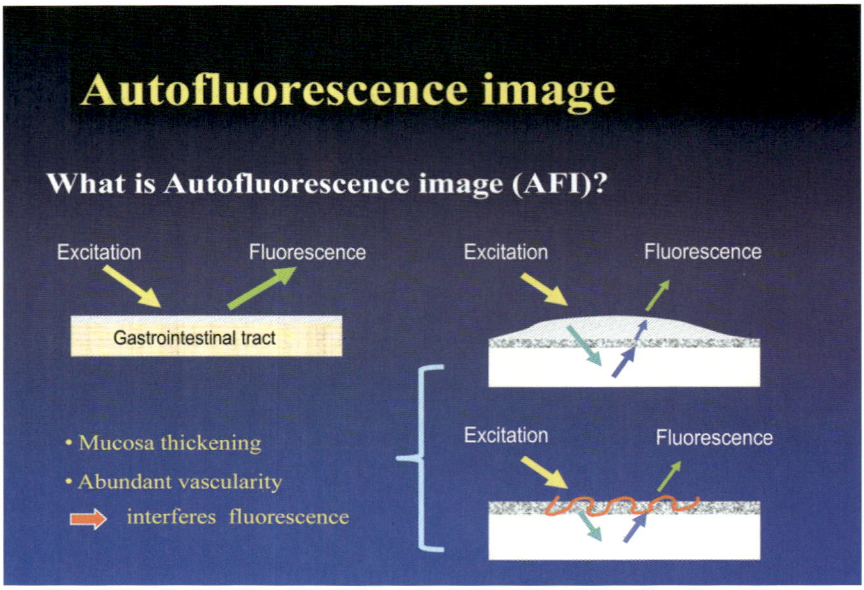

When the mucosa, which is the weakest fluorescent layer, is thickened, the light emission by fluorophores is decreased. Additionally abundant vascularity increases the light absorption by hemoglobin and decreases the scattering of the light, thus interfering with fluorescence.

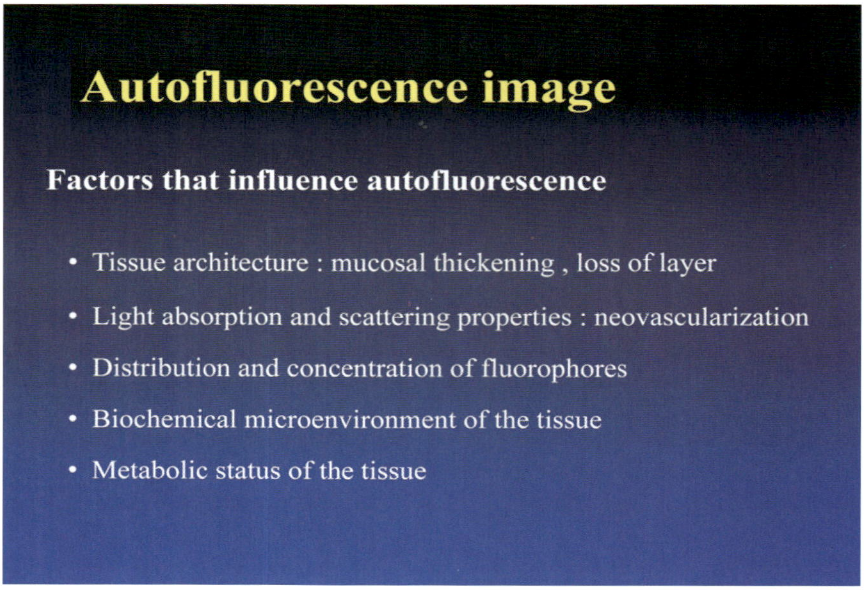

Factors that influence auto fluorescence are tissue architecture such as mucosal thickening, light absorption and scattering properties, such as neovascularization, distribution and concentration of fluorophores, the biochemical microenvironment and the metabolic status of the tissue.

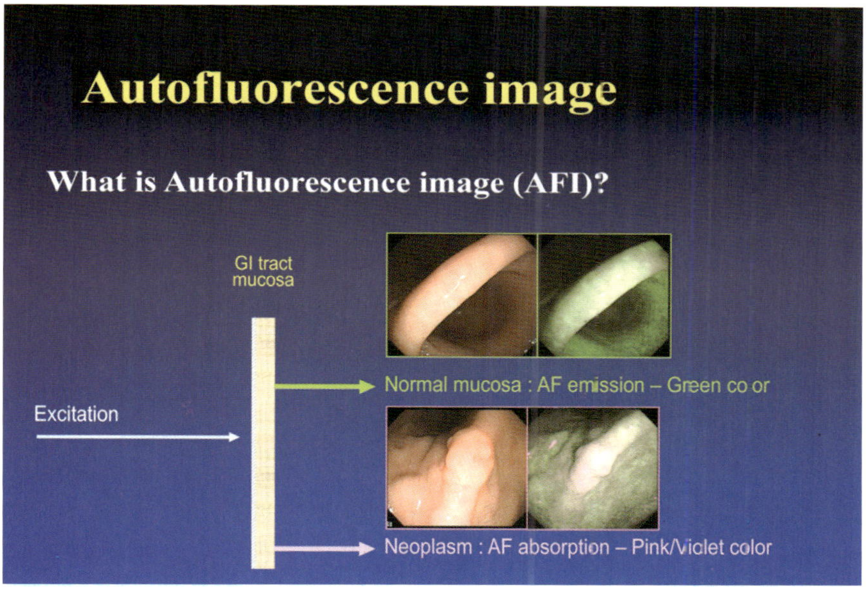

When normal mucosa is observed under AFI, the mucosa normally emits a green fluorescent color. However, when a neoplastic lesion is illuminated, due to the increase of tissue vascularity autofluoresence is decreased and the mucosa is observed as a pink or violet area.

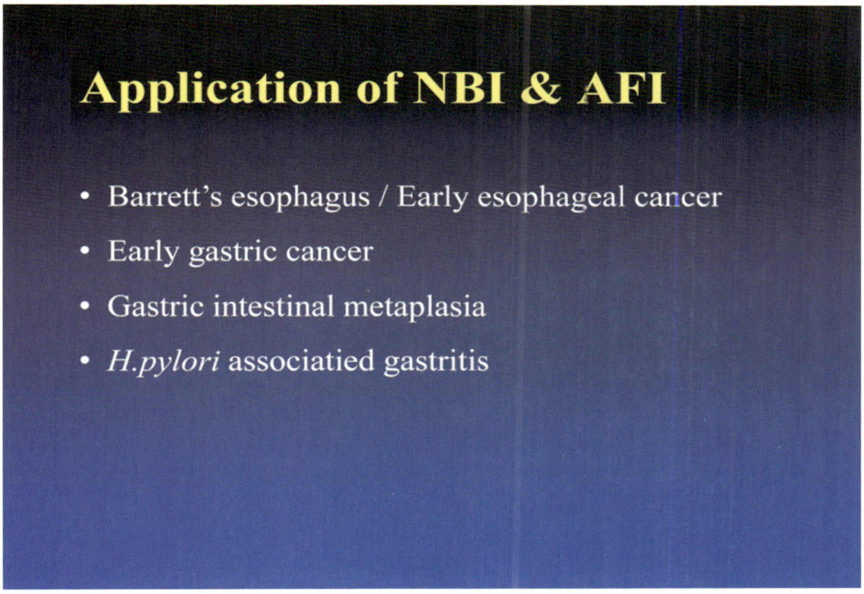

The applications of NBI and AFI are continuing to expand. Currently they are being used for the detection of Barrett' s esophagus, early esophageal cancer, early gastric cancer, gastric intestinal metaplasia and H. pylori associated gastritis.

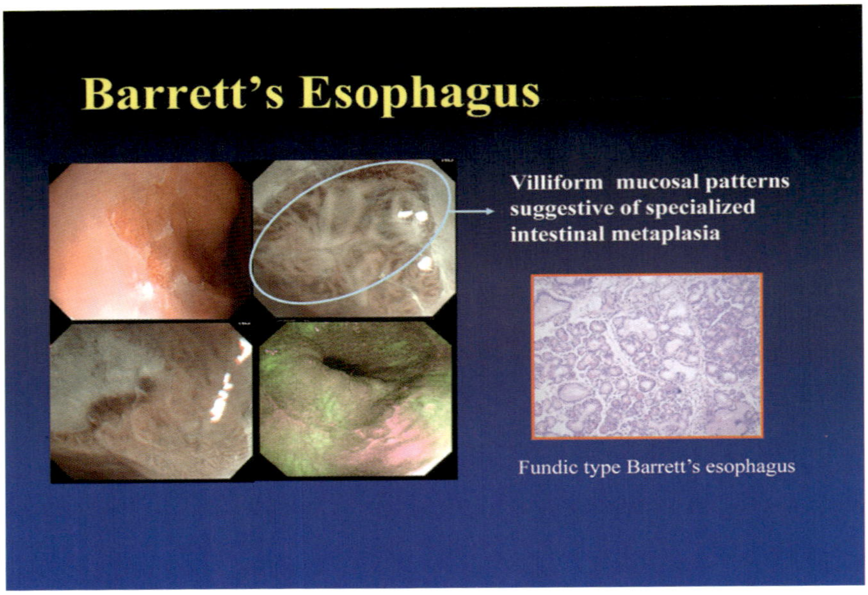

AFI can indentify abnormal mucosal patterns and magnifying NBI mode enables the endoscopist to confirm specific villous patterns simultaneously. Target biopsies using NBI and magnification help increase the diagnostic yield of biopsies.

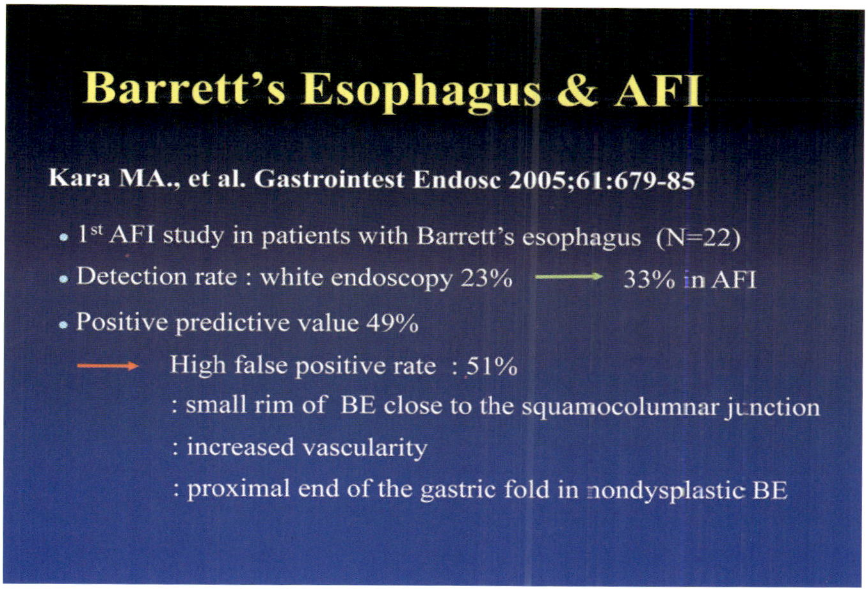

Although studies are limited, AFI increased the detection rate of high grade dysplasia or cancer from 23 to 33% in patients with Barrett' s esophagus. However, the false positive rate was high. Possible reasons for the high false positive rate are, a small rim of the BE immediately adjacent to the squamocolumnar junction often has a bluish color on AFI, which may lead to an increase in the false-positive rate of diagnosis. Second, areas with increased vascularity as seen by white light endoscopy exhibit a bluish color on AFI, Third, the gastric mucosa also appears blue/purple with AFI.

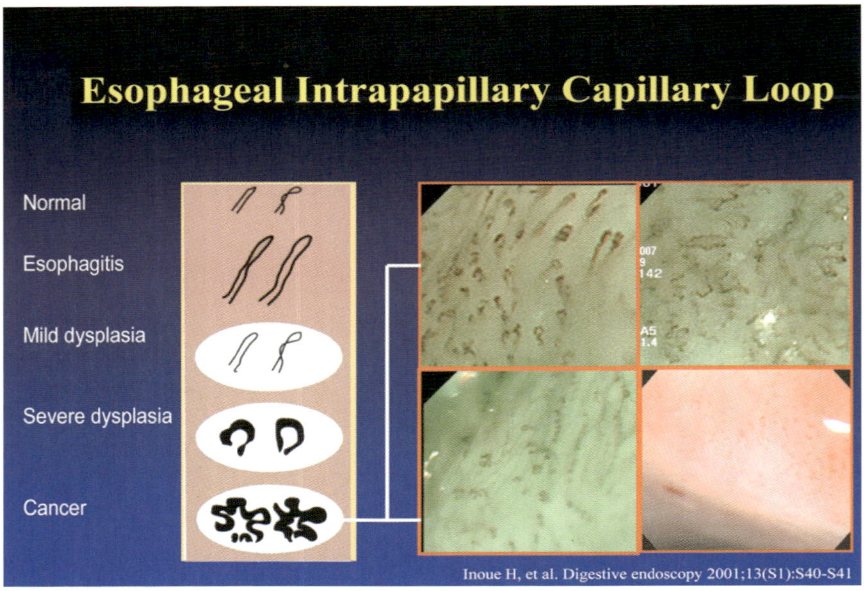

NBI can provide accurate images of the IPCL pattern in esophageal lesions.

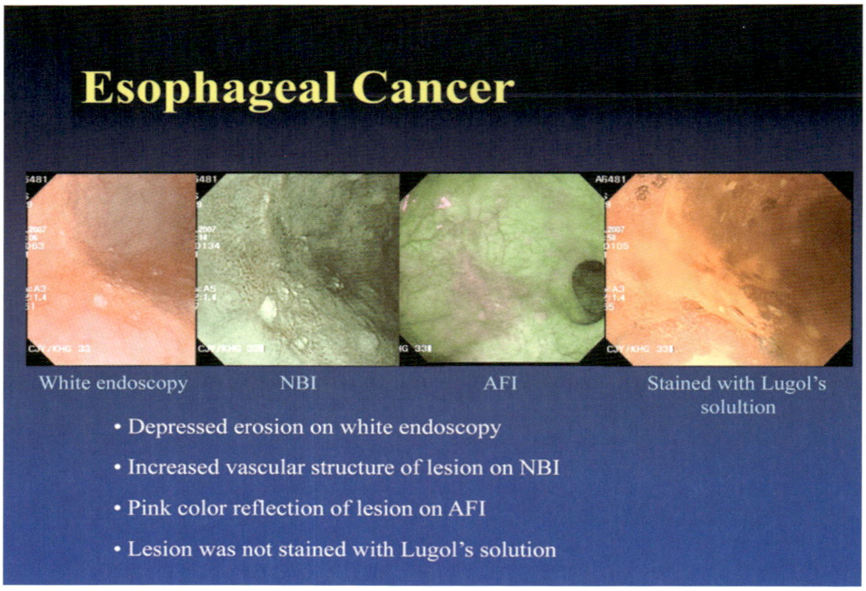

Conventional endoscopy, shows a superficial erosion on the midesophagus. In NBI mode, the lesion appears more definite, and with magnifying NBI, an elongated tortuous IPCL pattern can be observed. With AFI, the lesion is shown pink color as in contrast to the green normal mucosa. This lesion was not stained with Lugol' s solution

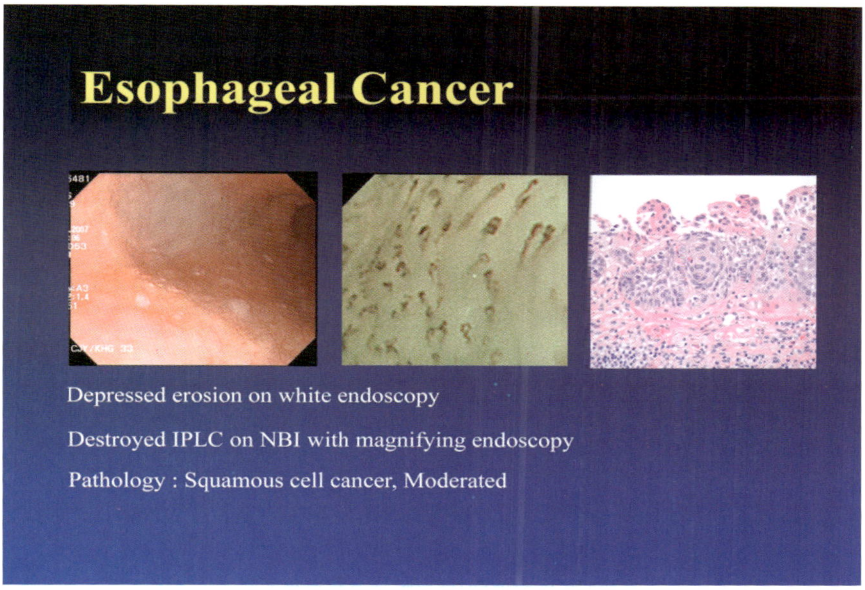

Tissue biopsy showed moderately differentiated squamous cell carcinoma. This patient eventually underwent endoscopic submucosal dissection and the pathologic report showed invasion of cancer cells up to the 3third mucosal layer which correlates to the IPCL pattern of classification for depth of invasion.

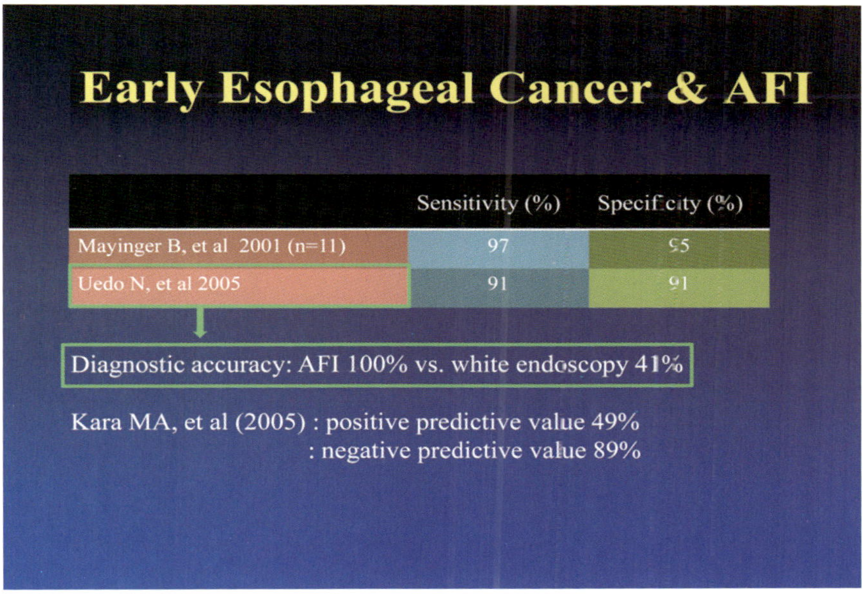

Reports demonstrate that AFI to superior to conventional endoscopy in both sensitivity and specificity for the detection of early esophageal cancer. One report showed that the negative predictive value of AFI was significantly greater than the positive predictive value (89% vs. 49%)

Esophageal Lesion & NBI

Author/Year	Pathologic confirm	Results	
		Sensitivity(%)	Specificity(%)
Sharma P, et al. 2006	Metaplasia	94	87
Sharma P, et al. 2006	Dysplasia	100	99
Kara MA, et al. 2006	Dysplasia	94	76
Goda K, et al. 2007	Adenocarcinoma	100	100

The sensitivity for NBI in detection of Barrett' s esophagus and early esophageal cancer varies. Most studies show a sensitivity greater than 90% and a specificity ranging from 76 to 100%. However most of these studies were small and further investigation is needed.

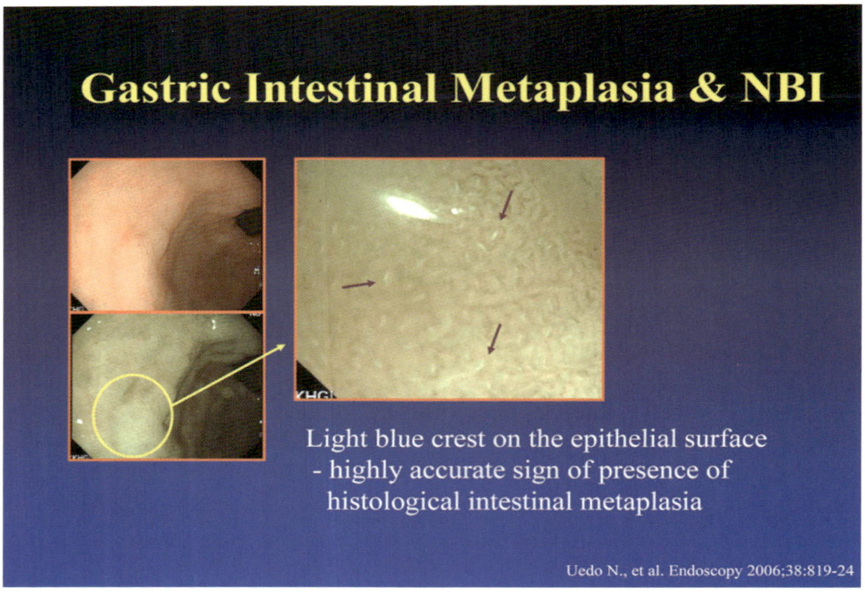

NBI can also detect intestinal metaplasia. The light blue crest on the epithelial surface with magnifying NBI has been reported to be a highly accurate sign of the presence of histological intestinal metaplasia.

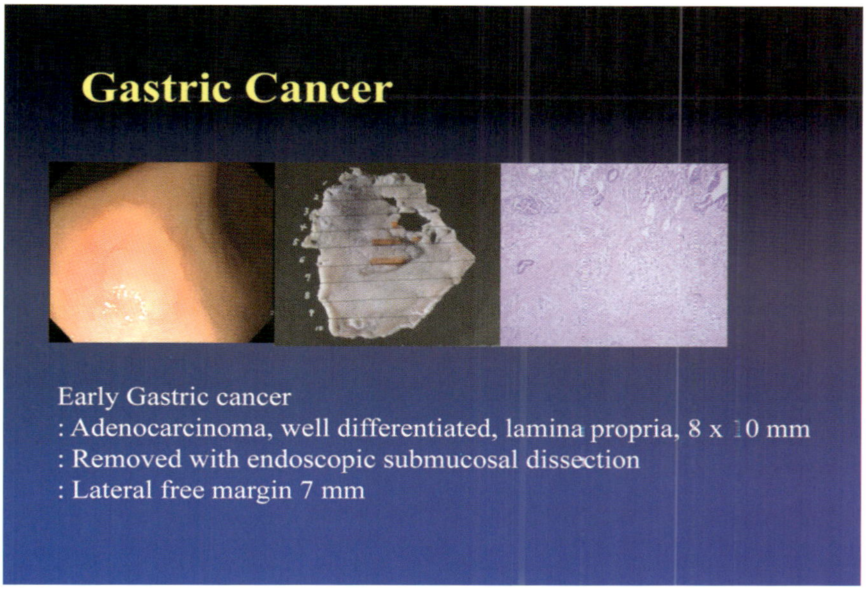

This case demonstrates the application of NBI and AFI in early gastric cancer. Endoscopy shows an elevated mucosal lesion on the anterior wall of the angle. After endoscopic submucosal dissection, the lesion was confirmed as adenocarcinoma invaded lamina propria.

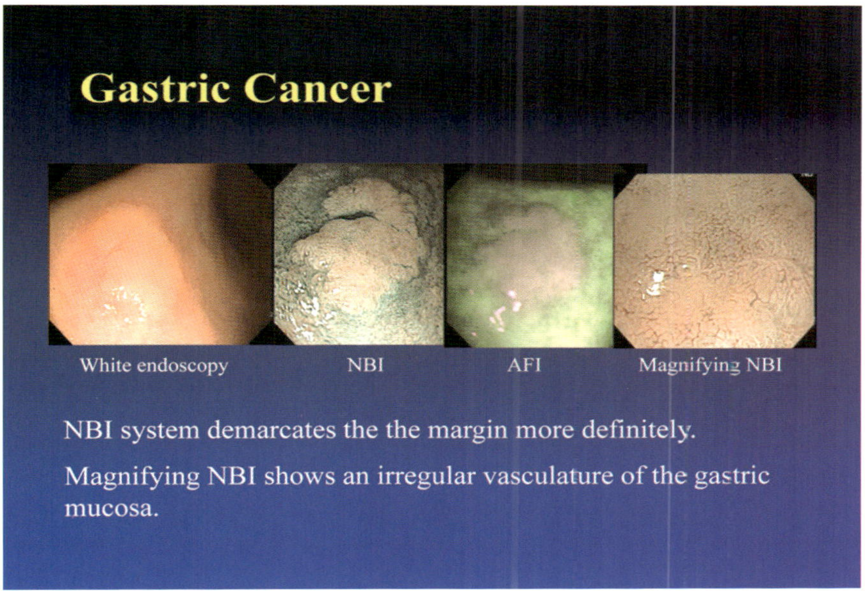

When observed with NBI, the margin of the lesion is much clearer than conventional endoscopy. With magnifying NBI, an irregular pit pattern and loss of the regular subepithelial capillary network was observed. When observed with AFI the lesion contrasted in pink.

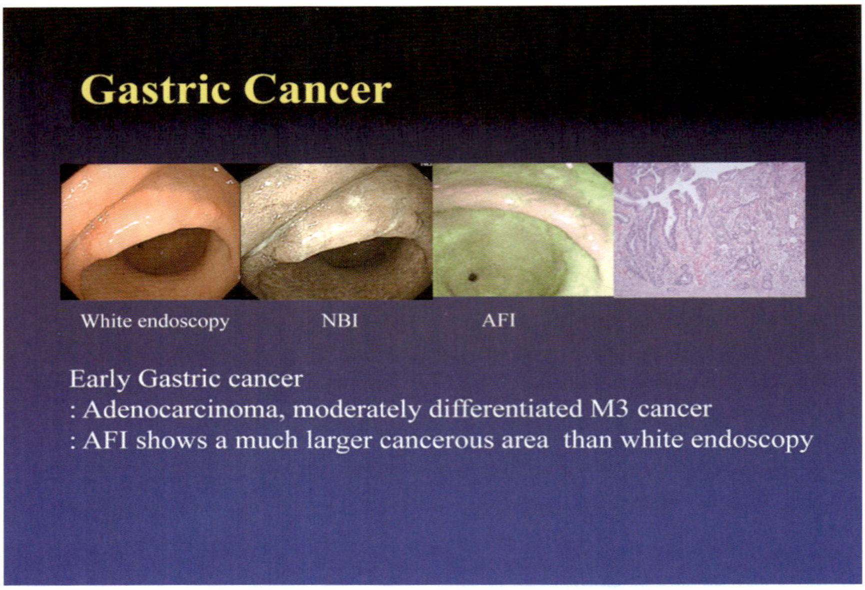

An elevated mucosal lesion is seen on the gastric angle by conventional endoscopy. An Irregular capillary network and irregular pit pattern are observed on the NBI magnifying mode. With AFI, the pink colored area is significantly broader than what was seen on conventional endoscopy. The patient underwent endoscopic submucosal dissection. The size of resected specimen measured 9 x 5 cm and the size of lesion was 72x44 mm. This case shows that AFI can assist in determinating the resection margin for endoscopic resection.

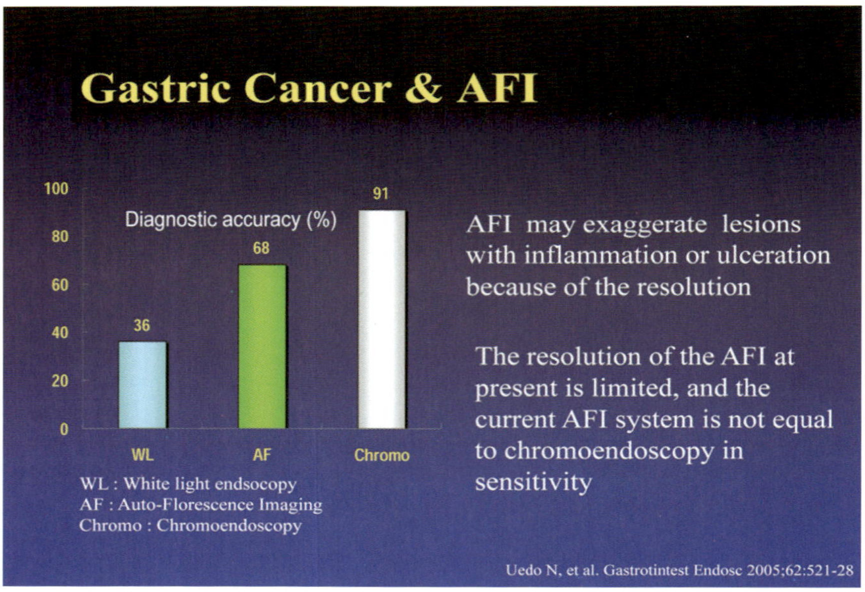

Current opinions are AFI may exaggerate lesions with inflammation or ulceration and the resolution of AFI at present is limited, and the current AFI system is not equal to chromoendoscopy in sensitivity.

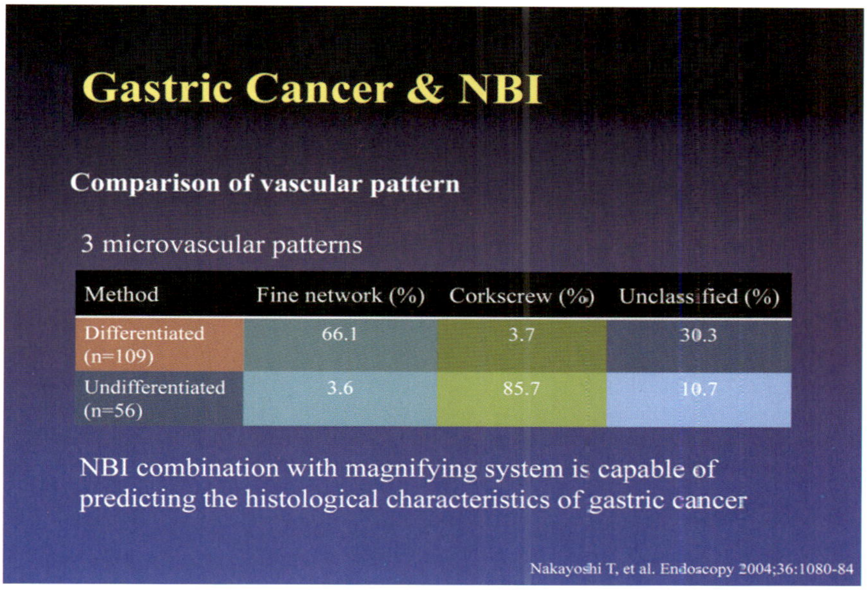

There are few studies of NBI and stomach cancer. NBI was mainly used in combination with magnifying endoscopy to identify the vascular pattern and thus the degree of differentiation.

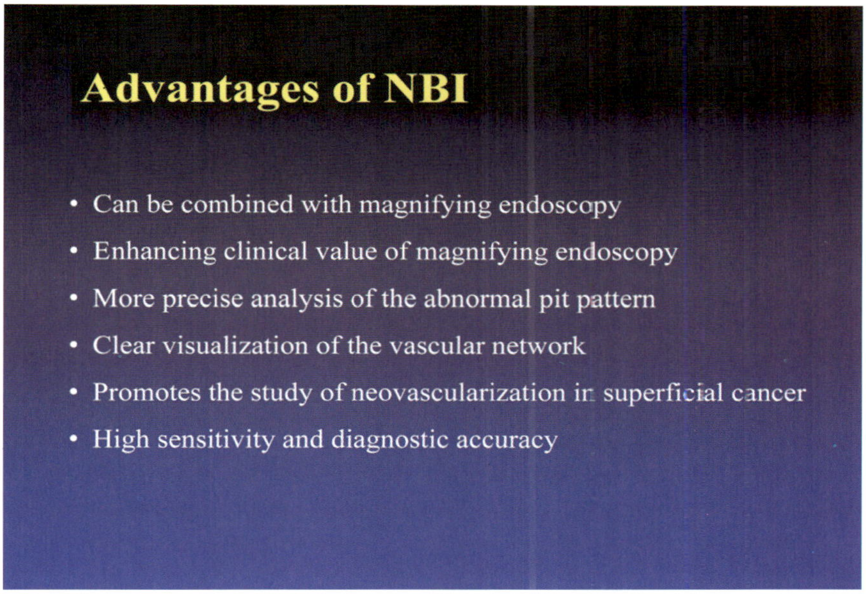

The advantages of NBI is it can be combined with magnifying endoscopy, it can enhance the clinical value of magnifying endoscopy, it can provide a more precise analysis of the abnormal pit pattern and it can provide a clear visualization of the vascular network. NBI also promotes the study of neovascularization in superficial cancer and has a high sensitivity and diagnostic accuracy.

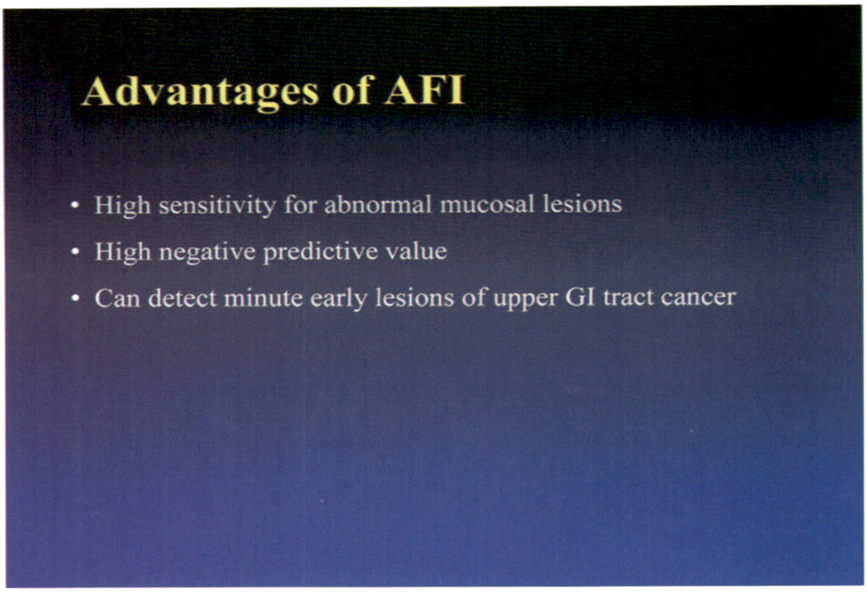

The advantages of autofluorescence imaging is the high sensitivity for abnormal mucosal lesions, the high negative predictive value and it can detect minute early lesions of upper GI tract cancer.

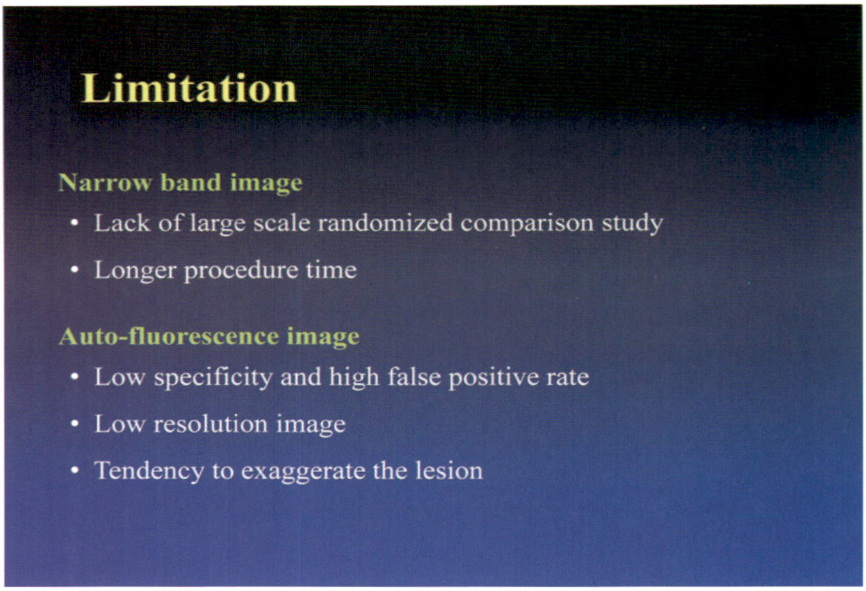

The limitations of NBI are the lack of large scale randomized comparison studies and a longer procedure time. The limitations of AFI are a low specificity and high false positive rate. Currently AFI has a low resolution image and tends to exaggerate lesions.

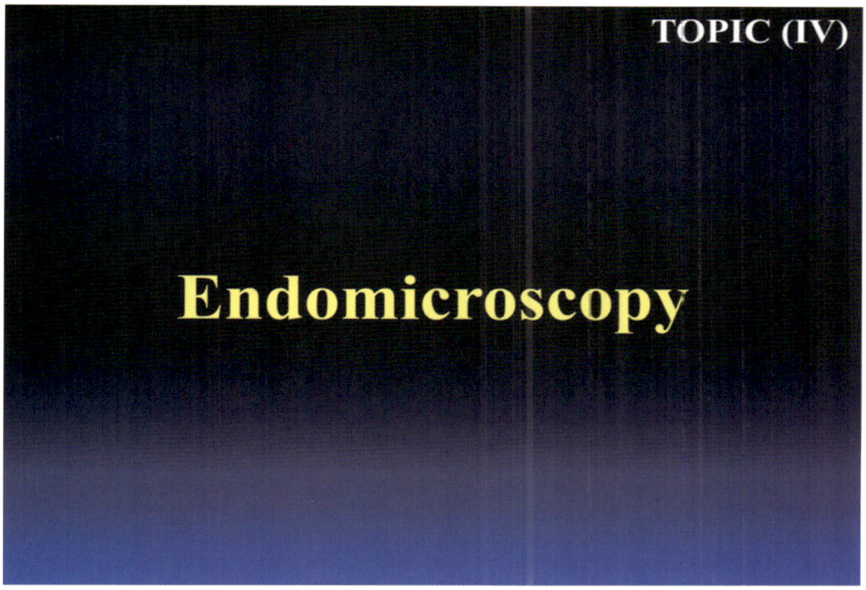

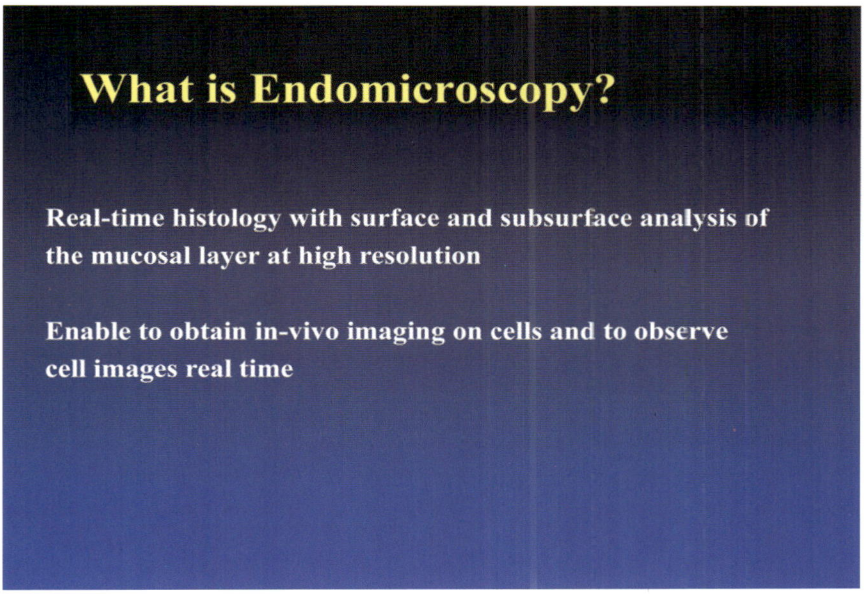

Endomicroscopy is real-time histology with surface and subsurface analysis of the mucosal layer at high resolution. Endomicroscopy is capable of obtaining in-vivo imaging of cells and to observe cell images real time.

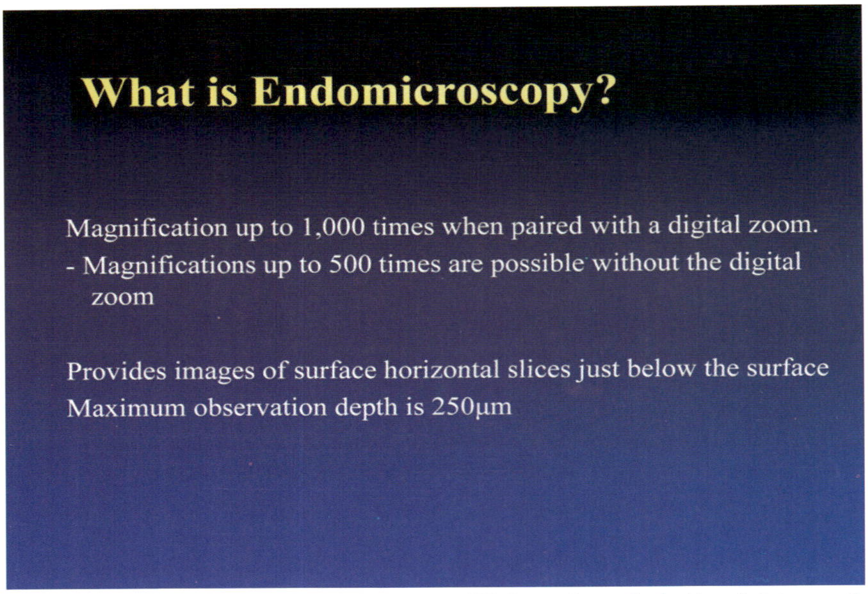

Endomicroscopy is capable of magnification up to 1,000 times when paired with a digital zoom. It provides images of surface horizontal slices just below the surface with a maximum observation depth of 250µm.

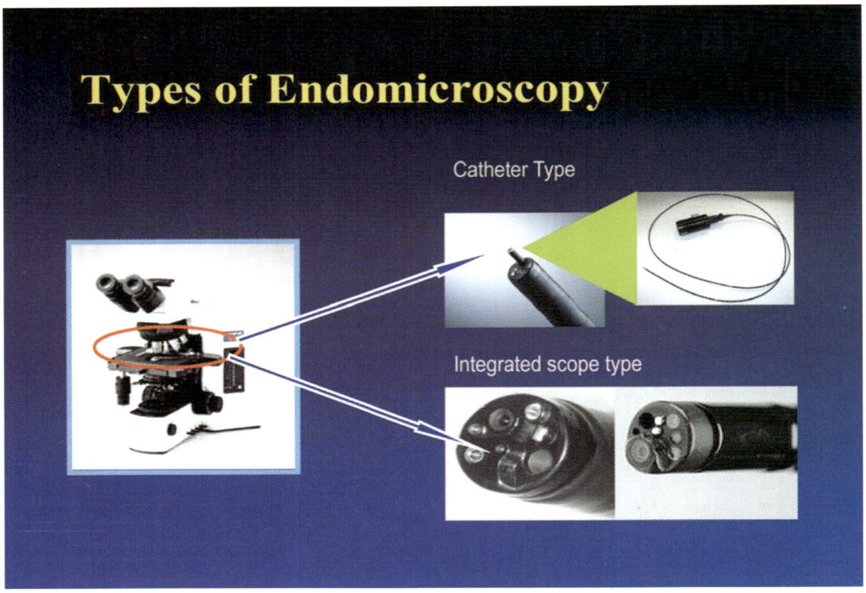

Currently there are two available types of endomicroscopy. The catheter type, similar to the miniprobe EUS, and the integrated scope type.

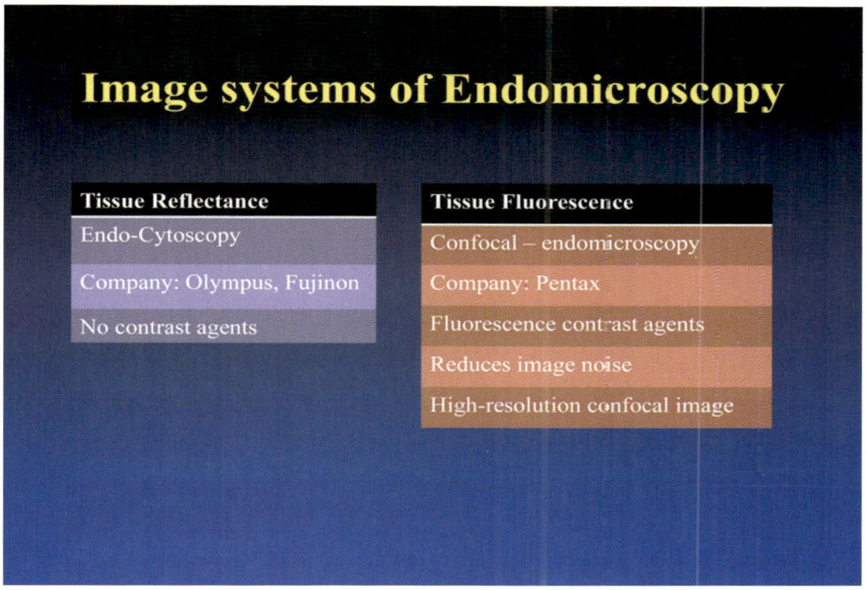

Two comparable imaging systems are also availabe. Endo-cytoscopy, is produced by Olympus and does not use contrast agents. And the Confocal-endomicroscopy, by Pentax which uses fluorescence contrast agents to provide high-resolution confocal images.

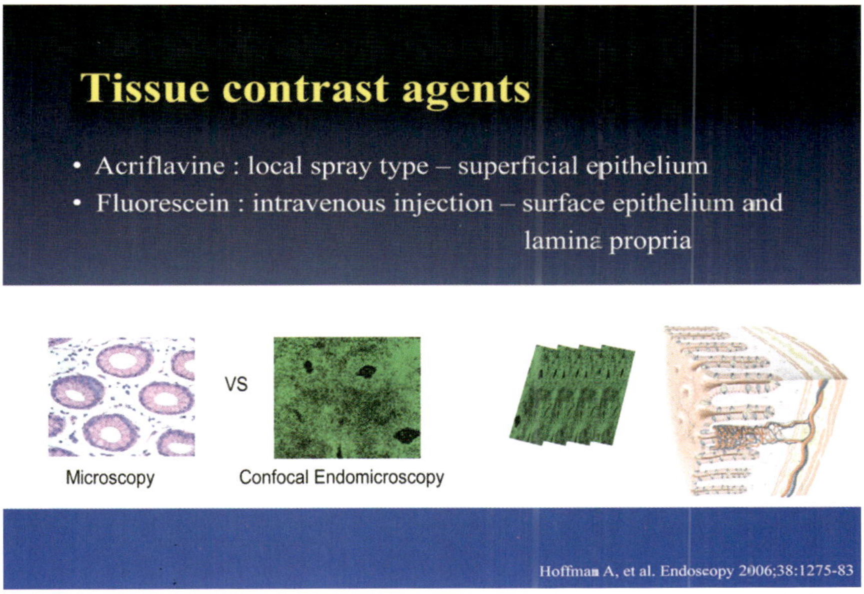

The contrast agents used for confocal endomicroscopy are acriflavine and fuorescein. Acriflavine is locally sprayed onto the surface where fluorescein is injected intravenously. Generally with acriflavine the superficial epithelium is mostly observed. With fluorescein deeped images upto the lamina propria can be observed.

Recent Focus of Endomicroscopy

- Detection of Barrett's esophagus and esophageal cancer
- Interobserver agreement between gastrologists and pathologists

Study of gastrointestinal tract mucosa with Confocal microscpy

Author	Method	Accuracy (%)	Sensitivity (%)	Specificity (%)
Alexander M, et al. 2007	Confocal fluloreseence	82.7	65	87.2
Inoue H, et al. 2000	Confocal Microscopy	89.7	85.7	92

The current clinical focuses of Endomicroscopy on the upper GI tract are detection of Barrett's esophagus and esophageal cancer, and interobserver agreement between endoscopists and pathologists. Recent reports shows high an accuracy rate, sensitivity and specificity for confocal endomicroscopy. Specificity had a tendency to be higher than sensitivity. Interobserver agreement varies with the experience of the investigator.

Endomicroscopy

Advantage

- Early detection of lesions that need pathologic confirmation
- Similar accuracy rate compared with pathologic diagnosis

Limitation

- Interobserver variability
- Resolution of photography

Advantages of endomicroscopy is early detection of lesions that need pathologic confirmation and the similar accuracy rate compared with pathologic diagnosis. Limitations are interobserver variability and the limited resolution of photography.

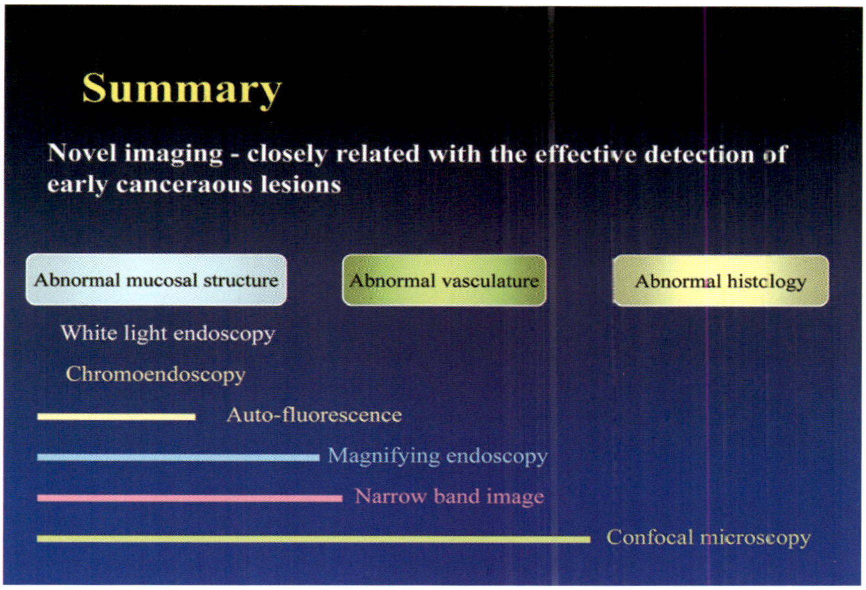

Novel imaging of upper gastrointestinal tract have been developed for effective detection of early cancerous lesions. Chromoendoscopy is useful for detection of abnormal mucosal patterns while AFI, NBI, and magnifying endoscopy not only detect abnormal mucosal patterns but also can detect abnormal vasculature.

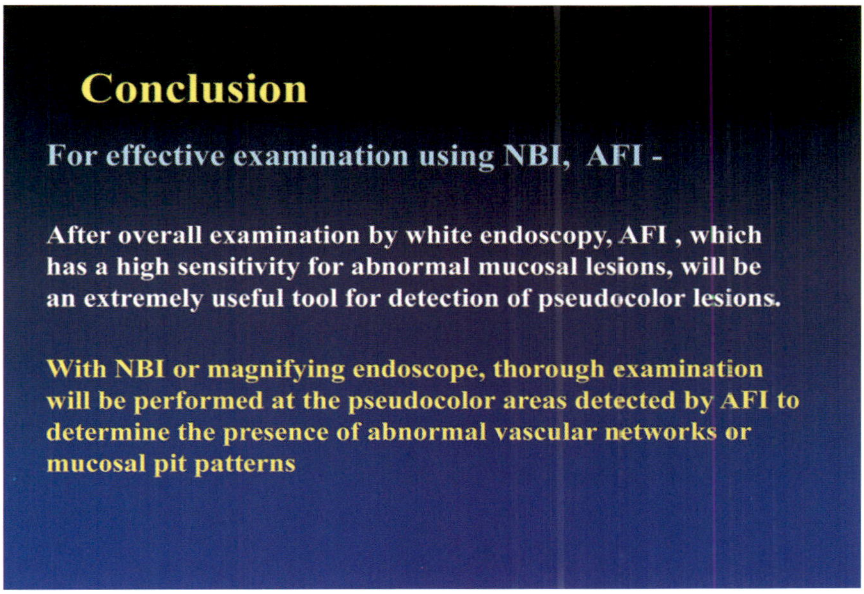

For effective examination using NBI and AFI, after overall examination with white endoscopy, AFI, which has a high sensitivity, will be an extremely useful tool for detection of abnormal mucosal lesions. With NBI or magnifying endoscope, thorough examination performed at the pseudocolor areas detected by AFI will assist the detection of abnormal vascular networks or mucosal pit patterns.

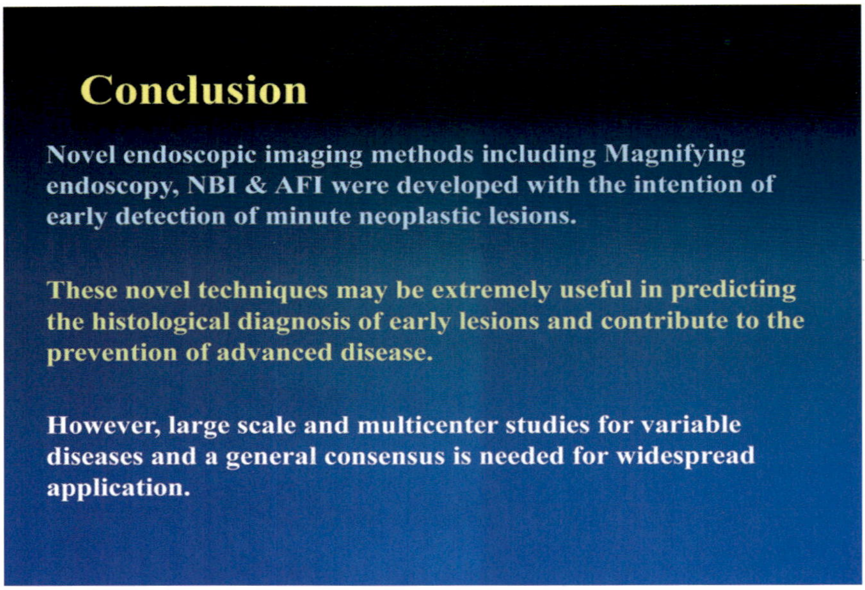

Novel endoscopic imaging methods including magnifying endoscopy, NBI & AFI were developed with the intention of early detection of minute neoplastic lesions. These novel techniques may be extremely useful in predicting the histological diagnosis of early lesions and contribute to the prevention of advanced disease. However, large scale and multicenter studies for variable diseases and a general consensus is needed for widespread application.

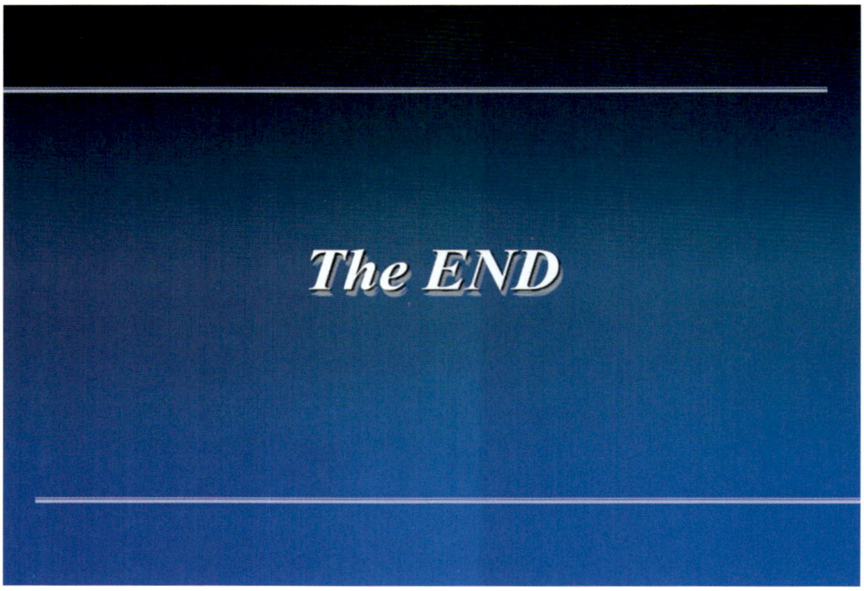

Novel imaging of upper gastrointestinal tract have been developed for effective detection of early cancerous lesions.

Chapter 5

Endoscopic Management of Variceal Hemorrhage in Cirrhosis

2009 ASGE Audiovisual Award Winner
Soung Won Jeong, M.D. Ph D.
Jae Young Jang, M.D. Ph D.
Joo Young Cho, M.D. Ph D.

Chapter 5

Endoscopic Management of Variceal Hemorrhage in Cirrhosis

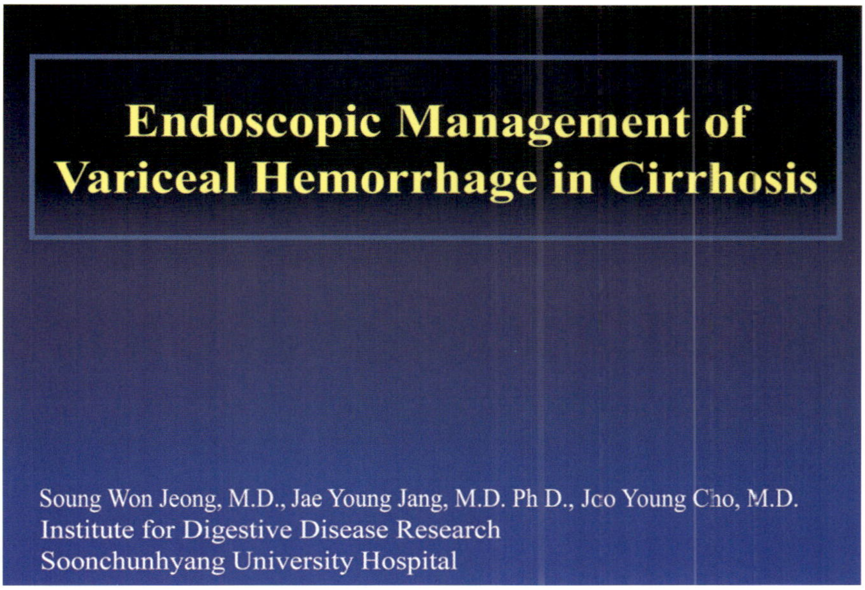

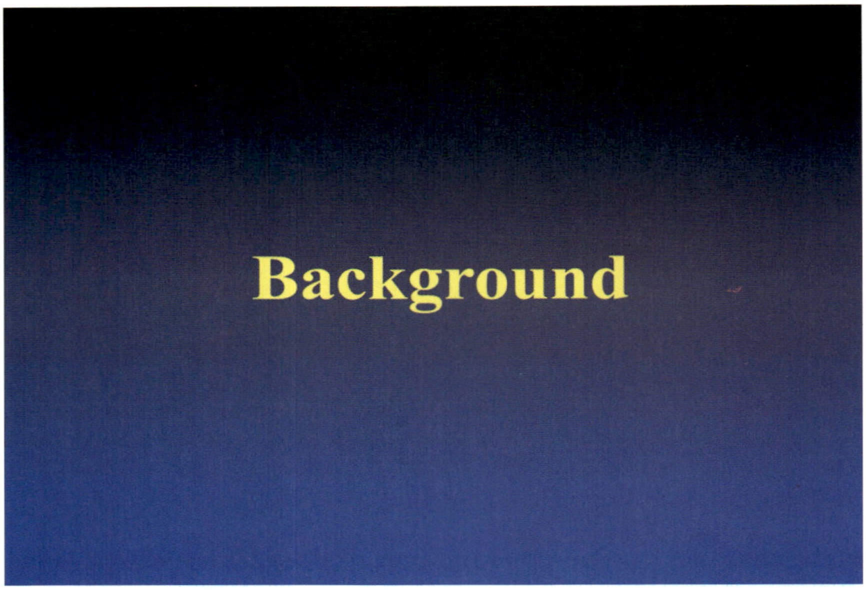

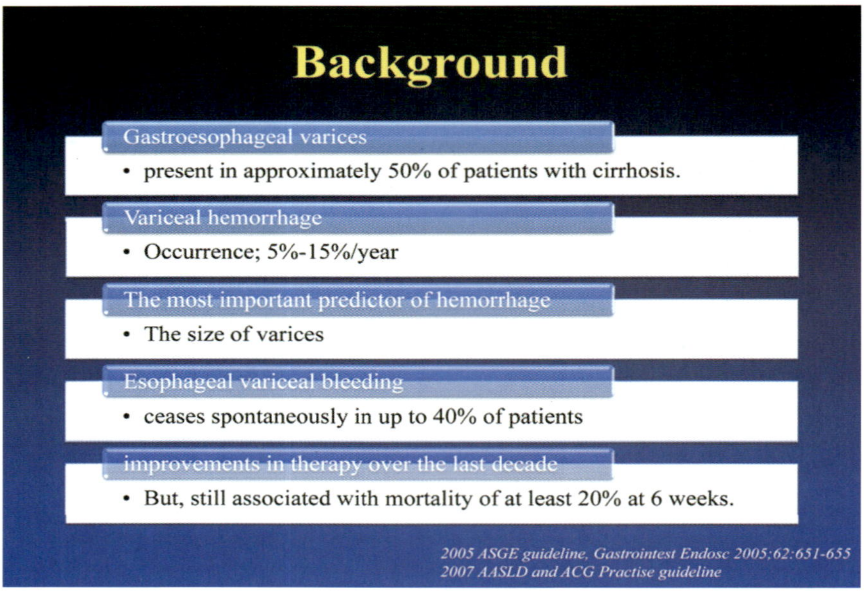

Gastroesophageal varices are present in approximately 50% of patients with cirrhosis.
Variceal hemorrhage occurs at a yearly rate of 5%-15% and the most important predictor of hemorrhage is the size of varices.
Although bleeding from esophageal varices ceases spontaneously in up to 40% of patients, and despite improvements in therapy over the last decade, it is associated with a mortality of at least 20% at 6 weeks.

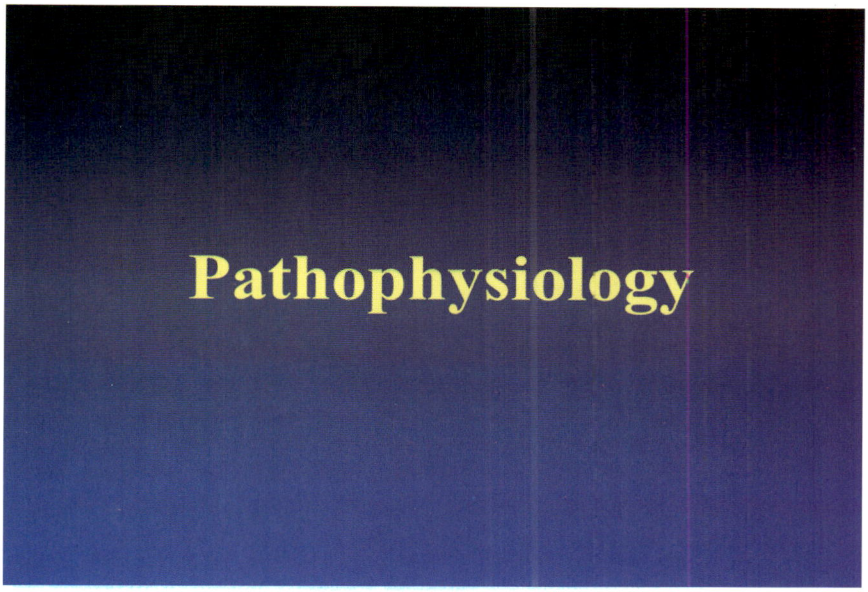

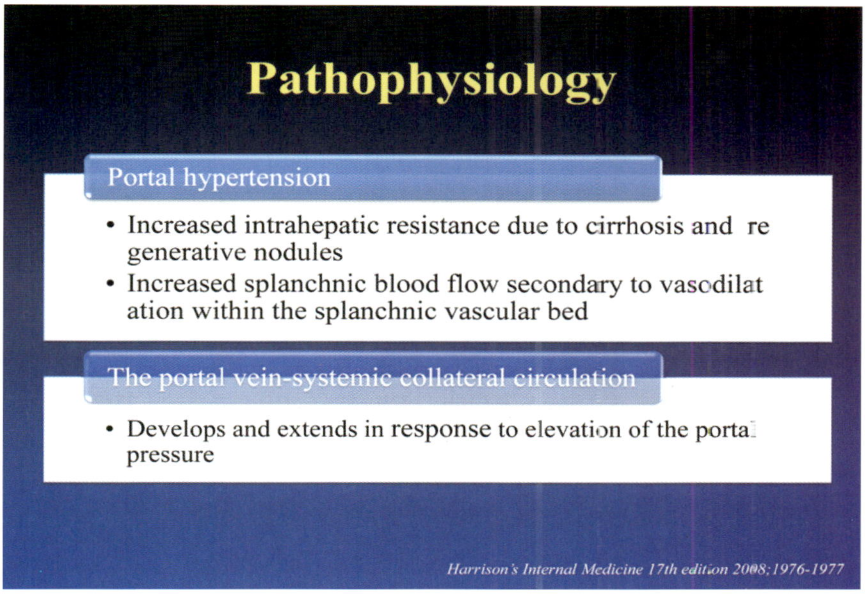

Portal hypertension is caused by two hemodynamic process

1> Increased intrahepatic resistance due to cirrhosis and regenerative nodules

2> Increased splanchnic blood flow secondary to vasodilatation with in the splanchnic vascular bed

The portal vein-systemic collateral circulation develops and extends in response to elevation of the portal pressure.

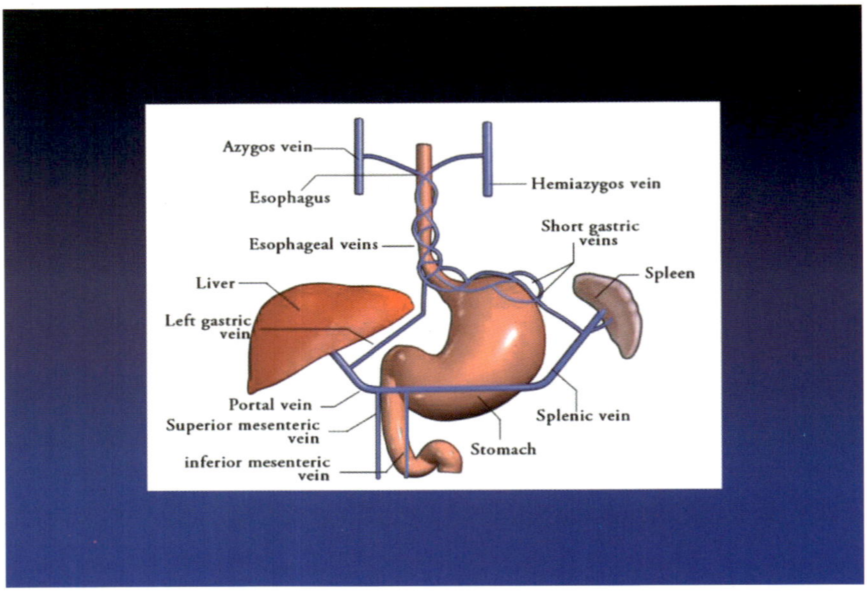

The portal vein is formed by the confluence of the splenic, superior mesenteric, and inferior mesenteric veins.

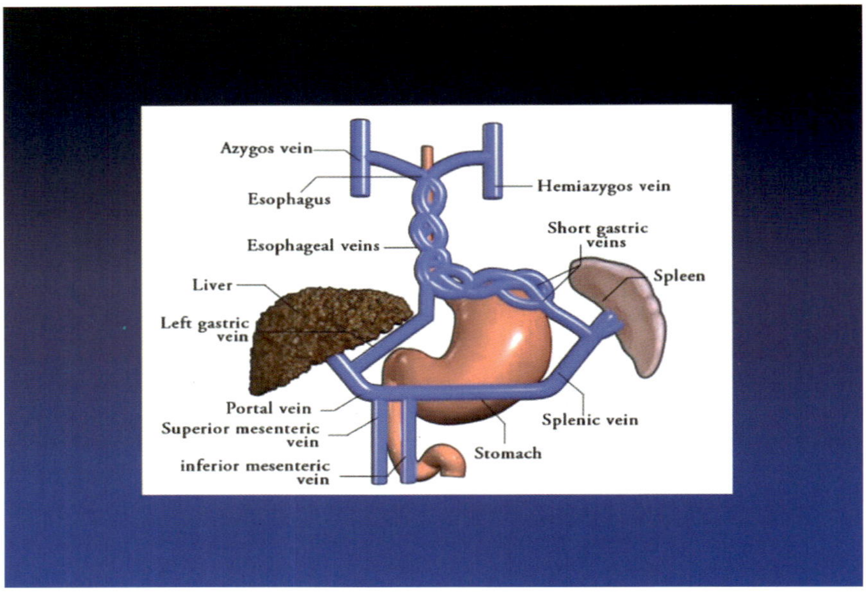

The portal system has numerous collaterals that interconnect with the systemic circulation and develops and expands in response to elevation of the portal pressure.

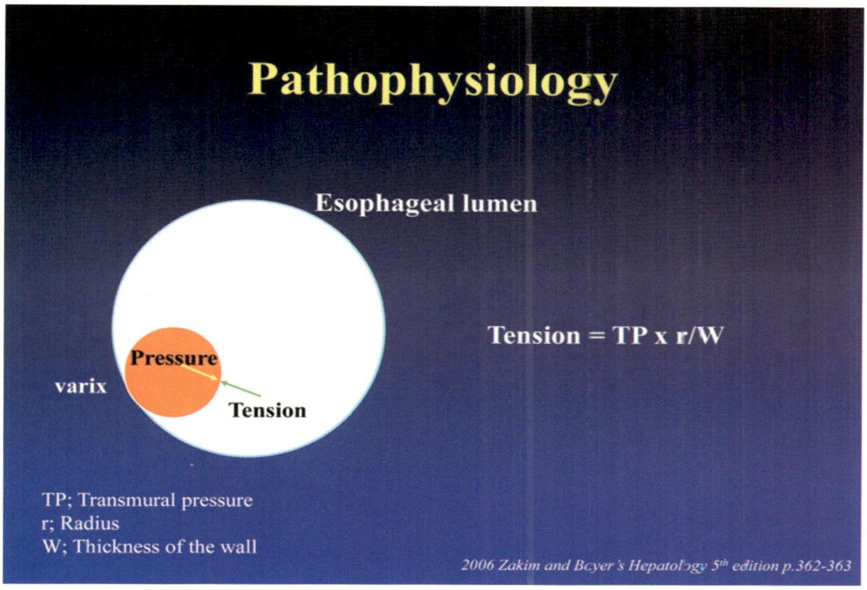

Tension(T) on varix wall is determined by transmural pressure(TP), radius(r) and thickness of the wall(W)

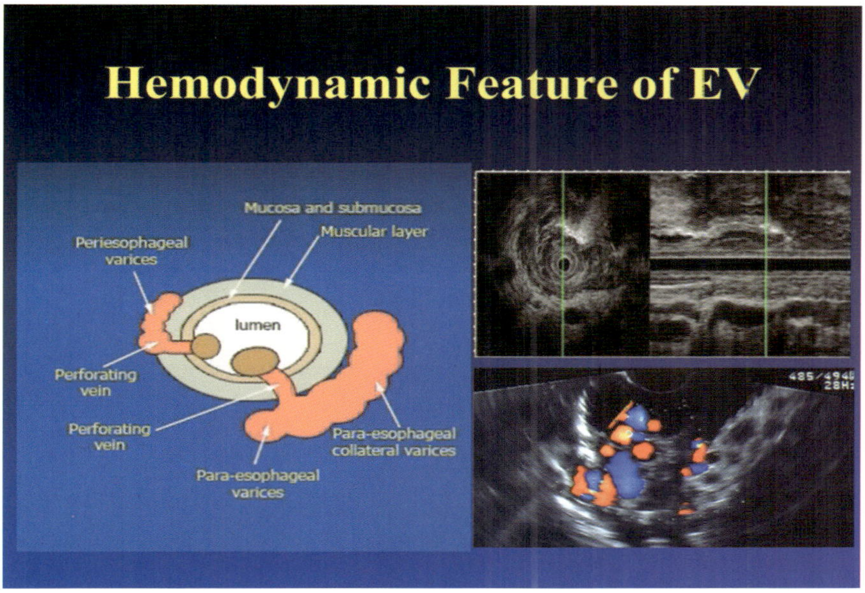

Varices in the esophaeal lumen arise from the para and peri esophageal collateral veins. Perforating veins connect the esophageal varices with peri-esophageal collateral veins and the connecting veins connect the peri-esophageal collateral veins with the para-esophageal collateral veins(para-ECVs) . Treatments results vary with the pattern of para and peri esophageal collateral veins

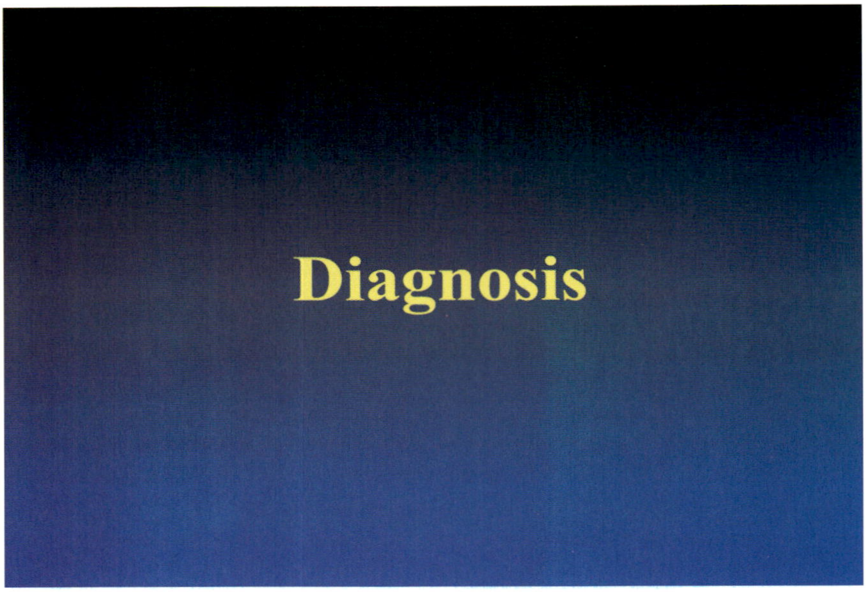

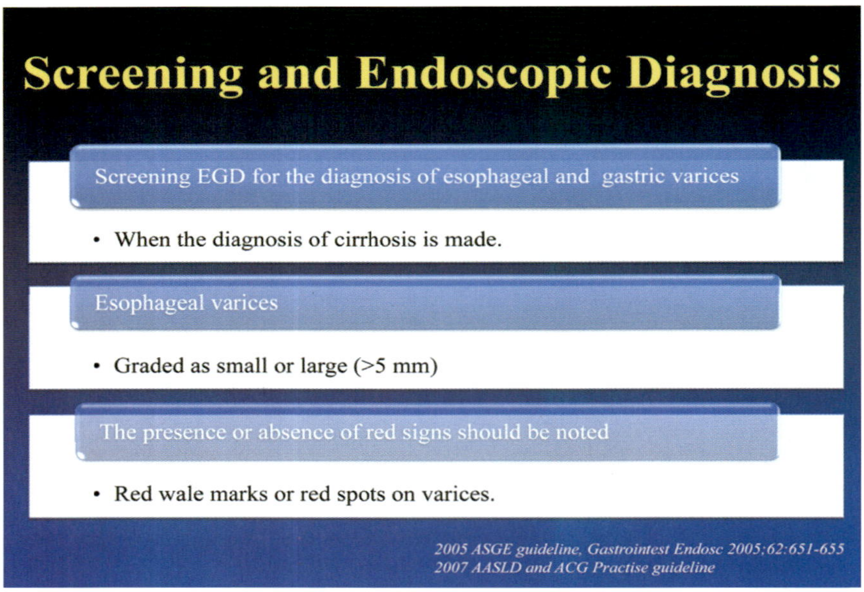

Screening esophagogastroduodenoscopy for the diagnosis of esophageal and gastric varices is recommended when the diagnosis of cirrhosis is made.

On EGD, esophageal varices should be graded as small or large (→5 mm) with the latter classification encompassing medium-sized varices when 3 grades are used (small, medium, large).

The presence or absence of red signs (red wale marks or red spots) on varices should be noted.

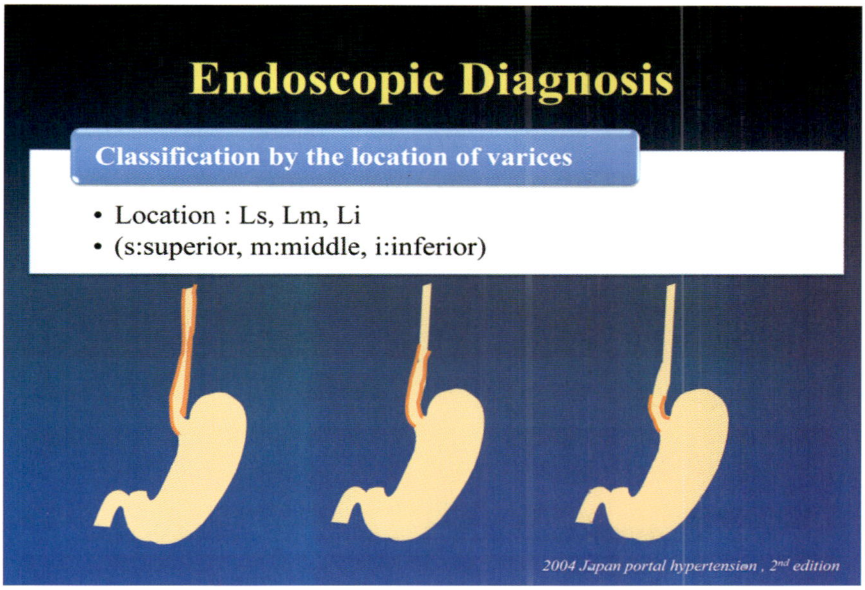

Endoscopy can classify varices by their location in the esophagus.
Ls, m and i respectively represents superior, middle and inferior location of the varix.

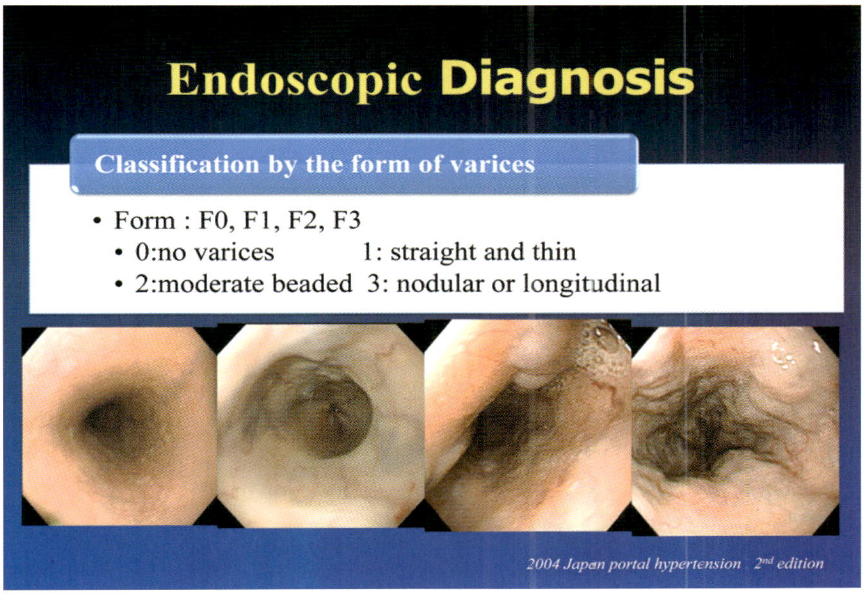

Varices are also classified by the form captured on endoscopy
F0 is no varices
F1 is straight and thin
F2 is moderate beaded
F3 is nodular or longitudinal

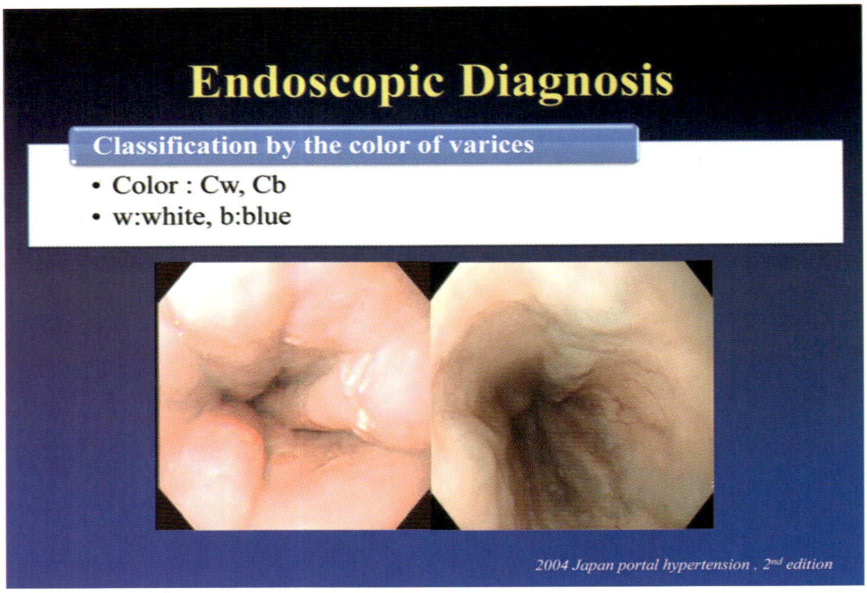

Varices can be classified by color as white or blue

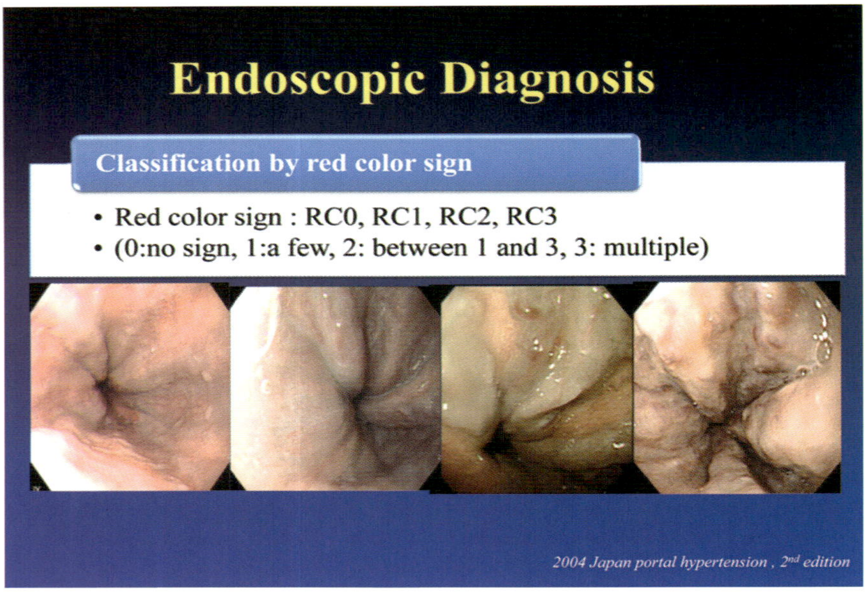

Varices can also be classified by the presence and degree of the 'red color sign'
A step wise increase in severity from RC0 no signs to RC3 multiple signs is used

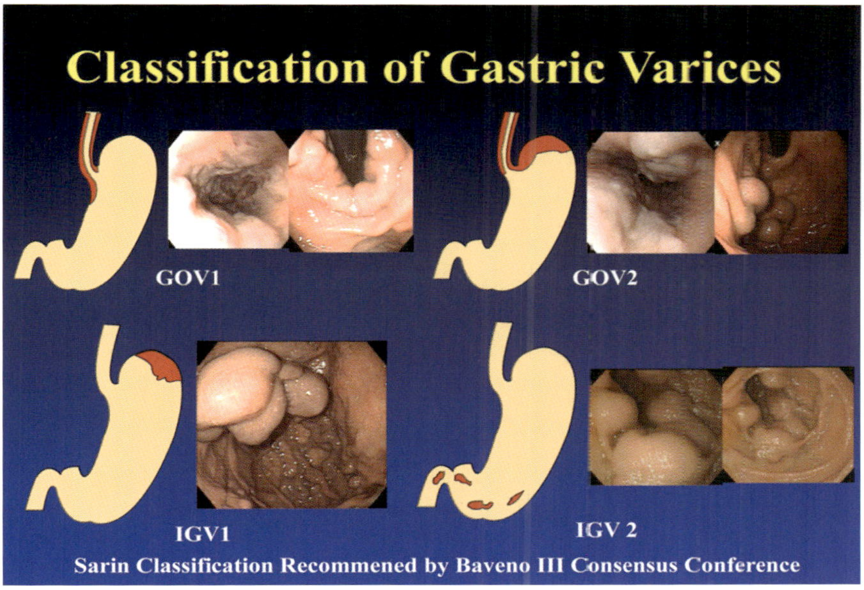

Gastric varices are classified using the Sarin classification
GOV1 are varices that are located in lower esophgus and pericardial area
GOV2 are varices that are located in fundal area
IGV1 are isolated gastric varices located in fundal area
And IGV2 are isolated gastric varices in the antrum, and duodenum

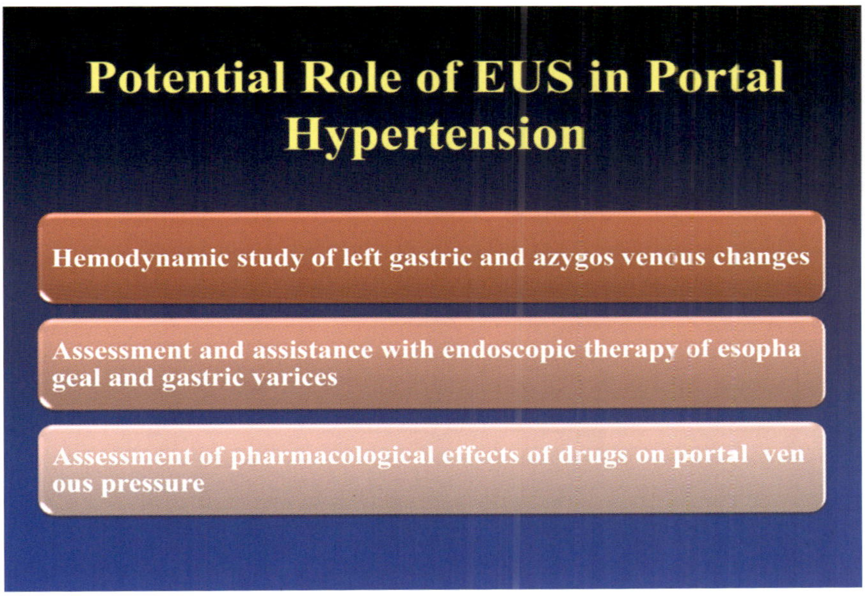

EUS can be used to evaluate portal hypertension.
It can be used to evaluate the hemodynamics of the left gastric and azygos veins, and assess and assist endoscopic therapy of esophageal and gastic varices.
EUS can also assess pharmocological effects of drugs on portal venous pressure.

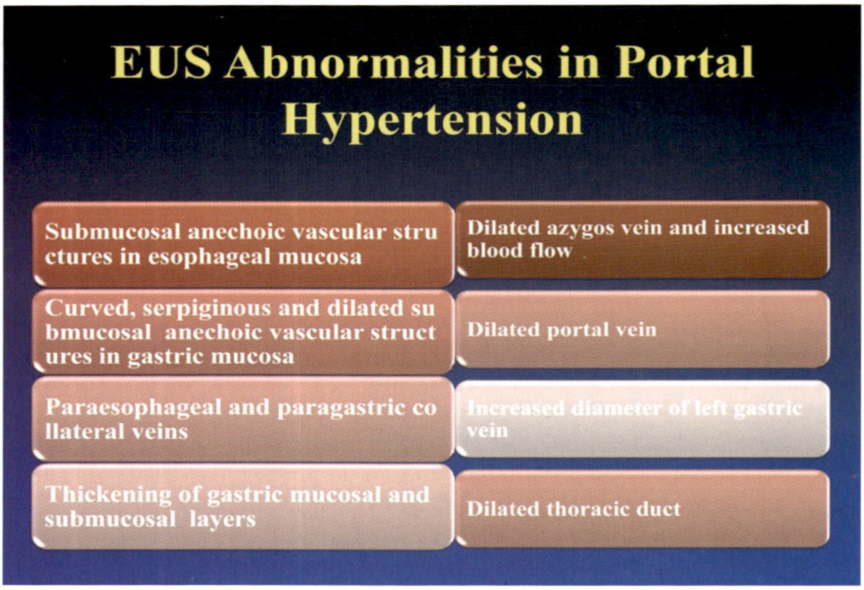

When portal hypertension is present, EUS can detect several abnormal changes.

The abnormal findings that may be detected are, submucosal anechoic vascular structures in esophageal mucosal, dilated azygos vein and increased blood flow, curved, serpiginous and dilated submucosal anechoic vascular structures in gastric mucosa, dilated portal vein, paraesophageal and paragastric collateral veins, increased diameter of left gastric vein, thickening of gastric mucosal and submucosal layers, and a dilated thoracic duct.

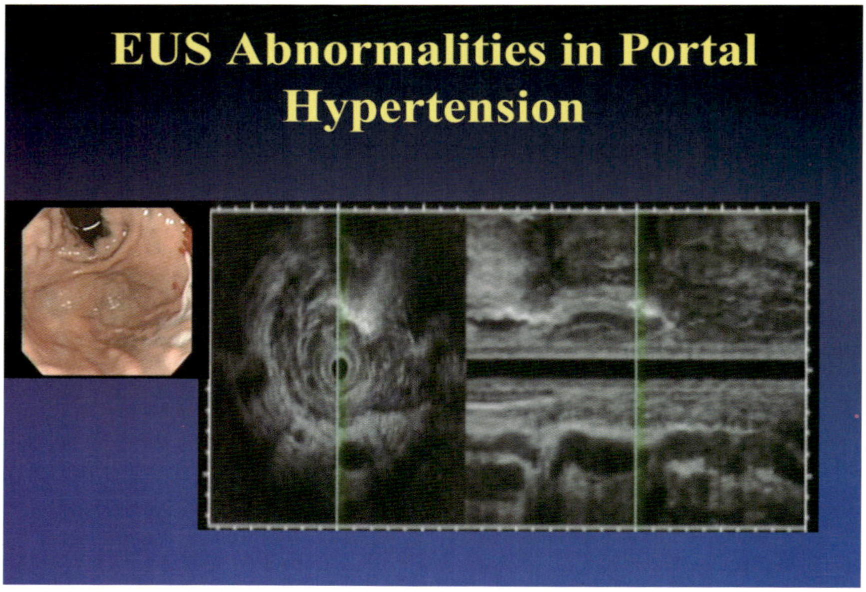

Using EUS, submucosal anechoic vascular structures in the esphageal mucosa are detected.

EUS can visualizes paraesophageal and paragastric collateral veins and assess and diagnosis esophageal and gastric fundal varices. We can also examine the para-esophageal collateral veins(para-ECVs) and the peri-esophageal collateral veins(peri-ECVs).

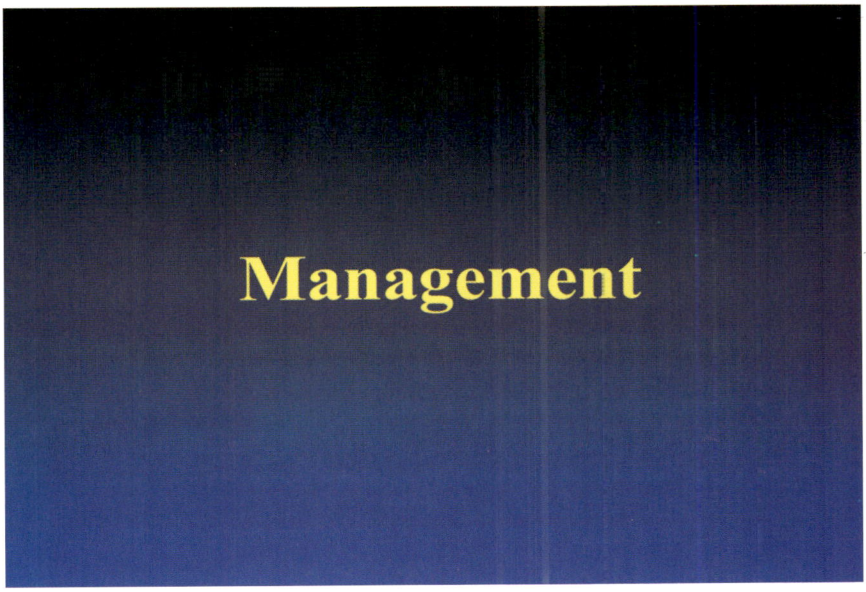
Management

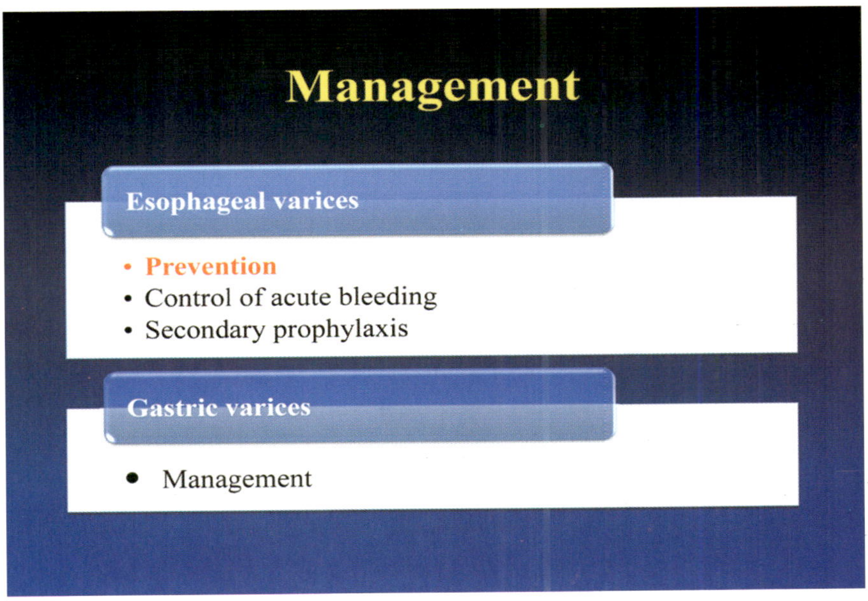
Management
Esophageal varices
• Prevention
• Control of acute bleeding
• Secondary prophylaxis
Gastric varices
• Management

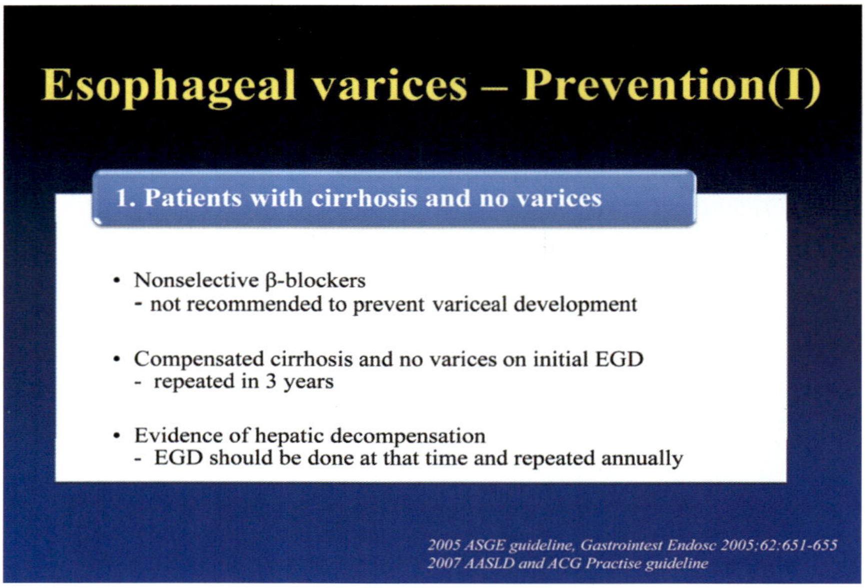

In patients with cirrhosis and no varices, nonselective β-blockers cannot be recommended to prevent variceal development

In patients with compensated cirrhosis and no varices on initial EGD, EGD should be repeated within 3 years.

If there is evidence of hepatic decompensateion, EGD should be done at that time and repeated annually.

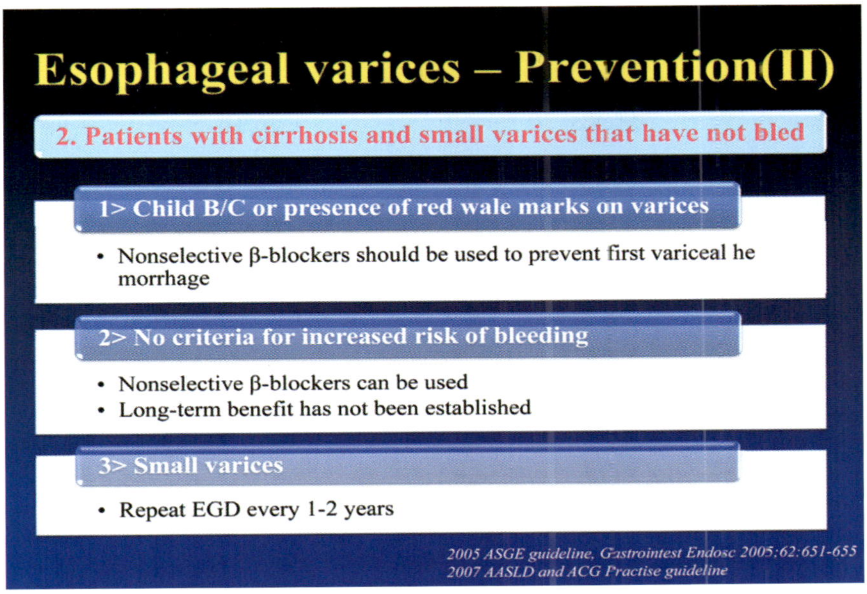

In patients with cirrhosis and small varices that have not bled, if the patient is Child B or C or has red wale marks on the varices, nonselective beta-blockers should be used to prevent first variceal bleeding.

If the patient has no criteria for increased risk of bleeding, non selective beta-blockers can be used. However, the long term benefit has not been established.

In patients with cirrhosis and small varices that have not bled and who are not receiving beta-blockers, EGD should be repeated every 1~2 years.

In patieuts with hepatic decompensation , EGD should be done at that time and repeated annually.

In patients with small varices who receive beta-blockers, a follow up EGD is not necessary.

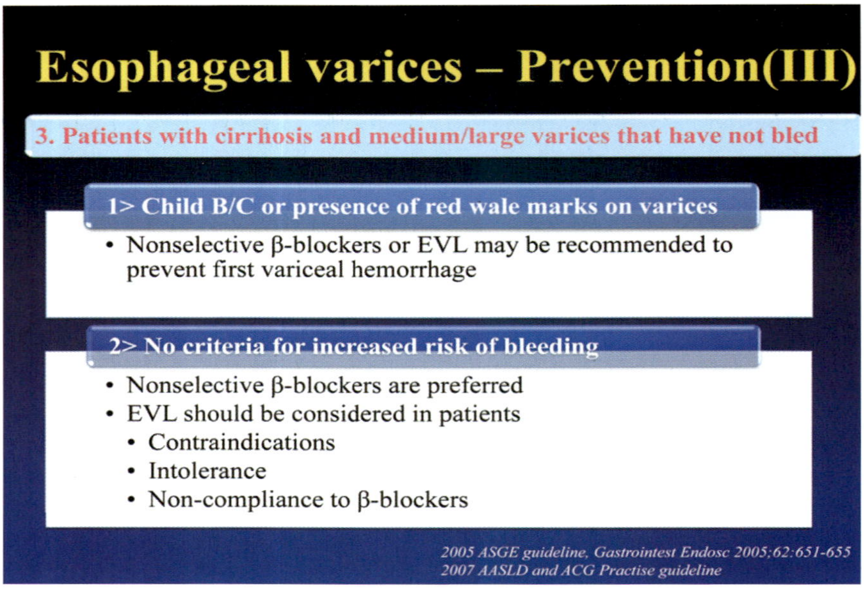

In patients with cirrhosis and medium or large varices that have not bled, if the patient is Child B or C or has red wale marks on the varices, nonselective beta-blockers or EVL may be recommended to prevent first variceal hemorrhage. If the patients have no criteria for increased risk of bleeding, nonselective beta blockers are preferred. However EVL should be considered if the patient has contraindications, or is intolerant or non-compliant to beta-blockers.

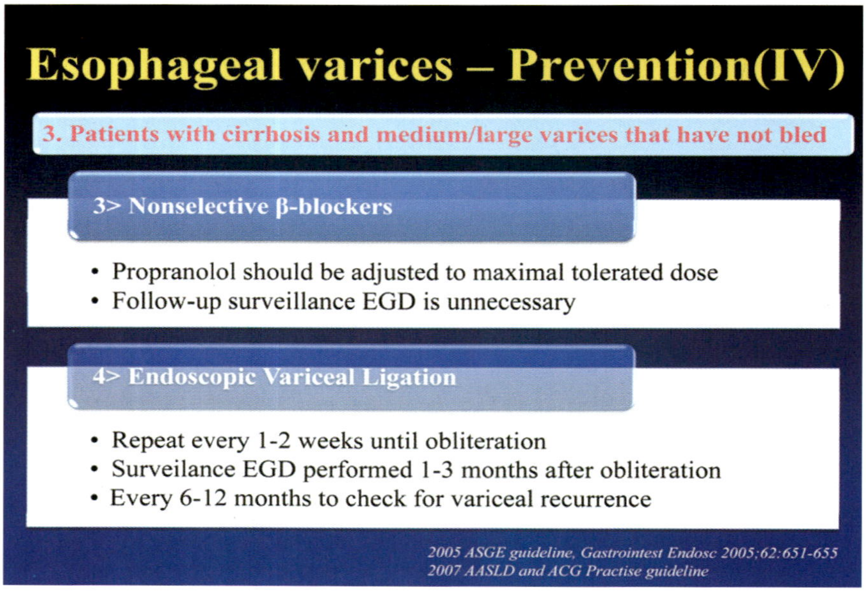

If the patients is placed on a nonselective β-blockers, propranolol should be adjusted to maximal tolerance dose and follow-up surveillance EGD is unnecessary. If the patient is treated with EVL, EVL should repeated every 1-2 weeks until obliteration is achieved. Surveilance EGD should be performed 1-3 months after obliteration and then every 6-12 months to check for variceal recurrence.

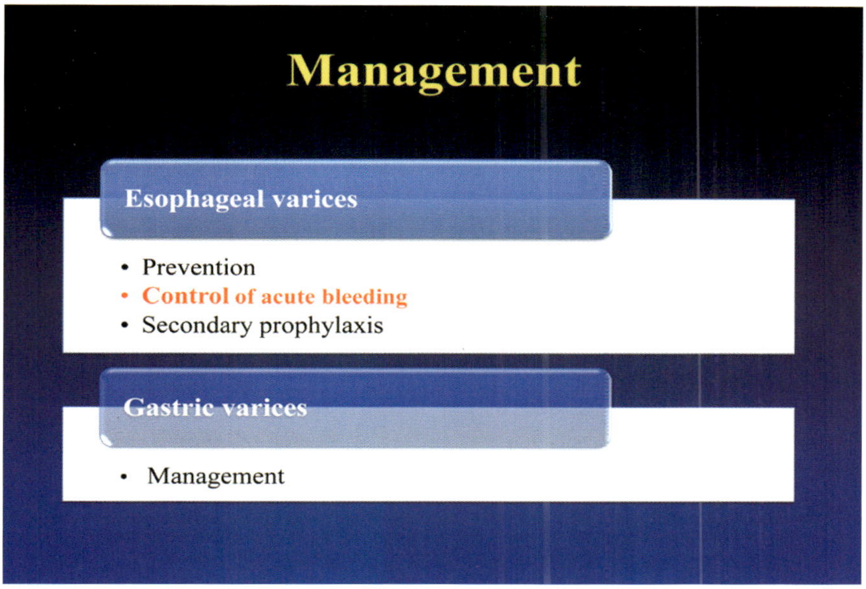

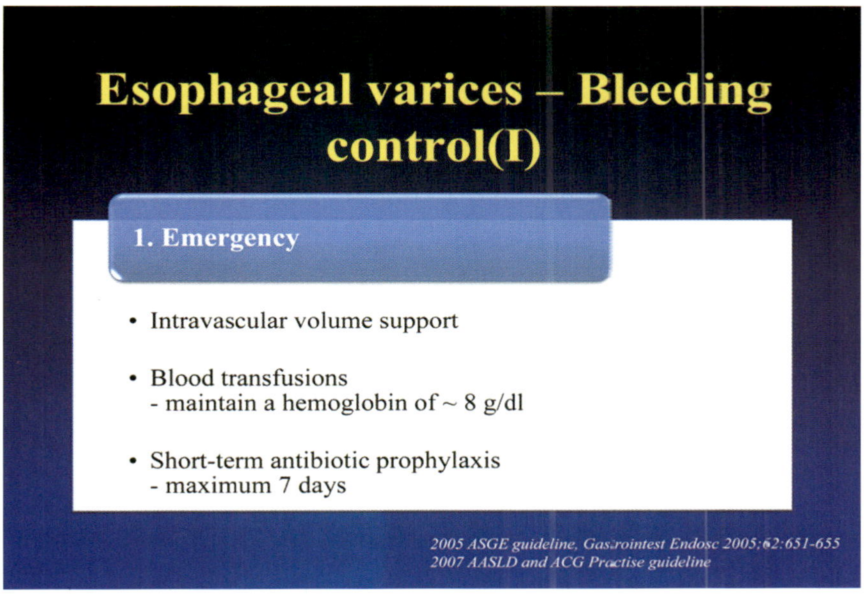

Acute GI hemorrhage in a patient with cirrhosis is an emergency that requires prompt attention with intravascular volume support and blood transfusions, being careful to maintain a hemoglobin of ~ 8 g/dL. Short-term(maximum 7 days) antibiotic prophylaxis should be initiated.

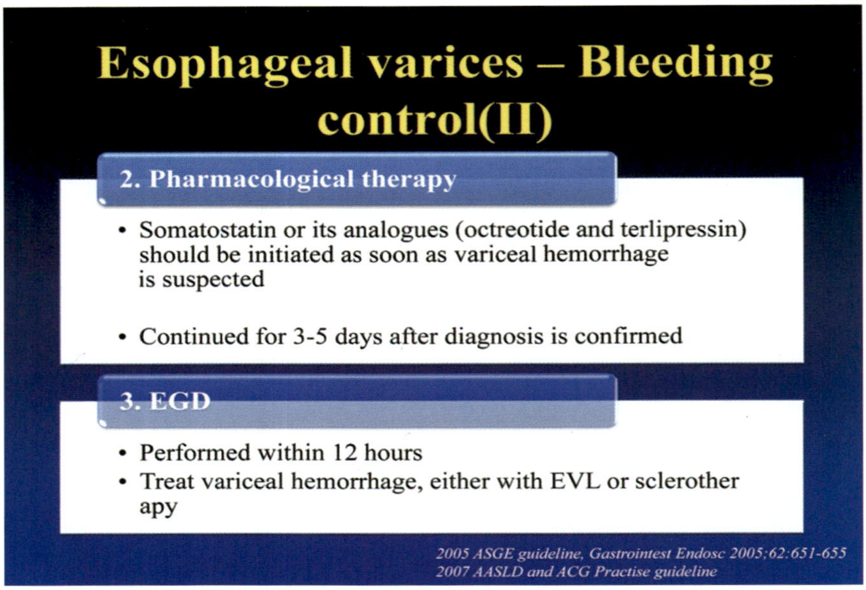

Pharmacological therapy (somatostatin or its analogues octreotide and terlipressin) should be initiated as soon as variceal hemorrhage is suspected and continued for 3-5 days after diagnosis is confirmed. EGD, performed within 12 hours, should be used to make the diagnosis and to treat variceal hemorrhage, either with EVL or sclerotherapy.

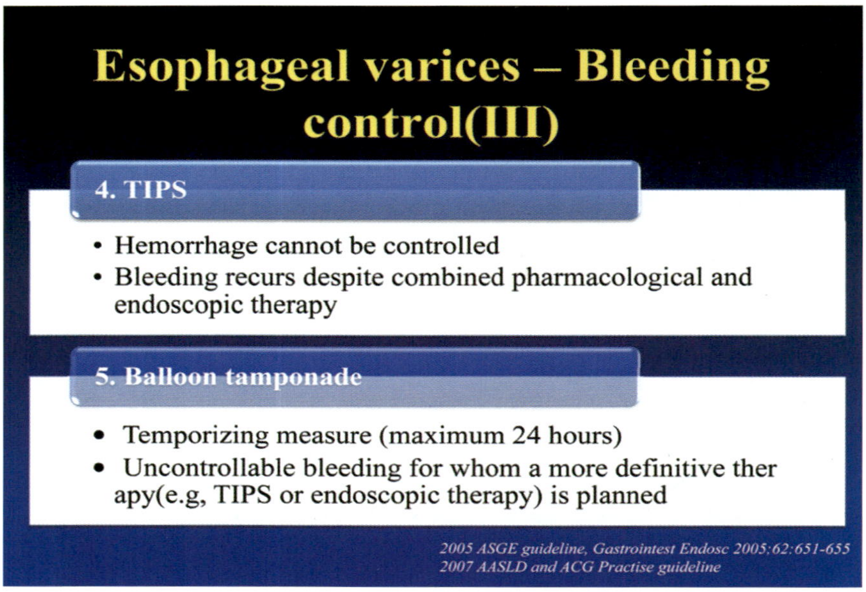

TIPS is indicated in patients in whom hemorrhage from esophageal varices cannot be controlled or in whom bleeding recurs despite combined pharmacological and endoscopic therapy. Balloon tamponade should be used as a temporizing measure(maximum 24 hours) in patients with uncontrollable bleeding for whom a more definitive therapy (e.g, TIPS or endoscopic therapy) is planned.

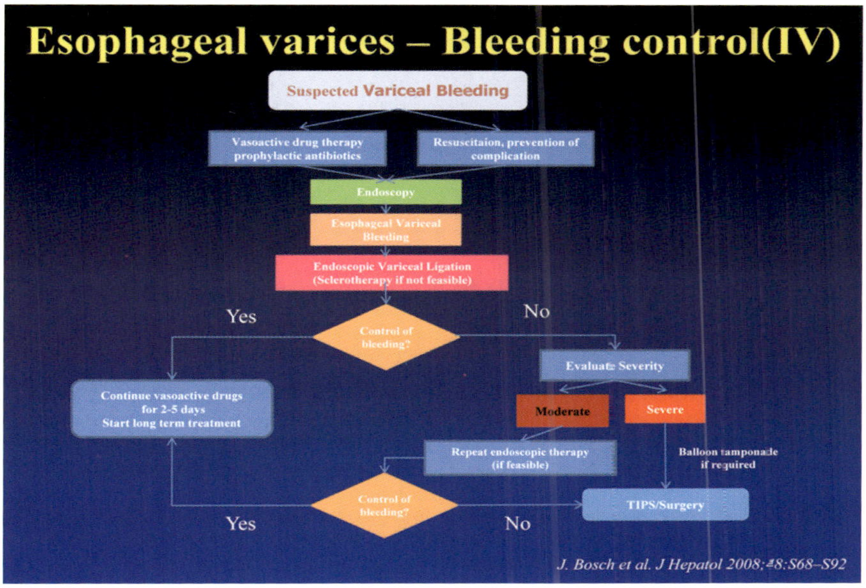

This is an algorithm for treatment of esophageal varices. When variceal bleeding is suspected, the current recommendation is to start early vasoactive drug therapy.

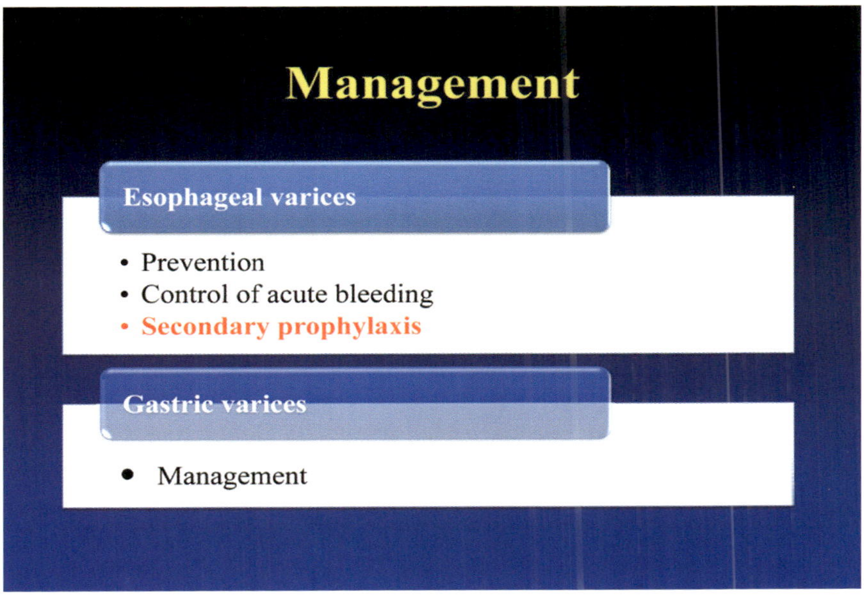

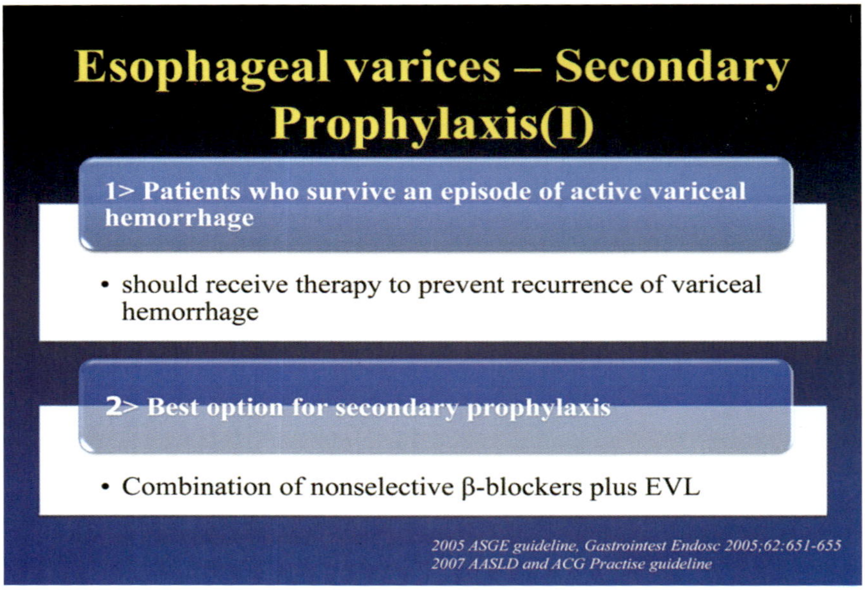

Patients with cirrhosis who survive an episode of active variceal hemorrhage should receive therapy to prevent recurrence of variceal hemorrhage (secondary prophylaxis). The best option for secondary prophylaxis of variceal hemorrhage is the combination of nonselective β-blockers plus EVL.

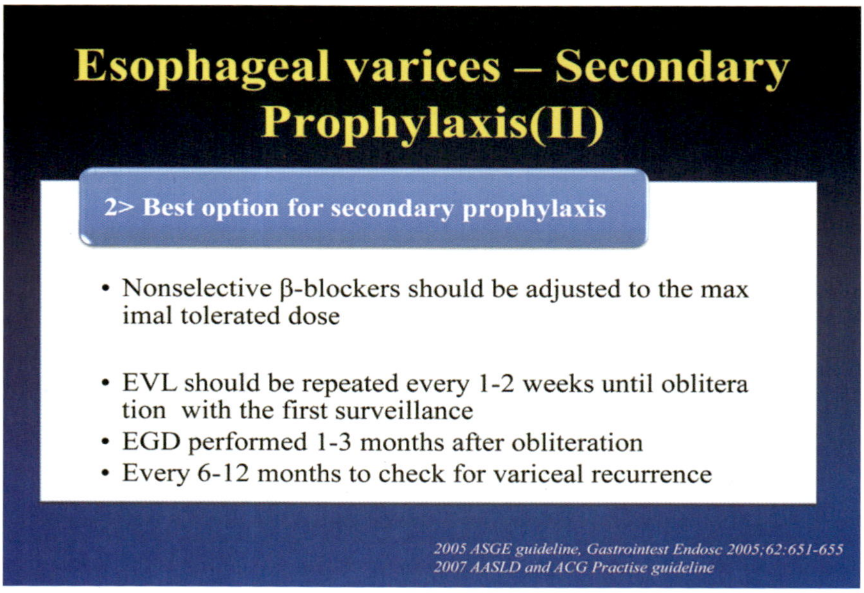

For optimal secondary prophylaxis nonselective β-blockers should be adjusted to the maximal tolerated dose. EVL should be repeated every 1-2 weeks until obliteration. The first surveillance EGD should be performed 1-3 months after obliteration and then every 6-12 months to check for variceal recurrence.

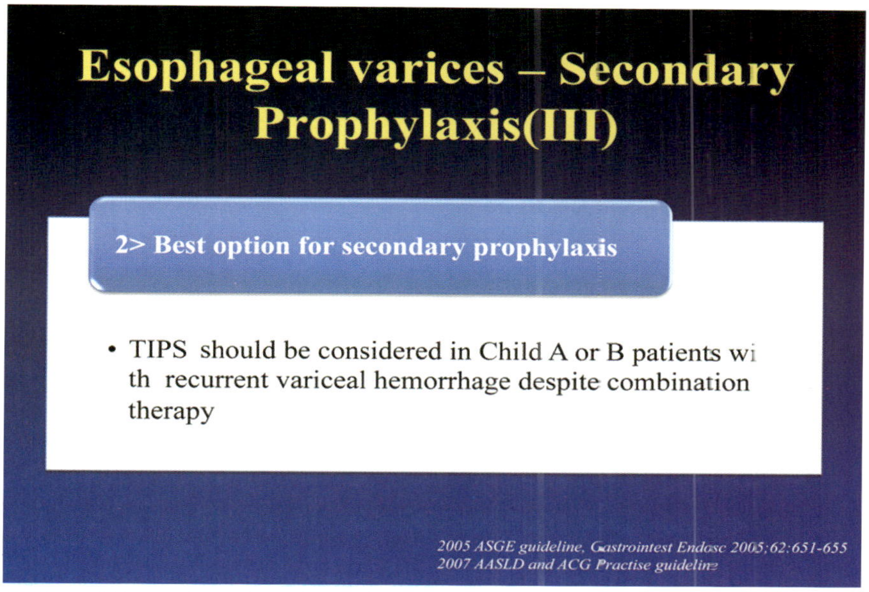

TIPS should be considered in patients who are Child A or B who experience recurrent variceal hemorrhage despite combination pharmacological and endoscopic therapy.

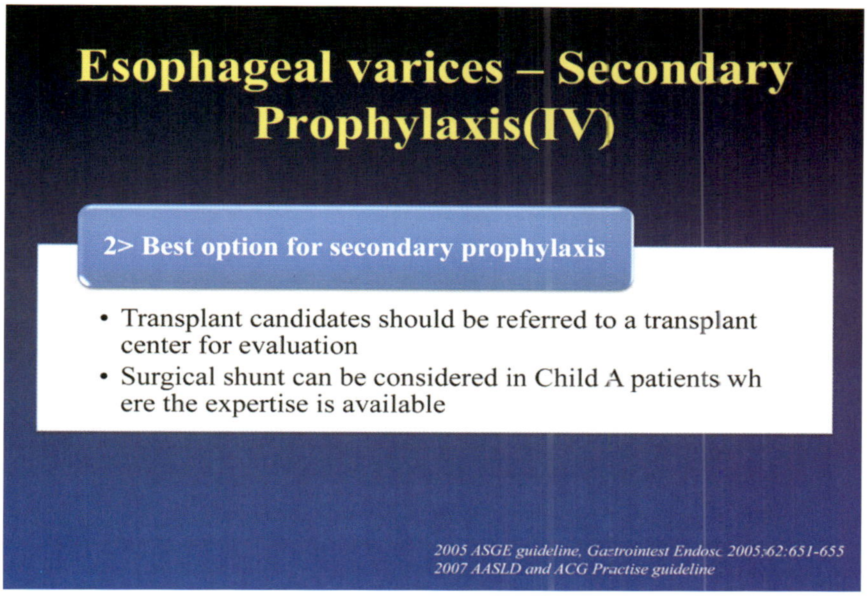

Patients who are otherwise transplant candidates should be referred to a transplant center for evaluation. A surgical shunt can be considered in Child A patients in centers where the expertise is available.

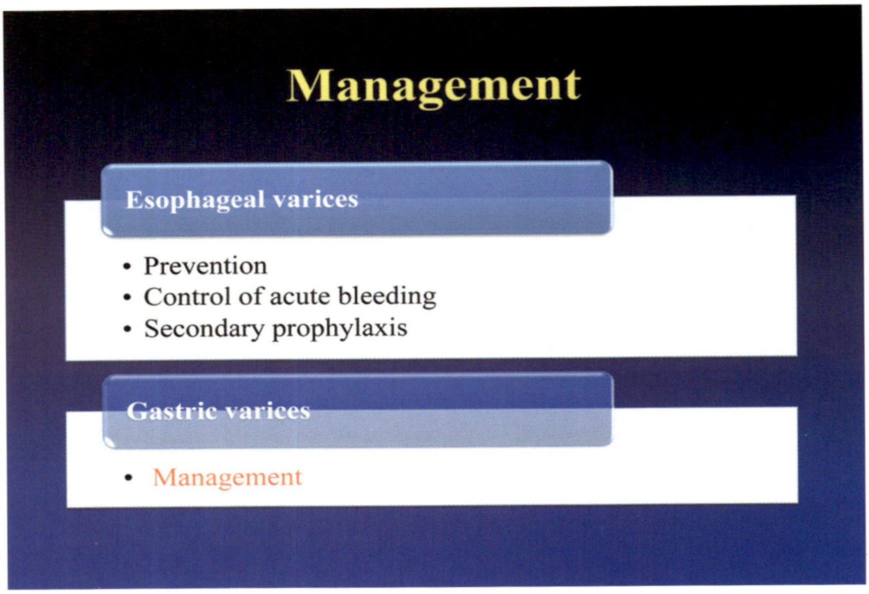

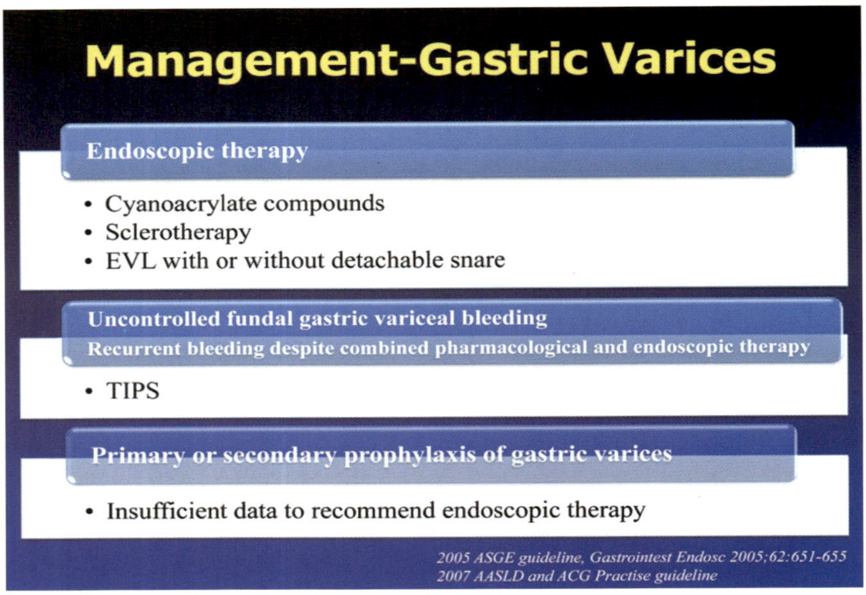

For management of patients with gastic varix bleeding, endoscopic therapy using cyanoacrylate compounds, sclerotherapy, or EVL with or without detachable snare should be tried. In patients with hemorrhage from fundal varices that cannot be controlled or in whom bleeding recurs despite combined pharmacological and endoscopic therapy, TIPS should be considered. Up to now there is insufficient data to recommend endoscopic therapy for primary or secondary prophylaxis of gastric varices.

Endoscopic treatment

Management

Esophageal varices

- MBL(Multi-Band Ligation) - Acute Variceal Bleeding
- MBL - Primary Prophylaxis
- Injection Sclerotherapy(5% etanolamine)
- Micellaneous
  - MBL plus APC(Argon Plasma Coagulation)
  - Mini-Detachable Snare Ligation
  - Stent

Gastric Varices

- Injection Sclerotherapy(N-butyl-2-cyanoacrylate)
- Detachable Snare, Clipping
- BRTO
- TIPS

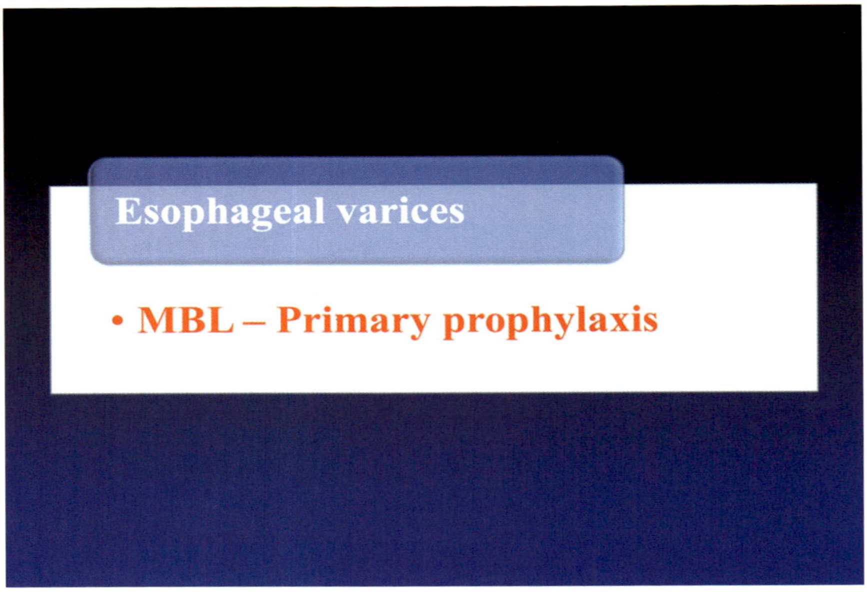

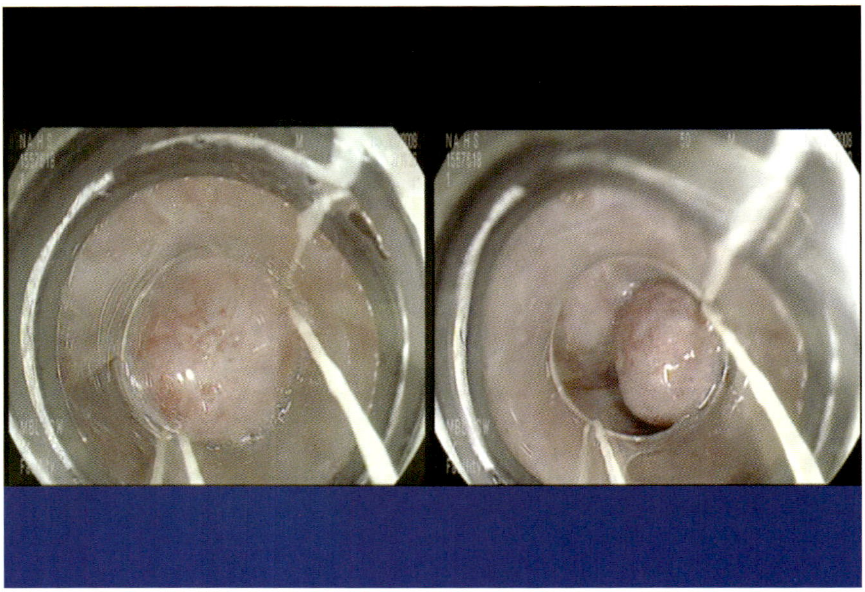

This is a cirrhotic patient with large esophageal varices. This patient had no prior history of variceal bleeding. However, red wale marks were apparent on the varices and we performed multi-band ligation to prevent future hemorrhage. As the endoscope approaches the varix negative pressure is applied sucking the varix and the surrounding mucosa into the multi-band equipped cap. A band is then deployed ligating the varix.

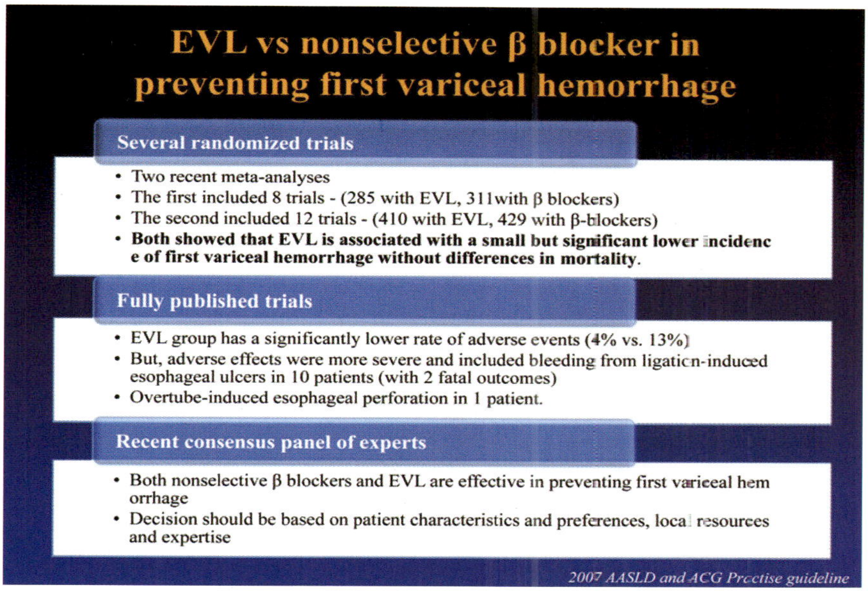

There is much debate on the optimal choice for preventing first variceal hemorrhage. Two recent meta-analysis, one including 8 trials and the other 12 trials, showed that EVL is associated with a small but significant lower incidence of first variceal bleeding without differences in mortality. Other report described EVL to have a significantly lower rate of adverse effects. However these adverse effects were more severe and included bleeding from ligation induced esophageal ulcers with 2 fatal outcomes.

Recent consensus is both nonselective betablockers and EVL are effective in preventing first variceal hemorrhage and decision should be based on patietn characteristics and preferences, local resources and expertise.

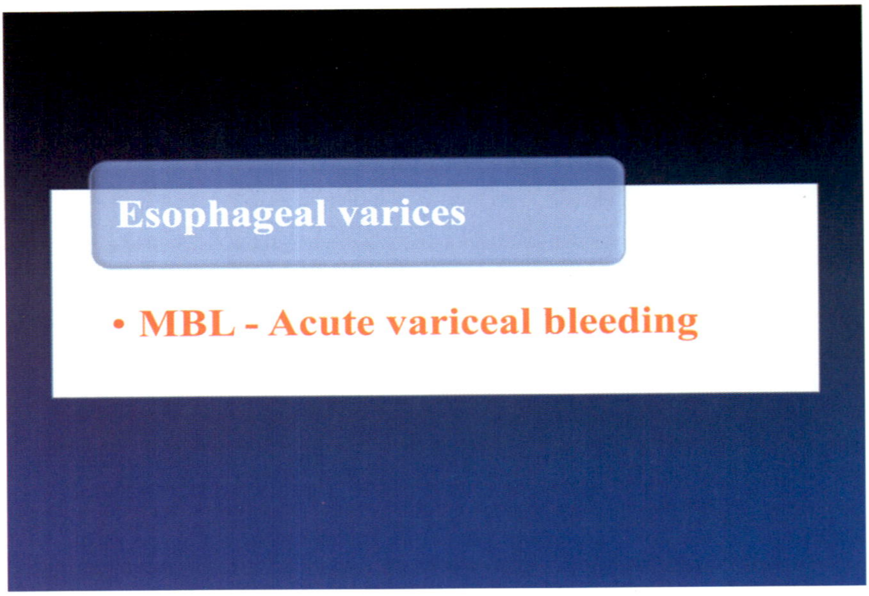

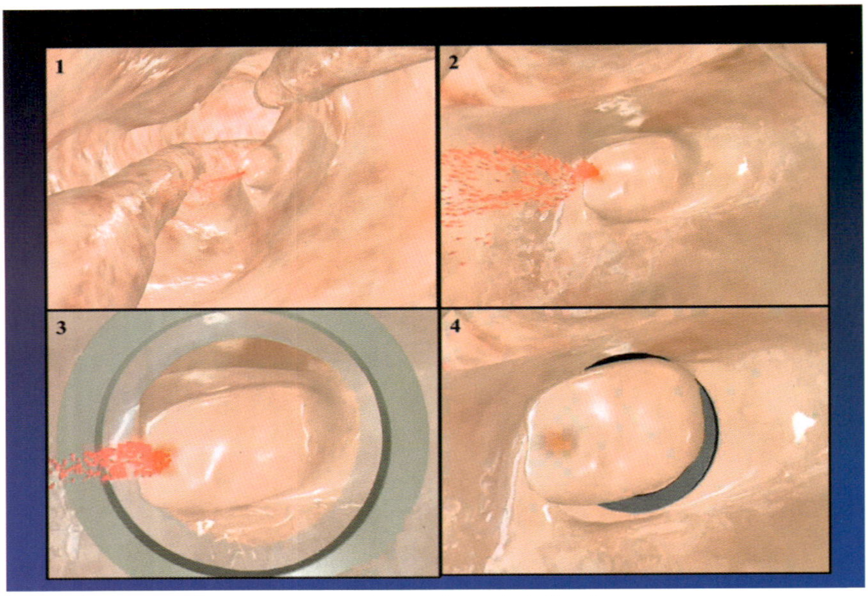

This simulation demonstrates multiband ligation of an actively bleeding varix.

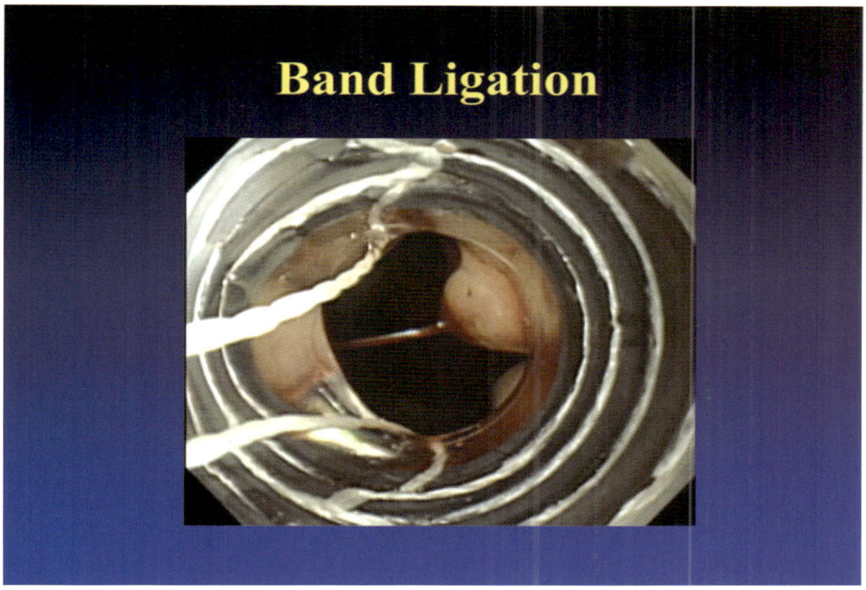

This is a cirrhotic patient with active variceal bleeding. As the endoscope is advanced, pumping variceal bleeding is seen through a ruptured varix.

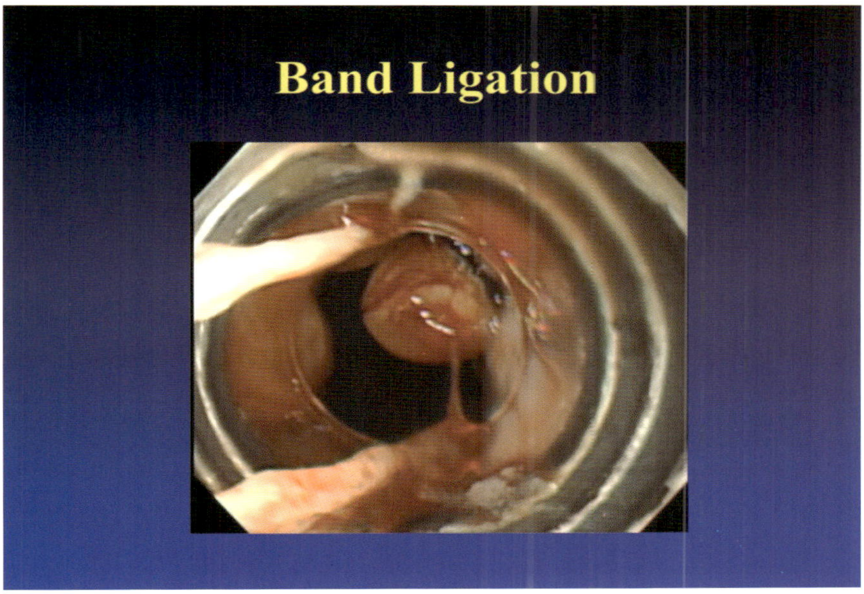

Ligation is successful and the bleeding completely stops.

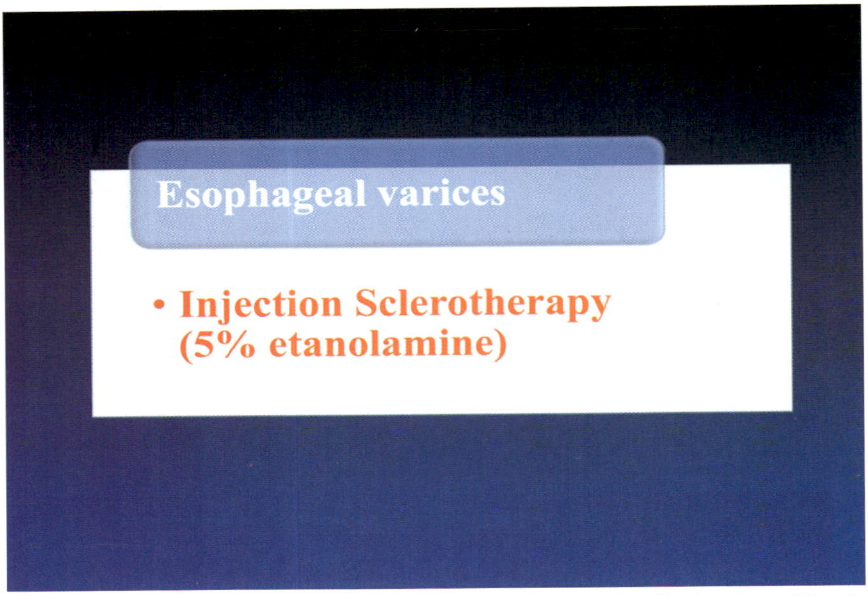

This video clip shows endoscopic injection sclerotherapy using 5% ethanolamine oleate. When it comes to varix, this made thrombi with enthothelial cell destruction.

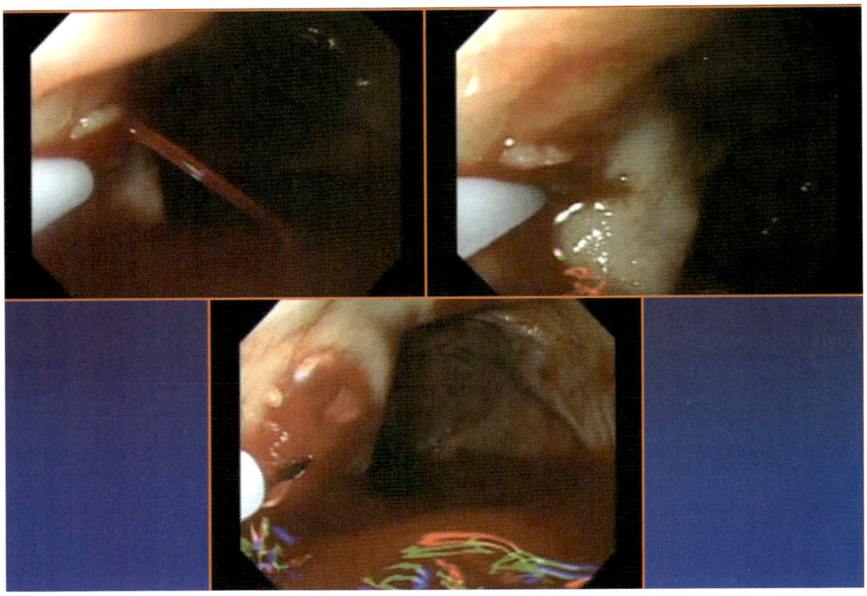

These figures show endoscopic injection sclerotherapy using 5% ethanolamine oleate. When the ethanolamine is injected into the varix, endothelial cells are damaged causing thrombi to form within the varix.

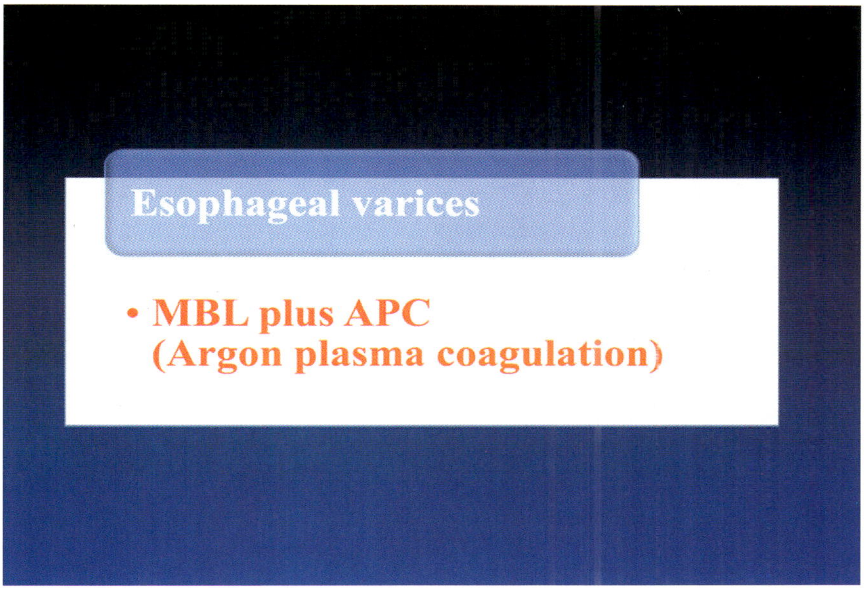

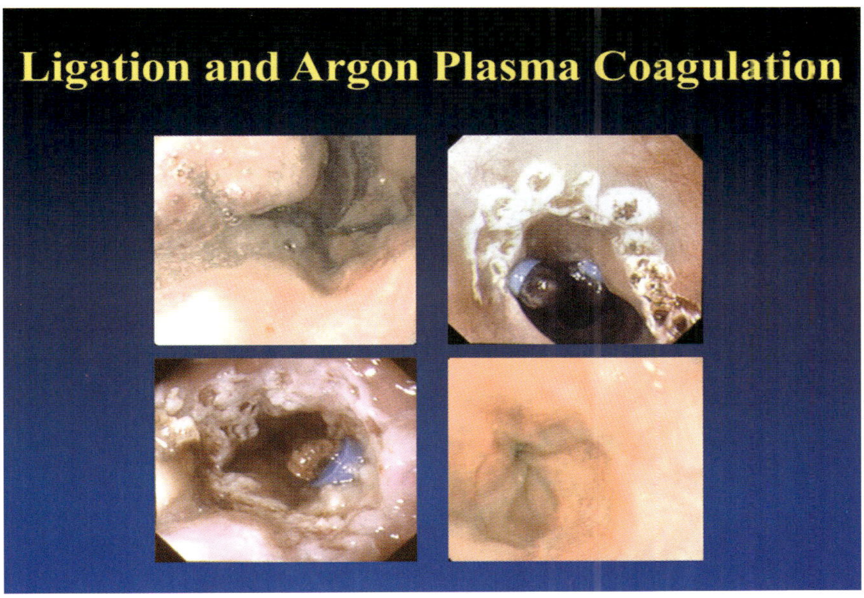

This series of figures show esophageal ligation and argon plasma coagulation. Esophageal varices are ligated with blue bands and multiple sessions of APC (argon plasma coagulations) is performed around the surrounding bands and mucosa.

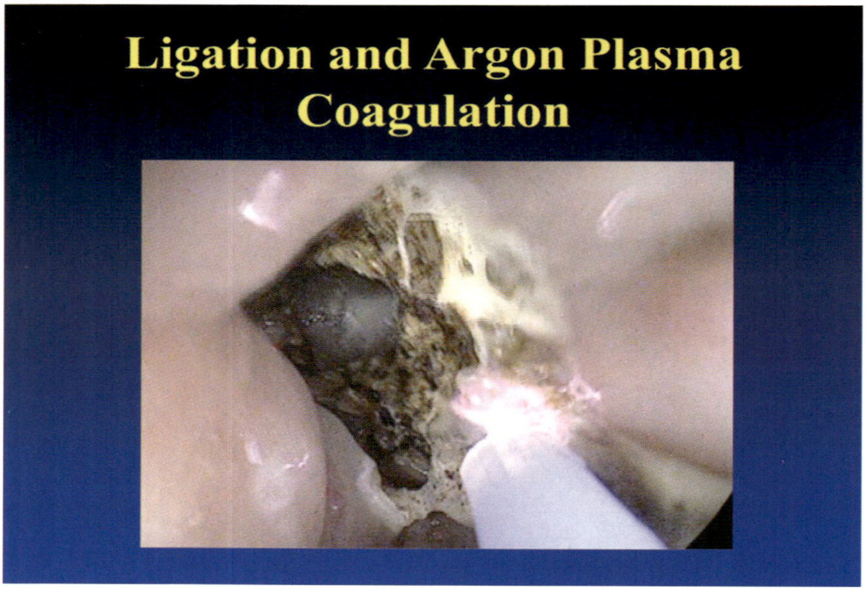

These figures show esophageal ligation and argon plasma coagulation. After MBL ligation of the esophageal varices and APC (argon plasma coagulations) is performed around the bands and remnant varices. Some authors belive that APC following MBL may reduce the rate of rebleeding.

Results

	Ligation plus APC (30 patients) n/%	Ligation alone (30 patients) n/%	P
Complications			
Pyrexia(38℃)	19/63.3	10/33.3	<0.05
Retrosternal pain	2/6.7	2/6.7	Ns
Dysphagia	9/30.0	8/26.7	Ns
Stricture	1/3.3	0/0.0	Ns
Recurrent bleeding	1/3.3	2/6.7	Ns

Nakamura S, et al. Endoscopy 2001; 33 (3): 210–215

One study compared the recurrent bleeding rate and complications of combined ligation and APC with therapy with ligation alone. The rate of rebleeding was not significantly different between the two groups. With regard to post-procedure complications, the incidence of pyrexia was significantly higher in the combined group (p 〈0.05), but there was no difference in the incidence of others complications such as retrosternal pain, dysphagia and strictures.

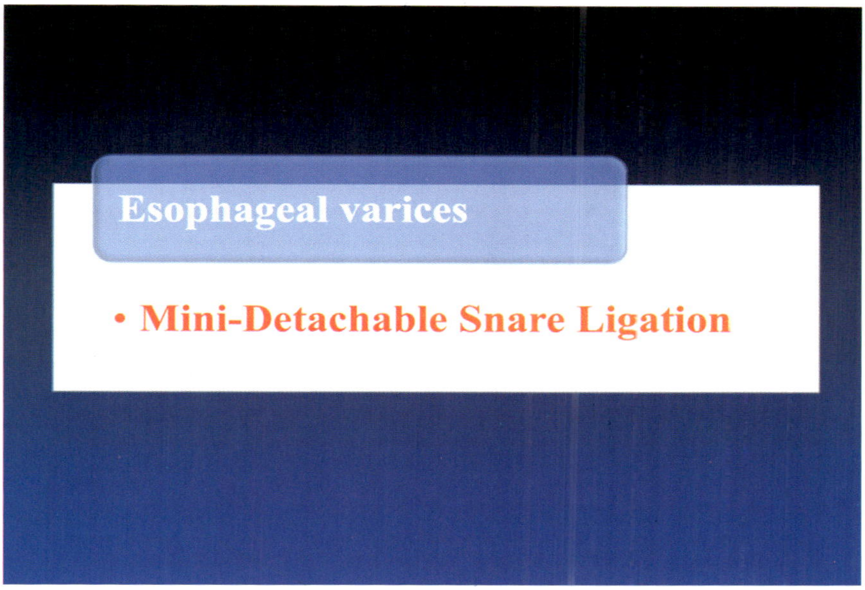

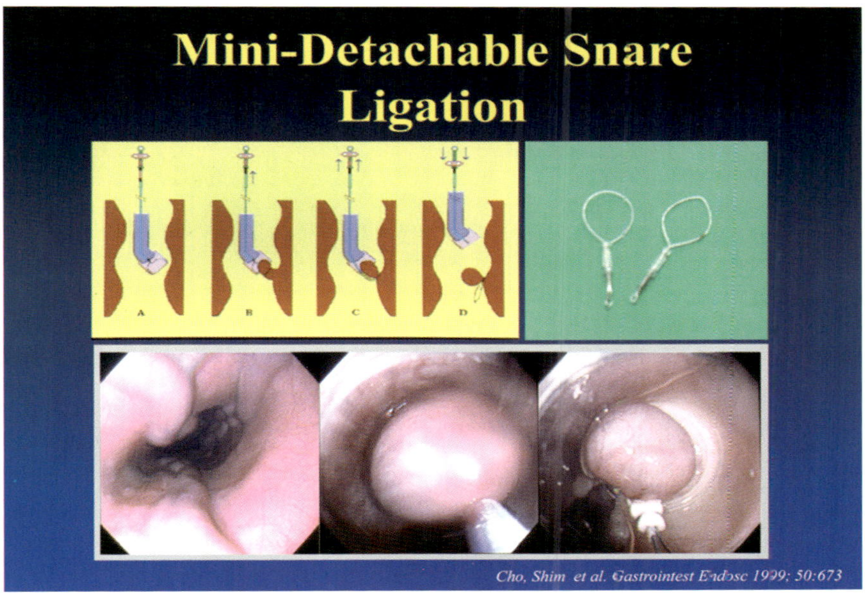

Mini-detachable snare varicel ligation utilized a mini-detachable snare atached to a cap on the tip of the endoscope. The snare can effectively entrap relatively large esophageal varices effectively by covering the varix with the cap and snaring the neck of varix with a mini-detachable snare.

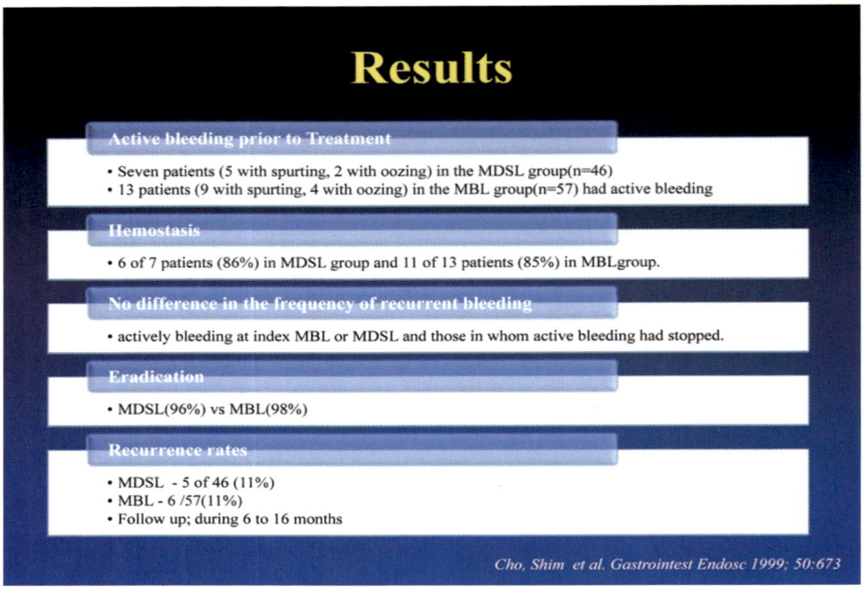

Data on the minidetachable snare for esophageal varices is limited. When compared with MBL, one report showed no significant difference in the rate of hemostasis, frequency of recurrent bleeding and recurrence rate.

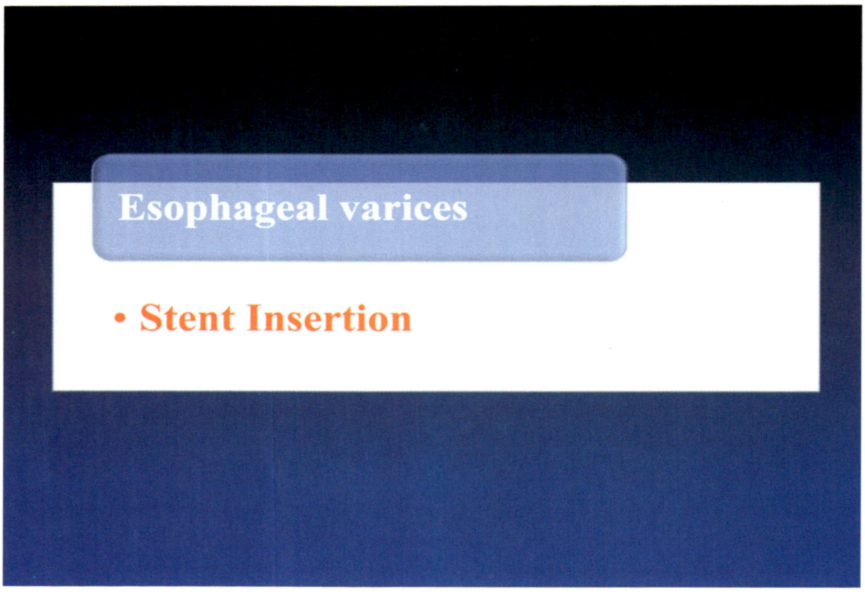

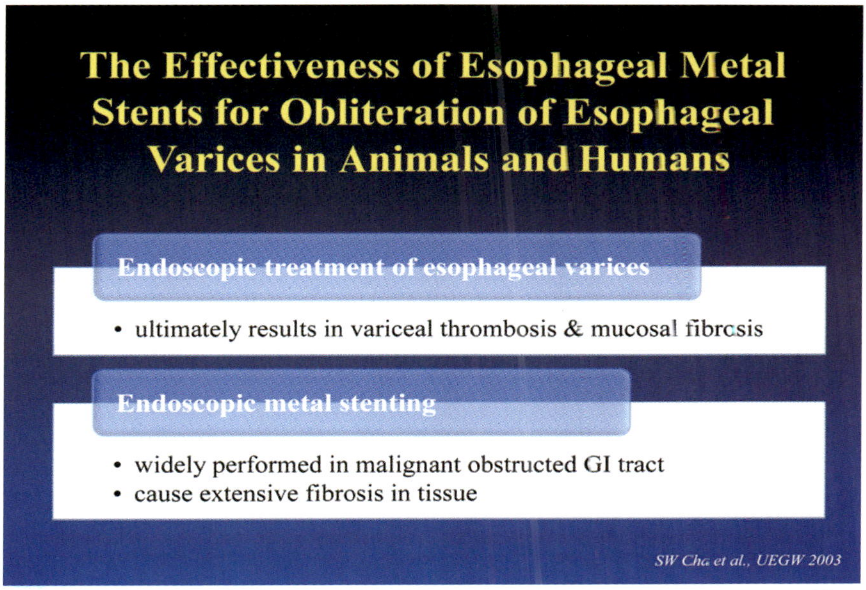

Endoscopic metal stenting is widely performed in malignant obstructions of the GI tract. After deployment these stents usually induce an extensive fibrous tissue reaction. The effect of metal stenting in esophageal varices ultimately results in variceal thrombosis and mucosal fibrosis.

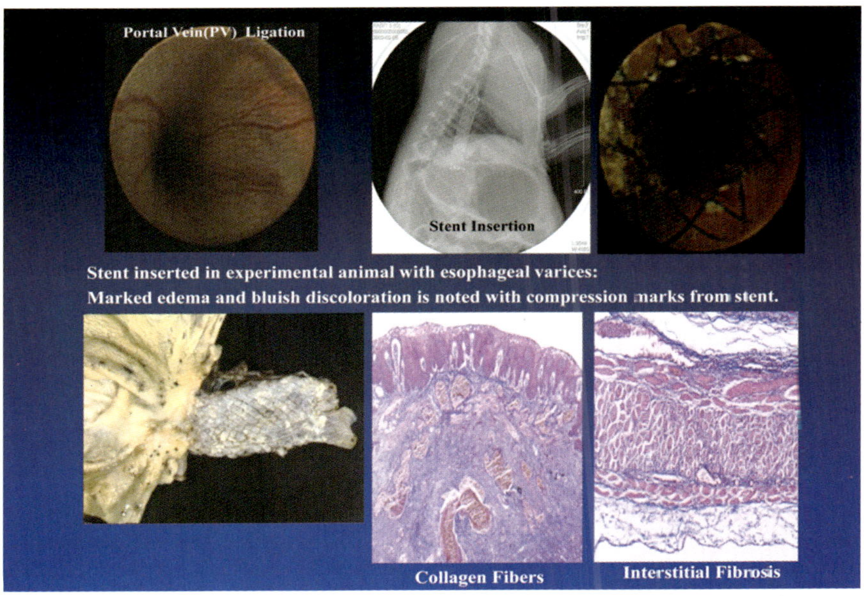

This series of figures show the endoscopic, post autopsy and pathologic findings of stenting in an experimental animal with esophageal varices. Marked edema and bluish discoloration is noted with a compression mark by the stent on post autopsy.
Pathological findings show dense collagen fibers and interstitial fibrosis of the underlying mucosa.

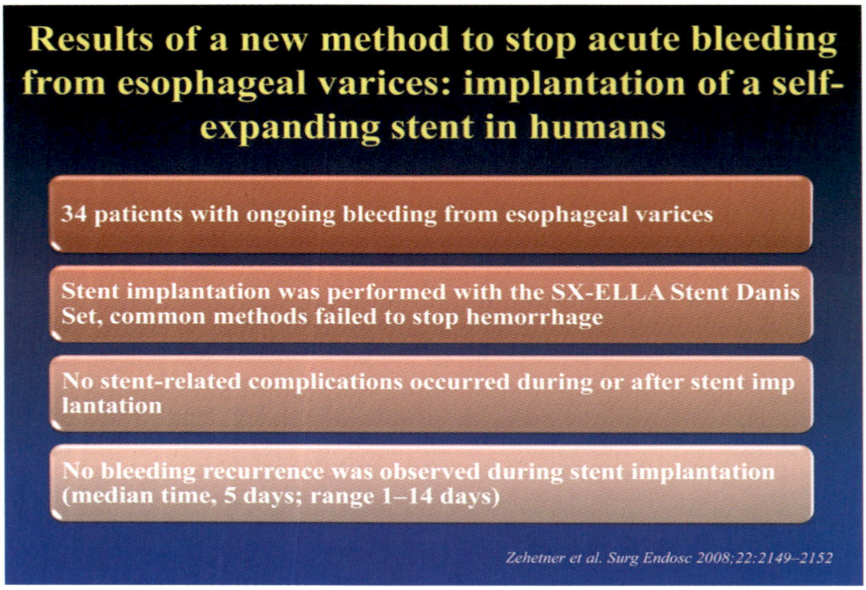

A recent study reported the outcome of self expanding metal stents for patients with onging bleeding form esophageal bleeding.

Stent implantation was perfomed in 34 paients with the SX-ELLA stent danis set. The mean duration of stents implantation was 5 days. And no rebleeding or stent related complciations were observed during stent implantation.

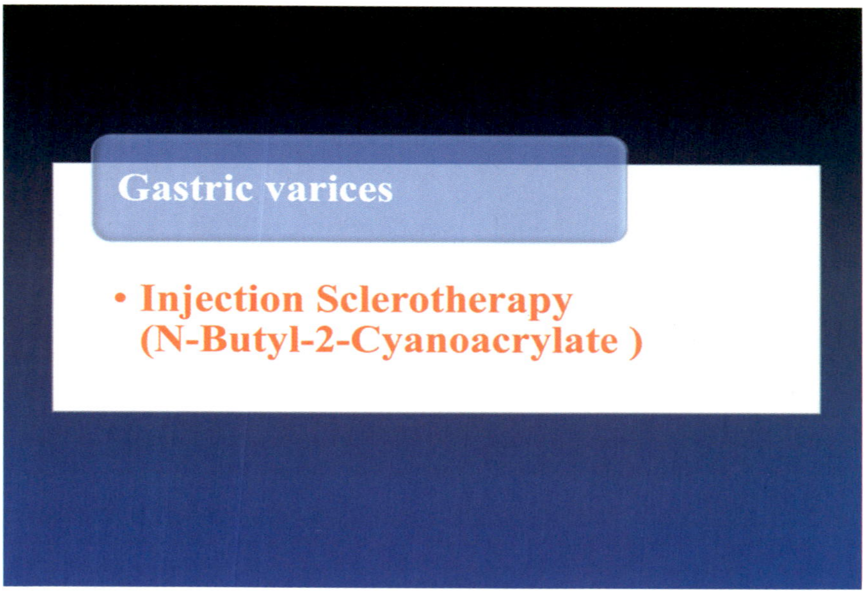

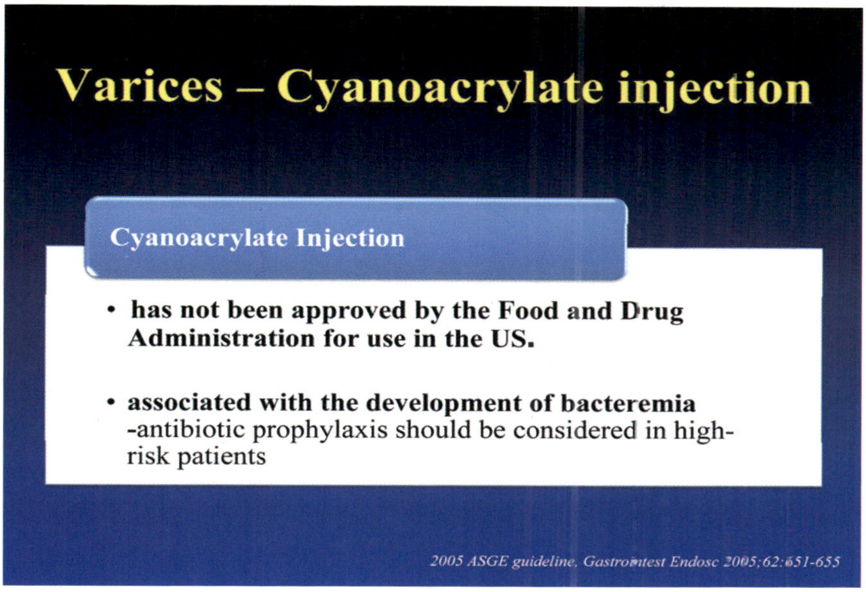

Injection sclerotherapy using cyanoacrylate injection has not been approved by the FDA for use in the US. Cyanoacrylate injection is associated with the development of bacteremia and antiboitic prophylaxis should be considered in high risk patients.

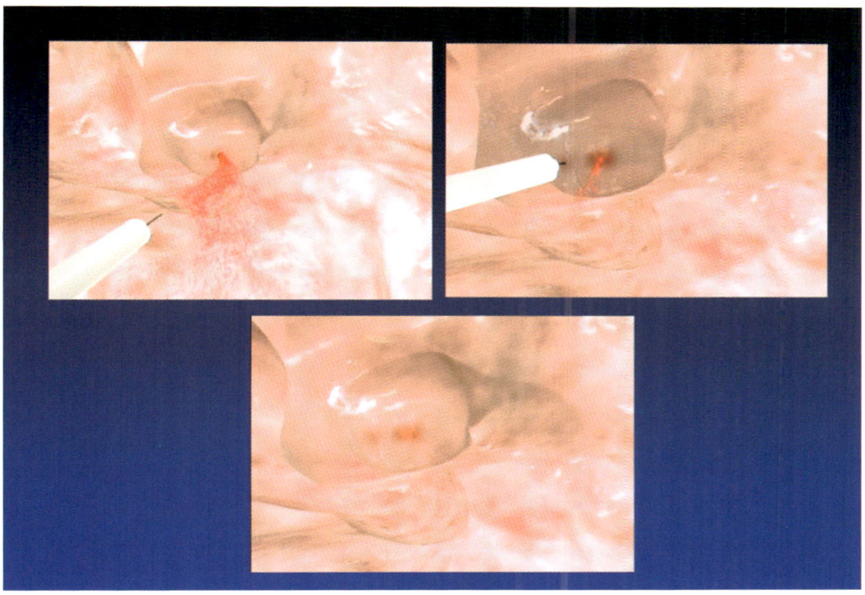

This is a simuation of cyanoacrylate injection therapy for fundal varices. As cyanoacrylate is injected, it immediately hardens on contact with the blood.

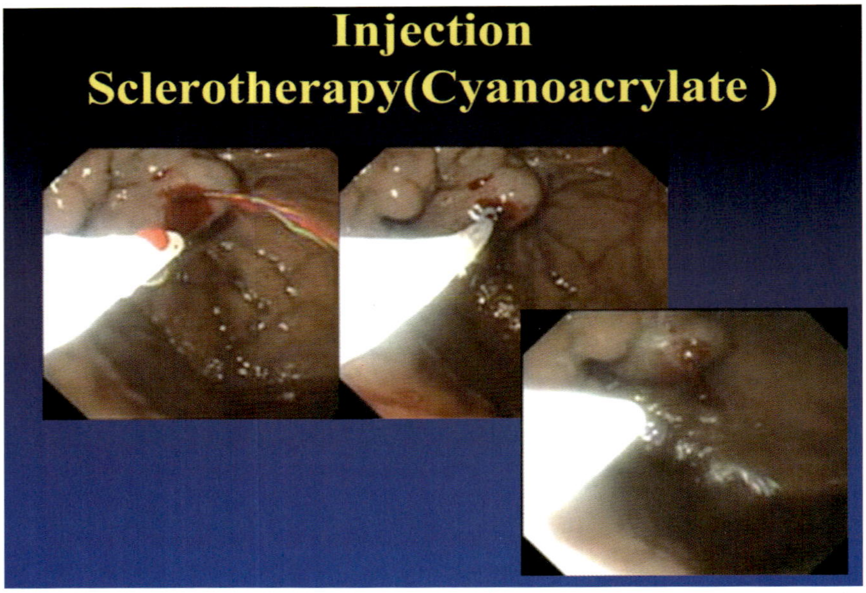

These figures show cyanoacrylate injection therapy performed on an actively bleeding gastric fundal varix. The varix is punctured and a mixed solution of cyanoacrylate and contrast is injected. When in contact with blood, the cyanoacrylate immediately crystalizes forming a harden plug. Proper delivery of cyanoacrylate can be confirmed real time by fluroscopy.

Outcome of N-butyl-2-cyanoacrylate injection for fundal gatric varices

	No.	Hemostasis (%)	Variceal Obliteration(%)	Recurrent bleeding(%)	Mortality rate(%)	Follow-up(mo)
D'Imperio, et al 1996	54	90.9	87	3.7	9.5	6
Kind, et al 2000	174	97.1	32.6	Early; 15.5 Late; 12.8	19.5	36
Lee, et al 2000	RI;54	96.3	79.6	7.4	1.9	14.8
	OD;47	95.7	-	12.8	6.4	
Huang, et al 2000	90	94.4	36.1	23.3	2.2	13
Lo, et al 2001	31	87	51	13	6	14
Seewald, et al 2008	131	100	100	Early;0 Late;6.9	6.1	25.8

RI, Repeat injection (with aim to obliterate varices)
OD, on-demand injection (when bleeding recurs).

Seewald et al. Gastrointest Endosc 2008;68:447-54

According to several studies, the hemostasis rate for cyanoacrylate injection for fundal varices was 87 to 100%. The rate of variceal obliteration and recurrent bleeding was variable. Mortality rate were also variable with one study reporting a mortality rate of as high as 19%.

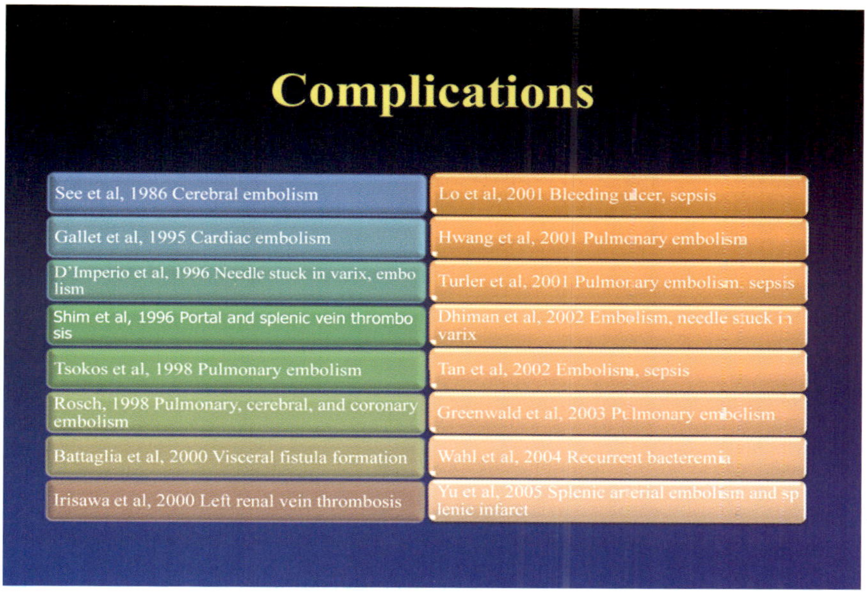

Complications following cyanoacrylate injection have been described in many case reports. Most of the complication were associated with sepsis and thromboembolism of the pulmonary and splenic vessels.

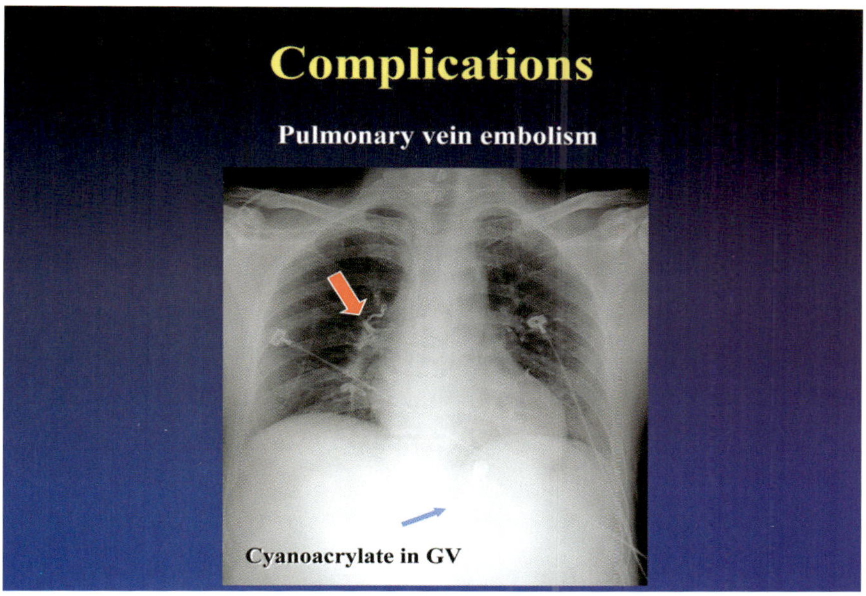

This is a chest X-ray of a patient who developed chest discomfort after cyanoacrylate injection for treatment of gastic fundal varices. Cyanoacrylate emboli can be seen in the pulmonary and splenic veins.

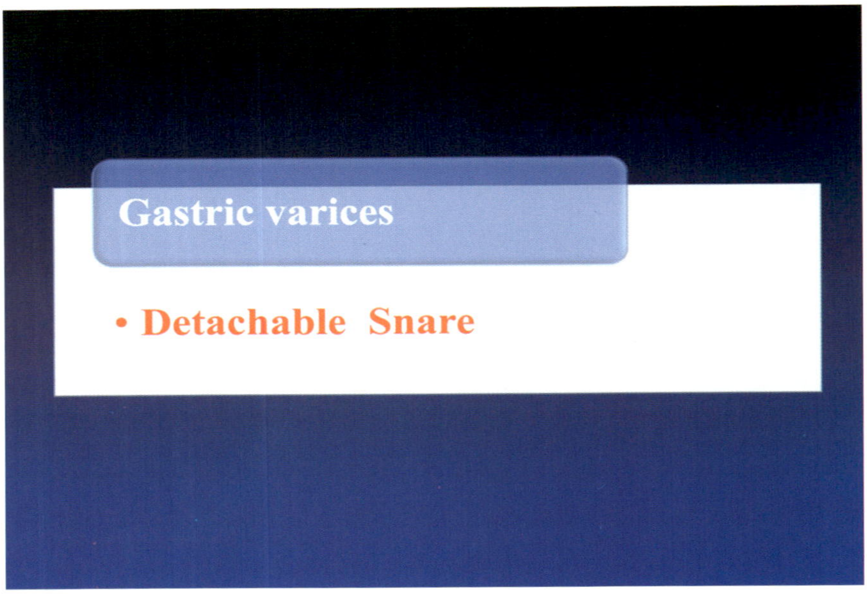

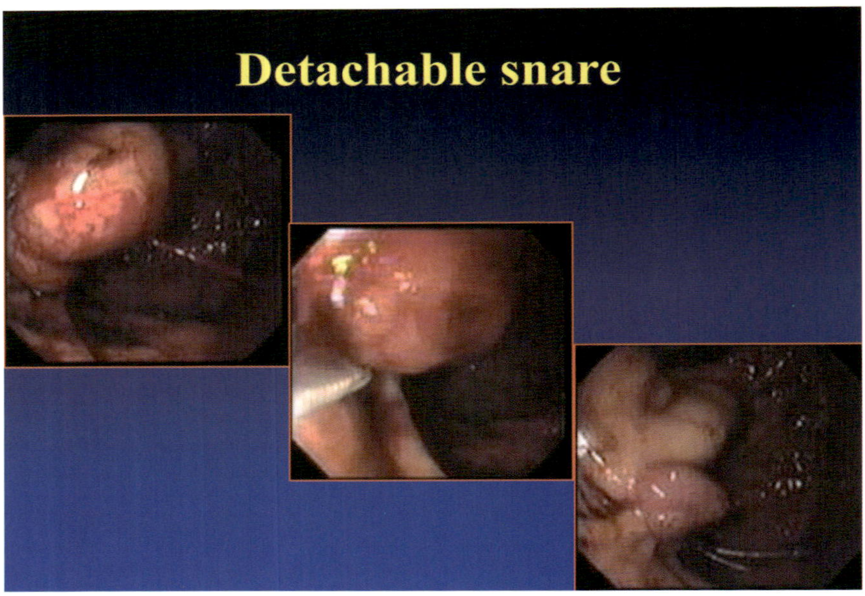

These figures demonstrate gastric varix ligation using a detachable snare. Ligation with a detachable snare is useful. An actively bleeding gastric varix is observed on the fundus. The snare is looped and tightened around the base of the varix. After the loop is tightened, the snare is detached. Following ligation, bluish congestion of the ligated varix is observed. If cyanoacrylate cannot be used or the amount of cyanoacrylate needed is excessive. Ligation with a detachable snare is useful.

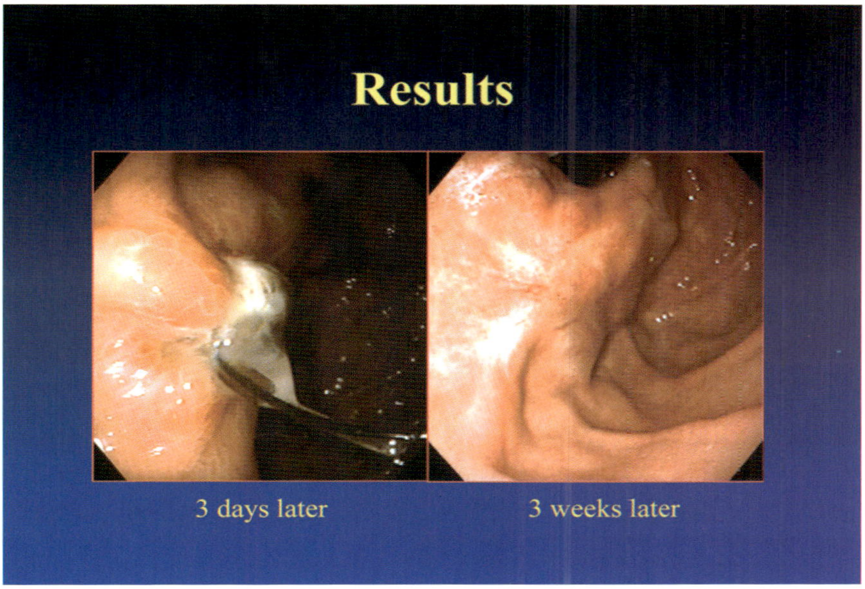

After 3 days of ligation, a post-ligation ulcer is seen with the detachable snare still in place. Three weeks later, the snare has been dislocated and a scar is observed on the fundus.

Gastric varices

- Hemoclip

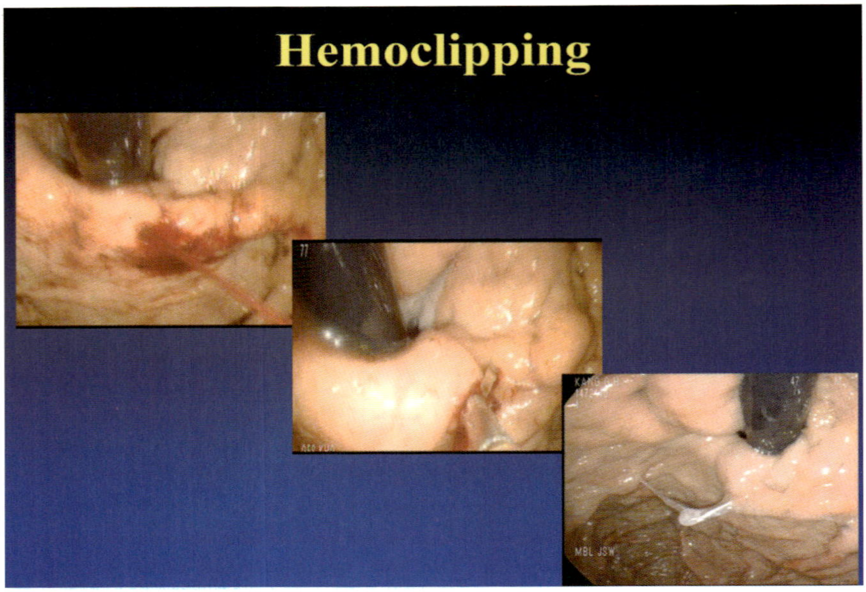

Hemoclip application, similar to surgical ligation of a bleeding vessls, can achieve prompt and permanent hemostasis. Limited number of studies showed good results for endoscopic hemostatic clipping for treating gastroesophageal varices. Hemostatic clipping also has the advantage of targeting vessels with minimal tissue damage. In this video clip, pumping variceal bleeding is stoped dramatically by one clip.

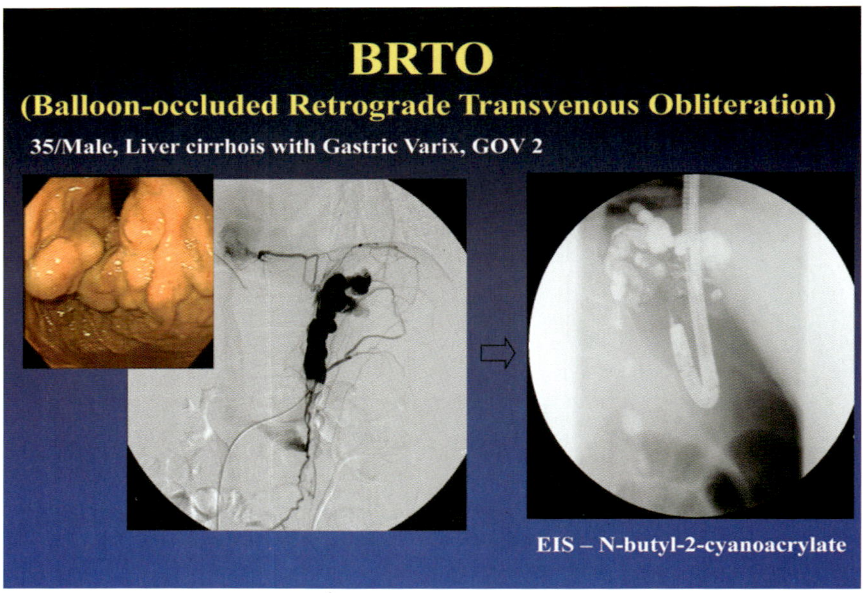

Balloon-occluded retrograde transvenous obliteration (BRTO), is a procedure effective for the treatment of large gastric fundal varices with a spontaneous splenorenal shunt and is also indicated for treating refractory portosystemic encephalopathy caused by large splenorenal shunt.

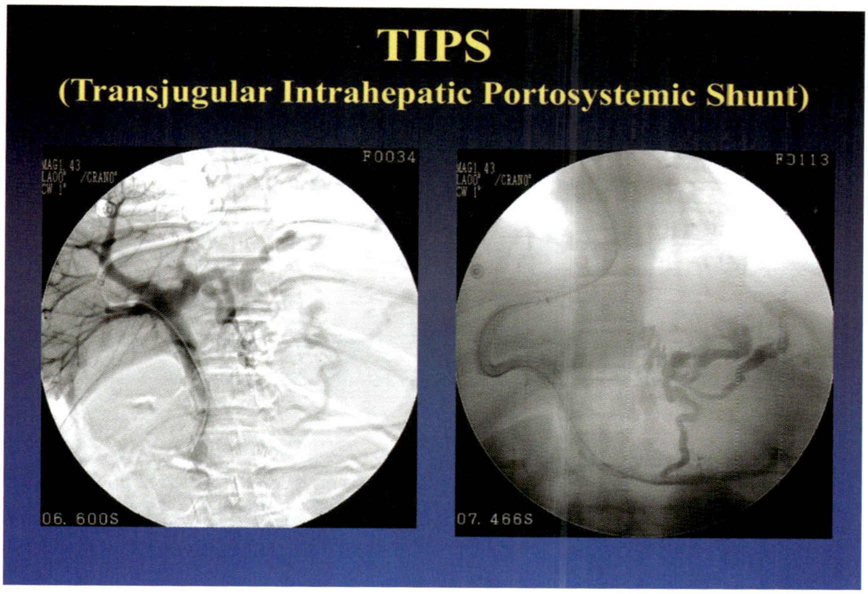

TIPS is an excellent salvage prodedure. TIPS should be considered in patients who are Child A or B who experience recurrent variceal hemorrhage despite combination pharmacological and endoscopic therapy.

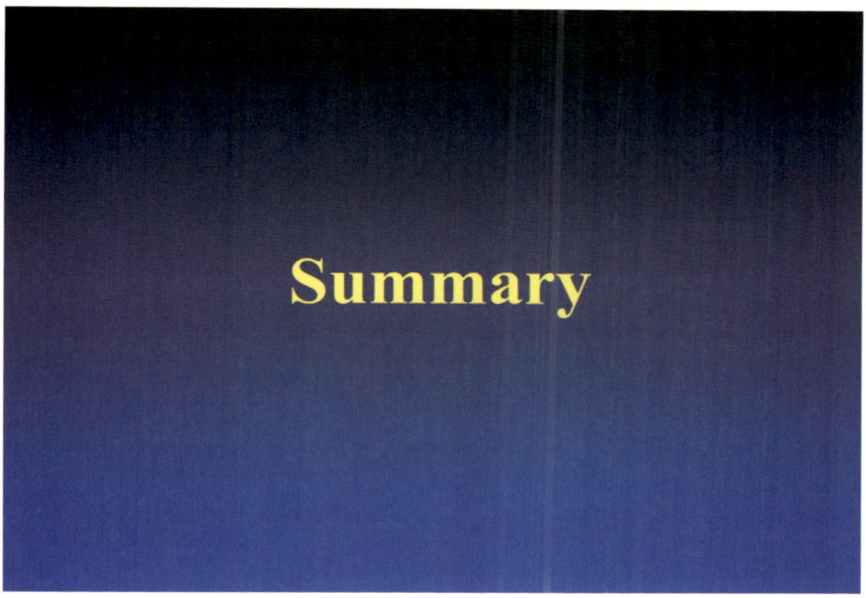

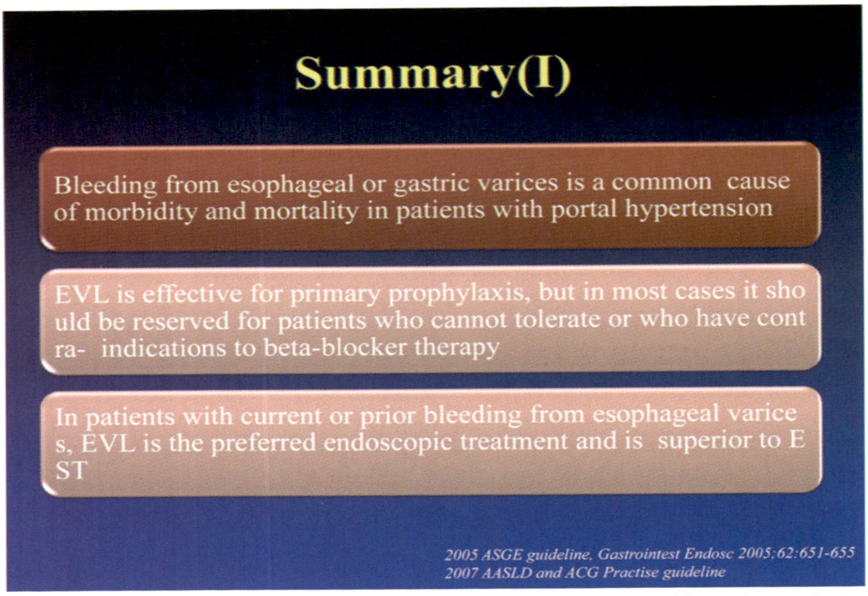

Bleeding from esophageal or gastric varices is a common cause of morbidity and mortality in patients with portal hypertension. EVL is effective for primary prophylaxis, but in most cases it should be reserved for patients who cannot tolerate or who have contraindications to beta-blocker therapy. In patients with current or prior bleeding from esophageal varices, EVL is the preferred endoscopic treatment and is superior to EST.

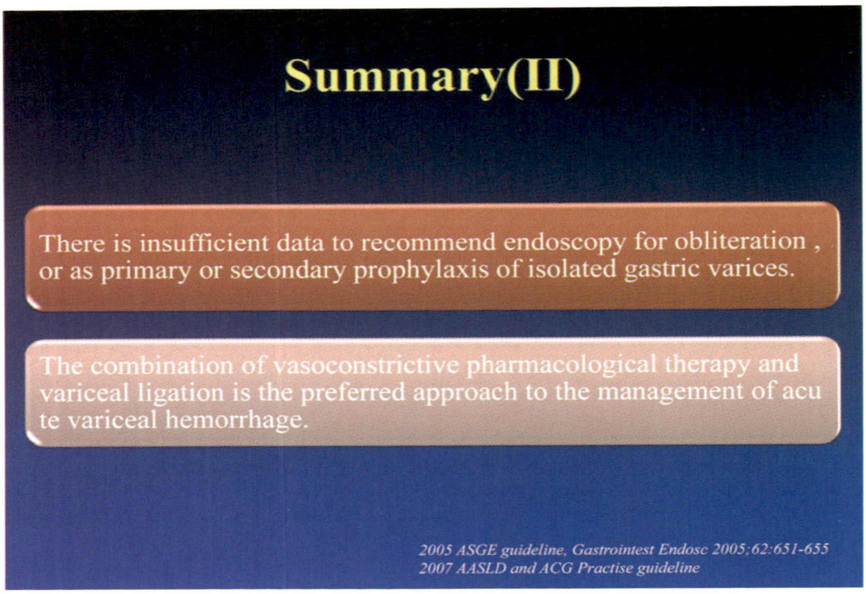

There is insufficient data to recommend endoscopy for obliteration, or as primary or secondary prophylaxis of isolated gastric varices. The combination of vasoconstrictive pharmacological therapy and variceal ligation is the preferred approach to the management of acute variceal hemorrhage.

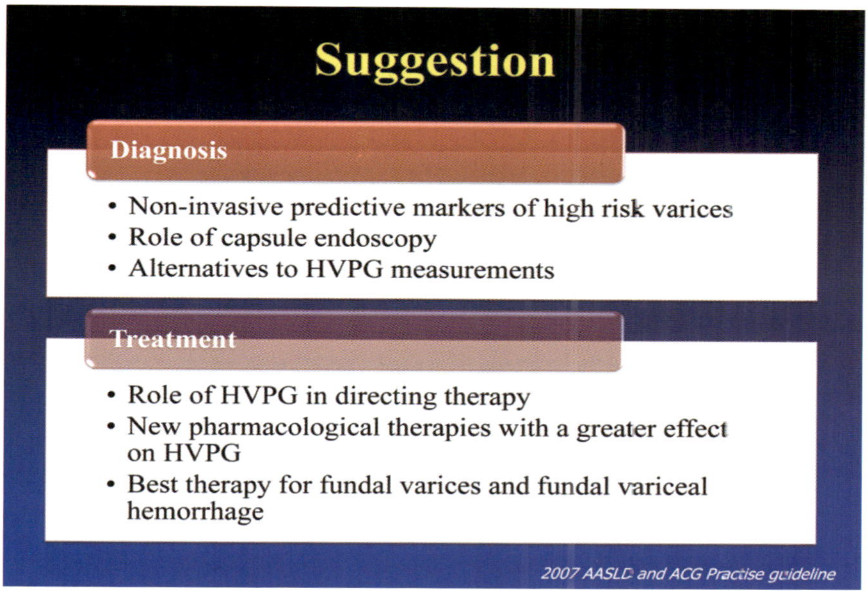

The following are important areas in the diagnosis and treatment of varices and variceal hemorrhage where additional research is needed.

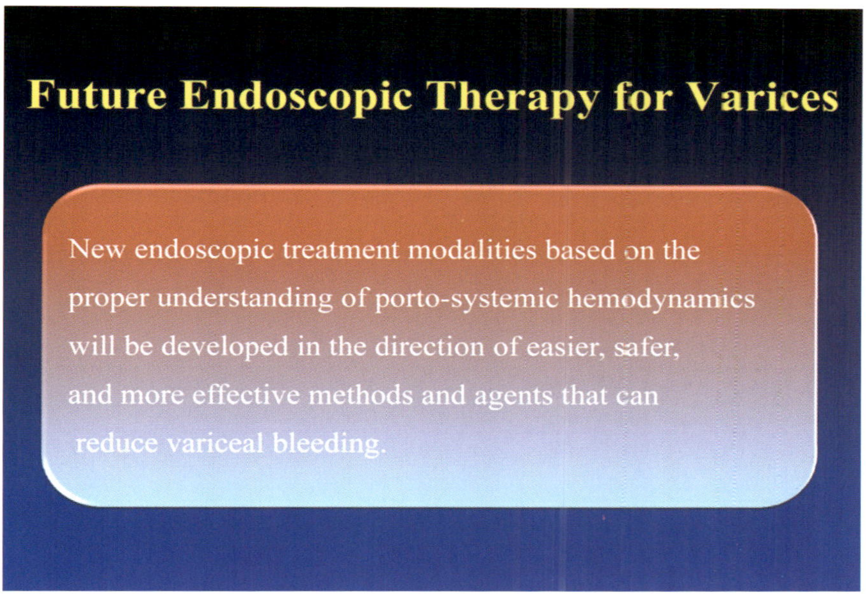

New endoscopic treatment modalities based on the proper understanding of porto-systemic hemodynamics will be developed in the direction of easier, safer, and more effective methods and agents that can reduce variceal bleeding.

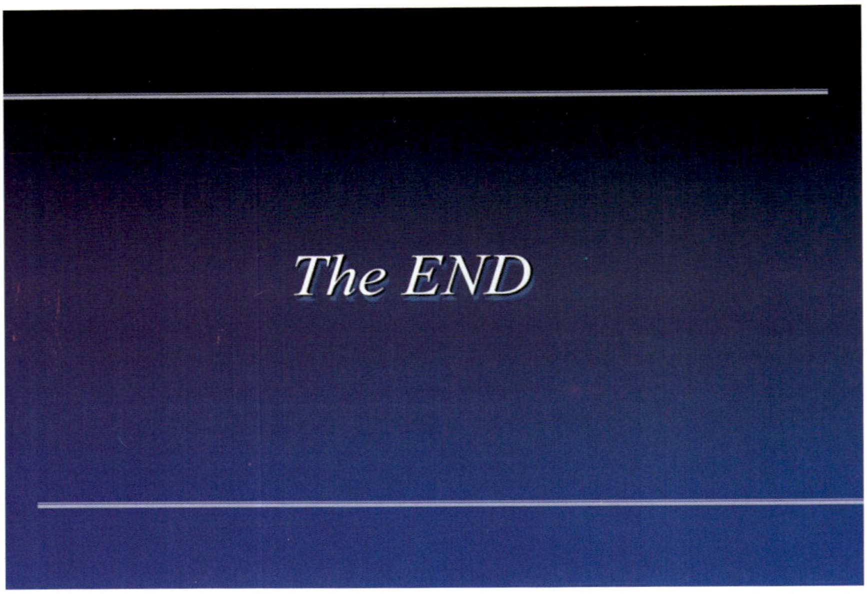

In patients with current or prior bleeding from esophageal varices, EVL is the preferred endoscopic treatment and is superior to EST. There is insufficient data to recommend endoscopy as primary or secondary prophylaxis of isolated gastric varices. New endoscopic treatment modalities based on the proper understanding of porto-systemic hemodynamics will be developed in the direction of easier, safer, and more effective methods and agents that can reduce variceal bleeding.

Chapter 6

Endoscopic Ablation Therapy of Gastrointestinal Disease

Educational Video Nominated for a 2009 ASGE Audiovisual Award

Youn Sun Park, M.D. Ph D.
Joo Young Cho, M.D. Ph D.

Chapter 6
Endoscopic Ablation Therapy of Gastrointestinal Disease

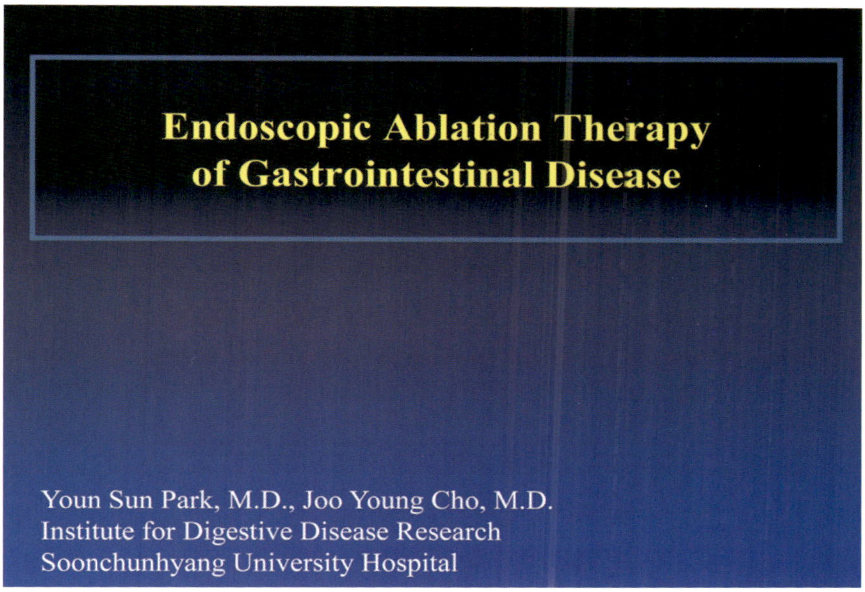

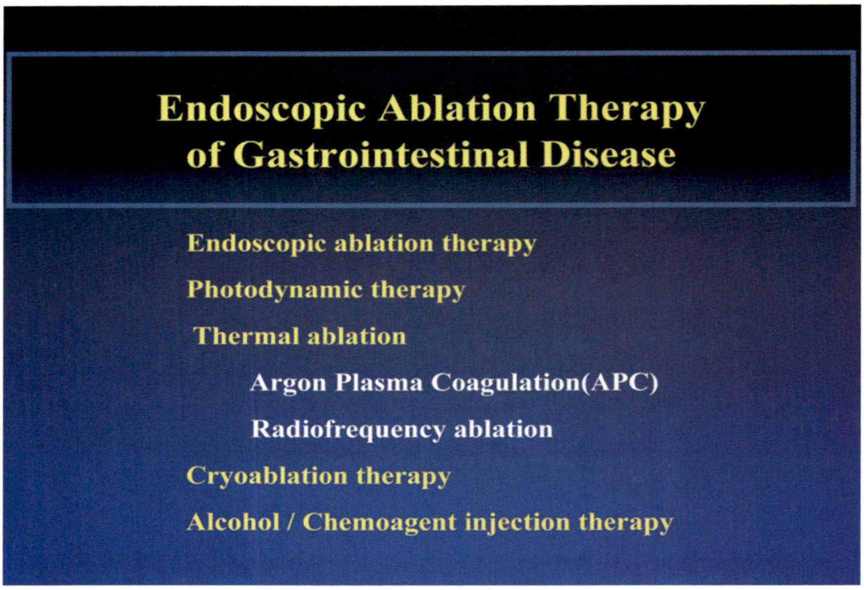

This chapter will focus on the various endoscopic ablation therapies that have been applied to gastrointestinal diseases including GI cancer and several benign GI lesions.

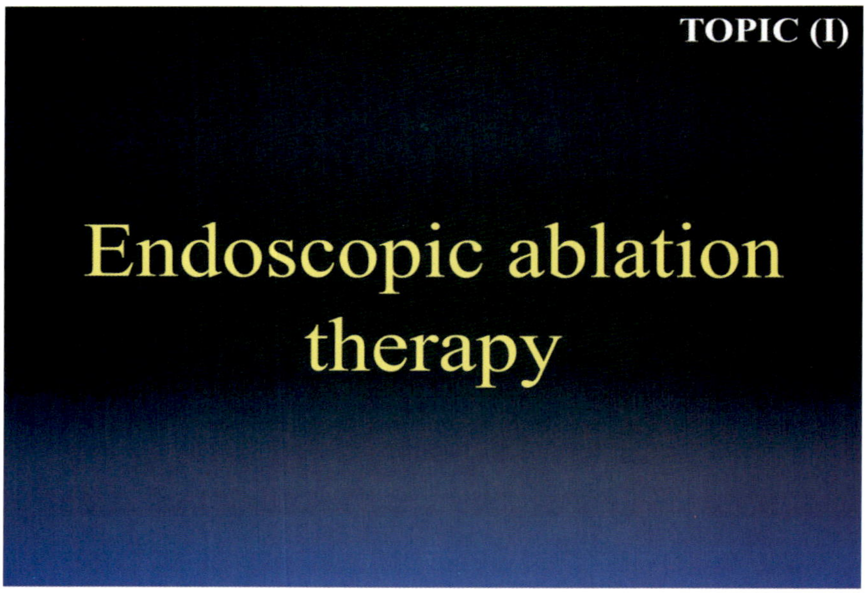

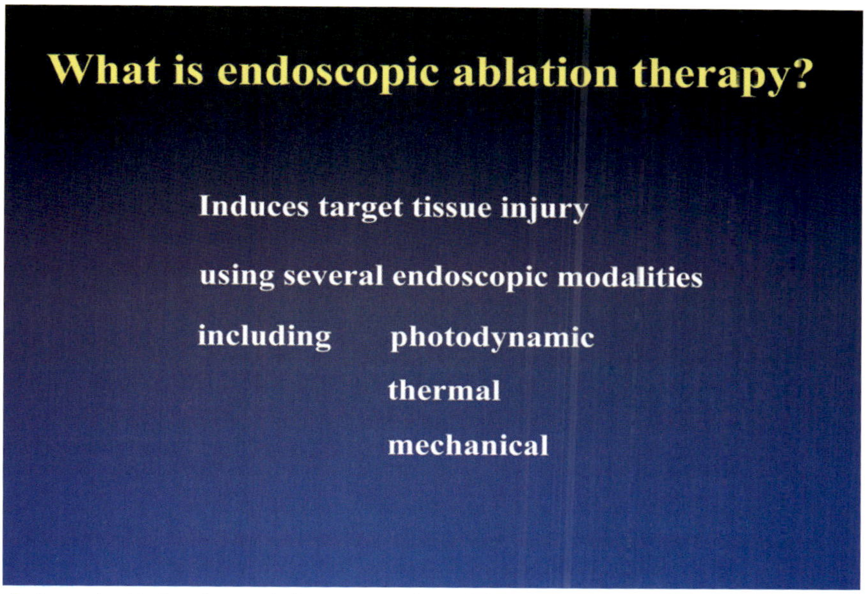

Endoscopic ablation therapy induces target tissue injury using several endoscopic modalities including photodynamic, thermal, and mechanical therapy.

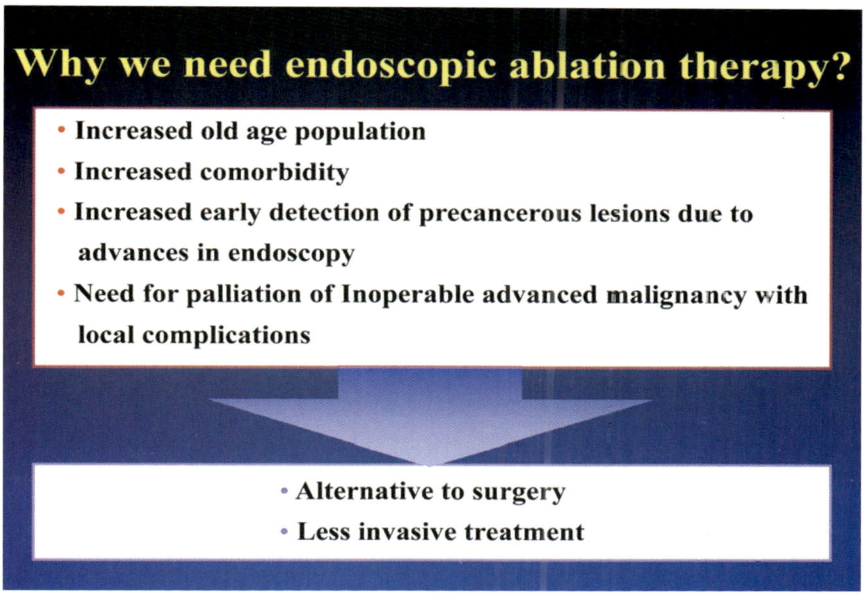

The need for endoscopic ablation therapy has arised due to the increasing old age population, comorbidity early detection of precancerous lesions, and need for palliation of inoperable advanced malignancies. Ablation therapy can serve as a minimal invasive alternative to surgery.

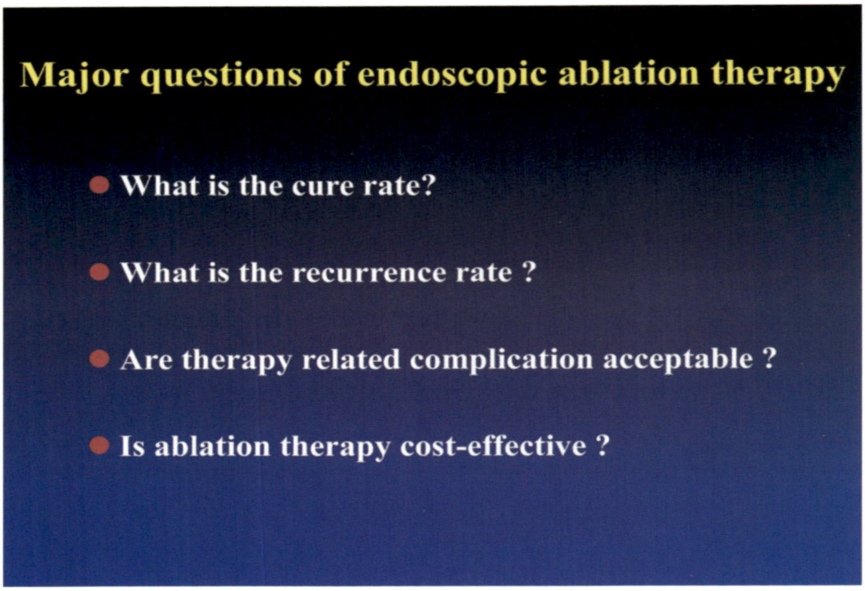

With the expansion of available modalities, multi-modality therapy, and the enlarged pool of candidate patients, many issues need to be resolved.

- What is the cure rate of disease?
- What is the incidence of recurrence of disease?
- Is complication rate acceptable?
- Is ablaton therapy cost effective?

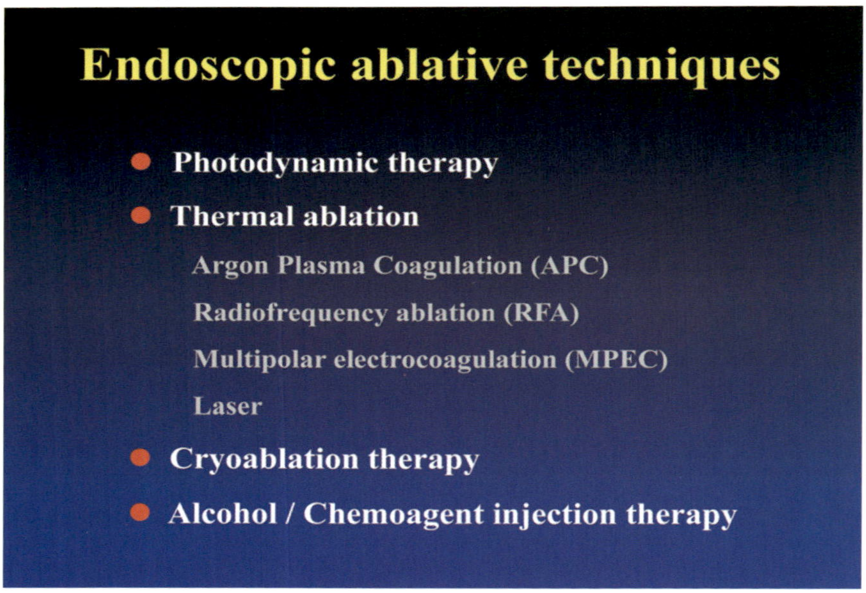

Endoscopic ablation therapies include several methods. Photodynamic therapy, radiofrequency ablation, argon plasma coagulation, multipolar electrocoagulation, laser, cryoablation therapy and alcohol / chemoagent injecton therapy.

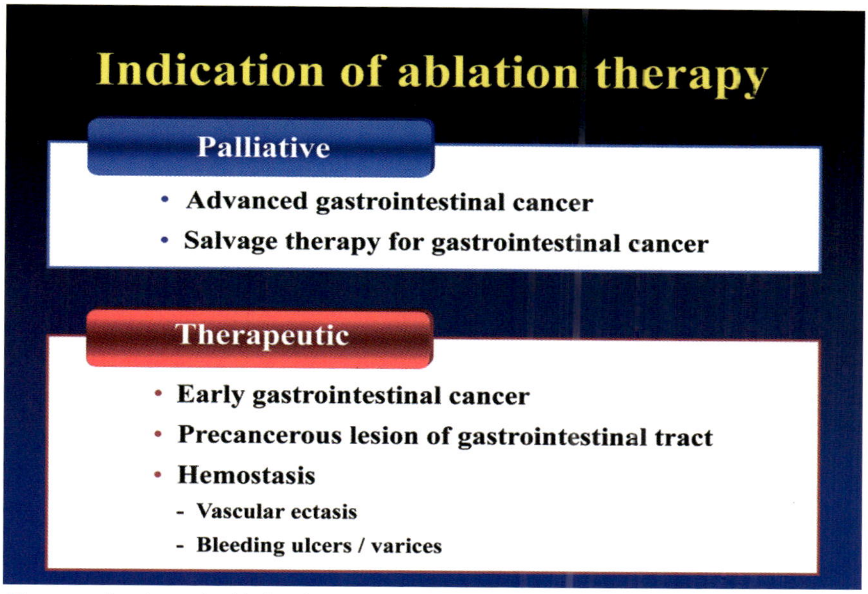

The uses of endoscopic ablation therapy can be broadly categorized as palliative or therapeutic. Palliative treatment for advanced gastrointestinal cancer or salvage therapy for gastrointestinal cancer, and therapeutic treatment for early gastrointestinal cancer, precancerous lesions and hemostasis of benign lesions.

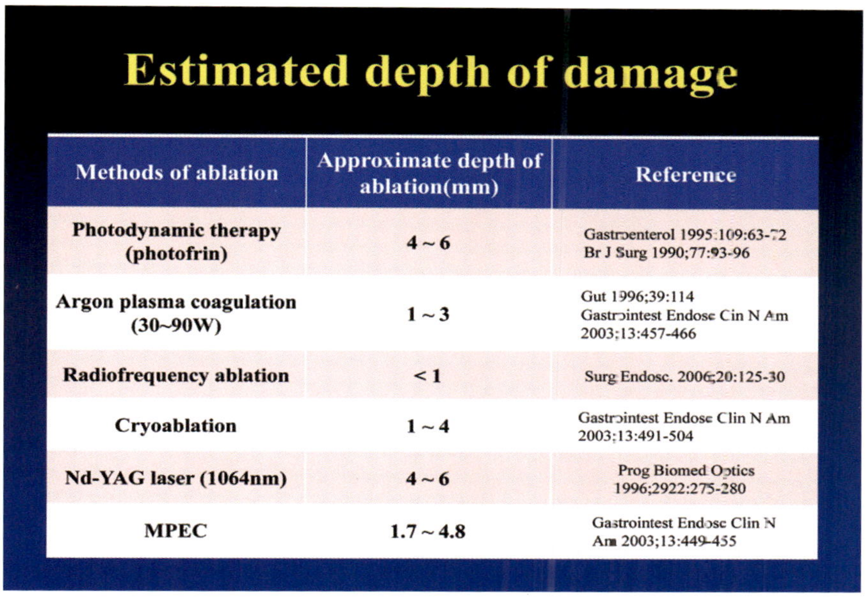

Estimated depth of damage

Methods of ablation	Approximate depth of ablation(mm)	Reference
Photodynamic therapy (photofrin)	4 ~ 6	Gastroenterol 1995;109:63-72 Br J Surg 1990;77:93-96
Argon plasma coagulation (30~90W)	1 ~ 3	Gut 1996;39:114 Gastrointest Endosc Cin N Am 2003;13:457-466
Radiofrequency ablation	< 1	Surg Endosc. 2006;20:125-30
Cryoablation	1 ~ 4	Gastrointest Endosc Clin N Am 2003;13:491-504
Nd-YAG laser (1064nm)	4 ~ 6	Prog Biomed Optics 1996;2922:275-280
MPEC	1.7 ~ 4.8	Gastrointest Endosc Clin N Am 2003;13:449-455

This table shows the estimated depth of tissue damage for various methods of endoscopic ablation therapy. The depth for radiofrequency ablation was less than 1mm.

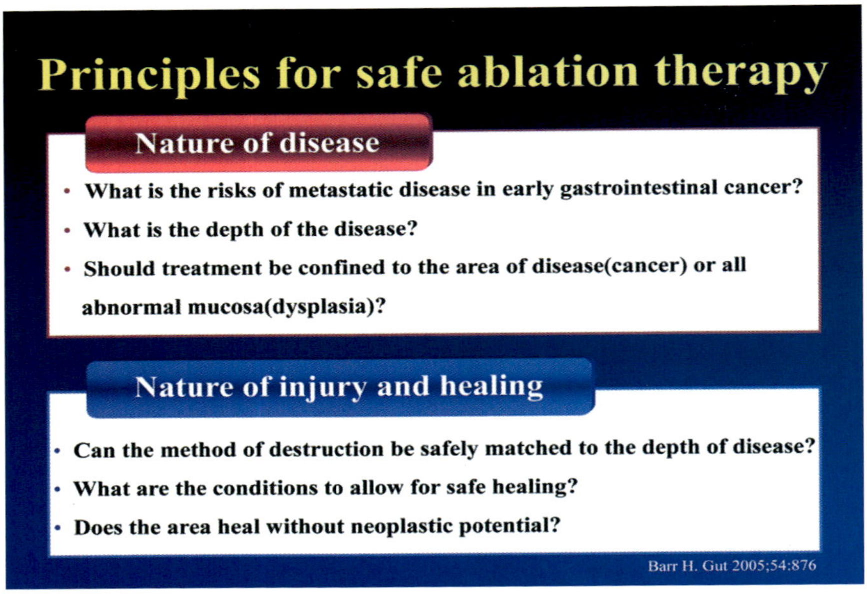

In order to set principles for safe endoscopic therapy, several questions must be addressed. Three relate to the nature of the disease and three to the nature of injury and healing

The nature of disease:

- What are the risks of metastatic disease in early gastrointestinal cancer?
- What is the depth of the disease?
- Should treatment be confined to the area of disease (cancer) or all abnormal mucosa (dysplasia)?

The nature of injury and healing:

- Can the method of destruction be safely matched to the depth of disease?
- What are the conditions to allow for safe healing?
- Does the area heal without neoplastic potential?

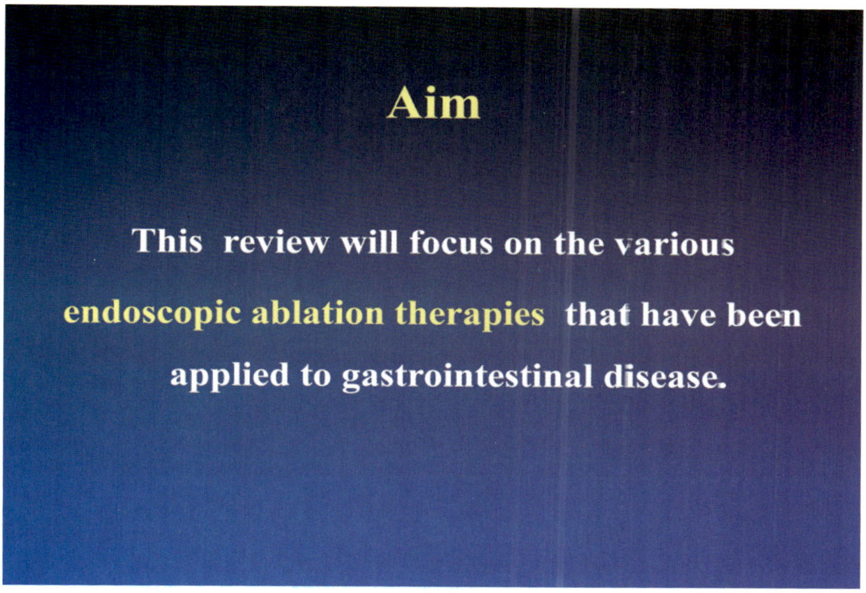
Aim
This review will focus on the various
endoscopic ablation therapies that have been
applied to gastrointestinal disease.

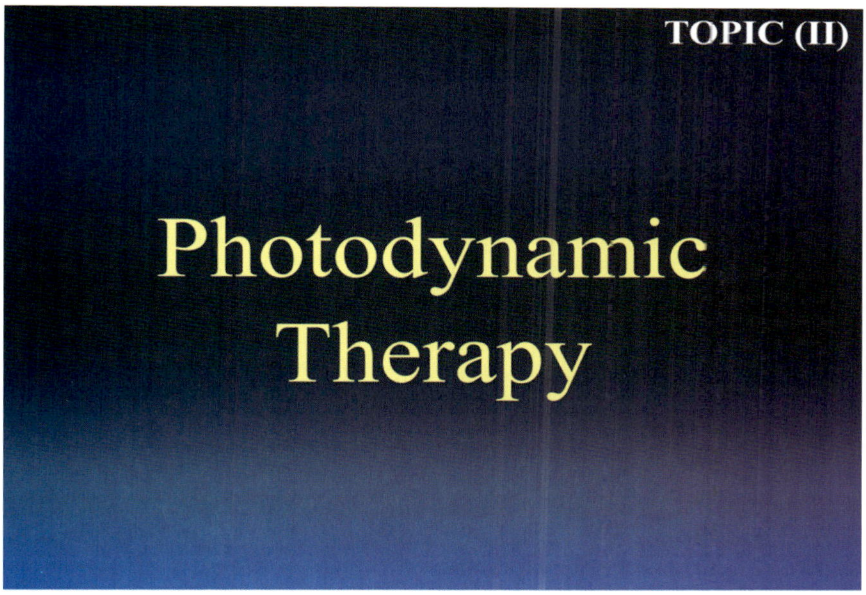
TOPIC (II)
Photodynamic
Therapy

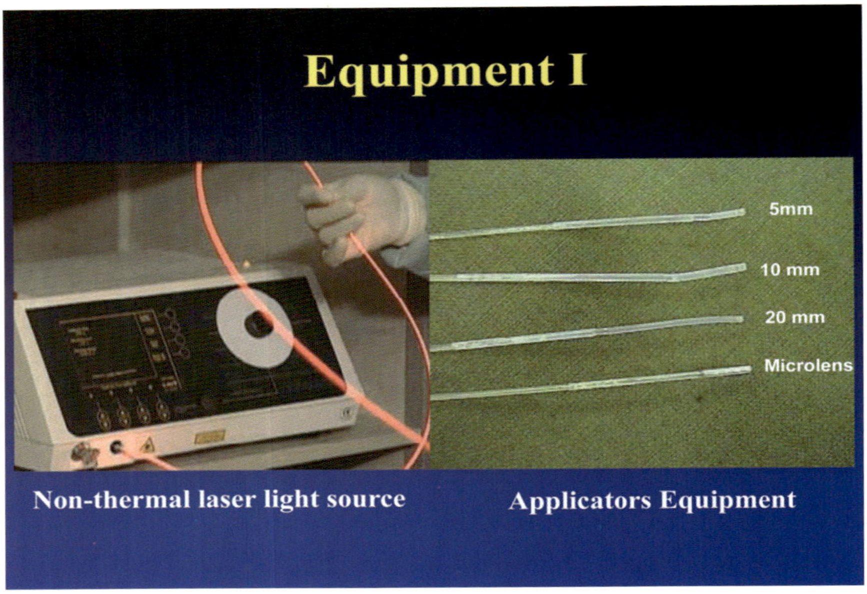

The essential components of PDT are a photosensitizing agent, a non-thermal laser light source, various applicator equipment and oxygen.

Equipment II

Photosensitizers in use		
Photosensitizer	**Peak wavelength (nm)**	**Comments**
5-Aminolaevulinic acid (5-ALA)	632	Limited tissue penetraion, can be taken orally, Low skin photosensitivity
Haematoporphyrin(HpD) / Photofrin	630	Instability at room temperature, long skin photosensitivity
Profimer sodium	630	Long skin photosensitivity (> 6 weeks)
Phthalocyanines (Pc)	675 ~700	Second-generation photosensitisers
Zn II Phthalocyanine	675 ~700	Strong light absorption and deep tissue penetration
Aluminum sulphonated Pc (AISPc)	675	High tumor selectivity and cytotoxicity, water insoluble
Benzoporphyrin derivatives	690	Low skin photosensitivity
Mesotetrahydroxyphenylchlorin (mTHPC)	652	High selectivity for tumor cells, suitable for irradiation with diode laser
Mono-L-aspartyl chlorin e6 (NPe6)	654	Low skin photosensitivity, limited clinical experience
Indocyanine green	790 ~ 805	No clinical experience reported (mostly used in cell cultures), little or no skin photosensitivity

Kubba AK. Digestion 1999;60: 1-10

This table lists the photosensitizers currently in use and their characteristics. The light wavelength and method of administration must be appropriate to initiate a photochemical reaction.

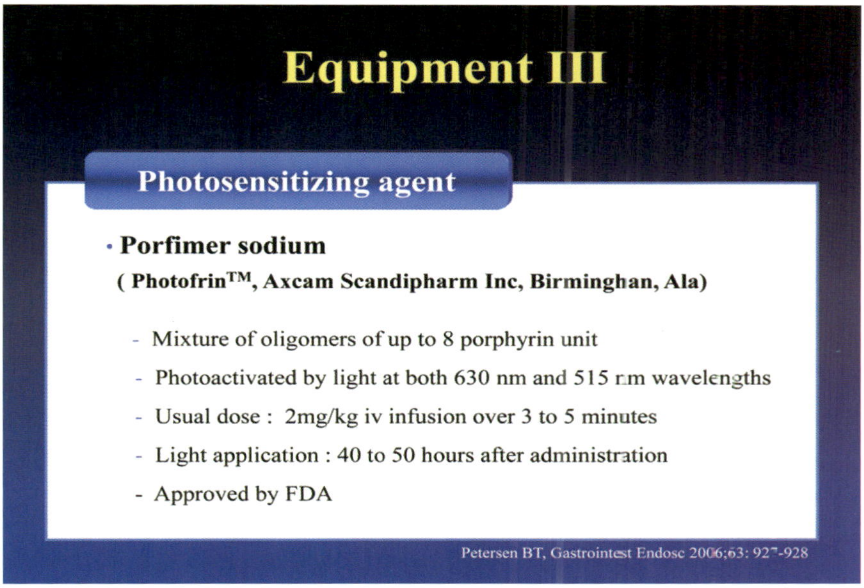

There is only one photosensitizer porfimer sodium (Photofrin™, Lederle Parenterals) approved by FDA. Porfimer sodium (Photofrin, Axcam Scandipharm Inc, Birmingham, Ala), is a mixture of oligomers of up to 8 porphyrin units and is photoactivated by light at both 630 nm and 515 nm wavelengths. It is a freeze-dried brownish powder, requiring reconstitution in 5% dextrose or 0.9% NaCl before use. After administration it is cleared from most tissues over 40 to 72 hours but retained for longer intervals in tumors, skin, and the reticuloendothelial system. Hence, light application is usually scheduled at 40 to 50 hours after administration.

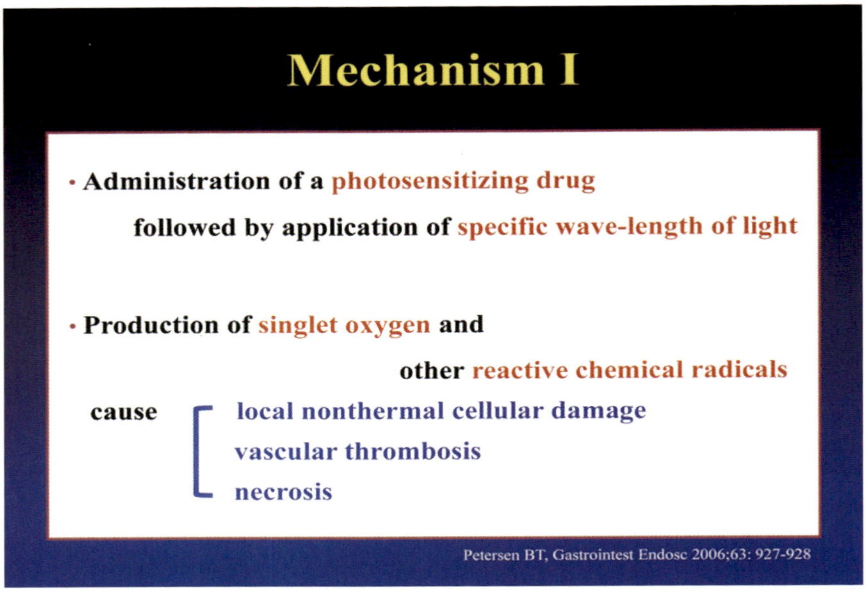

The basis for PDT is the propensity of some chemicals for photoexcitation when exposed to intense white or specific wavelength laser light. Upon light exposure, the production of singlet oxygen and other reactive chemical radicals cause local nonthermal cellular damage, vascular thrombosis, and necrosis, which evolve over hours to several days.

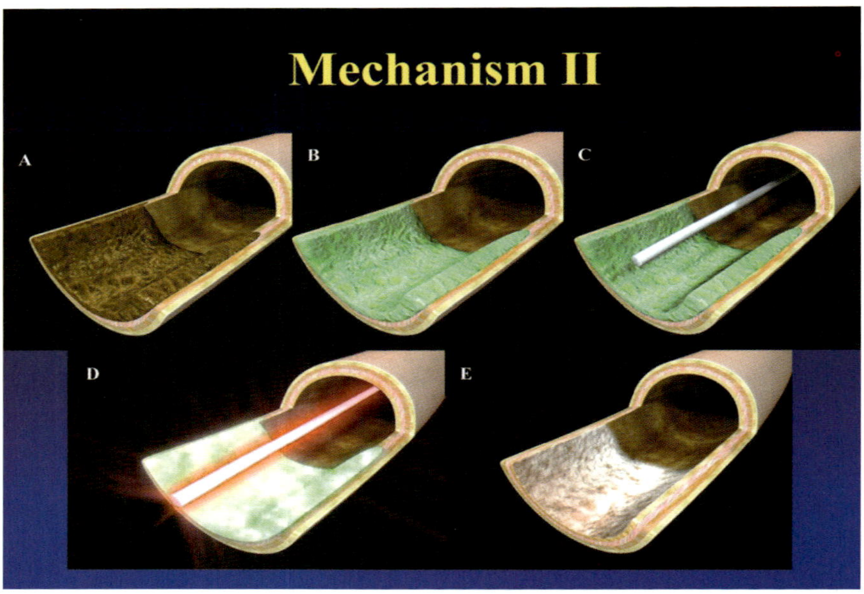

It employs administration of a photosensitizing drug (figure B) followed by insertion of application catheter through the working channel of the endoscope. When applicator catheter is placed in front of the target area (figure C), a specific wavelength of non-thermal laser light (figure D), leading to intracellular photoexcitation and injury(figure E). Photodynamic therapy (PDT) is an ablative treatment for rapidly proliferating tissues, including dysplastic and malignant lesions.

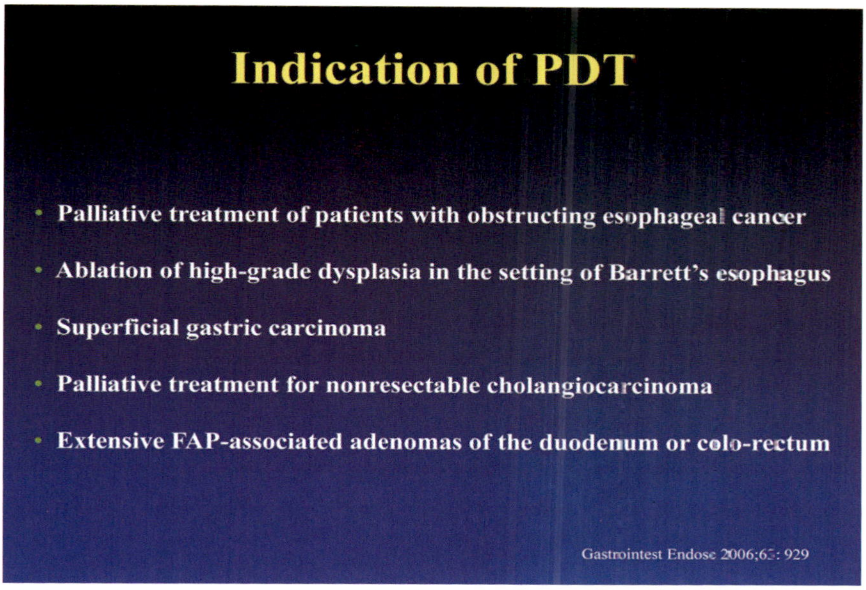

Photodynamic therapy using porfimer sodium (Photofrin II) is FDA cleared for palliative treatment of patients with completely or partially obstructing esophageal cancer, ablation of high-grade dysplasia in the setting of Barrett's esophagus in patients not undergoing surgery, and superficial gastric carcinoma, palliative treatment for nonresectable cholangiocarcinoma and extensive FAP-associated adenomas of the duodenum or colo-rectum.

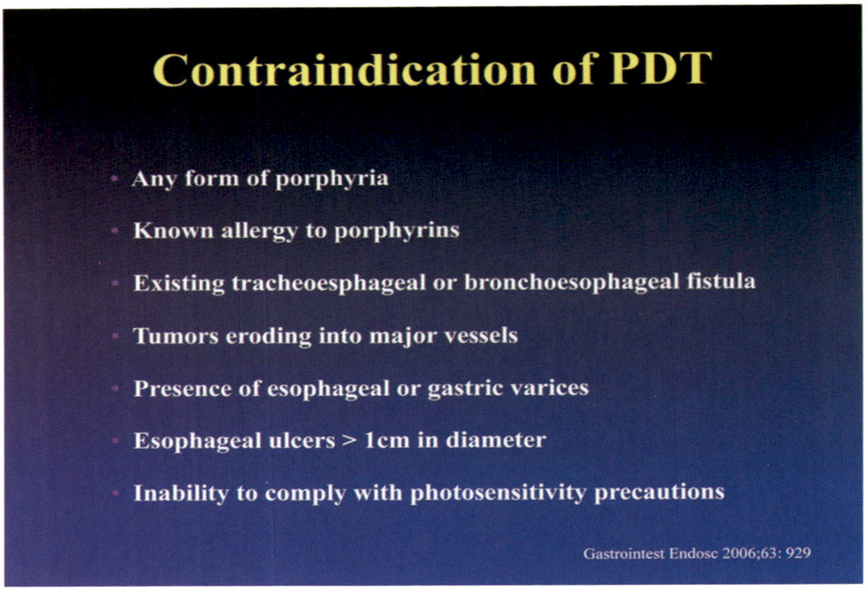

Contraindications include the presence of any form of porphyria or known allergies to porphyrins, existing tracheoesophageal or broncho-esophageal fistula, tumors eroding into major vessels, the presence of esophageal or gastric varices, esophageal ulcers →1 cm in diameter, and inability to comply with photosensitivity precautions.

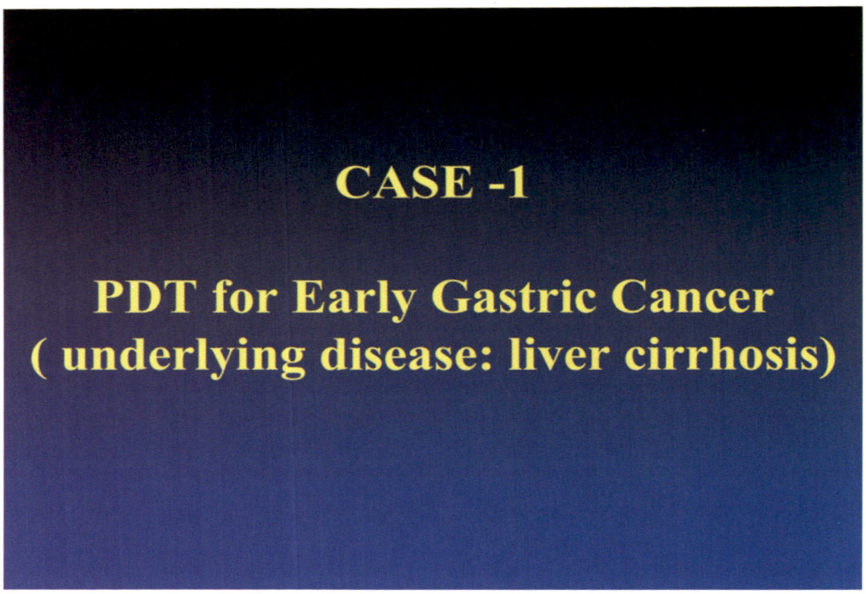

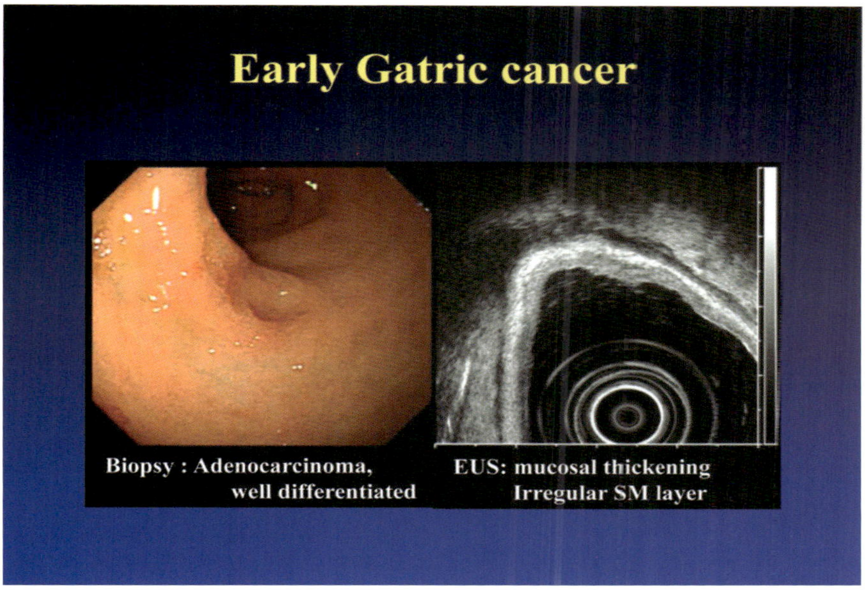

This is a 58 year male with liver cirrhosis on convention endoscopy a 1.2cm sized flat elevated lesion on the anterior wall of the antrum. Biopsies confirmed well differentiated adenocarcinoma. EUS showed mucosal thickening and an irregular SM layer. Surgery was deemed too high a risk, and PDT was performed.

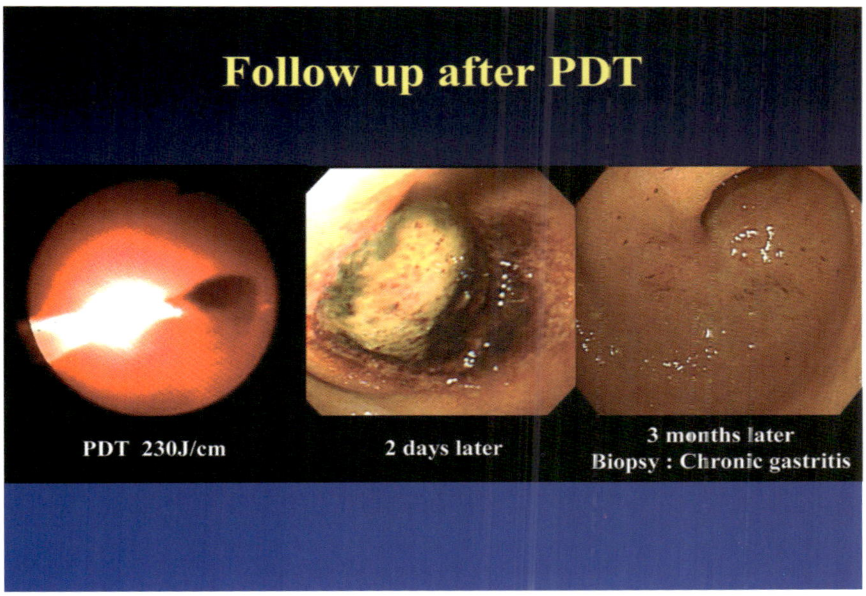

PDT energy was set at 230 Joule per square centimeter. Follow up endoscopy showed an post PDT ulcer at 2 days and a post PDT scar at 3 months. Biopsies of the scar showed chronic gastritis.

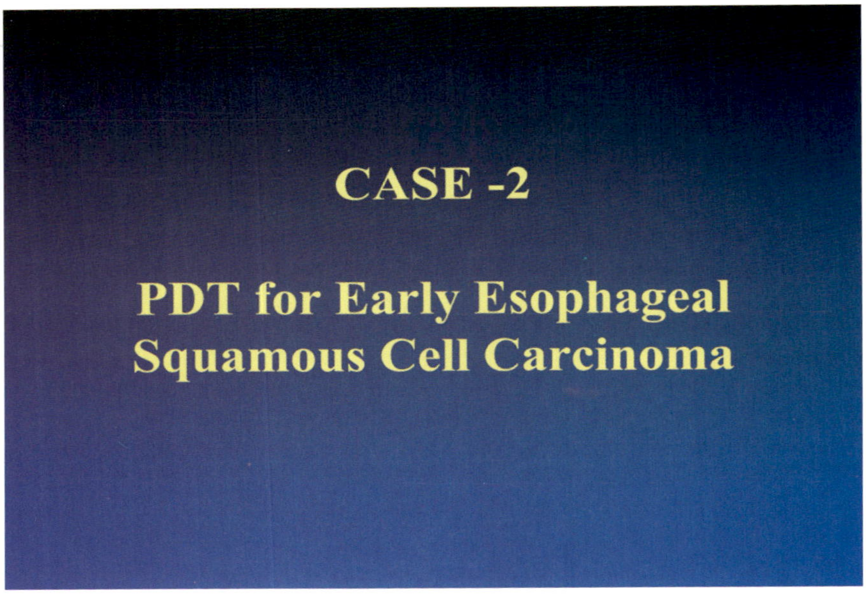

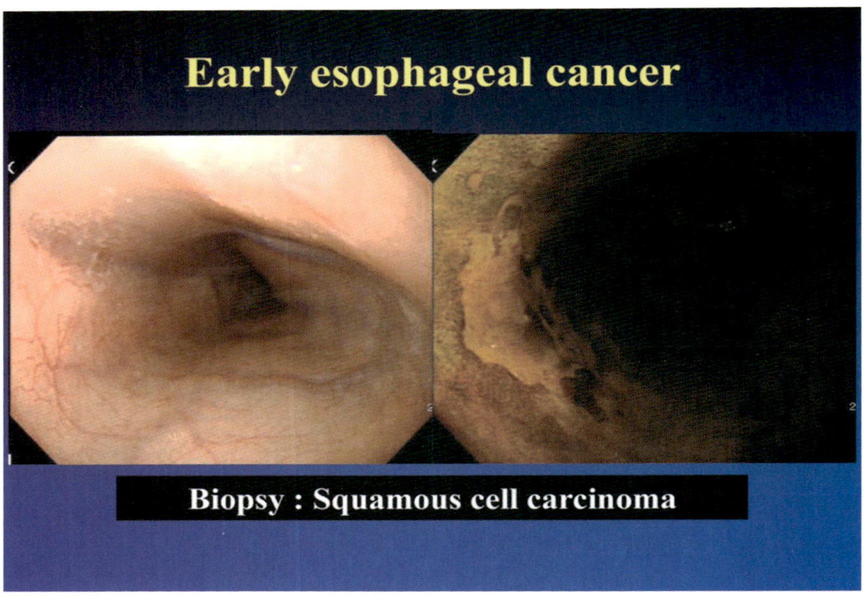

This is a 70 year old male who underwent total gastrectomy for gastric cancer 10 years ago. Follow up endoscopy detected irregular mucosal abnormalities 28cms from lower incisors which remained unstained after iodine spray. Biopsies of the lesion reveal squamous cell carcinoma.

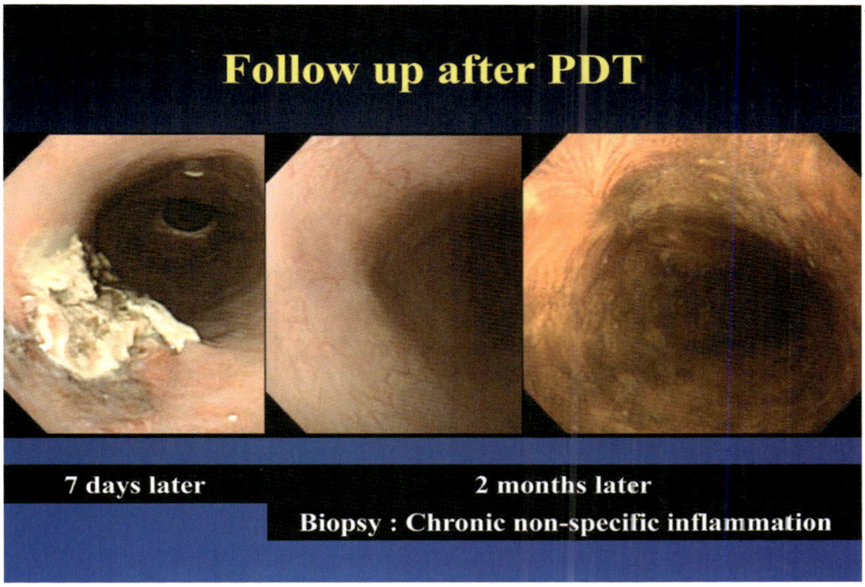

We decided to perform PDT. For adequate light illumination, a catheter is applied to the lesion. Energy was set at 180 Joule per square centimeter. 1 week later, an artificial ulcer is shown on the post-PDT area. Two months later, endoscopy showed a scarred lesion and the result of biopsy revealed chronic non-specific inflammation without tumor evidence.

PDT for High Grade Dysplasia in Barrett's Esophagus

Reference	Patients (n)	Photo sensitizer	Complete BE eradication (%)	HGD eradication (%)	Cancer detected following PDT	Stricture rate	F/U
Overholt BE et al (2007)	208	Photofrin®	NR	77	15	36	5 years
Overholt BE et al (2003)	80	Photofrin®	54	77	7.5	30	58.5 months
Panjehpour M et al (2000)	43	Photofrin®	42	96	0	33	9.8 months

Cx; complication, CR; complete response, F/U; follow up, BE; Barrett's Esophagus, NR; not reported

These reports show the results of PDT for HGD in Barrett' s esophagus. The overall rates of HGD eradication ranged from 77% to 96%. According to Overholt' s report, 5 year follow up of a randomized, multicenter, multinational, pathology-blinded HGD trial, a secondary outcome measure preventing progression to cancer showed a significant difference with about half the likelihood of cancer occurring in PDT group (15%). PDT is an effective therapy for ablating HGD in patients with Barrett' s esophagus and in reducing the incidence of esophageal adenocarcinoma.

PDT for Early Gastric Cancer

Reference	Patients (n)	Photo sensitizer	Pathology	Major Cx	CR	Mean follow up period
Rabenstein T et al (2008)	22	5-ALA	Bx : gastric cancer 10 : AC, WD 12 : SRC	0%	81.8%	56.2 months
Cheon YK et al (2006)	8	Photofrin®	1 : AC, WD 6 : AC, MD 1 : AC, PD	2 : epigastric pain 3 : skin photosensitivity reaction	87.5%	17.3 months
Ell C et al (1998)	22	mTHPC	16 : Intestinal type cancer 6 : diffuse Lauren's carcinoma	7 : skin photosensitivity reaction 16 : local pain	73%	12~20 months

5-ALA: 5-aminolevulinic acid, mTHPC: *meso*-tetrahydroxyphenylchlorin Bx; biopsy, Cx; complication, CR; complete response, F/U; follow up, AC; Adenocarcinoma, WD; well differentiated, MD; moderately differentiated, PD; poorly differentiated, SRC: signet ring cell carcinoma, NR; not reported

These reports show the results of PDT for Early gastric cancer. For small cancers(< 2cm) the 5 year survival is between 80~95%. The overall rates of CR ranging from 73% to 87.5% and The median follow up period ranging 12~56.2 months have been reported. Photodynamic therapy has proved to be effective for the treatment of type I, 2a, 2b early gastric cancer if less than 2 cm diameter.

Salvage PDT for Persistent Esophageal Cancer after Chemoradiation Therapy

Reference	Patients (n)	Photo sensitizer	Histology	Major Cx	CR	F/U (range)	Recur
Yano T et al (2005)	13	Photofrin®	Esophageal cancer	Stenosis (3) Fistula (1) Mediastinitis (1) Pericarial effusion (1)	62%	12months (3 ~ 19 months)	30.7%
Wolfsen HC et al (2006)	7	Photofrin®	SCC(2) AC(5)	Stenosis (7)	71.4%	30 months (12 ~ 50 months)	28.5%

Cx; complication, CR; complete response, F/U; follow up, AC; Barrett's Adenocarcinoma, SCC: squamous cell carcinoma

These reports show the results of salvage PDT for persistent esophageal cancer after chemoradiation therapy. Locally advanced esophageal cancer may not be completely eradicated after chemoradiation therapy (CRT) and further treatment options are limited. Complete response was reported to be 62-71%. The overall rates of recurrence ranging from 28.5% to 30.7% have been reported. These results show that salvage photodynamic therapy could be a promising curative intent treatment option with low morbidity and mortality rates.

Palliative PDT for Advanced Esophageal Cancer

Reference	Patients (n)	Photo sensitizer	Histology	Major Cx	CR/ PR	Dysphagia change	Median overall survival
Lightdale CJ et al (1995)	218	Photofrin®	AC (51%) SCC (49%)	Perforaton (1%) Pleural effusion (10%) Sun burn (19%)	8% / 26%	Dysphagia grade change : - 0.75	NR
Litle VR et al (2003)	215	Photofrin®	AC (83.2%) SCC (15.3%)	Perforation (2.3%) Stricture (2%) Pleural effusion (3%) Sun burn (6%)	NR	Dysphagia grade change : - 1	4.8 months
Moghissi K et al (2003)	84	Photofrin®	NR	Stricture (8%) Sun burn (5%)	7% / 92.8%	Esophageal diameter : 6.2 → 11.1 mm	9.5 months

Cx; complication, CR; complete response, PR; partial response, F/U; follow up, AC; Barrett's Adenocarcinoma, SCC; squamous cell carcinoma, NR; not reported

These reports show the results of palliative PDT for advanced esophageal cancer. CR ranged from 7% to 8% and dysphagia was significantly improved. The median overall survival ranged 4.8~9.5 months. These results show that PDT offers effective palliation for patients with obstructing esophageal cancer.

PDT for Advanced Rectal Cancer

Reference	Patients (n)	Photo sensitizer	CR	PR	NR	Follow up period
Dohmoto M et al (1996)	71	NR	35%	44%	21%	13 ~ 51 months
Nakamura T et al (2003)	2 cases	T2N0M0 Snare polypectomy → PDT (Hematoporphyrin drivative)	100%	NR	NR	Pt 1 : 25 months Pt 2 : 6 years

CR; complete response, PR; partial response, NR; no response, pt; patient, NR; not reported

In advanced rectal cancer, PDT has induced a reduction of tumor size and has been associated with a substantial relief of chronic tumor related pain. This effect may be useful in improving quality of life of inoperable patients.

TOPIC (III)

Thermal Ablation Therapy

Thermal ablation therapy

Argon Plasma Coagulation

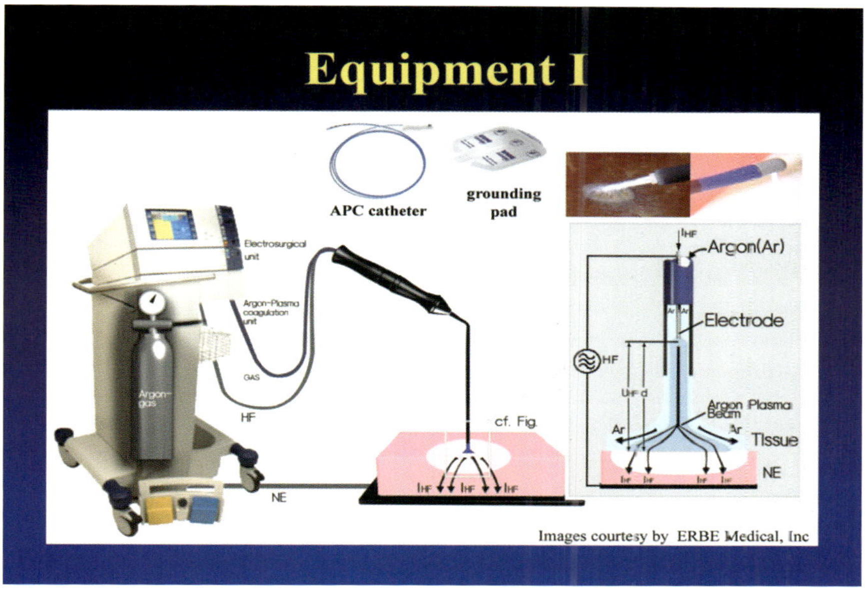

Argon plasma coagulator (APC) is a device intended for thermal coagulation of tissue. The APC apparatus includes a high-frequency monopolar electrosurgical generator, source of argon gas, gas flow meter, flexible delivery catheters, grounding pad, and foot switch to activate both gas and energy. The standard probes are 220 cm long, 300 cm probes can be specially ordered for use during push enteroscopy. Probes are available that direct the plasma parallel or perpendicular to the axis of the catheter. Electrons flow through a channel of electrically activated, ionized argon gas from the probe electrode to the targeted tissue. Current density on arrival at the tissue surface causes coagulation.

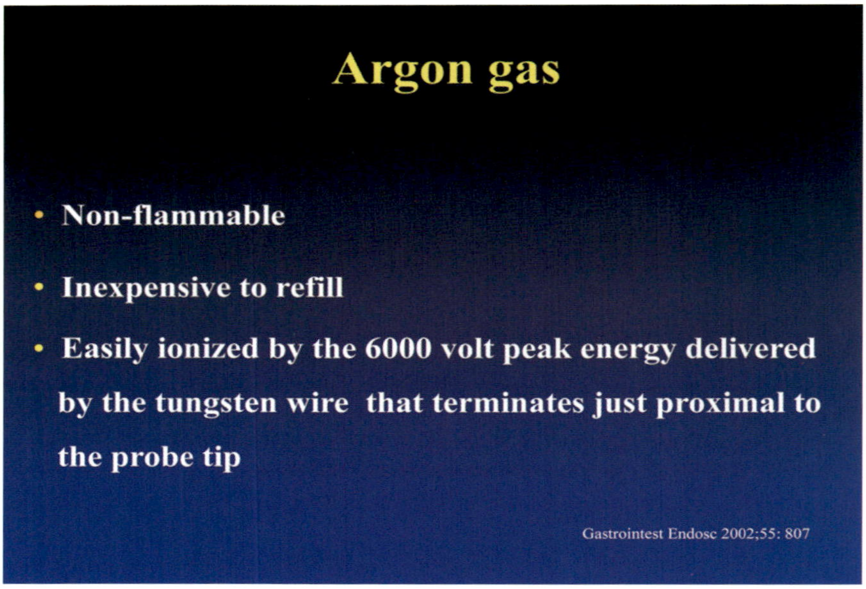

Argon gas is non-flammable gas, inexpensive to refill and easily ionized by the 6000 volt peak energy delivered by the tungsten wire that terminates just proximal to the probe tip.

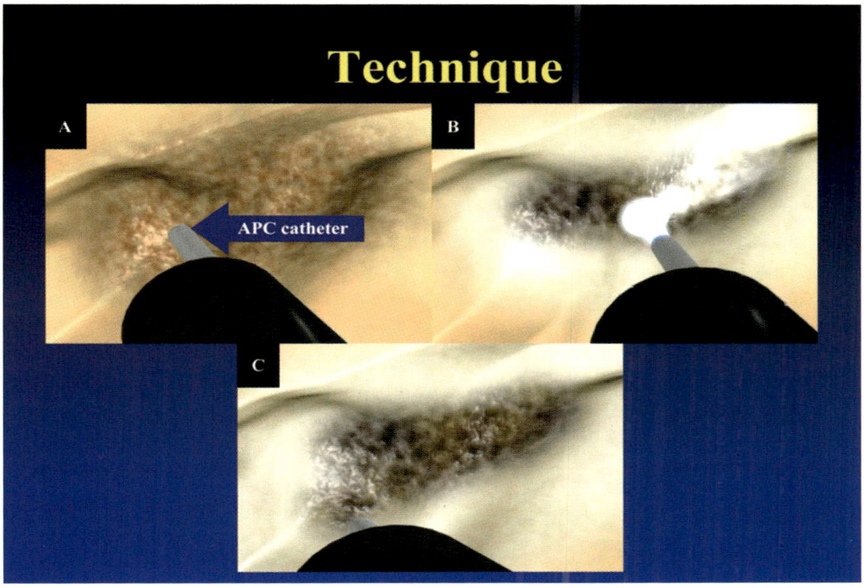

Under direct endoscopic visualization of the target lesion. The APC catheter is inserted through working channel of endoscope (figure A). The operative distance between probe and tissue ranges from 2 to 8 mm (figure B). Direct contact with the tissue should be avoided. The surface of the targeted tissue should be free of liquid (including blood). If the surface is not clear, a coagulated film develops leaving the tissue surface beneath inadequately treated. Deep thermal injury will allow argon gas to flow into the submucosa producing pneumatosis and even extraintestinal gas. The dissected gas usually resorbes rapidly.

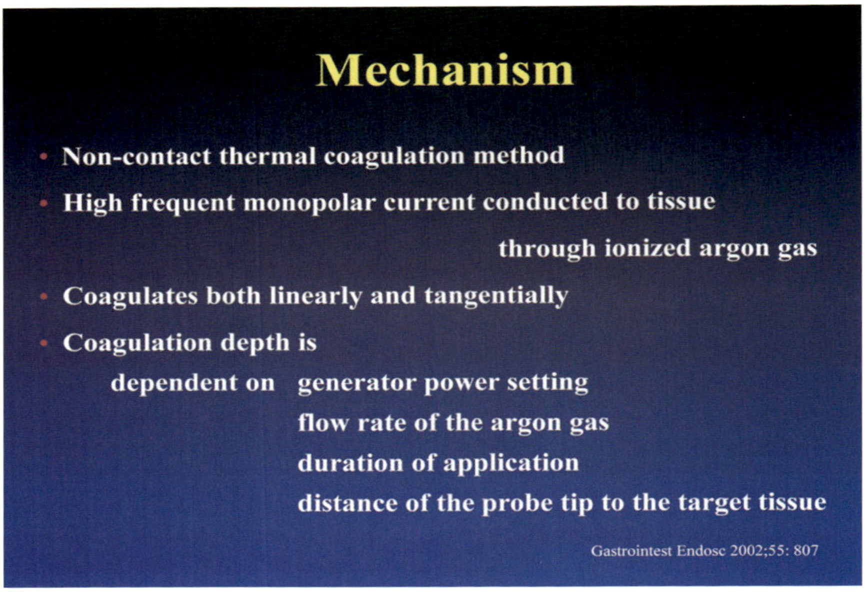

APC is non-contact thermal coagulation method that uses high-frequency monopolar current conducted to target tissues through ionized argon gas. APC coagulates both linearly and tangentially. Coagulation depth is dependent on the generator power setting, flow rate of the argon gas, duration of application, distance of the probe tip to the target tissue.

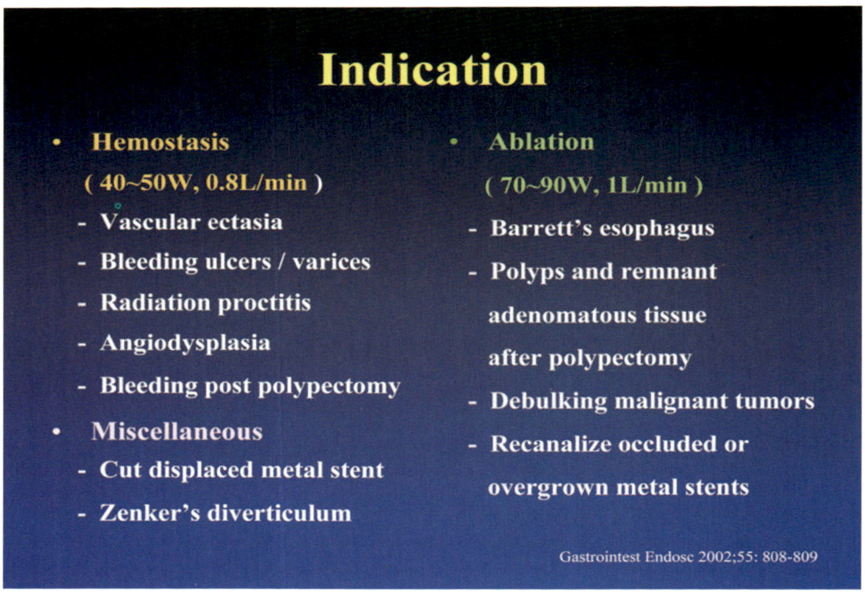

Argon plasma coagulation is used for hemostasis, ablation of Barrett' s esophagus, polyp or remnant adenomatous tissue after polypectomy, debulking malignant tumors, recanalization of occluded or overgrown metal stent and cutting of displaced metal stent or zenker' s diverticulum.

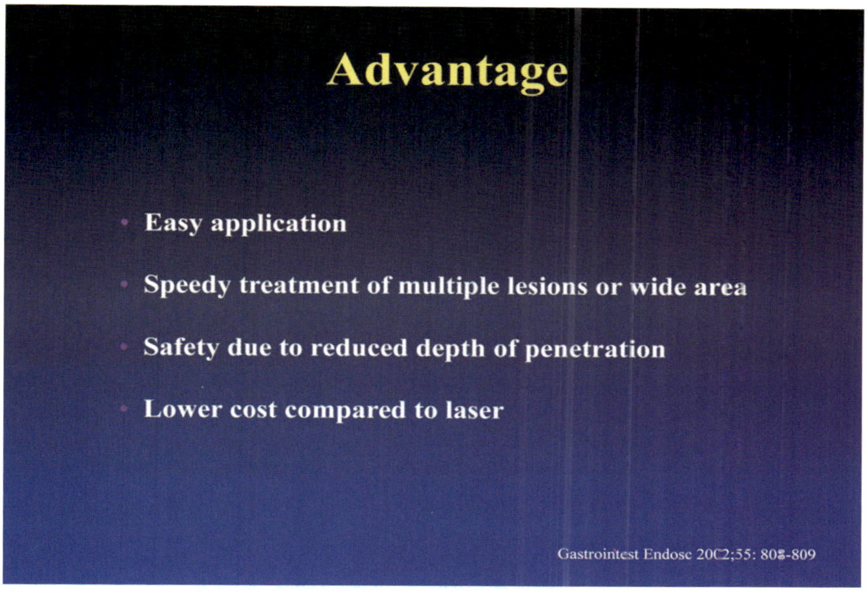

The advantages of APC are easy application, speedy treatment of multiple lesions or wide area, safety due to reduced depth of penetration, lower cost compared to laser.

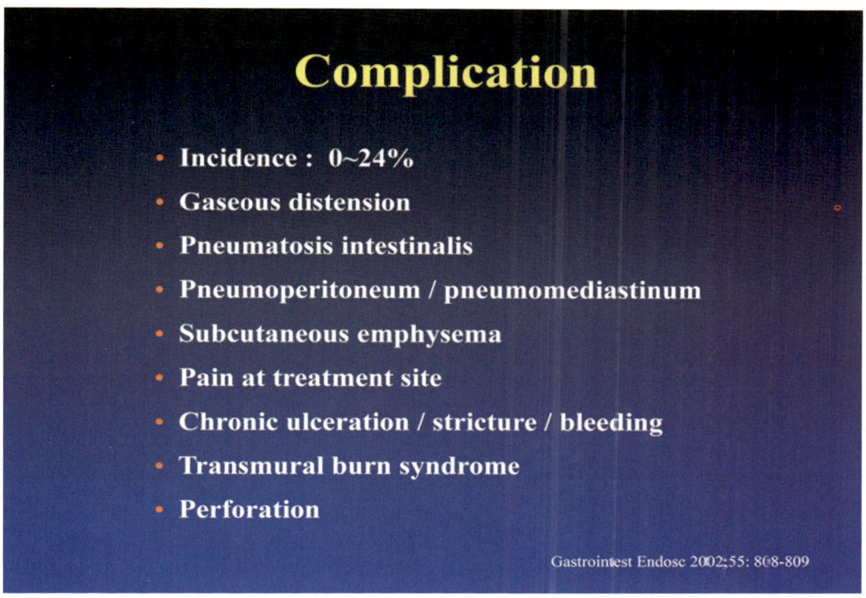

Reported complication rates range from 0% to 24% and include gaseous distension, pneumatosis intestinalis, pneumoperitoneum, pneumomediastinum, subcutaneous emphysema, pain at the treatment site, chronic ulceration, stricture, bleeding, transmural burn syndrome, perforation.

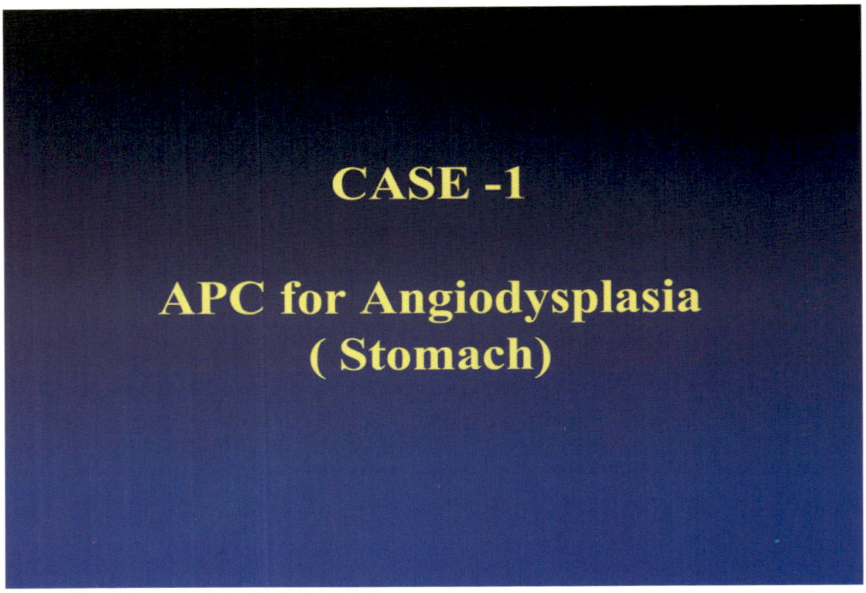

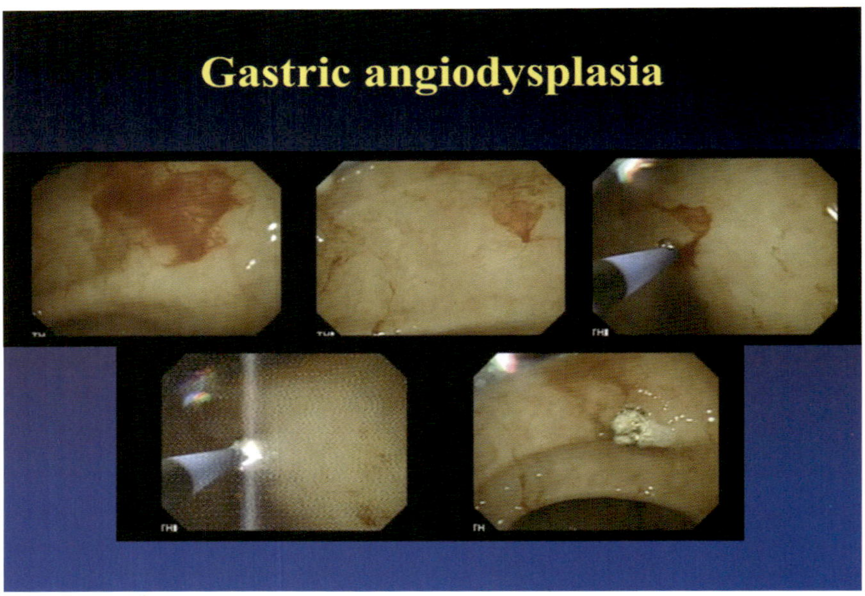

In this patent APC was performed on actively bleeding angiodysplasia of the stomach.

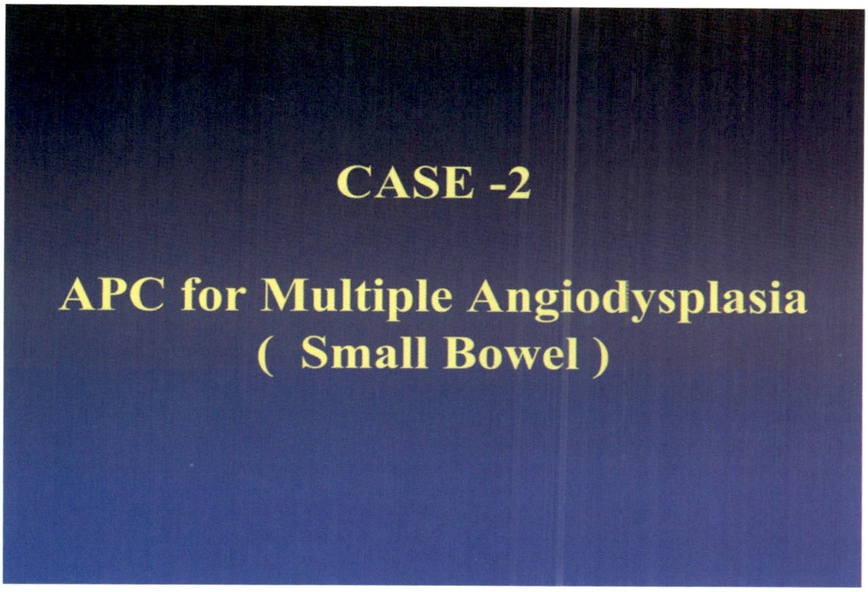

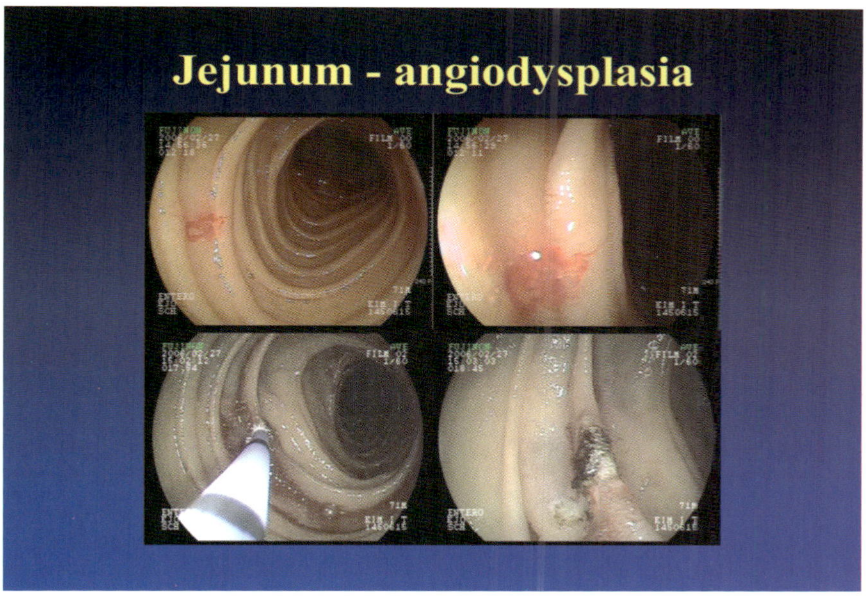

This is a 71 year old male complaining of melena. Conventional upper and lower endoscopy was unrevealing. Enteroscopy was performed and angiodysplasia was observed at the proximal jejunum. APC were used for treatments.

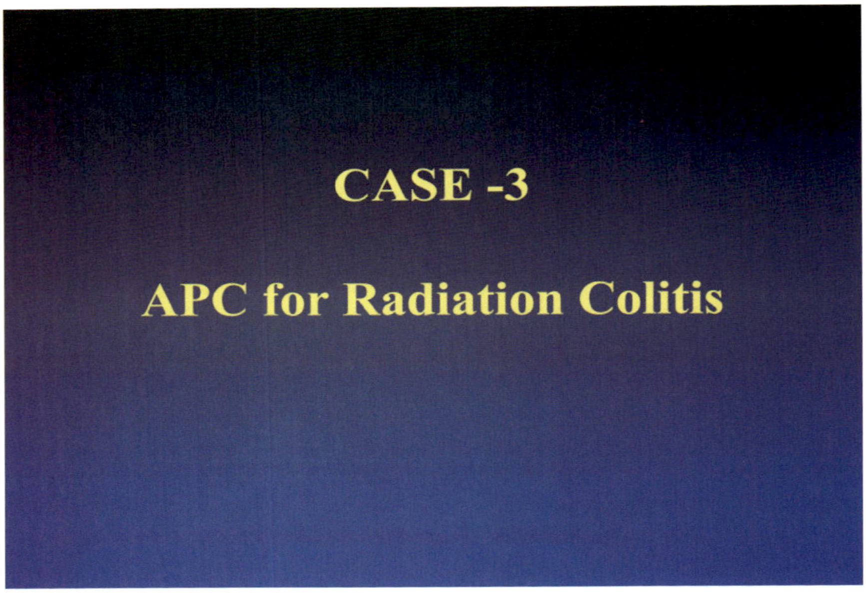

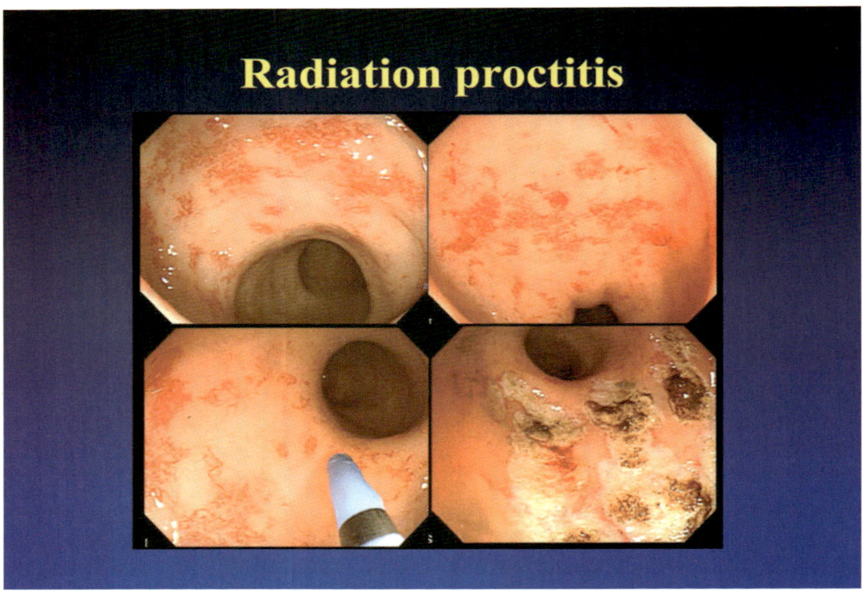

This is a 72-year-old female complaining of hematochezia. She had a past history of radiation therapy for cervical cancer. On colonoscopy diffuse and multiple angiodysplasia lesions were seen in the rectum APC was performed (flow 2L, 50W)

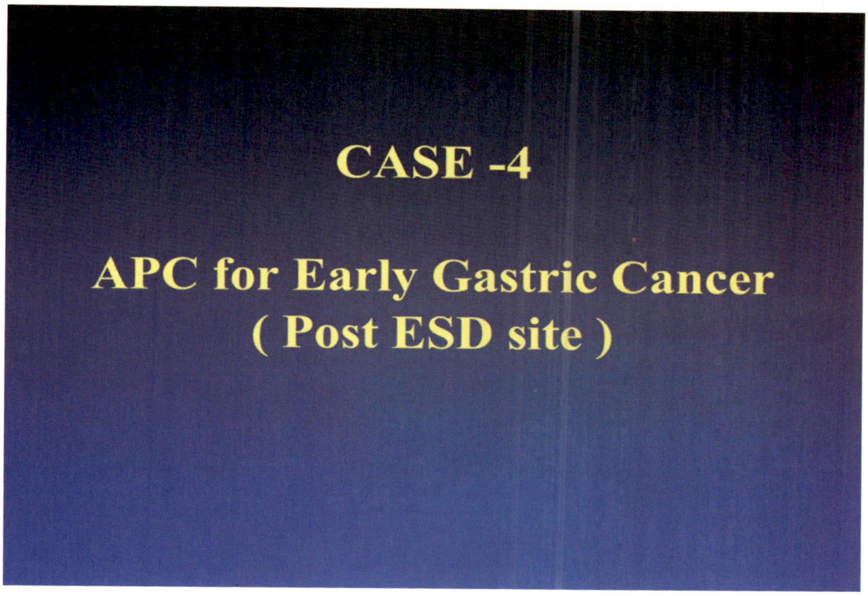

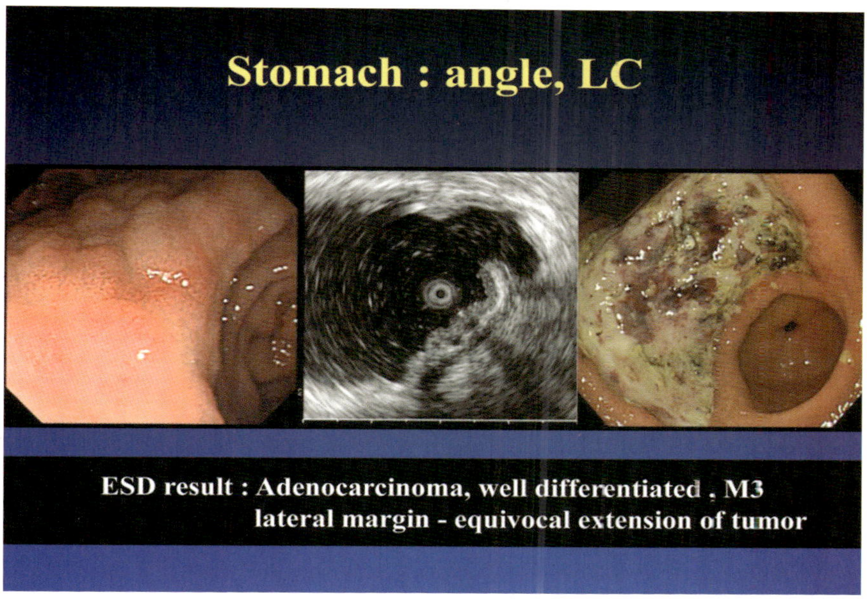

ESD was performed on this patient for EGC on the lesser curvature. Final pathologic result was adenocarcinoma, well differentiated, M3 and lateral margin was equivocal extension of tumor.

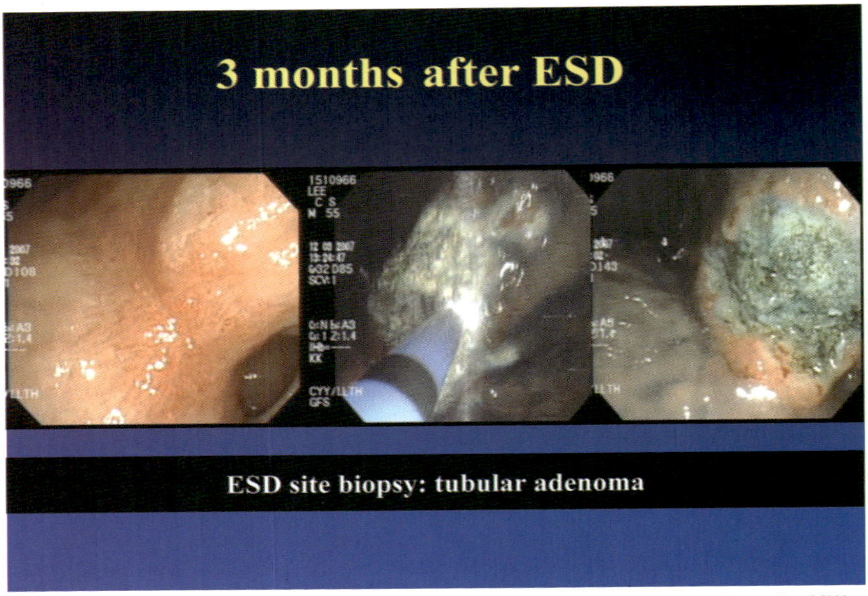

3 months after ESD, biopsies from the scar showed tubular adenoma. APC was performed at 80W.

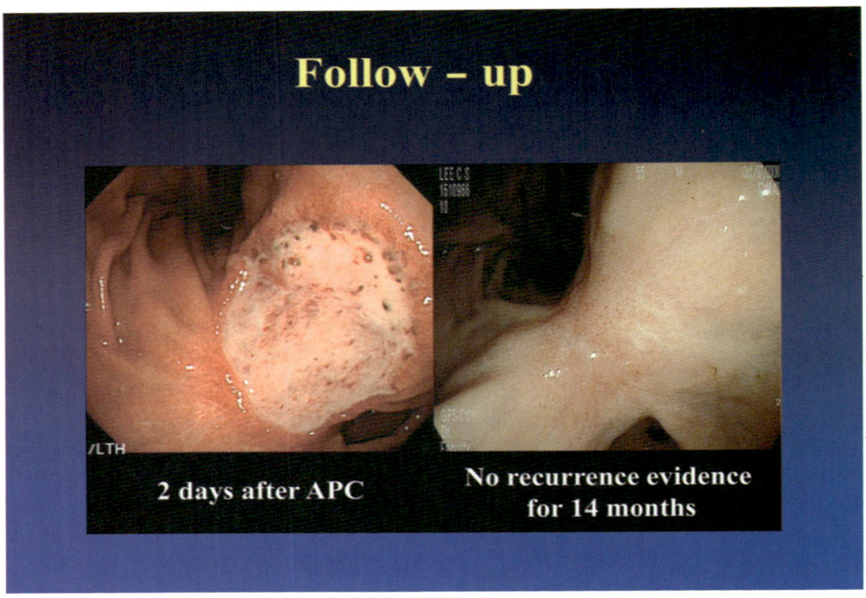

After 2 days, a post APC ulcer is seen on endoscopy. No recurrence was discovered during 14 months of follow up.

APC for Hemostasis

Reference	Patients (n)	Study disease	Major Complication	Session	Recurrence	F/U Period
Probst A et al (2001)	17	GAVE	NR	1~4	5 (29.4%)	30.4 months
Rolachon A et al Kaassis M et al Tam W et al (2000) Siliva RA et al Fantin AC et al (1999)	78	Radiation Proctitis	• Anorectal pain (2.5%) • Chronic rectal ulcer (2.5%) • Stricture (2.5%)	NR	5 (6.4%)	8~28 months
Cipolletaa L et al (1998)	21 : APC 20 :heater probe	Bleeding ulcer	• No major Cx • gastrointestinal distension (14%)	NR	3 (15%) vs 4 (21%)	NR
Nakamura S et al (2001)	30 : APC after ligation 30 : ligation only	Bleedng varix 1.5~2L 50~60W	• Pyrexia	2.9	8 (25.8%) vs 15 (50.4%)	18.5 months

GAVE: gastric antral vascular ectasia syndrome, Cx; complication, NR; not reported

These reports show the results of APC for hemostasis of several bleeding lesions. The overall rates of recurrence bleeding ranging from 6.4% to 25.8% and the median follow up period ranging 8~30 months. These results show that APC is safe and effective for patients with gastrointestinal bleeding.

APC for Barrett's Esophagus

Reference	Patients (n)	Length BE (cm)/grade	APC power & gas flow	Cx	CR recurrence	F/U Period
Madisch A et al (2005)	66	Mean 4cm (range:1~12cm)/ IM	90W 2L/min	NR	NR 3% / year	51 months
Pagani M et al (2003)	78	0.5~9cm / IM	60W 2L/min	1 stricture	72.34% NR	31.9 months
Pereira-Lima JC et al (2000)	33	Mean 4.05cm (range: 0.5~7cm) / 18 IM 14 LGD 1 HGD	65~70W 2L/min	5 pleural effusion 3 stricture	97% 3%	10.6 months
Attwood SE et al (2003)	29	HGD	70W 2L/min	1 perforation	76% NR	37 months

BE; Barrett's esophagus, IM; Intestinal metaplasia, LGD; low-grade dysplasia, HGD; high-grade dysplasia, Cx; complication, CR; complete response, NR; not reported

These reports show the results of APC for Barrett' s esophagus with/without dysplasia. Complete remission was 76% to 97% and the median follow up was 10.6~51 months. These results show that APC is safe and effective for Barrett' s esophagus.

APC for Colonic Polyps

Reference	Patients (n)	Study disease	APC power & gas flow	Complication	Complete response	F/U Period
Zlatanic J et al (1999)	30	Polyps and remnant adenomatous tissue after polypectomy	40W 0.8L/min	• Bleeding (16%) • Perforation (3.3%)	50% after 1 session 100% after 2 session	5.5~7.1 months
Brooker JC et al (2002)	21	Large, sessile colonic polyp after piecemeal resection 10 : APC 11 : no APC	45~55W 2L/min	1 : abdominal pain with minor rectal bleeding	APC group : 90% No APC group : 63.6%	12 months

These reports show the results of APC following colon polypectomy. The recurrence rate was substantially lower in patients who underwent APC after polypectomy. In patient with apparent complete endoscopic snare resection of large adenomas, APC may reduce recurrence.

APC for Early Gastrointestinal Malignancy

Reference	Patients (n)	Cancer type	APC power & Gas flow	Cx	Recurrence	F/U Period
Kitamura T et al (2006)	40	EGC Intestinal type 37 Duffuse type 3	60W 2L	4 (7.5%) - Perforation - Bleeiding - Subcutanetous emphysema	4 (10%)	52.4 months
Sagawa T et al (2003)	27	EGC Intramucosal invasion	60W 2L	No serious Cx	1 (3.7%)	30 months
Kawada K et al (2007)	48	Superficial esophageal squamous cell caricnoma	60W 2L	No major complication (No bleeding, perforation, stenosis)	NR	46 months
Nomura T et al (2007)	10	Superficial esophageal squamous cell carcinoma	60W 2L	No major complication (No bleeding, perforation, stenosis)	2 (20%) →0% after 2nd APC	28 months

EGC; Early gastric cancer, SCC ; Squamous cell carcinoma, Cx; complication, CR; complete response, NR; not reported

These reports show the results of APC for early gastrointestinal malignancy. APC was effective in both early gastric and early squamous esophageal cancer but the results were inferior to EMR and ESD. Therefore APC should be limited to cases of early cancer without metastasis in which EMR/ESD or operation has been deemed difficult.

APC for Advanced Gastrointestinal Malignancy

Reference	Patients (n)	Cancer type	APC power & gas flow	Complication	Recanalization rate	F/U Period
Hiendorff H et al (1998)	83	Cancer of Esophagus or Cardia	NR 2L	Perforation 7 (8%)	48 (57.8%) → 70 (84.3%) after 2nd APC	5.2 months
Dallal HJ et al (2001)	34 (repeated TTA) vs 31 (Stent)	Advanced esophageal cancer	50~65W NR	Perforation 2 (5.8%) T-E fistula 3 (8.8%) Septicemia 1 (2.9%)	79.4%	125 days vs 68 days

TAT ; thermal tumor ablation (Nd-YAG laser, argon diode laser, Argon plasma coagulation), NR: not reported

These reports show the results of APC for Advanced Gastrointestinal malignancy with luminal obstruction. The overall rate of recanalization was 79~84% and major complications occurred in less than 10% of patients. In one study patients treated by APC lived longer than patients with stent insertion.

Thermal ablation therapy

Radiofrequency Ablation

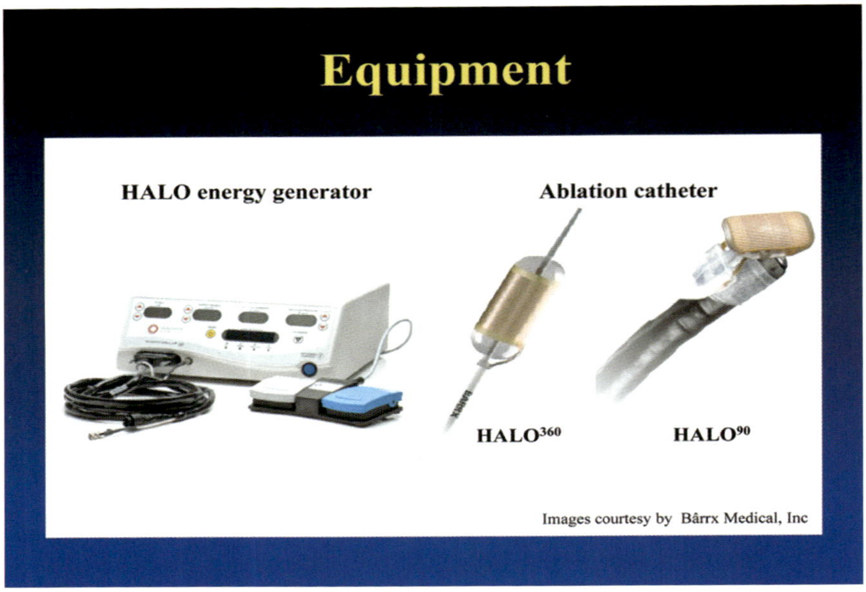

Components for Radiofrequency ablation are the HALO energy generator and the HALO 90 and 360 ablation catheters. The Halo 360 system uses a circumferential balloon ablation technique whereas the Halo 90 system can be used for focal ablation.

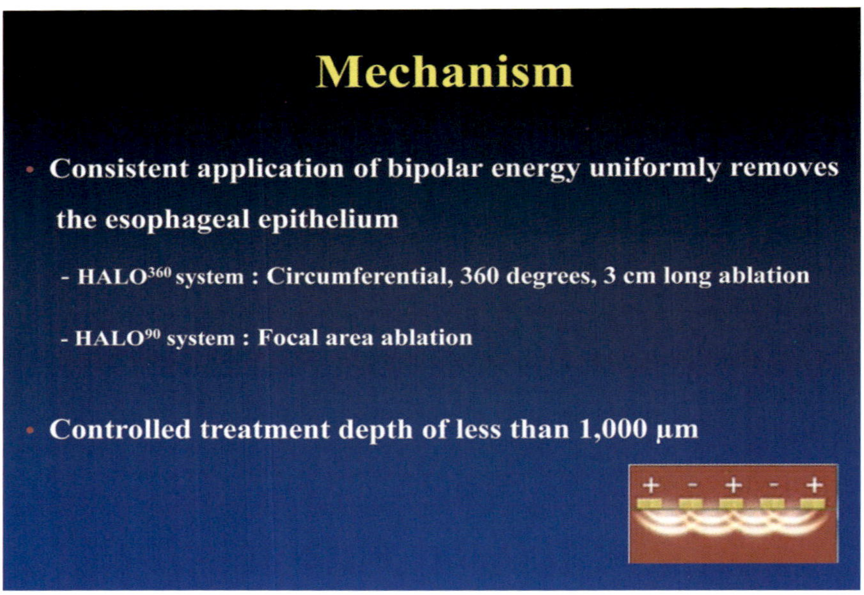

Consistent application of bipolar energy uniformly removes the esophageal epithelium, reducing potential for buried glands and improving patient tolerability. Bipolar electrode array geometry precisely controls the depth of ablation to < 1 mm.

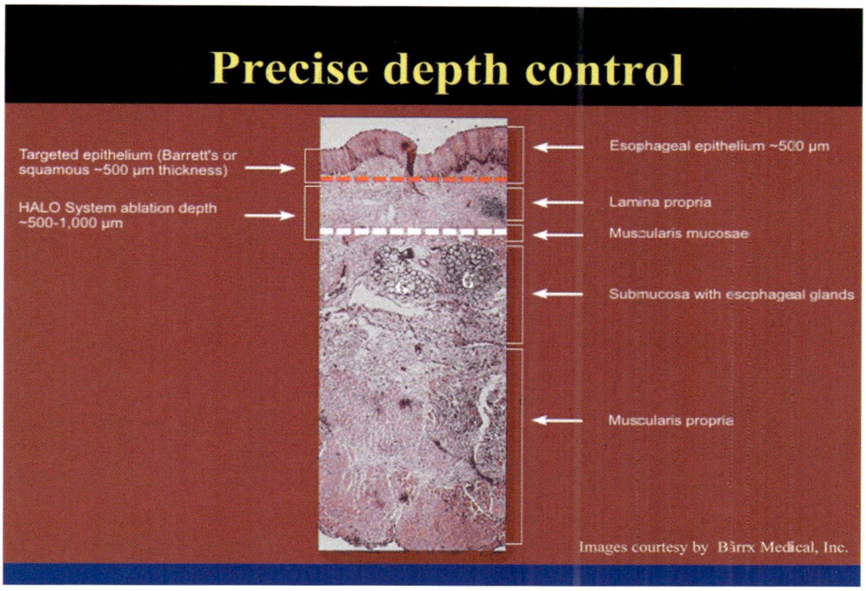

Barrett's epithelium is approximately 500 mm in thickness. The HALO energy generator and the HALO ablation catheter electrode array are designed to work in concert to achieve a uniform, superficial depth of ablation of ~1,000 mm. The therapeutic depth is limited to the muscularis mucosa with preservation of the submucosa.

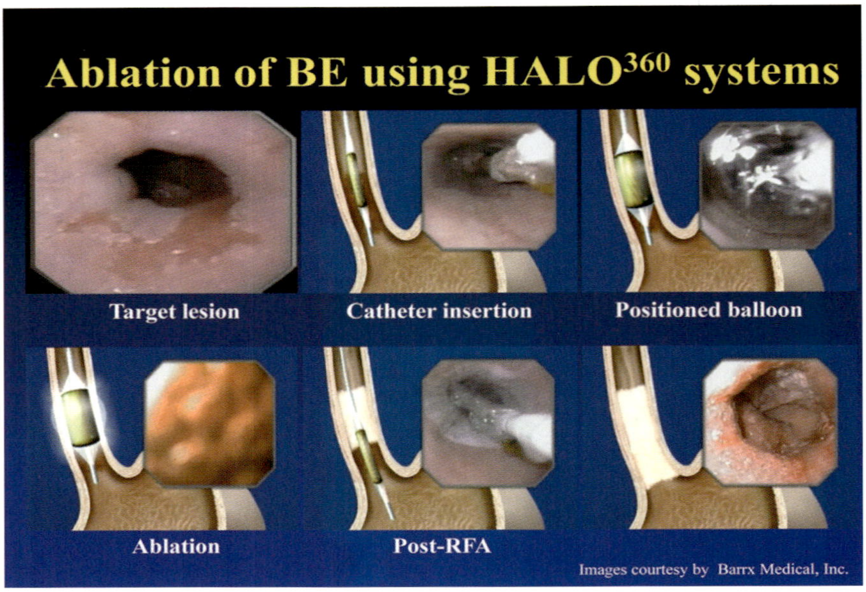

A sizing balloon is used to measure the inner diameter of the esophagus to select the appropriately sized ablation catheter. The sizing balloon is then removed and the treatment or HALO 360 ablation catheter is inserted. A HALO 360 ablation catheter is inflated within the area of the barrett' s tissue. This balloon is covered by a band of radiofrequency electrodes. The HALO 360 energy generator and the ablation catheter then work together to deliver a short burst of energy. This HALO 360 system ablate circumferentially, a 360 degrees, 3 cm long segment of Barrett' s tissue in ← 1 second. The result is uniformly ablated Barrett' s epithelium. The consistent ablation depth of ←1mm avoids damage to the underlying tissue layers.

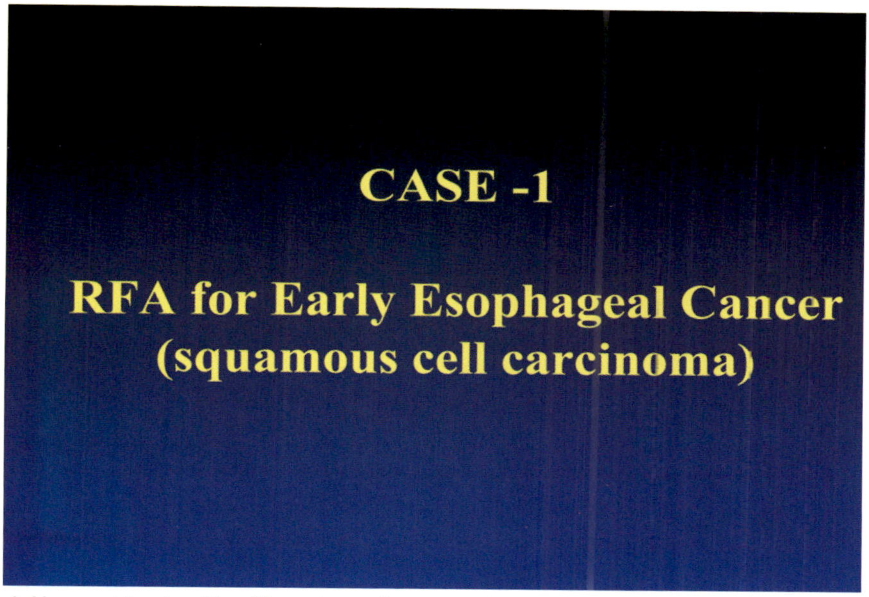

A 66-year-old male with a 35 mm large, flat-type early esophageal squamous cell cancer with surrounding high grade dysplasia.

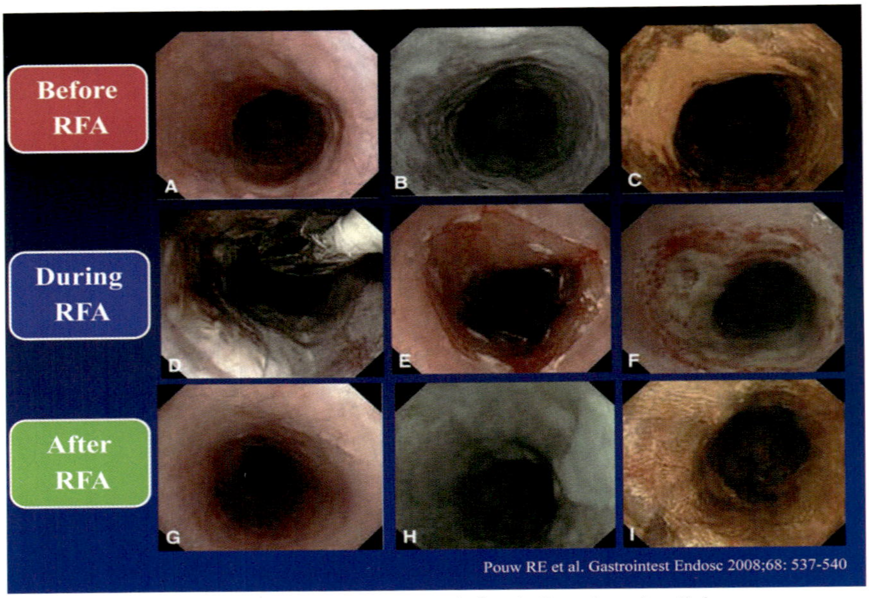

Figure 1. Endoscopic images before, during, and after balloon-based radiofrequency energy ablation of a widespread early squamous cell carcinoma and High-grade dysplasia of the esophagus. (A) A reddish, rough-appearing mucosal lesion between the 8 and 1 o'clock positions in the endoscopic view. (B) Narrow-band imaging revealed abnormal intrapapillary capillary loops. (C) The lesion is clearly demarcated as an unstained lesion on Lugol's chromoendoscopy. (D) Treatment effect immediately after the first balloon-based RF energy ablation. (E) After the second ablation passed, a 3 cm-long circumferentially ablated segment is seen. (F) Confluent superficial necrosis, without deep ulcerations or bleeding, 3 days after treatment. (G, H, I) Four months after treatment, a normal-appearing squamous esophagus is seen on high-resolution white-light endoscopy and narrow-band imaging, and no unstained lesions are seen after Lugol's chromoendoscopy.

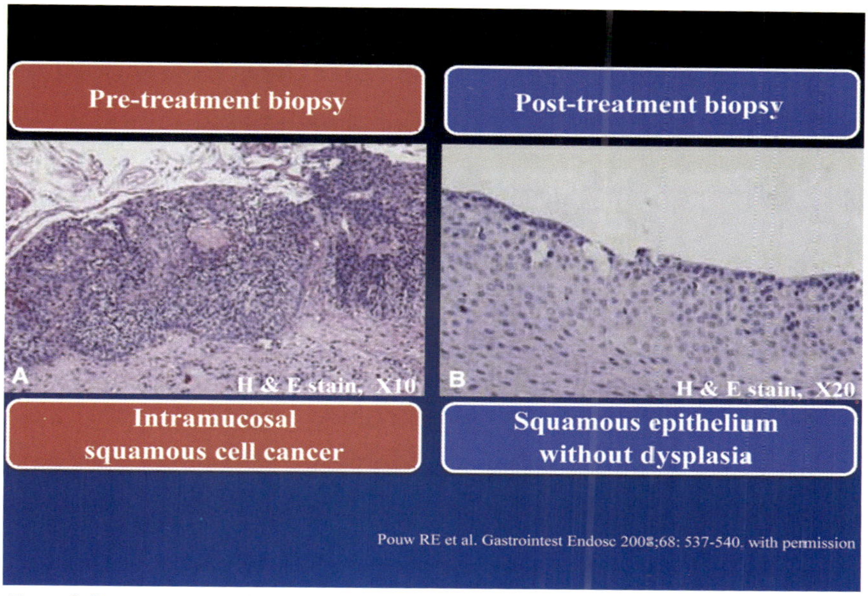

Figure 2. Pre-treatment and post-treatment histology images of a widespread early squamous cell carcinoma and HGD of the esophagus, treated with balloon-based RF energy ablation. (A) Pre-treatment biopsy (H&E, orig. mag. ×10) showing an intramucosal squamous cell cancer limited to the epithelial layer (M1). (B) Post-treatment biopsy (H&E, orig. mag. ×20) showing squamous epithelium without dysplastic changes.

RFA of Barrett's Esophagus

Reference	Patients (n)	Study device	Histology	Major Cx	Session	CR	F/U
Sharma VK et al (2008)	100	$HALO^{360}$	BE without dysplasia	No stenosis No buried glandular mucosa	1.5	70%	1 year
Fleischer DE et al (2008)	70	$HALO^{360}$ $HALO^{90}$	AC (83.2%) SCC (15.3%)	No stenosis No buried glandular mucosa	1.5 3.4	70% 98%	1 yaer 2.5 year

Cx; complication, CR; complete response, F/U; follow up, BE; Barrett's esophagus

These reports show the results of endoscopic radiofrequency ablation of Barrett's esophagus. At 1 year, a CR for BE was achieved in 70% of patients. Stepwise circumferential and focal ablation resulted in complete eradication in 98% of patients at 2.5-year follow-up. RFA of nondysplastic BE can be performed with no subsequent strictures or buried glands and with complete elimination of BE up to 98% at 2.5-year follow-up.

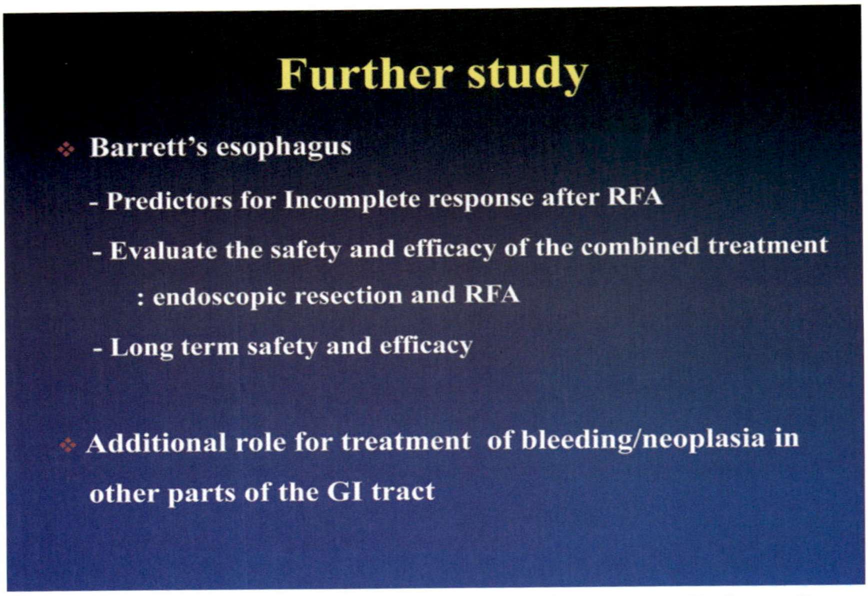

RFA has been used effectively for the treatment of Barrett' s esophagus. Further studies on predictors for incomplete response, the safety/efficacy of the combined treatment and long term safety/efficacy are needed as well as evaluation of the additional role for treatment of bleeding/neoplasia in other parts of the GI tract.

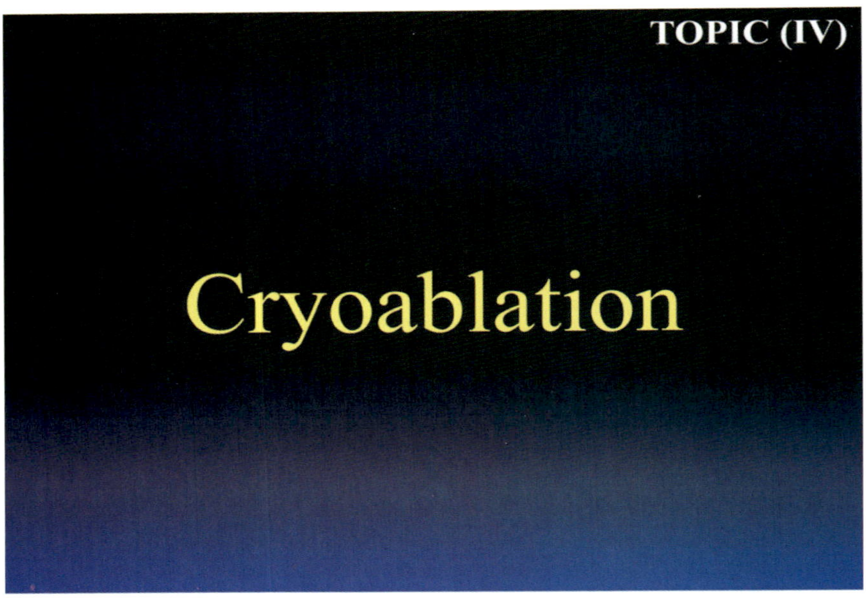

Cryoablation using liquid nitrogen sprayed through a low pressure device has recently been described to be effective and safe in the treatment of Barrett's esophagus including high-grade dysplasia.

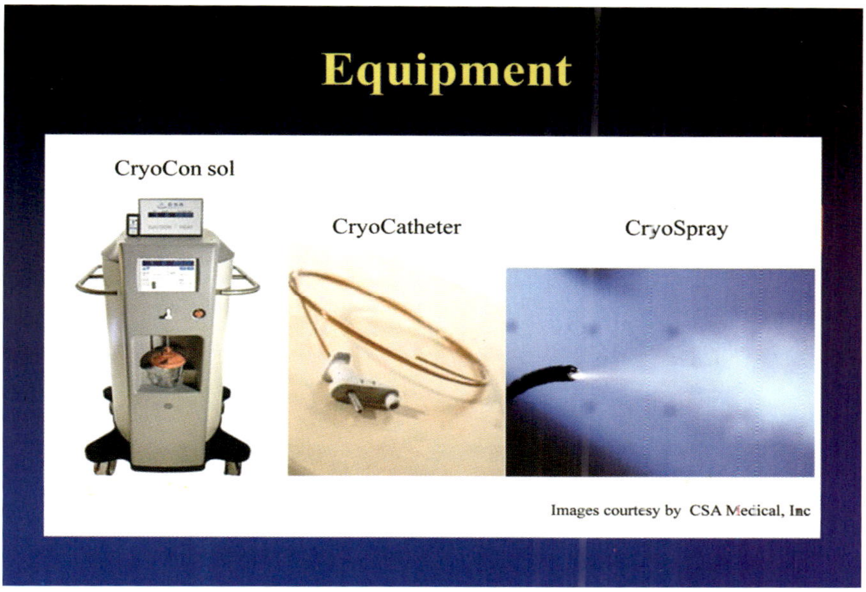

Cryoablation therapy is one of the newer ablative techniques. It is a low pressure system using liquid nitrogen spray. The components of the low-pressure spray cryoablation device are a liquid nitrogen tank, an electronic con sol for monitoring and control of cryogen release, a dual foot pedal for control of cryogen release and heating of the catheter, and a multi-layered 7-9 F open-tipped catheter for spraying super-cold nitrogen gas through an upper endoscope.

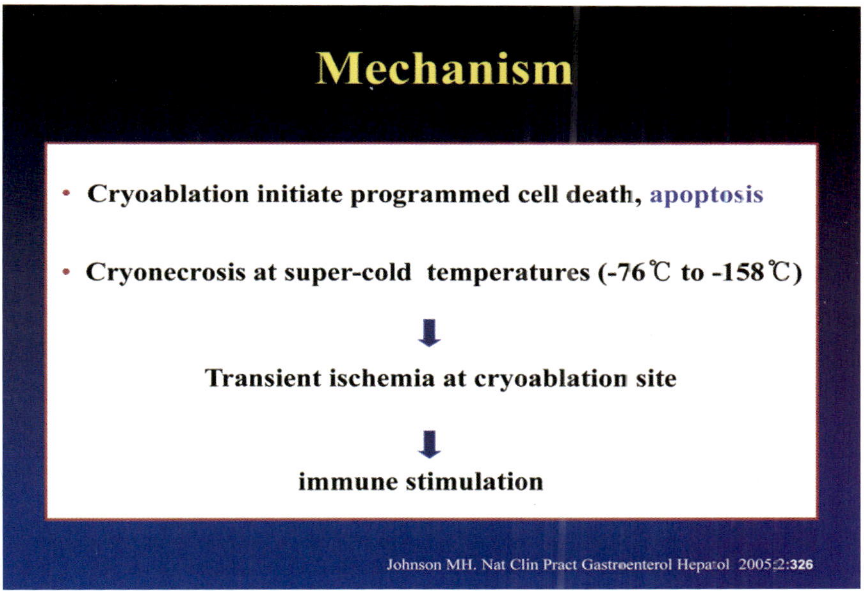

The mechanism of action underlying the injury caused by cryoablation is unique for an ablative technique. Cryoablation induces apoptosis and causes cryonecrosis at super-cold temperatures (-76 ° C to -158 ° C), which results in transient ischemia at the cryoablation site and can cause immune stimulation.

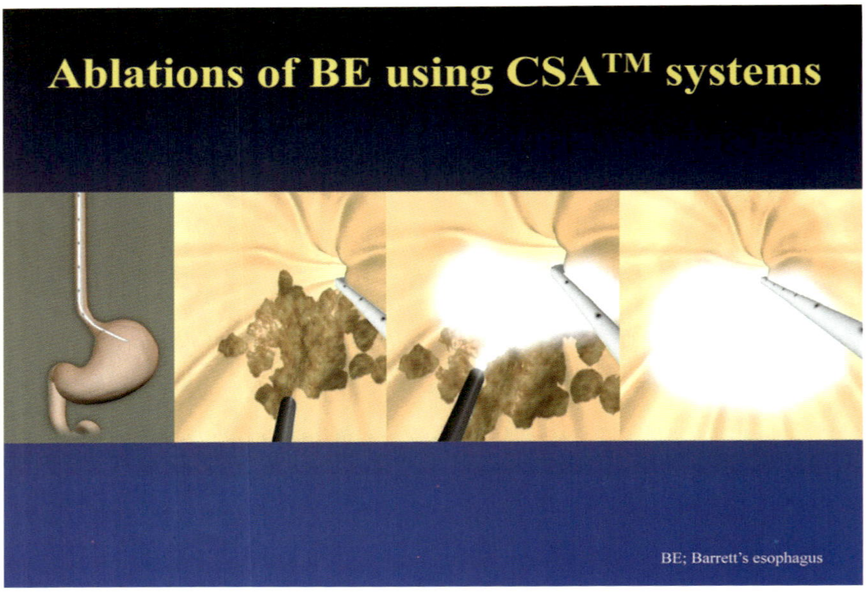

After endoscopic confirmation of the target lesion the endoscope is removed, and a modified orogastric tube is inserted to evacuate gas. After cryodecompression the cryospray catheter is inserted through the working channel of the endoscope and it is advanced to the targeted treatment area. Liquid nitrogen enters the catheter at low pressure and freezes the tissue upon contact. After Cryogen flow is discontinued the treatment area is allowed to thaw and reperfuse followed by a repeated cycle of cyroablation is performed.

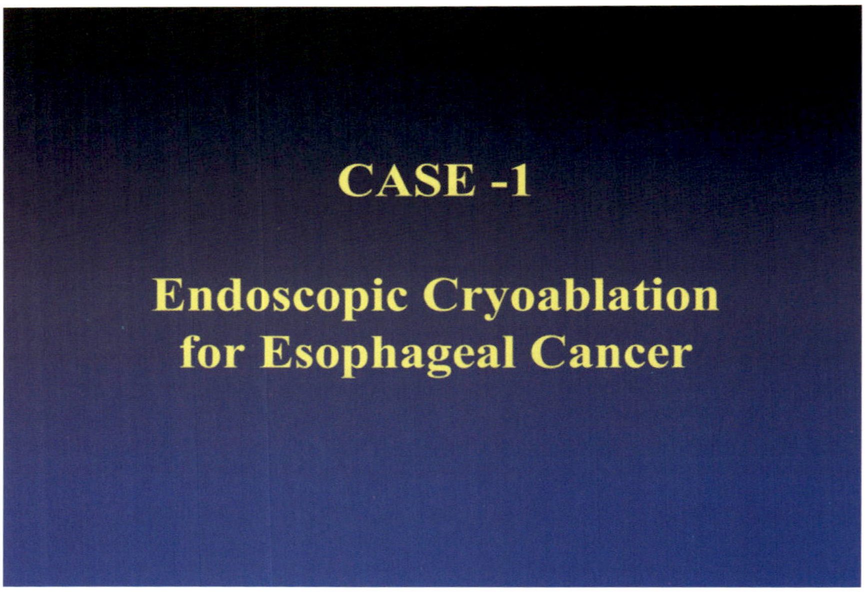

This case report describes the cryoablation in a patient with recurrent esophageal cancer for palliative treatment that has resulted in complete remission for 2 years.

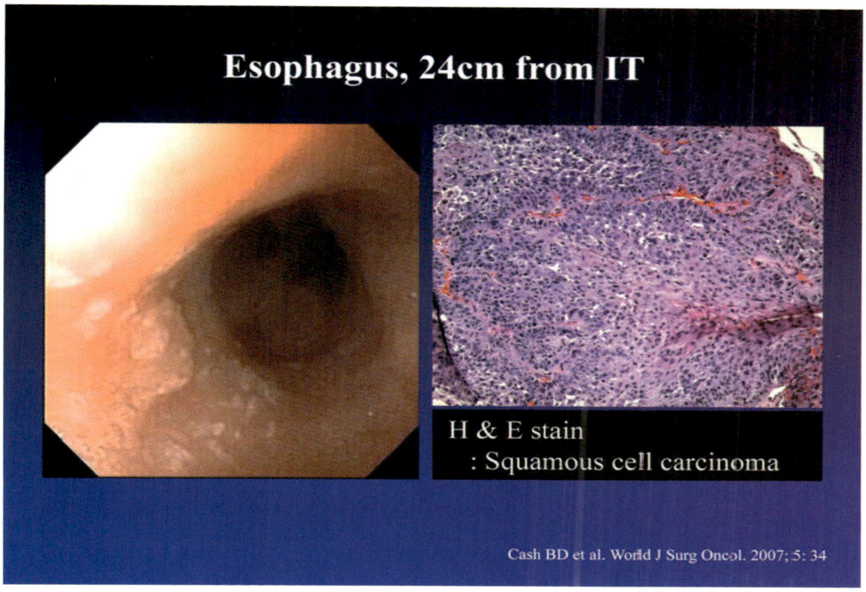

A 73-year-old African American male with history of squamous cell carcinoma (SCCA) of the esophagus treated with radiotherapy. On presentation, a new lesion at 24 cm was discovered and biopsies showed moderately differentiated SCCA. This new lesion was above the prior field of radiotherapy. The patient was deemed neither a surgical nor RT candidate based on significant cardiac comorbidities and maximum dose radiation therapy with his prior treatments. Palliative treatment options were explored.

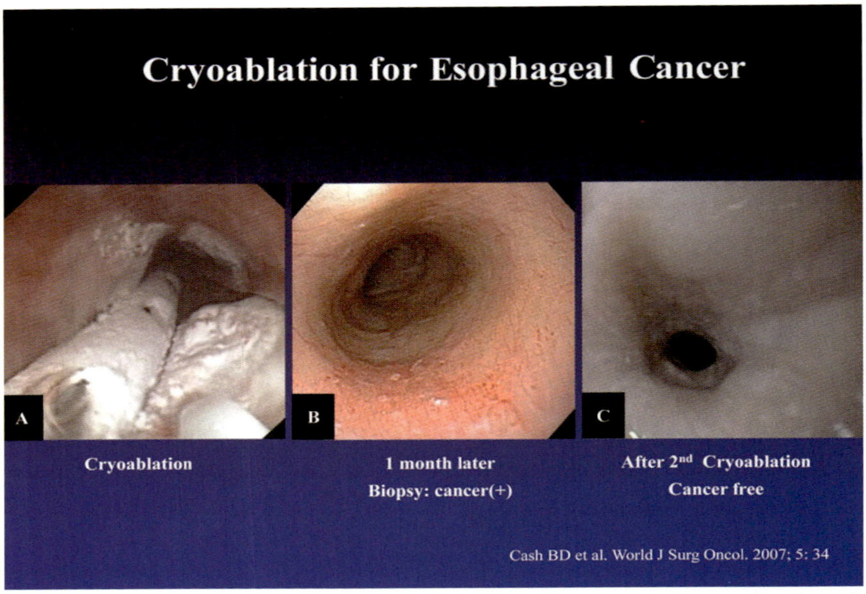

The patient's 2 cm long, hemi-circumferential SCCA was treated with two 30 seconds pulses of cryoablation under direct endoscopic visualization on an outpatient basis. Each session was separated by a 20 to 30 second thaw.

Figure A. Cryoablation of the SCCA. On the left is the cryo decompression tube. In the right for corner is the cryo catheter.

Figure B. One month latter a follow-up EGD revealed endoscopic resolution of the tumor, but biopsies remained positive for moderately differentiated SCCA.

Figure C. Fibrotic stricture which developed after the second cryospray ablation treatment. Biopsies at the cancer site 6 weeks after the second cryoablation and bimonthly in the subsequent 12 months of follow-up were completely negative for dysplasia or neoplasia.

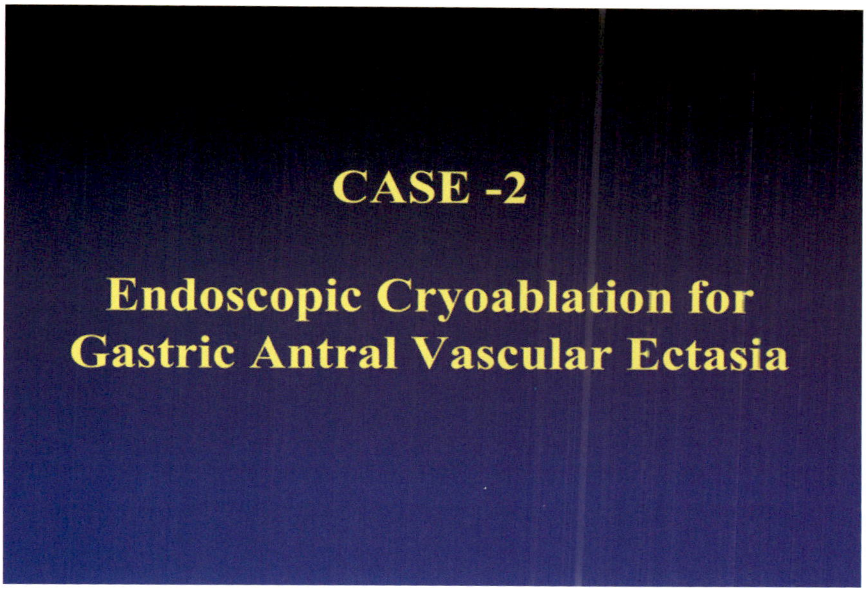

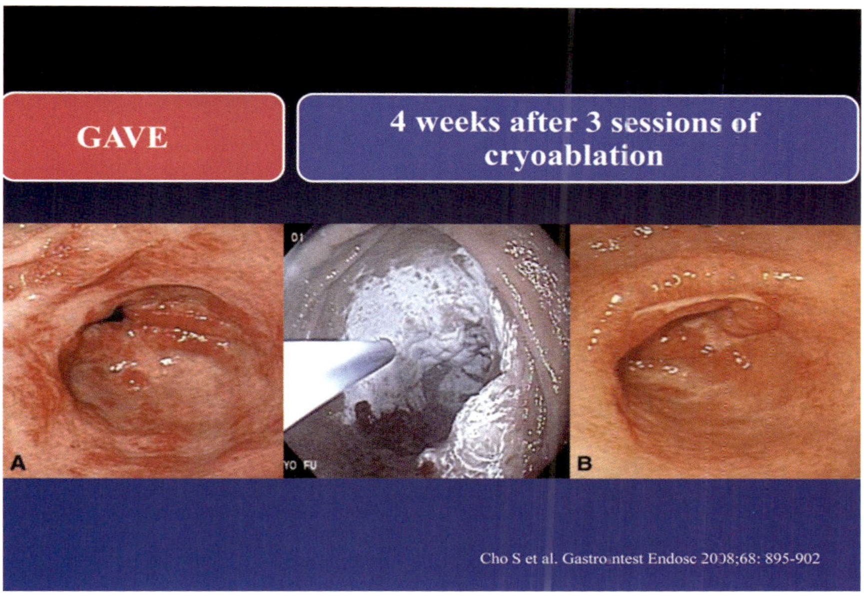

Figure 5. A, A "striped" pattern of GAVE (gastric antral vascular ectasia) in the gastric antrum before treatment with cryotherapy figure. Figure B, The same patient at a follow-up endoscopy 4 weeks after 3 sessions of cryoablation, demonstrating complete endoscopic response and associated minor scarring and superficial ulcerations.

The Outcomes of Cryoablation in BE & Esophageal Cancer

Reference	Patients (n)	Histology	Major complication	Session	Response	F/U
Johnston MH et al (2005)	11	BE 3 IFD 2 LGD 5 HGD 1	0 %	4.2 (1 ~ 8)	CR : 64%	6 months
John Dumot et al (2007, DDW)	14	AC 13 SCC 1	1: gastric perforation in patient with Marfan's syndrome	3.5	CR + PR - HGD 90% - IMC 75%	

BE; Barrett's esophagus, IFD; indefinite for dysplasia, LGD; low grade dysplasia, HGD; high grade dysplasia, AC; adenocarcinoma, SCC; squamous cell carcinoma , IMC; intramucosal cancer,, CR; complete response, PR; partial response, F/U; follow up

These reports show the results of endoscopic cryoablation therapy of Barrett' s esophagus. Based on preliminary studies, low-pressure spray cryoablation of BE under direct endoscopic visualization is safe and easy to perform. No complication occurred. It's relative risk of patient discomfort, it's simplicity and it's demonstrated efficacy make it modality that should be further explored in the ablation of GI mucosal lesion such as BE and perhaps early esophageal cancer.

TOPIC (II)

Alcohol/Chemoagent Injection Therapy

This topic will focus on the endoscopic resections that have been applied to early esophageal cancer including early neoplasia in Barrett' s esophagus.

List of Injection Agent

Injection agent	Component	Dosage
Alcohol	Ethanlol 99.5%	• 0.5~2mL/site • Weekly interval
Cisplatin / Epinephrine injectable gel	• Basis of the gel-matrix : Biocompatible, biodegradable, purified bovin collagen forms • Cisplatin 4ug/uL • 1:10,000 Epinephrine	• Cisplatin dose : 1mg/cm^3 ~ 6mg/cm^3 • Maximum total dose of cisplatin 380mg • Gel was prepared in a syringe upto 2 hours before use. • Weekly interval • Intratumoral injection : 22~25 gauge needle

Croffie J et al. Gastrointest Endosc 2007;66: 1-6
Harbord M, et al. Gastrointest Endosc 2002;55:644-551

The list of agents used for injection therapy. The cisplatin (4ug/uL) and the vasoconstrictor epinephrine (1:10,000, 0.1mg/mL) gel provides high concentrations of the cisplatin in the target area for an extended period, which maximizes local efficacy and minimizes systemic absorption and toxicity. The gel matrix flows readily through 22 to 25 gauge needles.

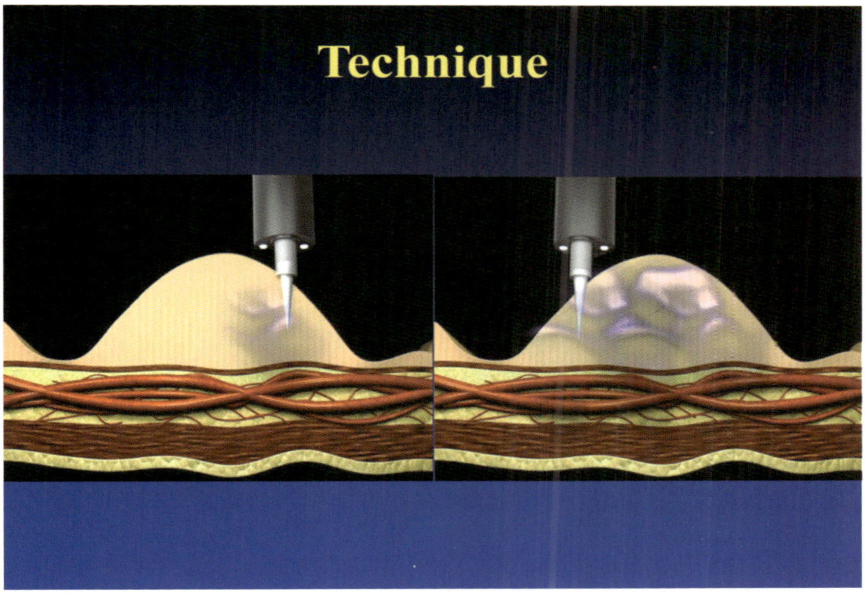

The most useful indication of injection therapy is likely to be bulky tumors in any part of the esophagus, especially where the tumor is attached predominantly to one side of the wall

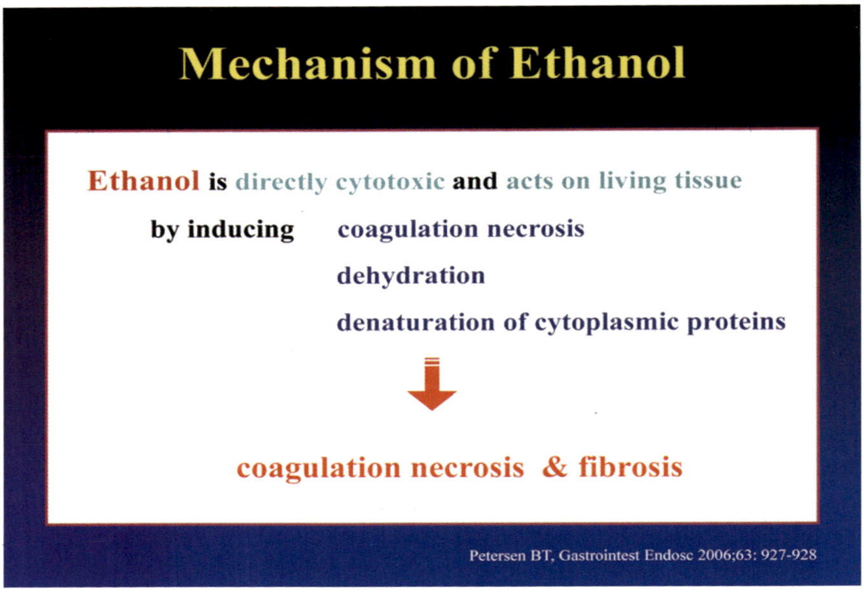

Ethanol is directly cytotoxic and acts on living tissue by inducing coagulation necrosis, dehydration, and denaturation of cytoplasmic proteins with consequent coagulation necrosis followed by fibrosis. Ethanol also enters the microcirculation and induces necrosis of endothelial cells and platelet aggregation with consequent thrombosis of small vessels, followed by ischemia of tumor tissue. Once injected alcohol can only drain away from the injection sites along lines of least resistances within the tumor or via lymphatic or blood vessels.

Alcohol/Chemoagent Injection Therapy of Advanced Esophageal Cancer with Dysphagia

Reference	Patients (n)	Disease	Injection material	Major Cx	Session	Response	Median survival
Harbord M et al (2002)	18	Advanced esophageal cancer - SCC 7 - AC 11	Cisplatin/epinephrine Injection gel - cisplatin 4ug/uL - 1:10,000 epinephrine 0.1mg/mL - maximum: 10uL for each session	1 : T-E fistula	Upto 6 injections (weekly interval)	• PR 8 (44.4%) • SD 7 (38.8%)	• <10cm^3 : 10 mo. • > 10cm^3 : 3 mo.
Monga SP et al (2000)	9	AC 13 SCC 1	Cisplatin/epinephrine Injection gel	1: gastric perforation in patient with Marfan's syndrome	3~8	Dysphagia↓ : 8	4 mo.
Güitrón A Et al (1996)	6	Advanced Esophageal cancer	Ethanol	0 %	6	Dysphagia↓ : 6	10.2 mo.

SCC; squamous cell carcinoma , AC; adenocarcinoma, T-E fistula; tracheo-esophageal fistula, Cx; complication, PR; partial response, SD; stable disease,, F/U; follow up,, mo. ; months

The aim of therapy for advanced esophageal cancer is relief of dysphagia with minimal treatment-related morbidity. Although data is limited results suggest that endoscopic injection of cisplatin/epinephrine gel or ethanol is a simple procedure that helps palliate dysphagia in patients with advanced esophageal cancer.

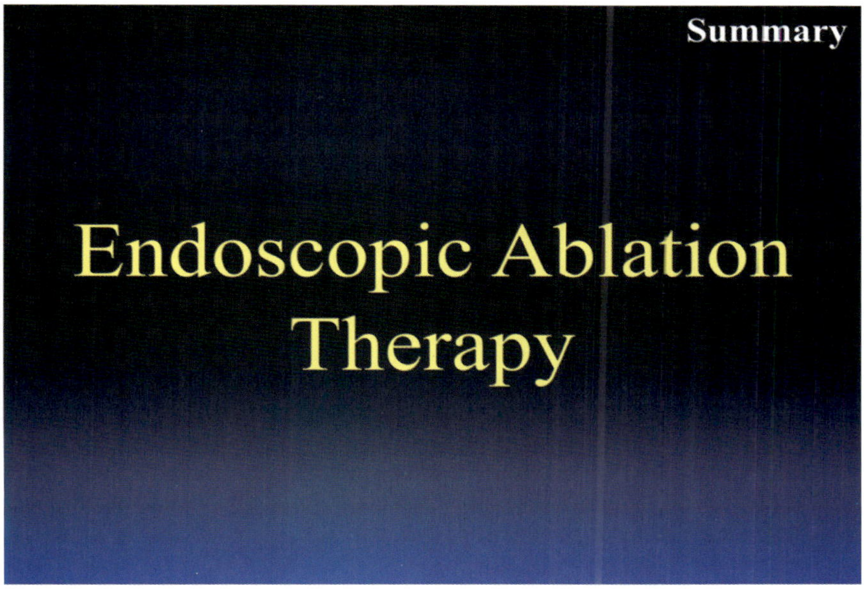

In summary, increasing numbers of early eosphageal neoplasias are being detected, so that endoscopic treatments with a curative intent play an increasing role.

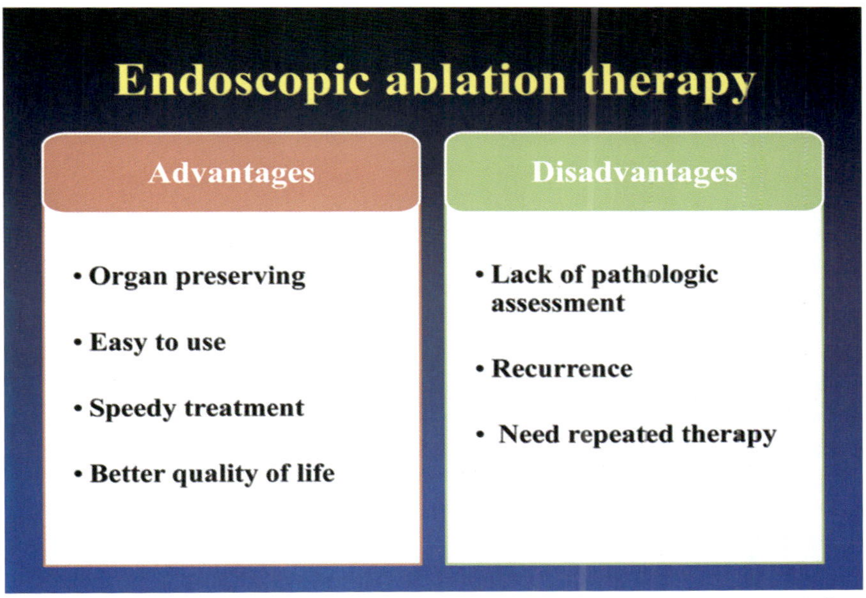

The advantages of ablation therapy are that it' s organ preserving, easy to use, a relatively fast treatment, and enables better quality of life. However, lack of pathologic assessment of the lesion, possibility of recurrence and repeated therapy are disadvantages.

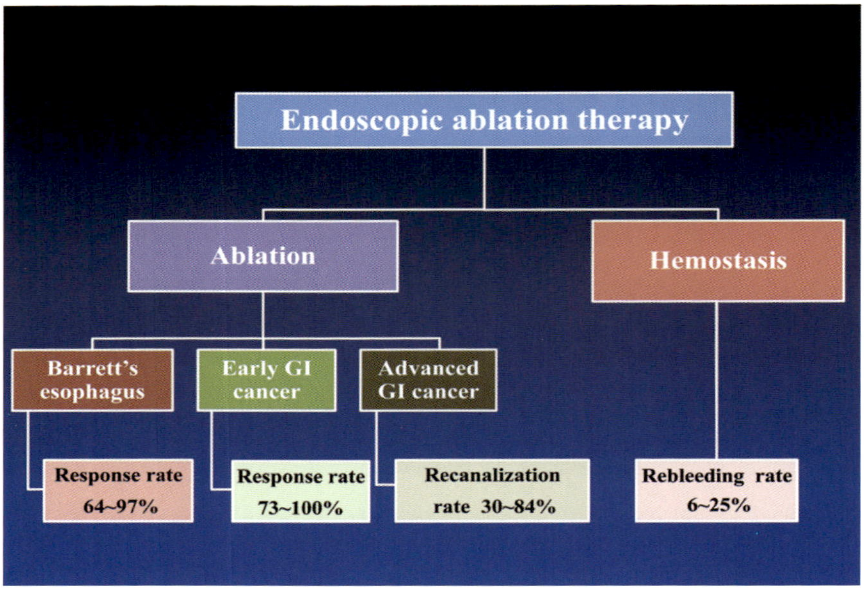

Endoscopic ablation therapy is used either for hemostasis or ablation of specific tissue. The response rates for BE, Early GI cancer are 64-97% and 73-100%. The rate of recanalization in advanced GI cancer is 30-84% and the rebleeding rate following hemostasis is 6~25%.

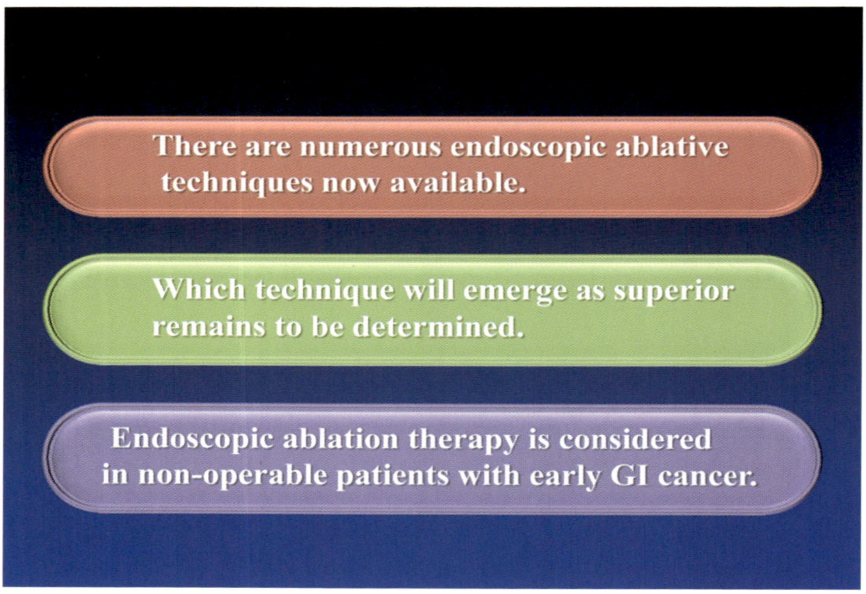

In summary, there are numerous endoscopic ablative techniques now available. Which technique will emerge as superior remains to be determined. Endoscopic ablation therapy is considered in non-operable patient with early gastrointestinal cancer.

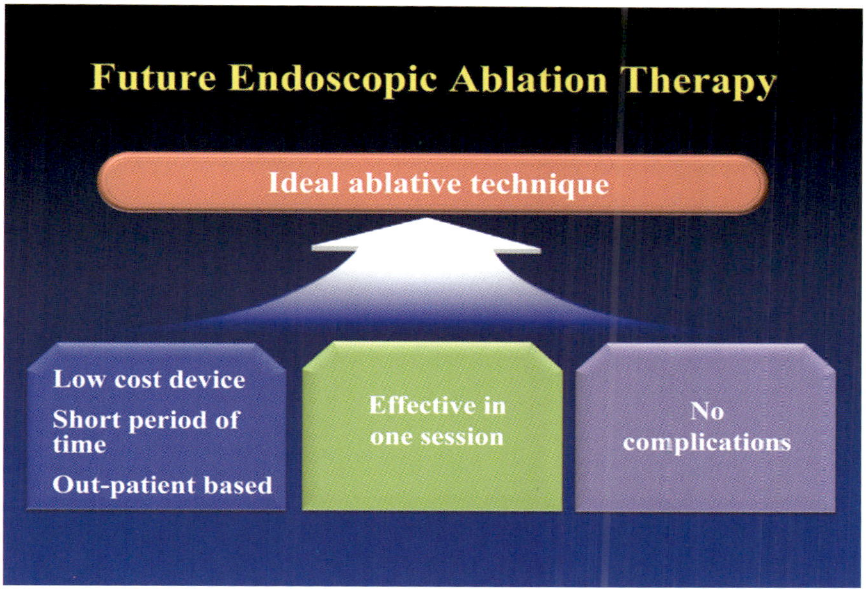

The ideal endoscopic ablation technique should be low cost, able to perform over a short period of time, out-patients based, effective in one session and have no complications.

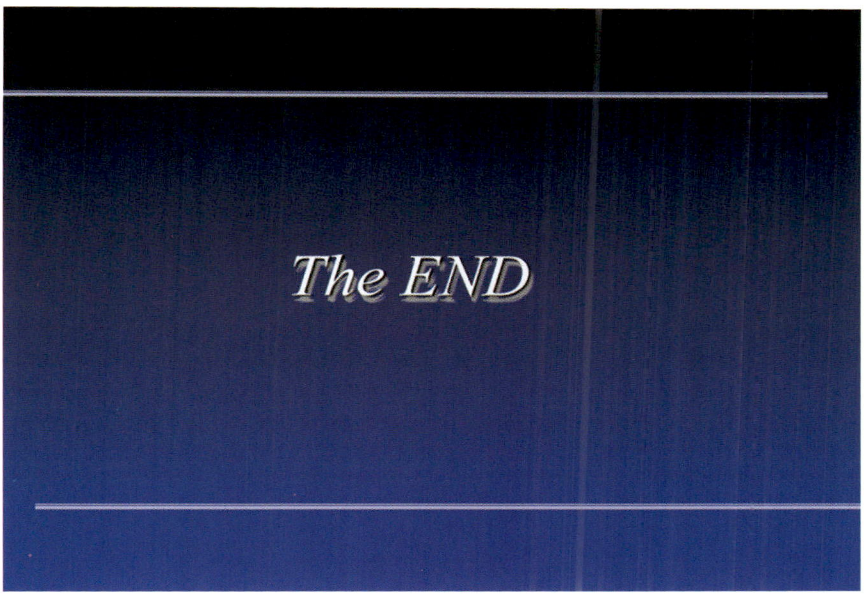

Chapter 7

Therapeutic Endoscopy for Strictures of the Upper Digestive Tract

2010 ASGE Audiovisual Award Winner

Tae Hee Lee, M.D.
Joo Young Cho, M.D. Ph D.

Chapter 7 Therapeutic Endoscopy for Strictures of the Upper Digestive Tract

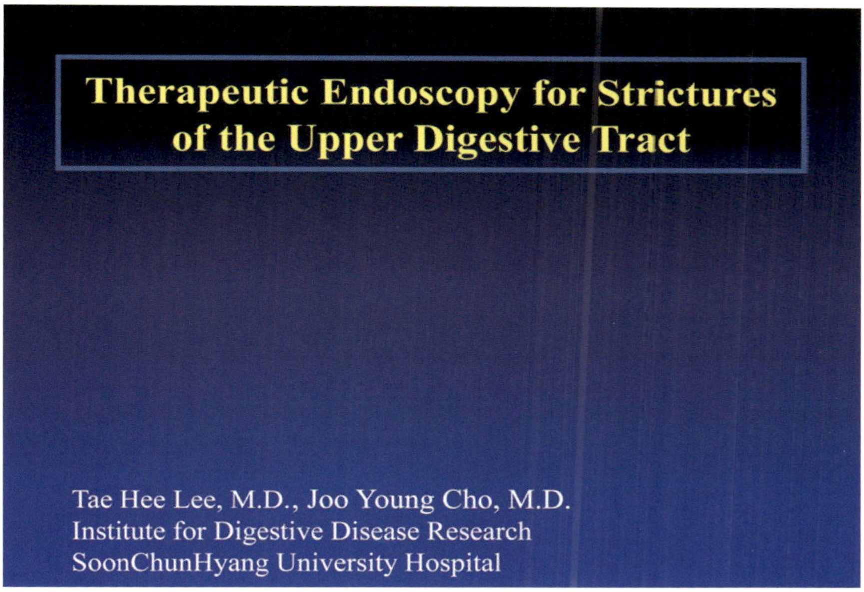

Strictures of the upper GI tract are not uncommonly encountered in the clinical practice and can pose a challenge to the gastroenterologist. It is important to know what techniques and instruments are indicated for different situations. This review will focus on the various endoscopic treatments that have been applied to strictures of the upper gastrointestinal tract. This chapter will focus on the various endoscopic treatments that have been applied to strictures of the upper gastrointestinal tract.

Therapeutic Endoscopy for Strictures of the Upper Digestive Tract

Esophageal strictures

- Dilation therapy
- Stenting therapy
- Incisional therapy

Gastric outlet obstruction

- Dilation therapy
- Stenting therapy

TOPIC (I)

Esophageal strictures

Gastric outlet obstruction

Esophageal Strictures-Etiologies-

Common causes of esophageal strictures/obstruction
Gastroesophageal reflux disease (peptic); most common form
Schatzki's ring
Esophageal cancer
Radiation therapy
Esophageal surgery
Eosinophilic esophagitis
Sclerotherapy
Caustic injury
Photodynamic therapy

Gastrointest Endosc. 2006 May;63(6):755-60

The most common cause of esophageal strictures is peptic strictures, resulting from reflux esophagitis. Today with the widespread use of proton pump inhibitors, the incidence is decreasing; however, in the past nearly 80% of esophageal strictures were associated with gastroesophageal reflux disease. Other causes are Schatzki' s rings, esophageal cancer and injury to the esophagus from surgery or other forms of treatment.

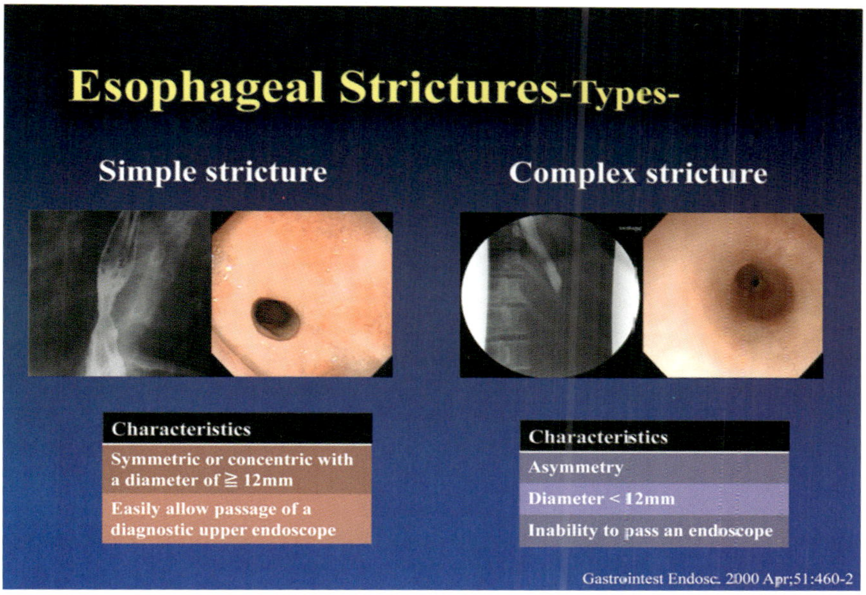

Esophageal strictures can be structurally categorized into simple and complex strictures. Simple strictures are symmetric or concentric with a diameter greater than 12 mm, and easily allow passage of a diagnostic upper endoscope. Complex strictures have one or more of the following features: asymmetry, diameter less than 12 mm or inability to pass an endoscope.

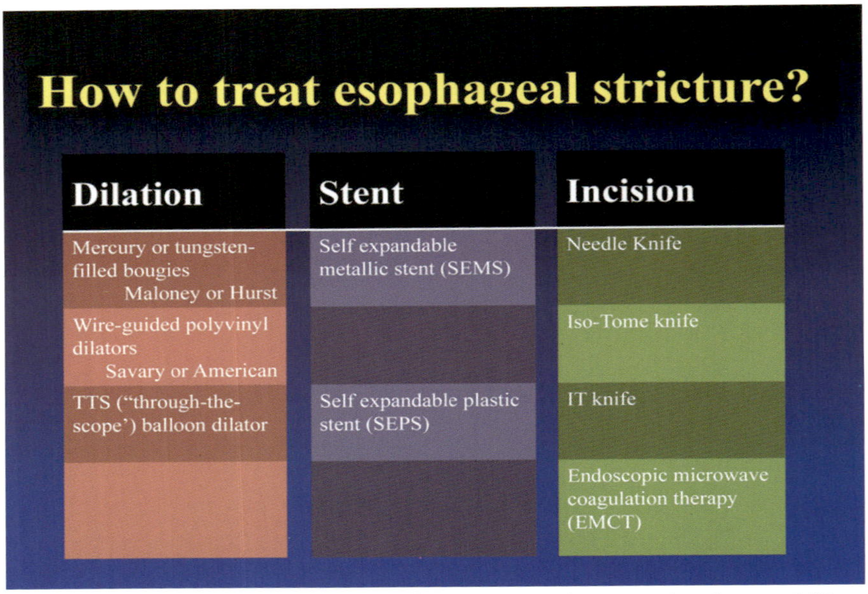

Today endoscopic treatment of esophageal strictures is largely narrowed to three modalities, Dilation therapy, stent therapy and incisional therapy.

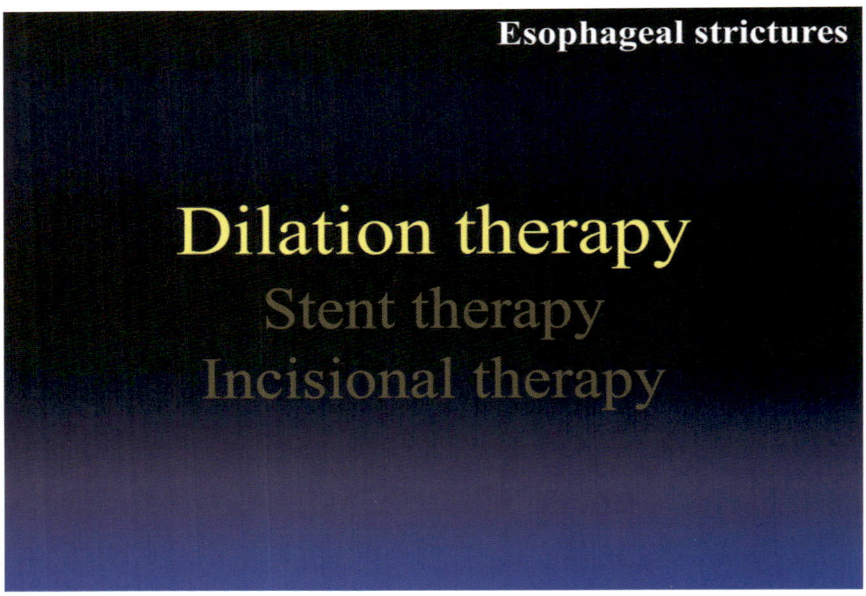

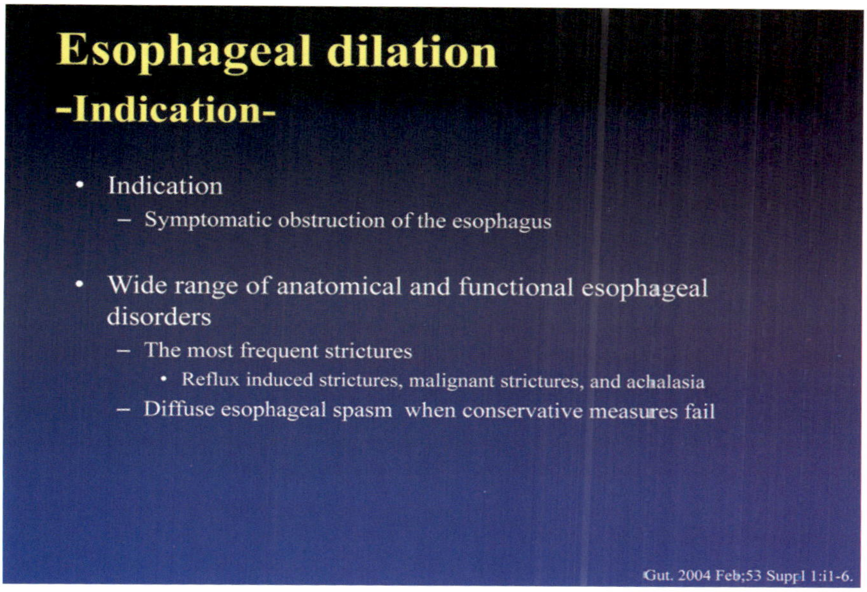

Esophageal dilatation is indicated in the treatment of symptomatic obstruction of the esophagus. Obstruction may develop as a consequence of a wide range of anatomical and functional esophageal disorders. Reflux induced strictures, malignant strictures, and achalasia are the most frequent indications but patients with anastomotic, sclerotherapy, radiation, and corrosive induced strictures, and those with rings and webs frequently require dilatation. Patients with diffuse esophageal spasm and other motility disorders may occasionally require dilatation of the lower esophageal sphincter when conservative measures fail.

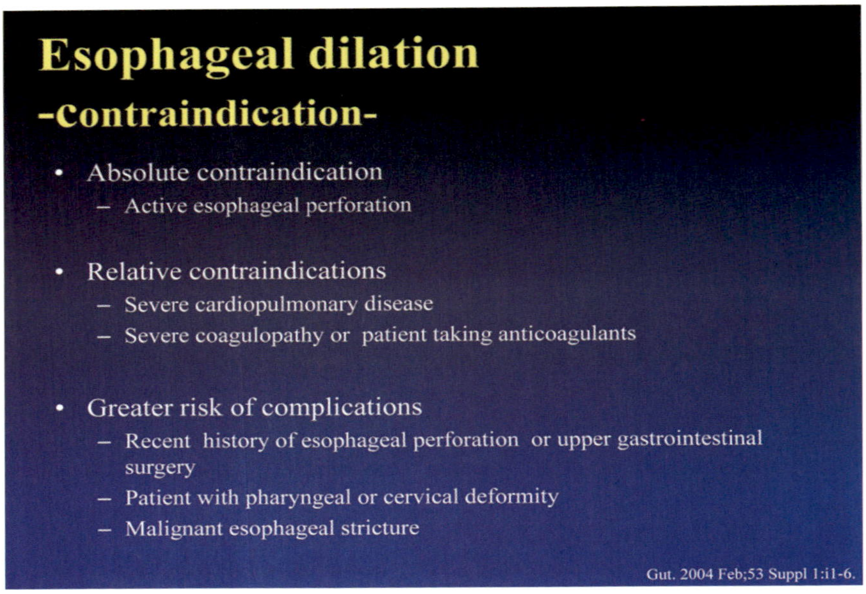

Active esophageal perforation is an absolute contraindication to esophageal dilatation as it may extend the esophageal defect and promote mediastinal contamination. Severe cardiorespiratory disease is a relative contraindication to all endoscopic procedures. The balance of risks and benefits should be individualized and carefully considered. Major bleeding is uncommon following oesophageal dilatation but is more likely in patients with severe coagulopathy and in those taking anticoagulant drugs. The procedure should be undertaken with caution in those who have suffered recent perforation or undergone recent upper gastrointestinal surgery. The risks of dilatation are likely to be greater in patients with pharyngeal or cervical deformity and in those with large thoracic aneurysms. The risks of a perforation are greater during dilatation of malignant disease of the esophagus.

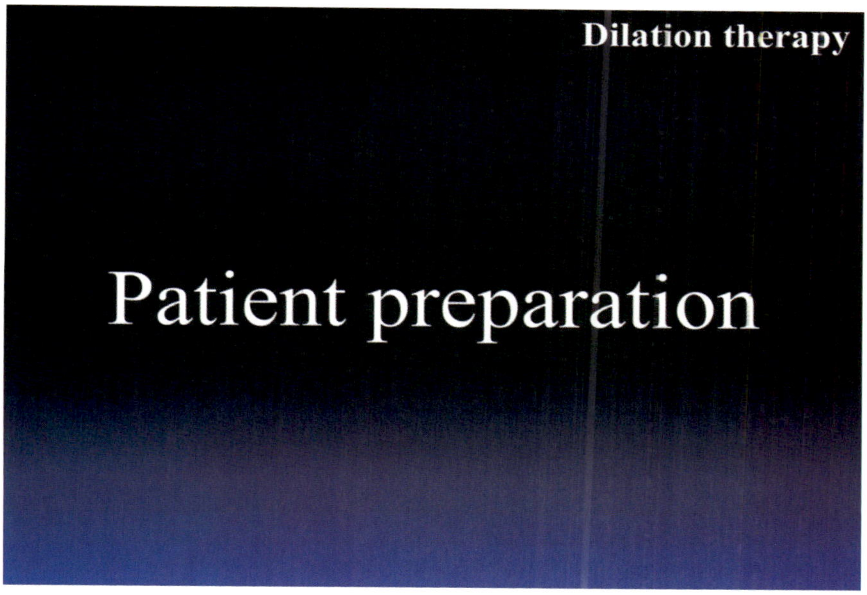

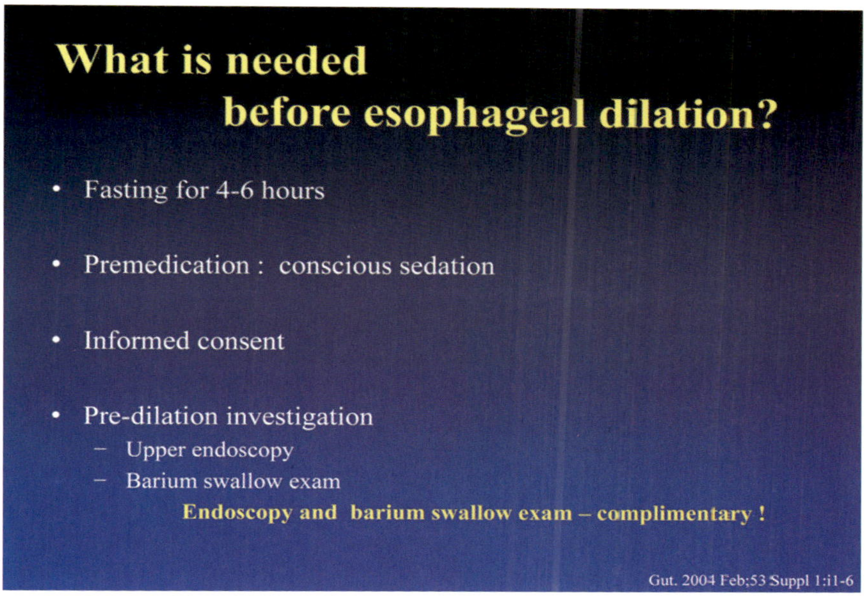

All patients should be fasted at least 4-6 hours prior to procedure. Endoscopy and contrast radiology are both helpful and are often complimentary.

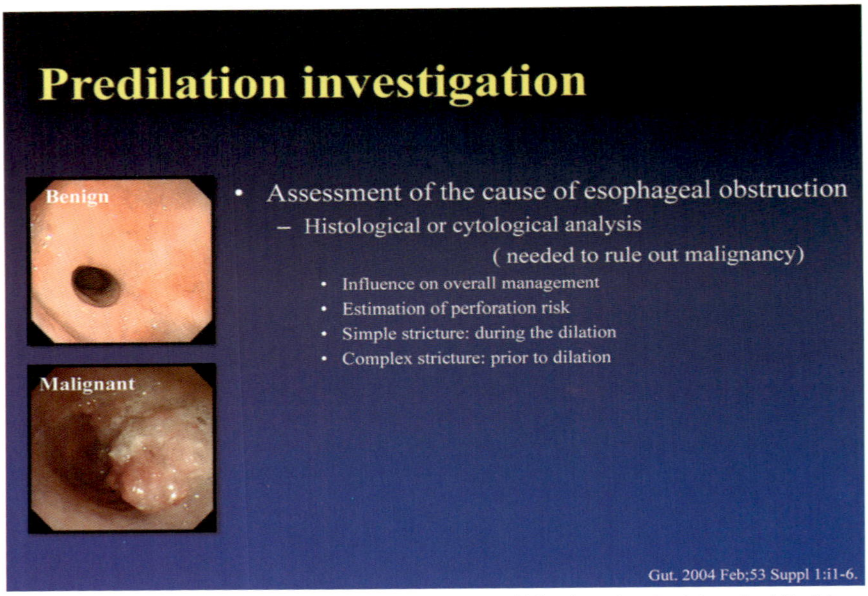

The cause of esophageal obstruction should be carefully assessed. Biopsies or brush cytology should be taken for analysis. A tissue diagnosis is desirable, prior to dilatation, as it will influence overall management and the estimation of perforation risk. In patients with short, simple, benign looking strictures however, it is common practice for biopsies to be taken and dilatation performed during the same examination. When the stricture is tight or when the endoscopic features suggest malignancy, the results of biopsies are best awaited unless the patient has absolute dysphagia.

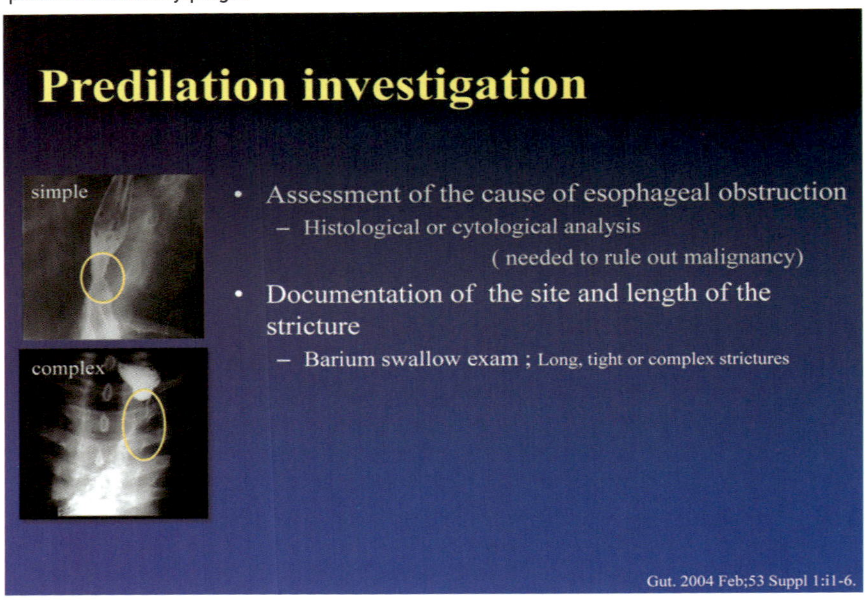

When a stricture prevents passage of the endoscope, a barium swallow examination will provide useful anatomical detail. This is helpful in patients with long, tight, or complex strictures in whom dilatation may be technically difficult and associated with greater risks.

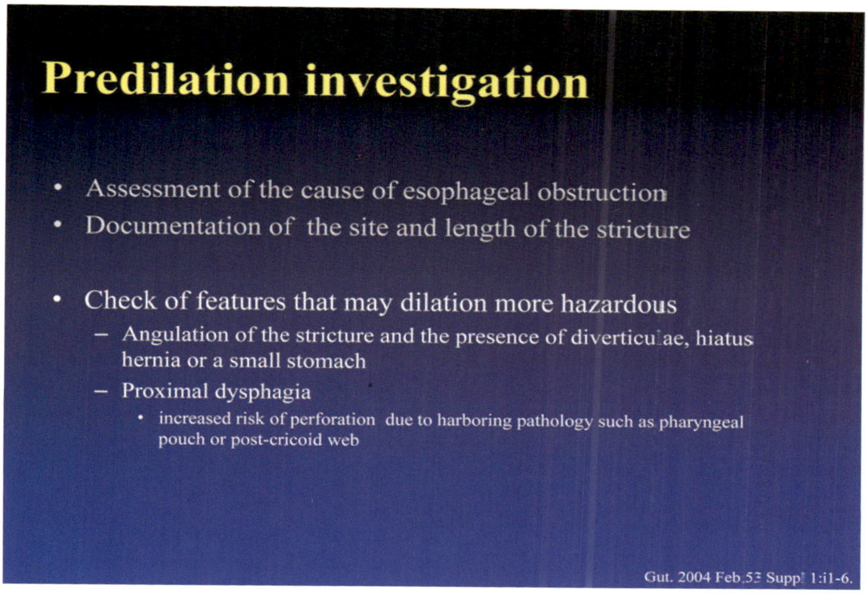

Features that may make dilatation more hazardous, such as angulation of the stricture and the presence of diverticulum, a hiatus hernia, or a small stomach, should also be noted. It should be remembered that patients with proximal dysphagia may be harboring conditions which increases the risks of perforation such as a pharyngeal pouch, or a post-cricoids web and in these circumstances endoscopy should only be undertaken by an experienced endoscopist.

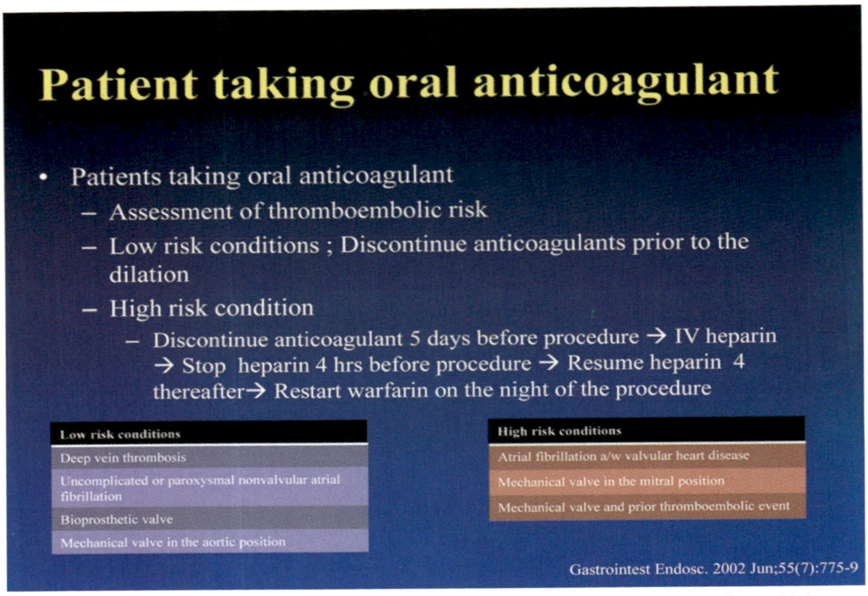

In patients taking oral anticoagulants, dilatation has the potential to produce bleeding, which may be difficult to control. It is therefore advisable that patients at low risk of thromboembolic events should discontinue anticoagulants prior to the dilatation. A preprocedure prothrombin time should be performed. In patients at high risk of thromboembolic events, oral anticoagulants should again be discontinued prior to the procedure. Monitoring should be undertaken and intravenous heparin started once oral anticoagulation becomes subtherapeutic. Heparin should be discontinued 4-6 hours before dilatation and resumed 4?6 hours thereafter. Anticoagulants are generally resumed on the night of the procedure.

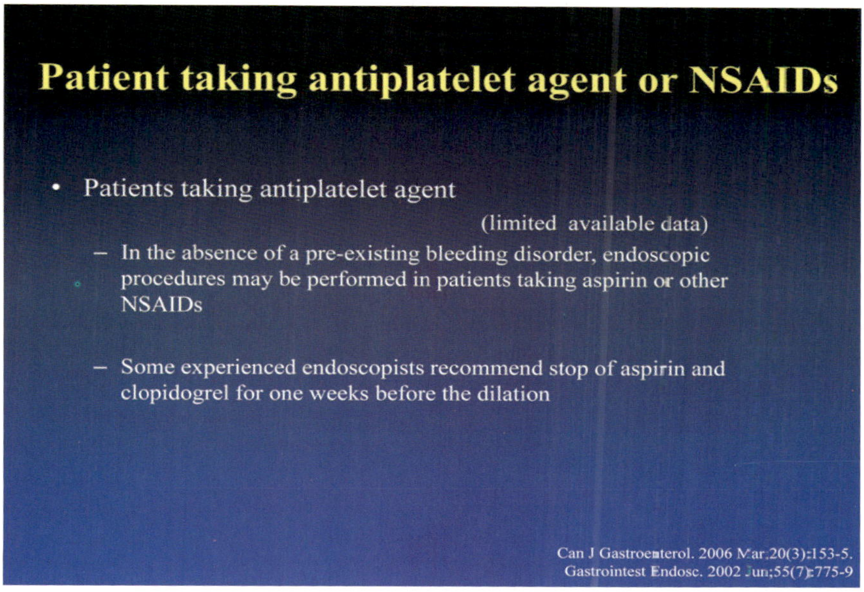

Limited data that is available suggests that aspirin and nonsteroidal anti-inflammatory drugs do not increase the risk of significant bleeding after therapeutic endoscopy. In the absence of a pre-existing bleeding disorder, endoscopic procedures may be performed in patients taking aspirin or other NSAIDs.

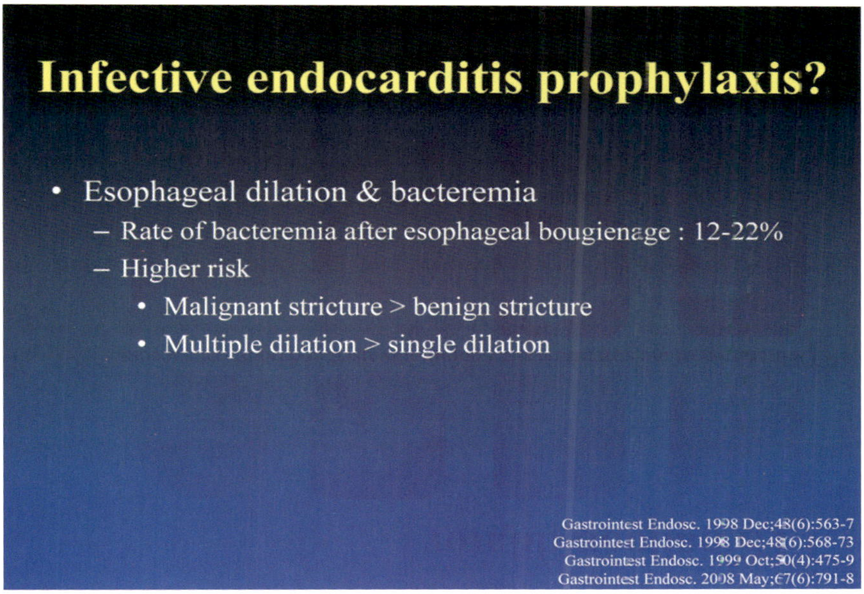

In 3 prospective studies, the rate of bacteremia after esophageal bougie dilatation was demonstrated to be 12% to 22%. Bacteremia may be more frequent with the dilation of malignant strictures than with benign strictures. Bacteremia may also be more frequent with the passage of multiple dilators rather than with a single dilation.

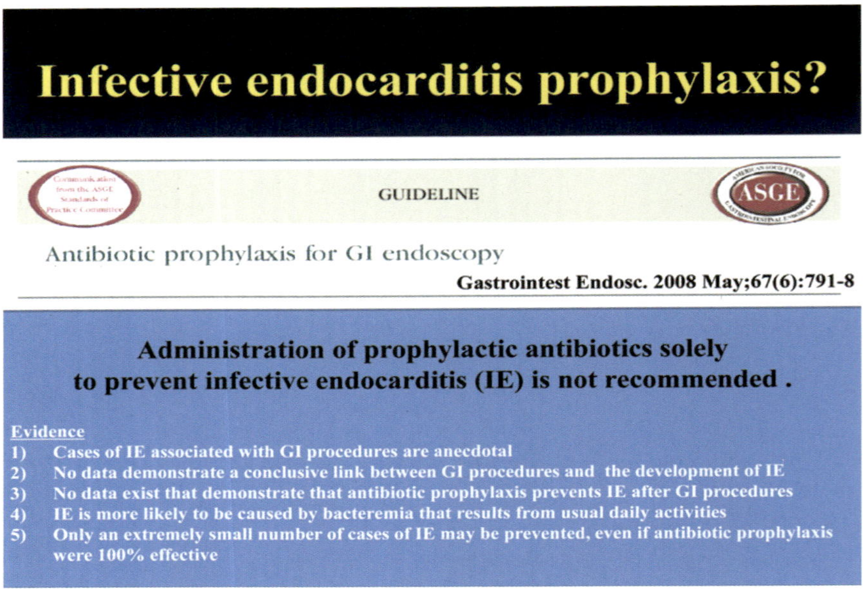

However, the 2008 ASGE guidelines, did not recommend administration of prophylactic antibiotics solely to prevent infective endocarditis, based on the following evidence.

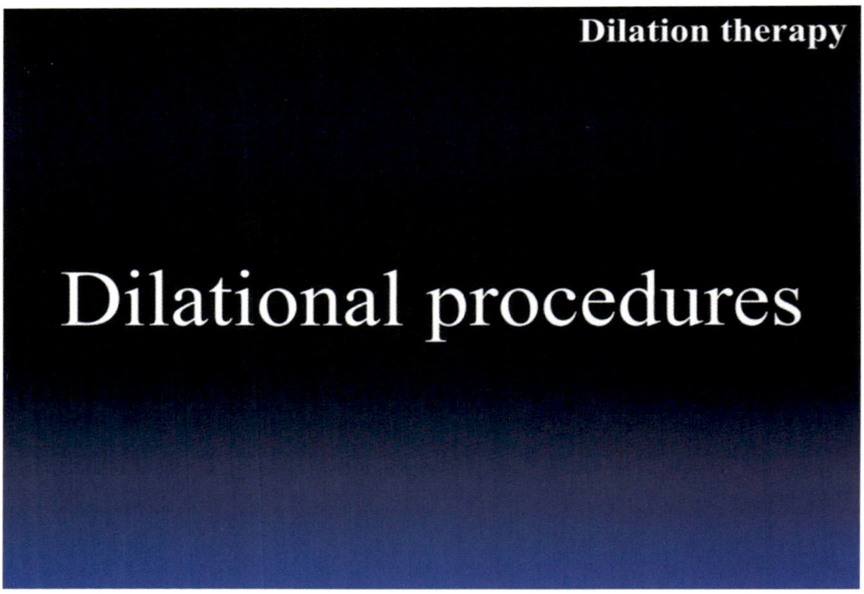

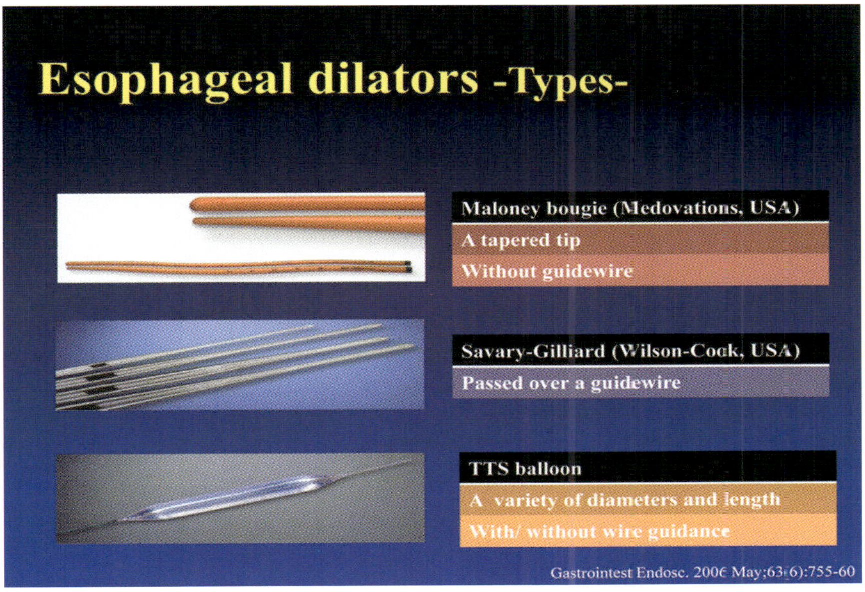

The Maloney bougie is the most commonly used bougie dilator. Made of rubber and filled with mercury or tungsten, it has a tapered tip and is freely passed without a guidewire. The Savary-Gilliard bougie is a tapered thermoplastic dilator and is passed over a guidewire. There are a variety of available TTS balloon dilators available in either single or multiple diameters that may be passed with or without wire guidance.

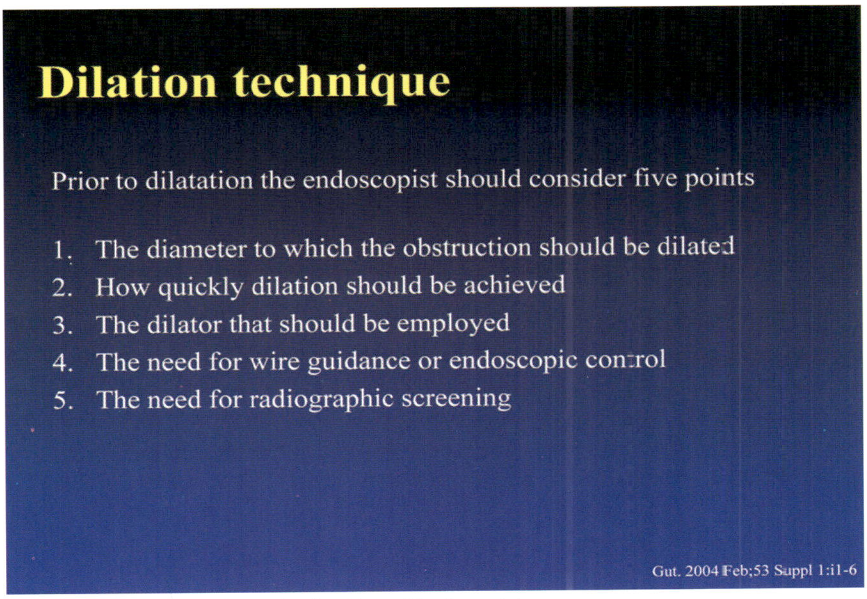

Prior to dilatation the endoscopist should consider five points.

1. The diameter to which the obstruction should be dilated
2. How quickly dilatation should be achieved
3. The dilator that should be employed
4. The need for wire guidance or endoscopic control
5. The need for radiographic screening

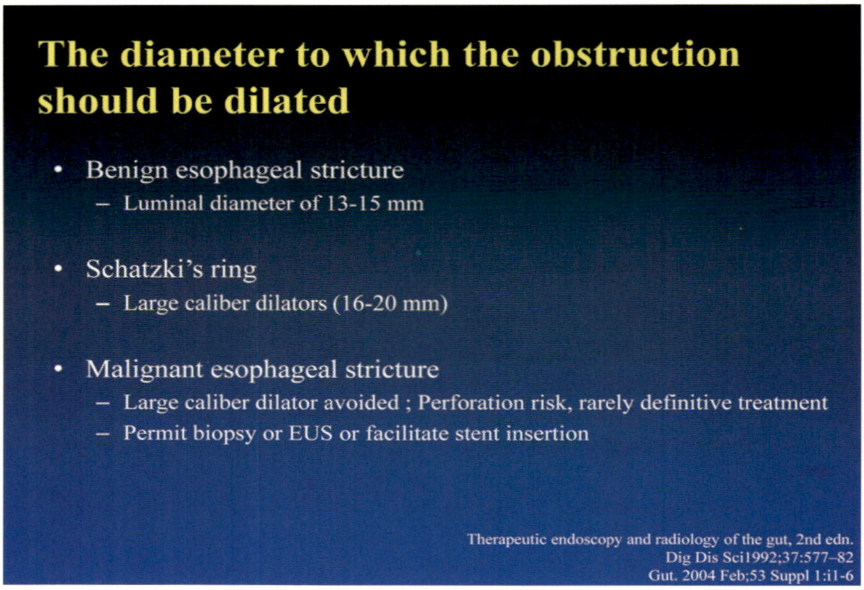

In patients with benign peptic strictures, the results of dilatation appear best when a luminal diameter of 13-15 mm is achieved. Large caliber dilators (16-20 mm) are advised in the treatment of patients with Schatzki' s rings. In patients with malignant oesophageal disease however large caliber dilators are best avoided as perforation is more likely and dilatation is rarely the definitive treatment. Modest dilatation, sufficient to permit biopsy or endoscopic ultrasound or facilitate stent insertion, is the safest approach.

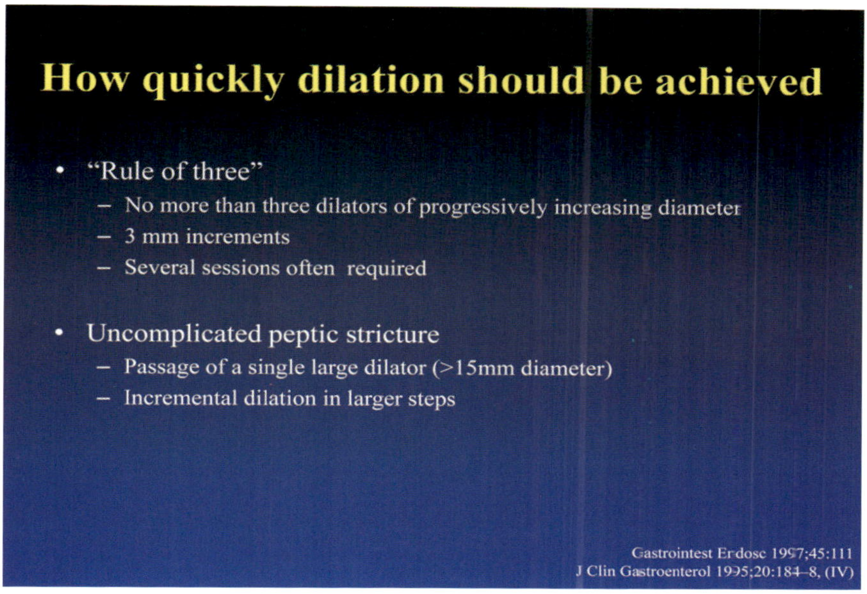

Traditionally, it has been suggested that no more than three dilators of progressively increasing diameter (3 mm increments) should be passed in a single session to reduce the risk of perforation ("rule of three"). Several sessions were therefore often required to achieve adequate dilation. Recent experience suggests that the passage of a single large dilator (>15 mm diameter) or incremental dilatation in larger steps may be safely employed in many patients with uncomplicated peptic strictures. However, it should be borne in mind that these observations were uncontrolled and it would be wise to employ a cautious approach in patients with tight, tough, or complex strictures.

The dilator that should be employed

	Maloney	Savary-Gilliard	TTS balloon
Mechanism	Longitudinal and radial forces (push dilators)		Radial forces (balloon dilator)
Techniques	Blindly or under fluoroscopic control	Over a guidewire	Through the scope
Perforation	Blind passage of Maloney dilators > with Savary or TTS balloons*		

*A large hiatal hernia, a tortuous esophagus or complex strictures

Gastrointest Endosc. 2000 Apr;51:460-2
Gastrointest Endosc. 2006 May;63(6):755-60

The risk of esophageal perforation may be higher with blind passage of Maloney dilators than with Savary or TTS balloons, particularly in patients with a large hiatal hernia, a tortuous esophagus, or those with complex strictures.

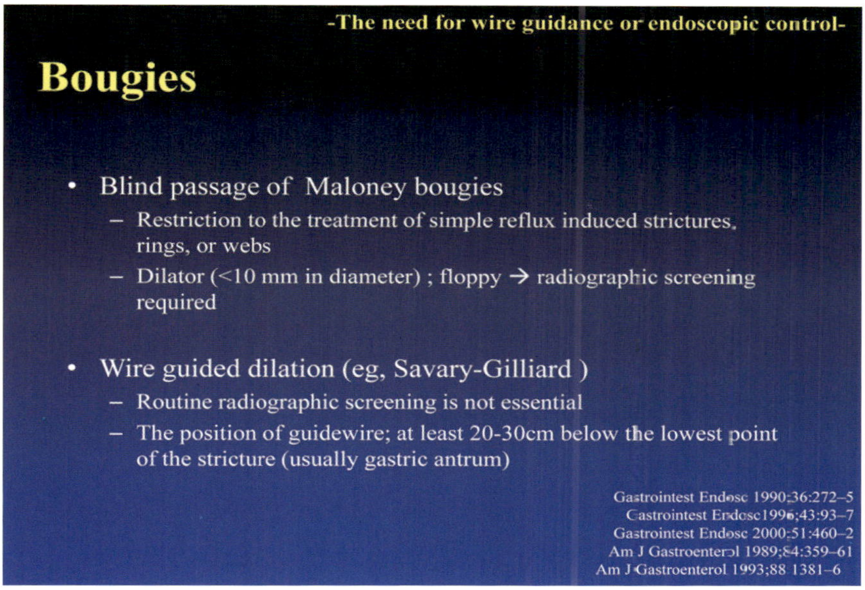

The unguided passage of weighted bougies should be restricted to the treatment of patients with simple reflux induced strictures, rings, or webs. Weighted bougies are not suited for the management of tight strictures. Wire guided dilatation gives greater assurance that the dilator is following the line of the oesophageal lumen, thus reducing the risk of perforation. Routine radiological screening was previously recommended when undertaking wire guided dilatation but this is not essential when the anatomy is well defined, axial alignments are maintained, and the wire passes easily into the stomach. The guidewire should be placed at least 20-30 cm below the lowest point of the stricture, usually in the gastric antrum.

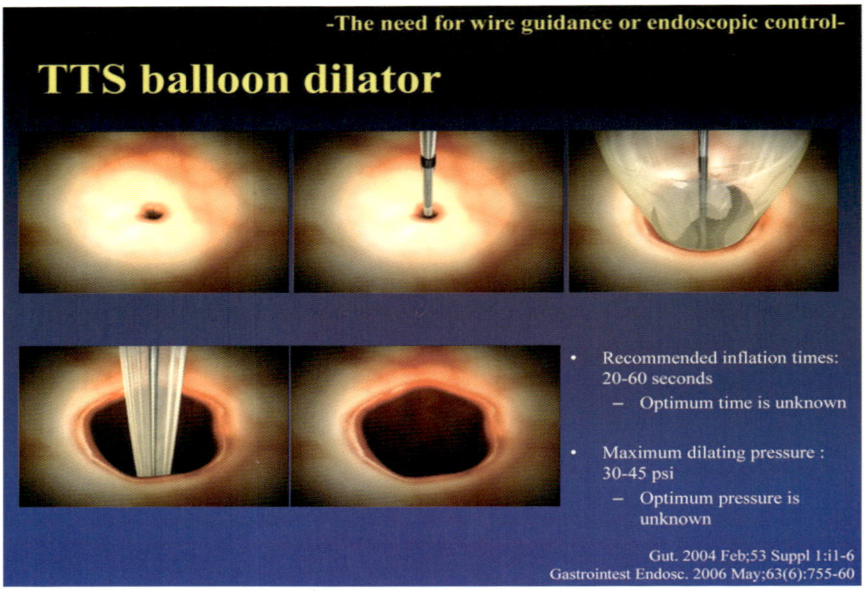

Through the scope balloon dilatation is performed under direct endoscopic visualization. An adequate channel size and lubrication facilitate easy passage. The balloon should be centered at the tightest point of the stricture. Recommended inflation times range from 20 to 60 seconds but the optimum time is unknown. Maximum dilating pressures vary in relation to balloon size and range between 30 and 45 psi but again, the optimum pressure is unknown.

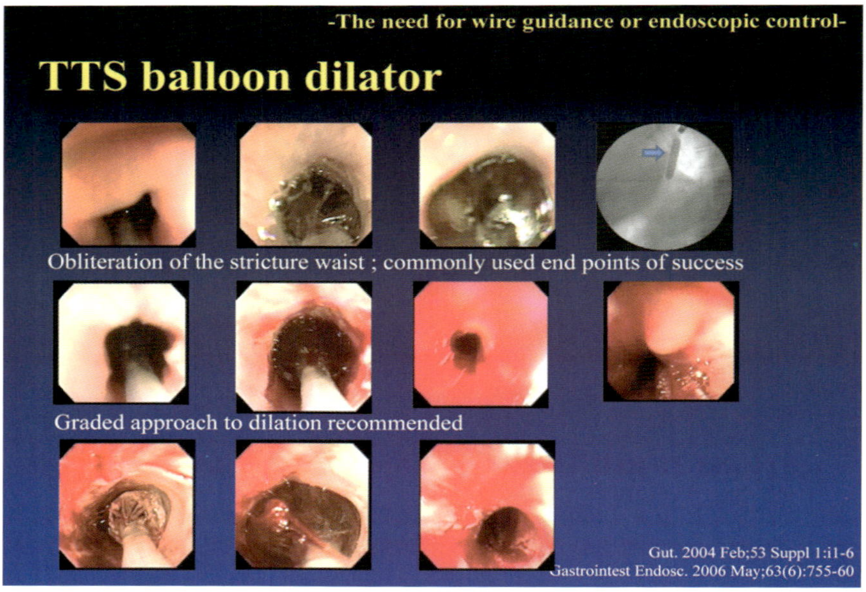

A graded approach to dilatation is recommended by some with obliteration of the stricture waist seen during radiographic screening or endoscopic assessment of stricture dilatation as commonly used end points of success. Through the scope balloon dilatation has the additional advantage that it allows dilatation of the proximal part of a stricture. This may be helpful when a guidewire will not pass.

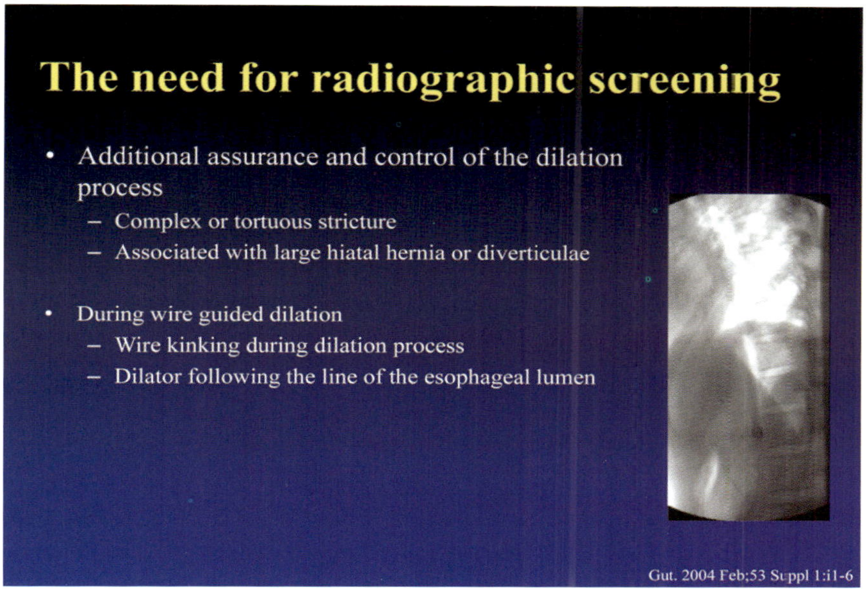

The use of radiographic screening gives additional assurance and control of the dilatation process. Radiographic screening is particularly helpful when the stricture is tortuous or complex or associated with a large hiatus hernia or diverticulae. It may also be of value when the guidewire meets with resistance during passage through the stricture or when an adequate length of wire cannot be passed distal to the stricture. Although comparative trials are not available, the selective use of radiological screening appears safe and effective and is supported by extensive clinical experience. During wire guided dilatation, it ensures that the wire has passed the stricture, that kinking of the wire has not occurred within or distal to the stricture and that, during the dilatation process, the dilator is following the line of the oesophageal lumen.

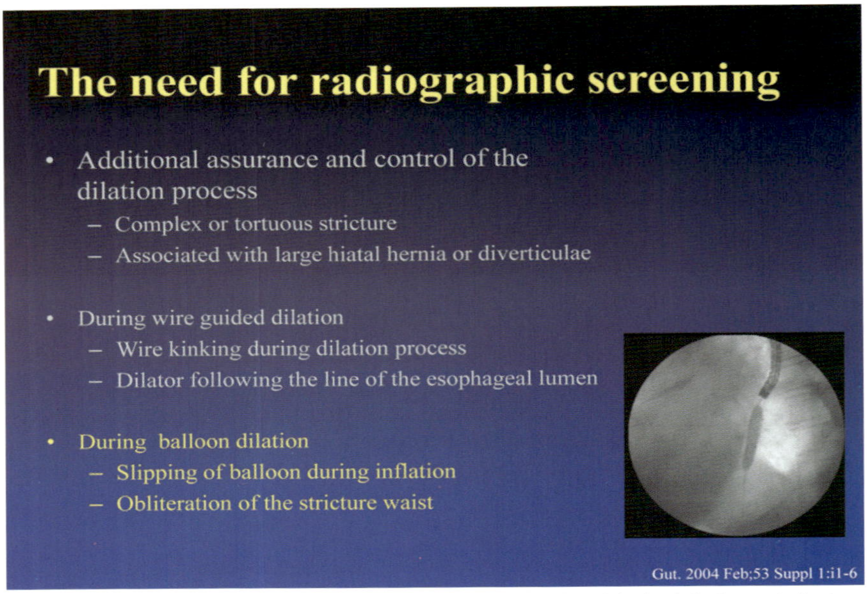

During balloon dilatation, it indicates whether the balloon has slipped during inflation and whether obliteration of the stricture waist has occurred.

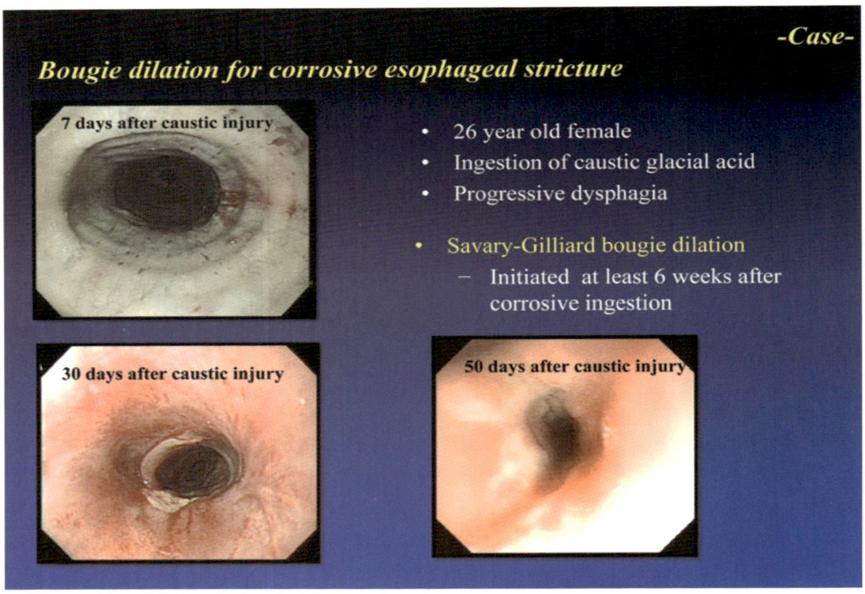

A 26-year-old female swallowed an acidic caustic solution. The patient developed dysphagia. 50 days after caustic injury a stricture is seen in the mid esophagus.

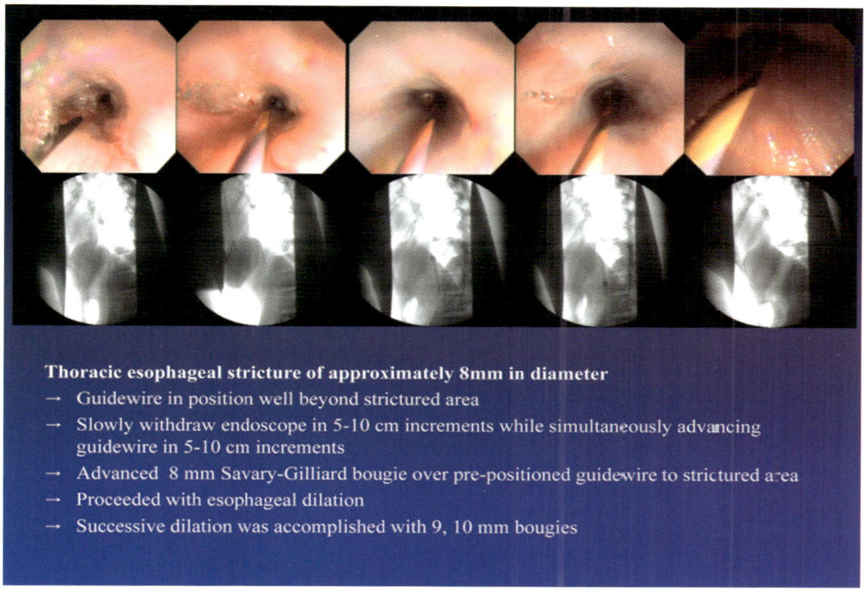

Bougie dilation for corrosive strictures is usually initiated at least 6 weeks after corrosive ingestion. Endoscopy showed a stricture approximately 8mm in diameter. A lubricated guidewire was introduced through the accessory channel and the tip was placed in antrum for stability. The endoscope was withdrawn slowly in 5-10 cm increments while simultaneously advancing the guidewire in comparable length. An 8 mm Savary-Gilliard bougie was advanced over the pre-positioned guidewire to the strictured area because the first dilation performed should be approximately the diameter of the stricture. Dilation is considered to have been performed when there is a moderate or significant amount of resistance. If there is no resistance dilation has not been performed. Excessive force is not necessary and should not be used. It is reasonable to follow the 'rule of three', performing up to three dilations that meet resistance per session. Successive dilation was accomplished with 9, 10 mm bougies.

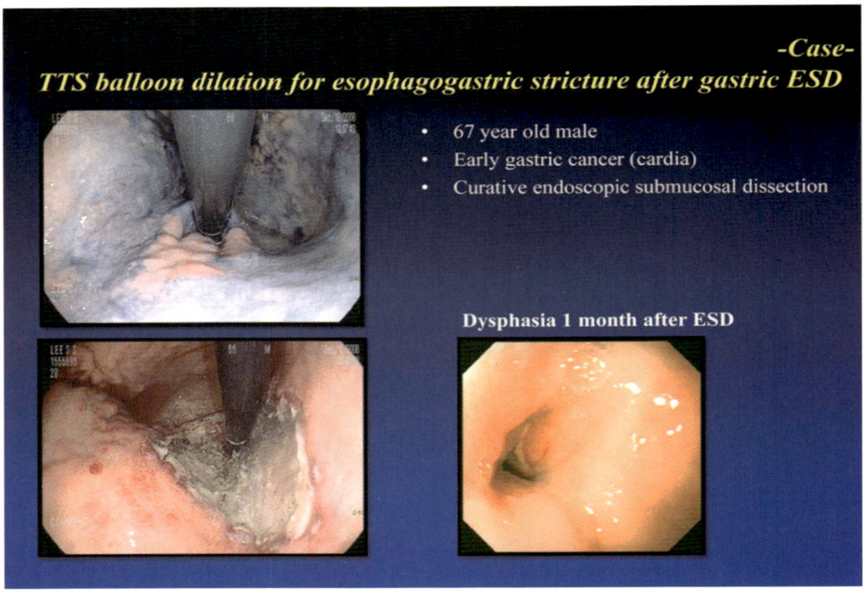

This is a 67-year-old male who was diagnosed with early gastric cancer at the gastric cardia. ESD was successfully performed. However this patient eventually developed dysphagia 1 month after ESD and endoscopy showed that a stricture developed at the gastroesophageal junction.

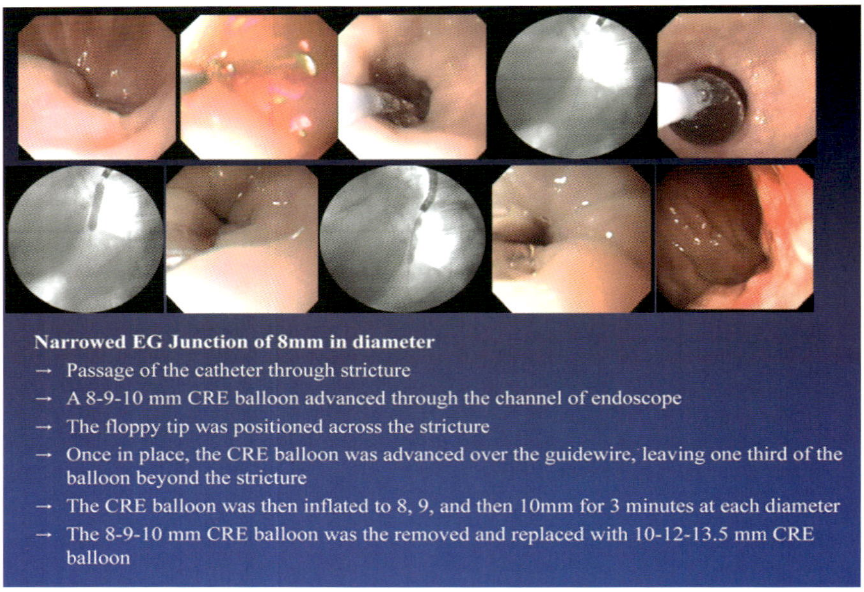

Under direct endoscopic visualization the CRE balloon catheter is passed through the stricture. The 8-9-10 mm CRE balloon is advanced through the channel of endoscope. The floppy tip was positioned across the stricture once in place, the CRE balloon was advanced over the guidewire, leaving one third of the balloon beyond the stricture. The CRE balloon was then inflated 8, 9, and then 10 mm for 3 min at each diameter.

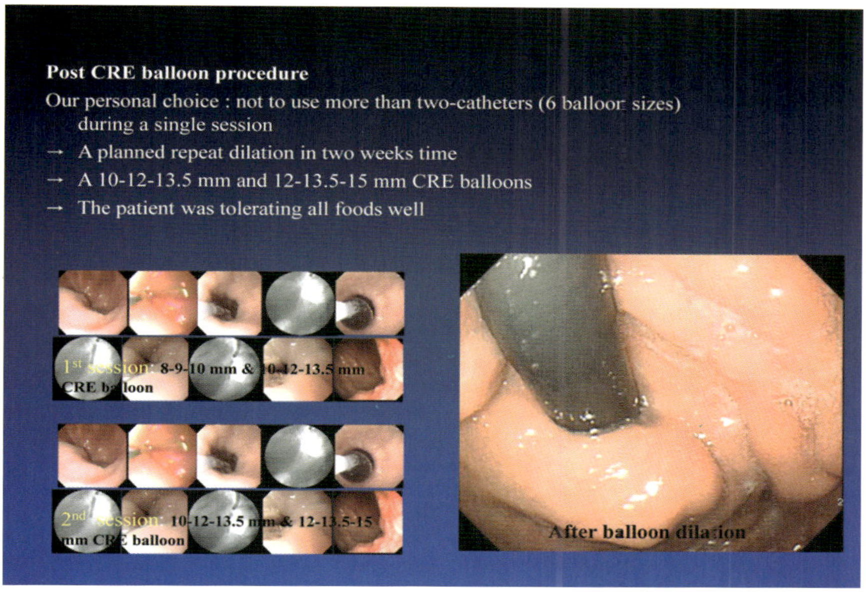

When to repeat dilation depends on the degree of stenosis and success of the initial procedure. The procedure should be repeated within two weeks for high-grade strictures. A planned repeated dilation was performed in two weeks time. We chose not to use more than two-catheter during a single session, for the second dilation a 10-12-13.5 mm and 12-13.5-15 mm CRE balloons were used. Following dilation, the patient eventually tolerated all foods well.

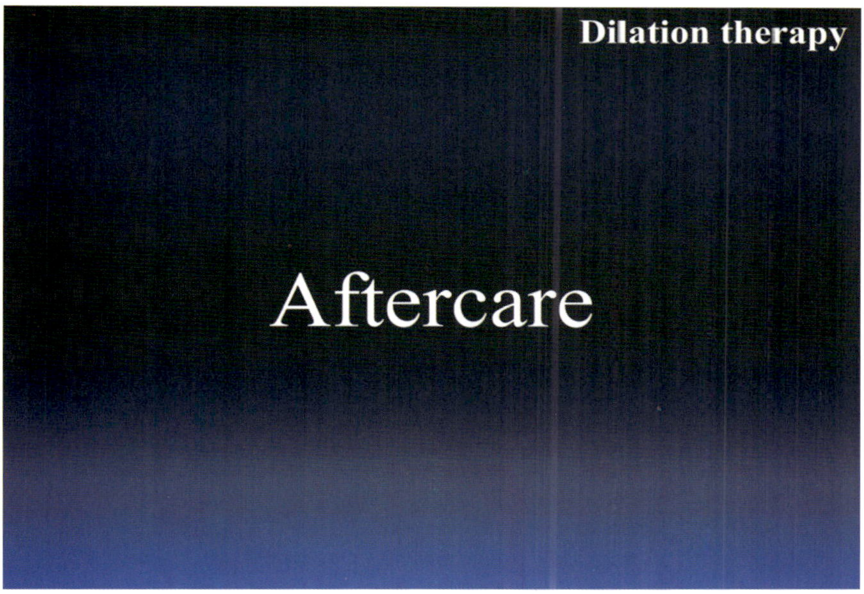

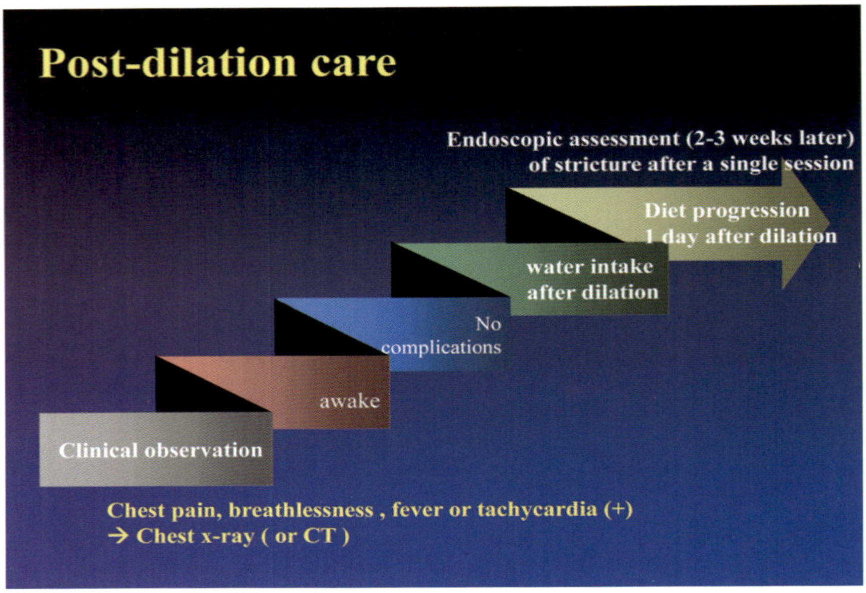

Patients should be closely observed after oesophageal dilatation. Chest x-ray is not essential but should be performed urgently in patients who develop pain, dyspnea, fever, or tachycardia. We recommended the patient to initially drink water, if the patient was awake and alert and had no evident complications. We advanced the diet carefully in a stepwise pattern. Endoscopic assessment of the stricture was performed 2 weeks after a single session.

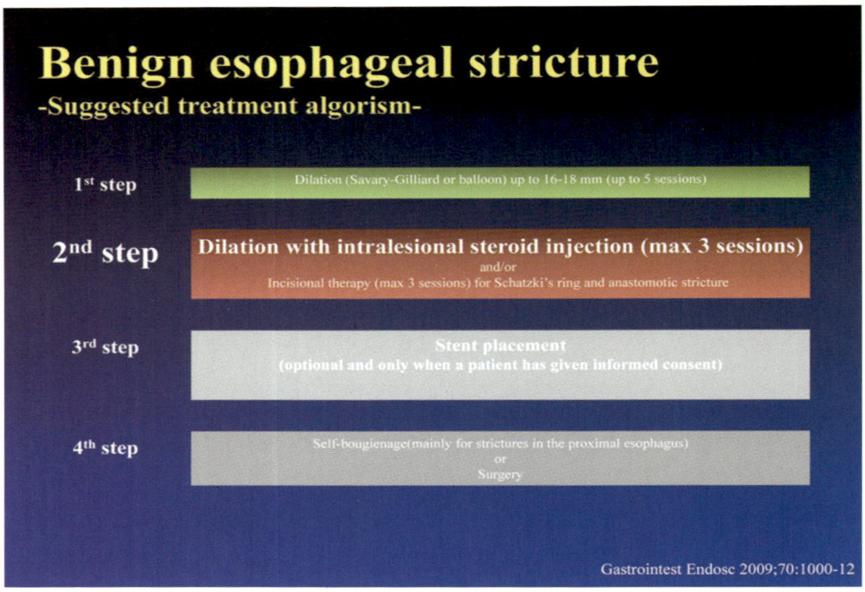

Benign esophageal strictures can be dilated with a savary-gilliard bougie or TTS balloon for up to 5 sessions, If the stricture is refractory to treatment, Dilation with intralesional steroid injection can be attempted. Stenting is optional and should only be considered when the patient has given informed consent.

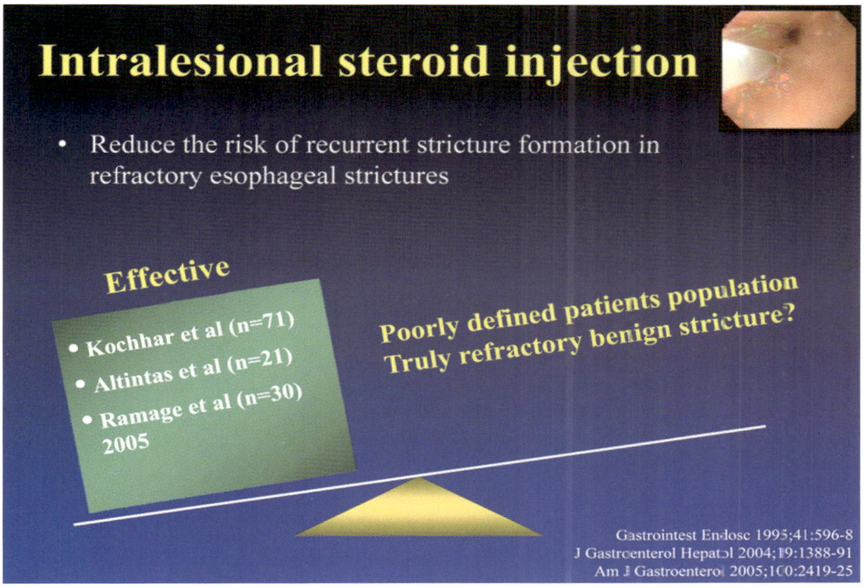

There is evidence that intralesional steroid injection prior to dilation reduces the risk of recurrent stricture formation in refractory benign esophageal strictures. However, this comes from studies with poorly defined patient populations in which it was not clear whether the patients truly had refractory benign esophageal strictures.

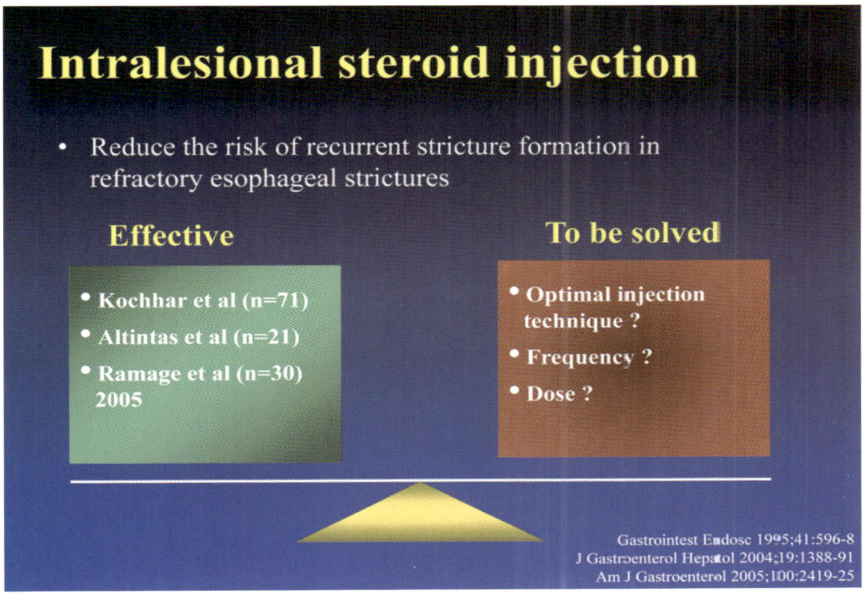

It also remains to be defined what the optimal injection technique and frequency is, and at what dose, steroids should be injected.

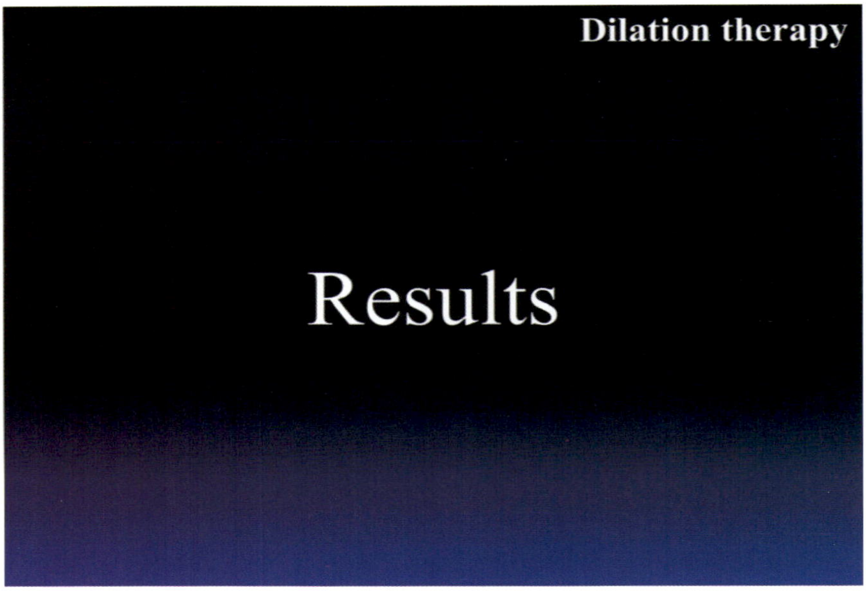
Dilation therapy
Results

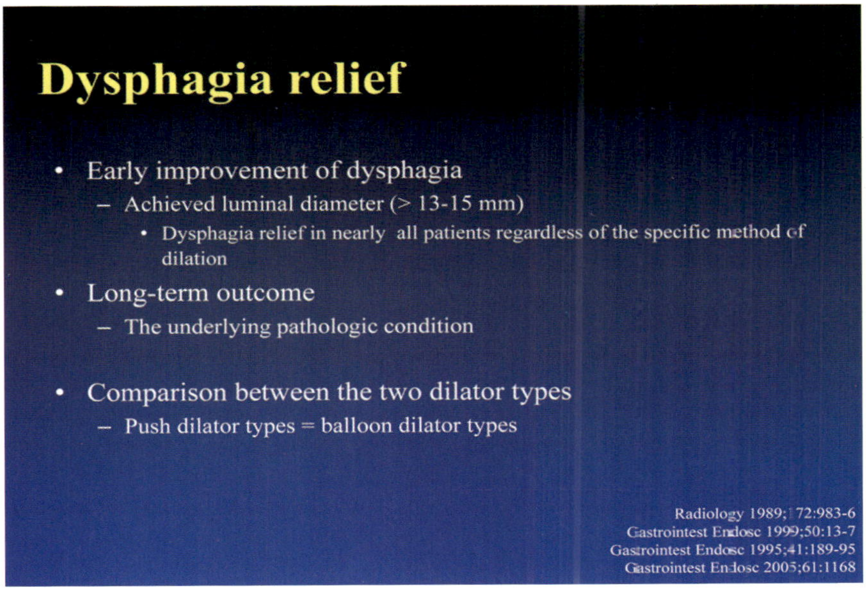

Regardless of the specific method of dilation, early improvement in the ability to swallow is achieved in virtually all patients; however, longer-term outcomes are influenced by the underlying pathologic condition. If a luminal diameter of at least 13 to 15 mm can be achieved, nearly all patients will be relieved of dysphagia. In patients with benign peptic strictures, a graded stepwise dilating approach between 13 and 20 mm yields relief in 85% to 93%. Bougie-type dilators exert not only radial forces as they are passed but also longitudinal forces as the result of a shearing effect. Longitudinal forces are not transmitted with balloon dilators because the entire dilating force is delivered radially and simultaneously over the entire length of the stenosis rather than progressively from it's proximal to distal extent. Despite these differences, no clear advantage has been demonstrated between the two dilator types.

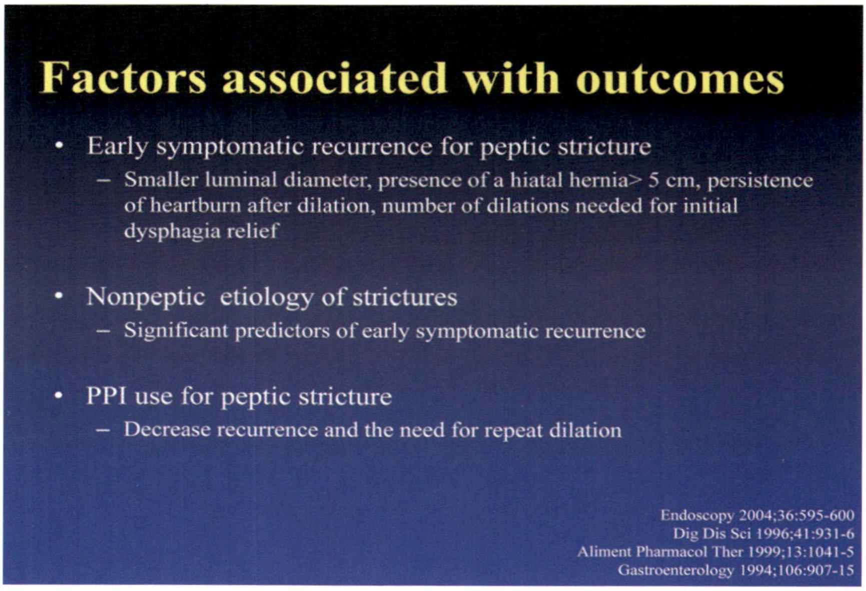

Several clinical features are associated with outcome. For peptic strictures, smaller lumen diameter, presence of a hiatal hernia >5 cm, persistence of heartburn after dilation, and number of dilations needed for initial dysphagia relief were significant predictors of early symptomatic recurrence. A multivariate analysis revealed that a nonpeptic etiology of strictures was a significant predictor of early symptomatic recurrence within 1 year of initial dilation. Patients with peptic strictures should be treated with PPI therapy. Compared with histamine receptor antagonist therapy, PPI use decreases stricture recurrence and the need for repeated stricture dilation.

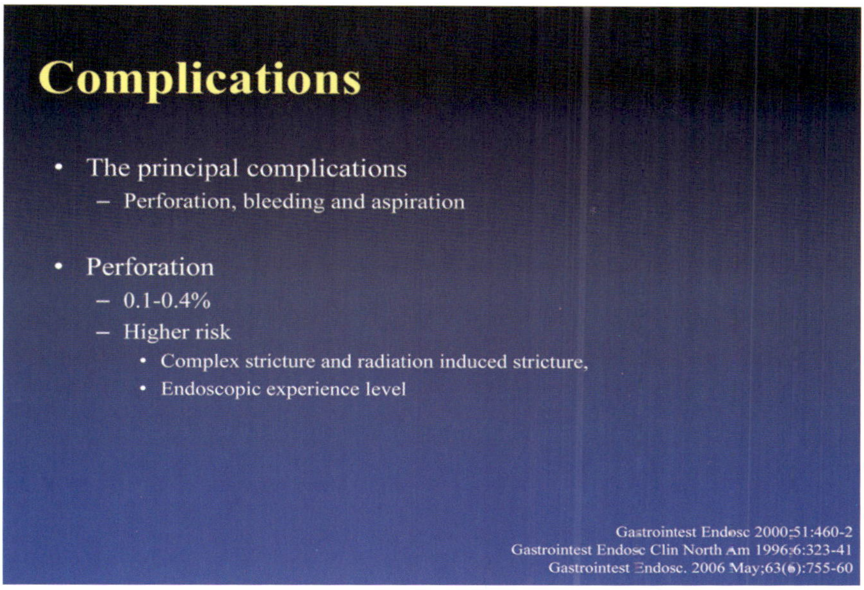

The principal complications of esophageal dilation are perforation, bleeding, and aspiration. The perforation rate for esophageal strictures after dilation has been reported to be 0.1% to 0.4%. The risk of perforation is lower in simple strictures and higher in more complex strictures. Perforation may be more common and severe with radiation-induced strictures. And the perforation rate may be influenced by the endoscopist' s experience level.

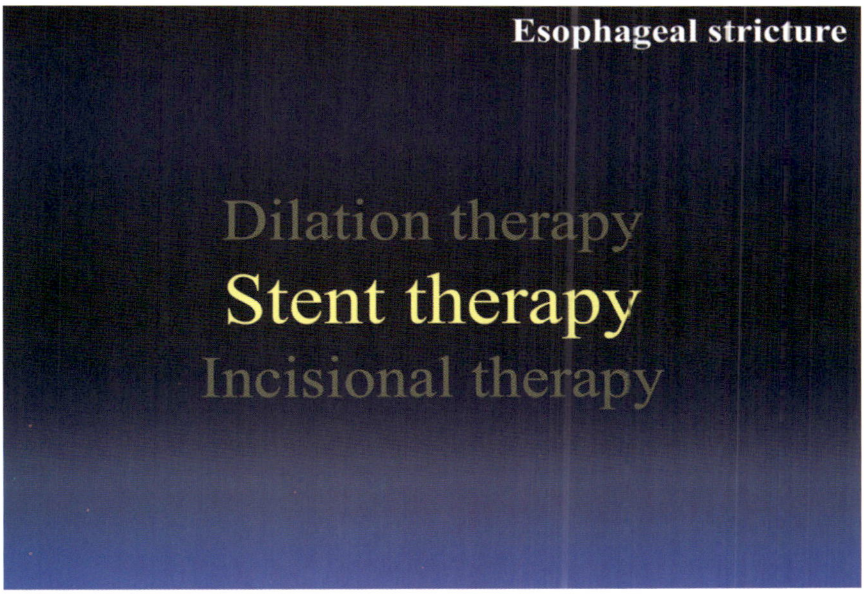

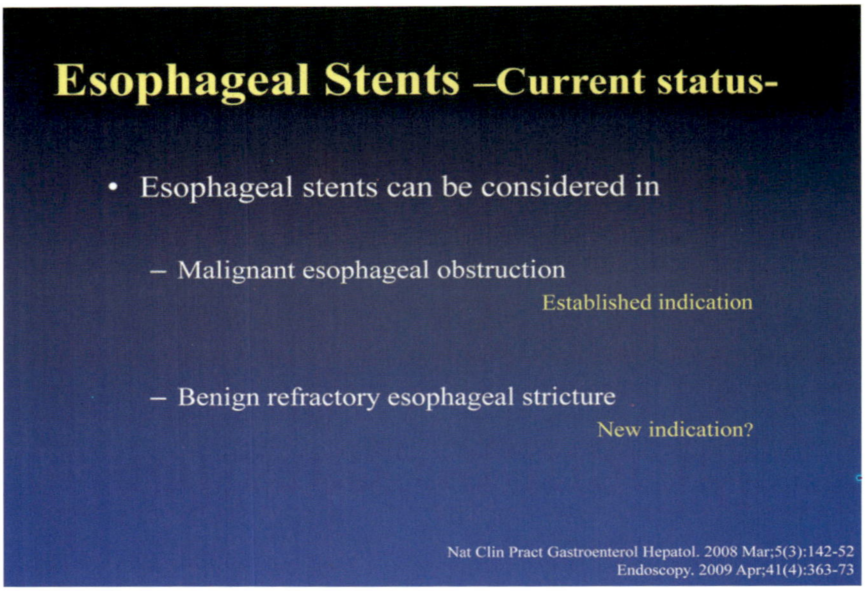

Esophageal stents scan be considered in malignant esophageal obstruction and benign refractory esophageal strictures.

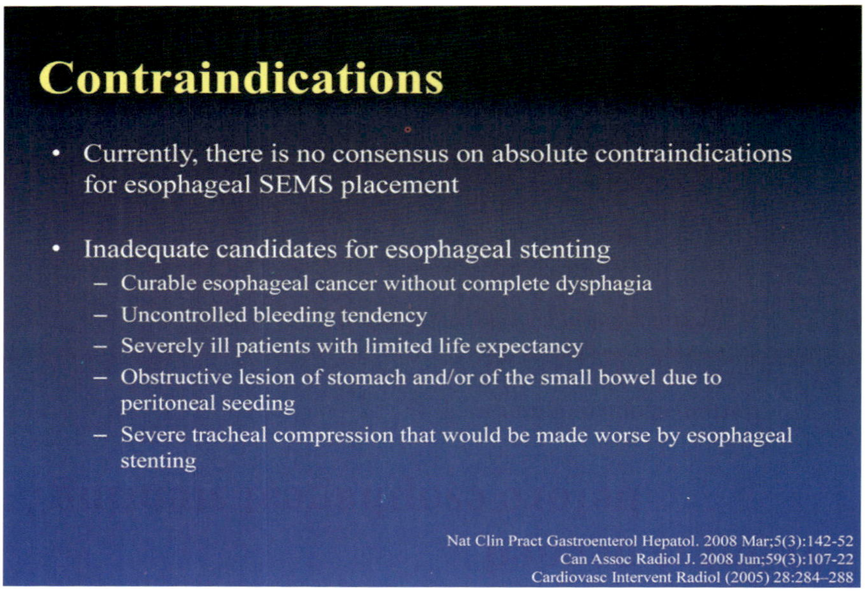

Currently, there is no consensus on absolute contraindications for esophageal SEMS placement. Inadequate candidates for esophageal stenting includes curable esophageal cancer without complete dysphagia, uncontrolled bleeding tendency, severely ill patients with limited life expectancy, obstructive lesion of stomach and/or of the small bowel due to peritoneal seeding, or severe tracheal compression that would be made worse by esophageal stenting.

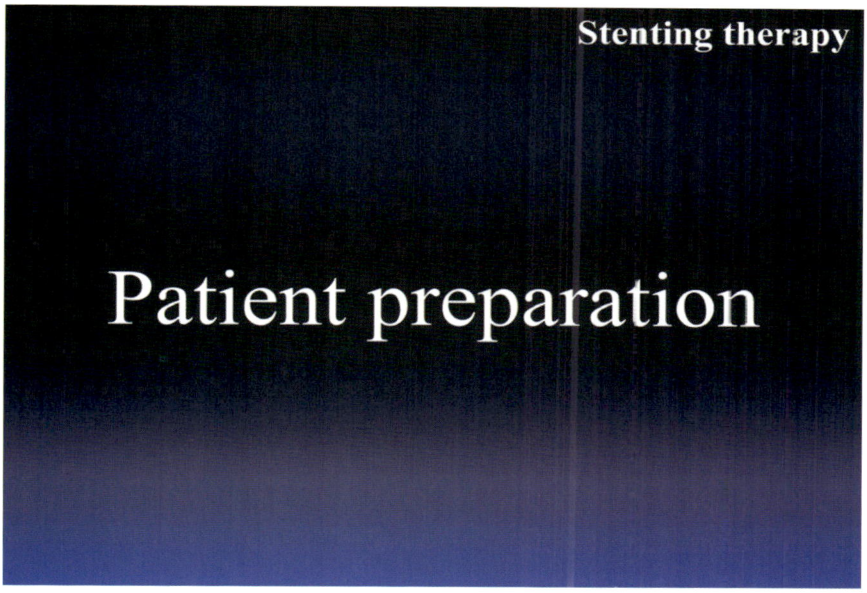

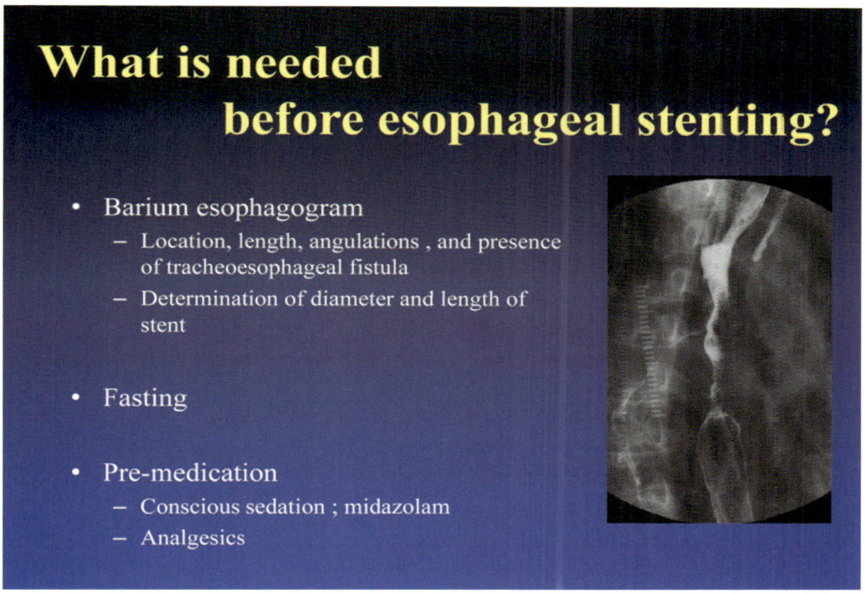

Before stent placement, it may be helpful to obtain a barium esophagogram to define stricture location, length, angulations, and presence of tracheoesophageal fistulas. It can provide useful information regarding the diameter and length of the stent to be employed.

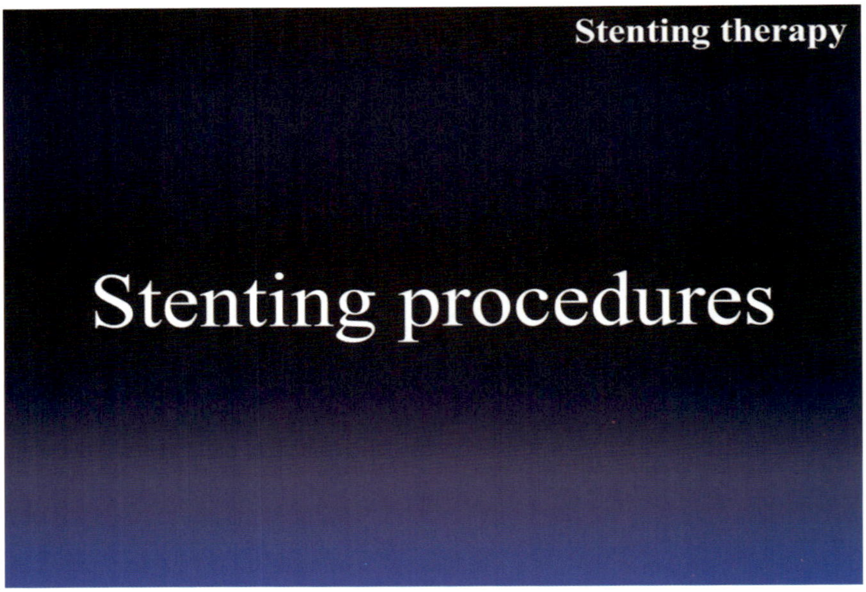

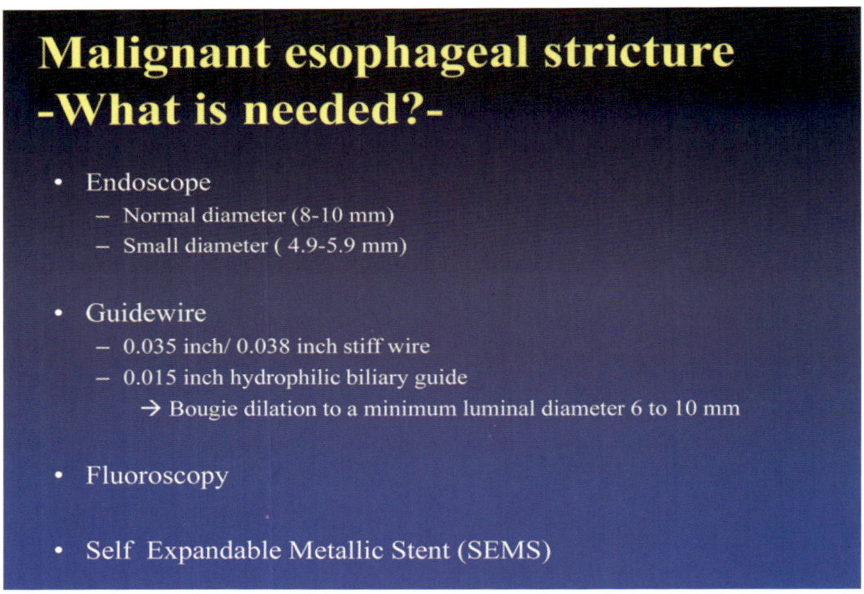

Small caliber endoscopes (nasogastroscope, Olympus XP 160; 5.9 mm diameter) can easily pass through the stricture, offering a simple and safe evaluation of the lesion. We usually use 0.035 or 0.038 inch stiff wire. But if the stricture is extremely tight or tortuous we use a hydrophilic biliary guide wire preloaded through a standard biliary catheter. Once the guide wire has been passed through the stricture under fluoroscopic monitoring, bougie dilation is performed to a minimal luminal diameter of 6 to 10 mm that will permit deployment.

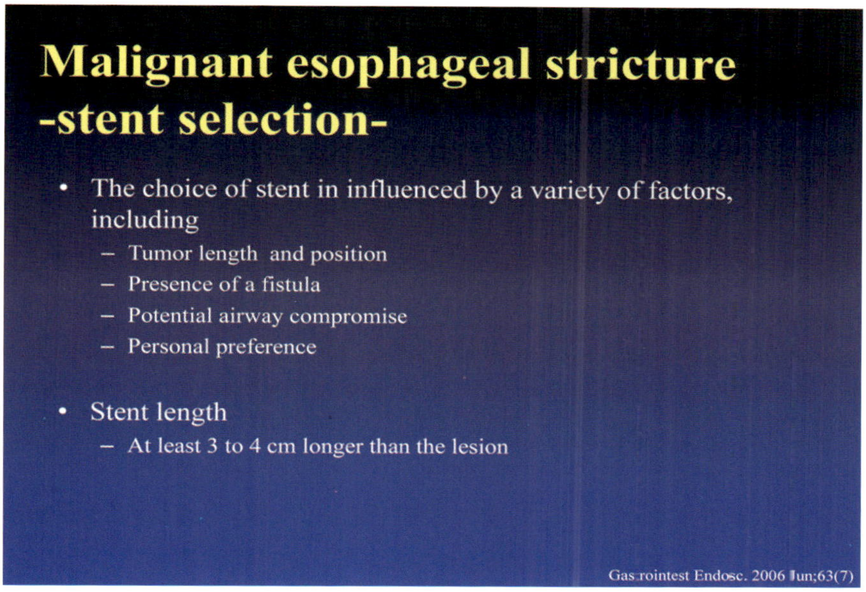

The choice of stent for an individual is influenced by a variety of factors, including tumor length and position, and presence of a fistula, potential airway compromise, and personal preference of the physician inserting the stent. The diameter and length of the stent should be determined after measuring and monitoring the length of the stricture using fluoroscopy or endoscopy. The length of the stent chosen should be at least 3 to 4 cm longer than the obstruction, to allow an adequate margin of stent on either side of the obstruction.

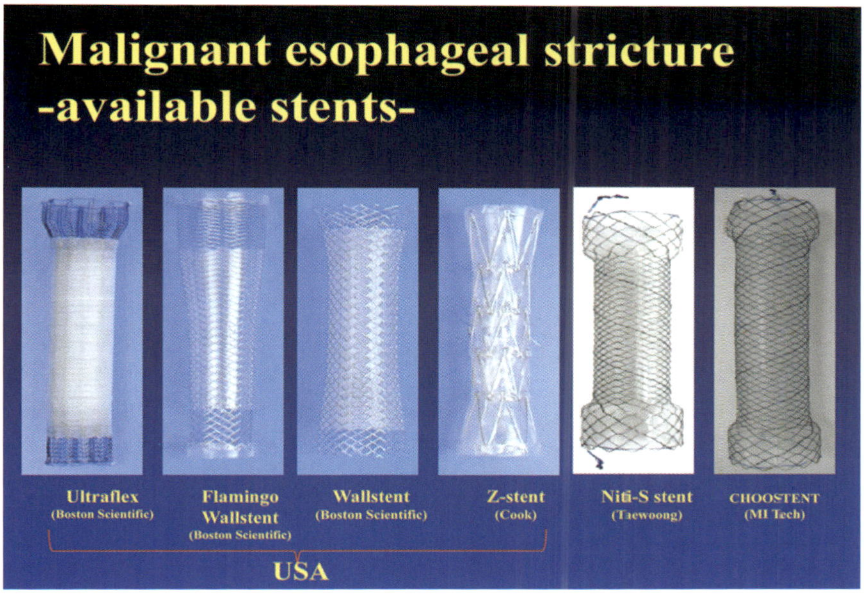

Self-expandable metallic stents (SEMS) are composed of a variety of metal alloys with varying shapes and sizes depending upon the individual manufacturer. All stents appear to be equally effective in palliating obstructive symptoms. None of the currently available stents are small enough to pass through the endoscope.

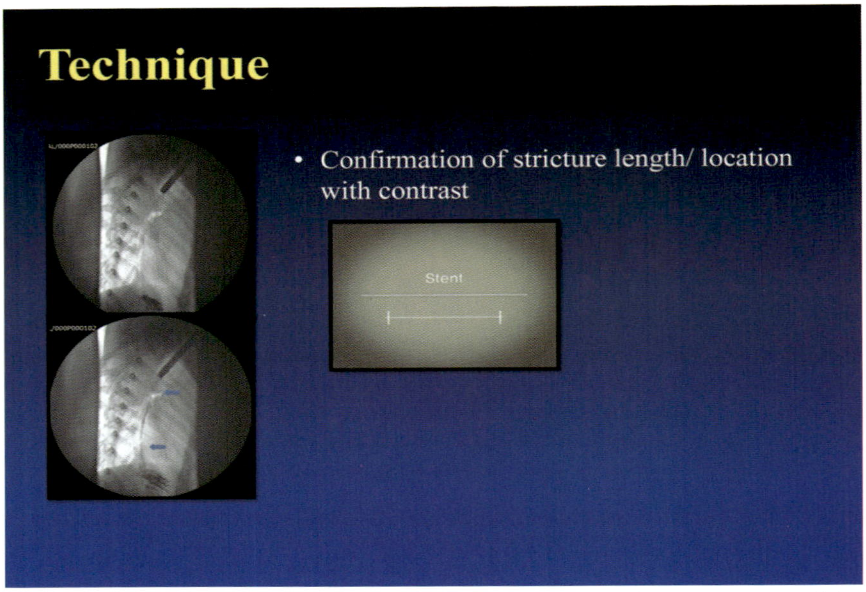

Fluoroscopy is used to confirm the length and location of the stricture. Once the length of the stricture has been determined, the length of the stent can be chosen.

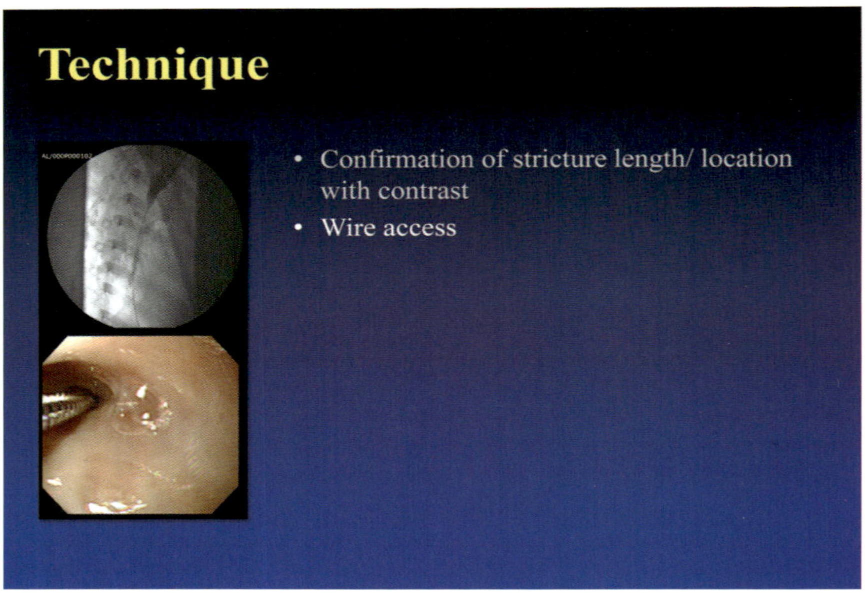

After determination of the stricture length and location a guidewire is introduced through the stricture.

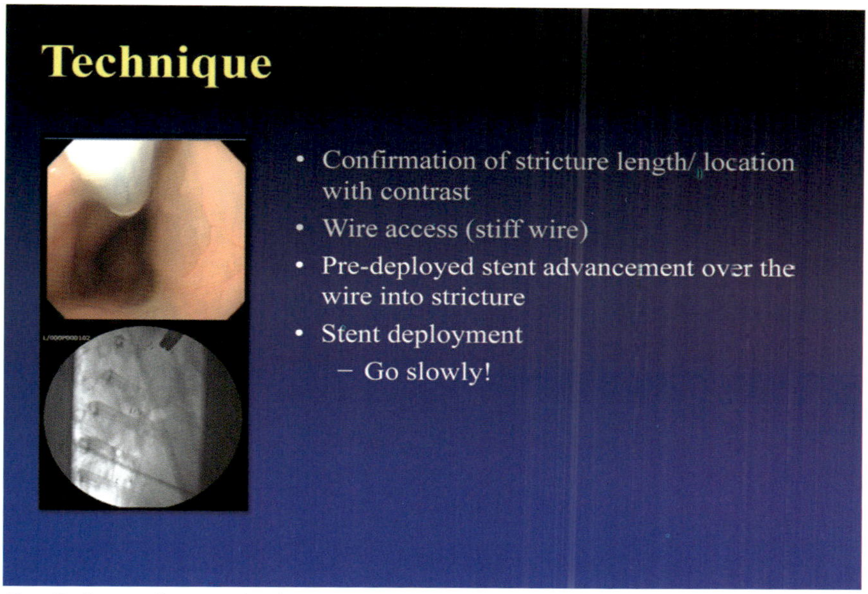

Pre-dilation may increase the risk of perforation; however there is currently no consensus on how many sessions of pre-dilation can be performed before the risk of perforation increases. If the endoscope can be passed with minimal difficulty through the obstruction, this can be attempted without pre-dilation. Once the guidewire is in place a pre-deployed stent is advanced over the wire into the stricture. It is important to realize that some stents are available as proximal release devices (deployment proceeds in a proximal-to-distal sequence), while others deploy in distal-to-proximal sequence. The distal release stents are used for stent placement in the mid and upper esophagus while proximal release stents are used for gastro-esophageal junction lesions. Deployment should be performed slowly.

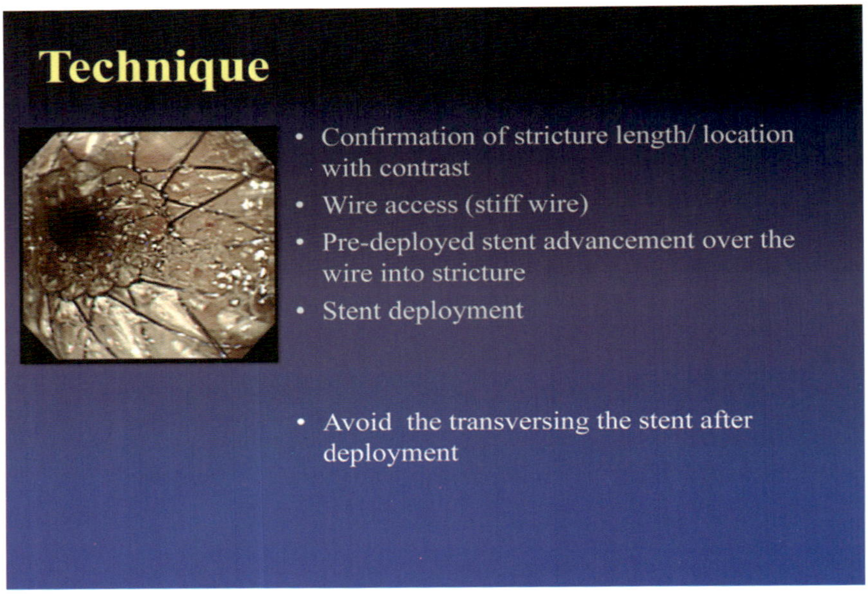

After deployment, the endoscope is passed into the proximal portion of the stent, but not through the stent, to assess stent position relative to the tumor while avoiding dislodgement.

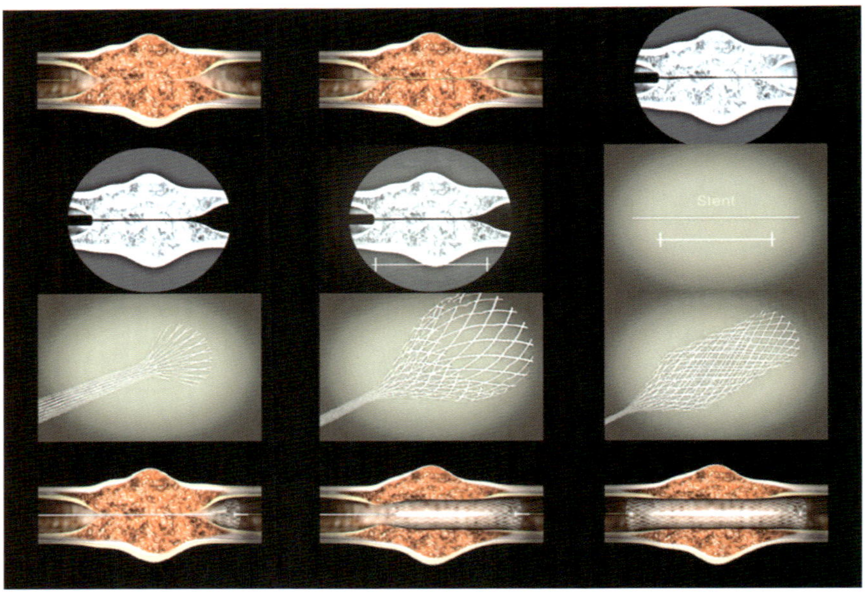

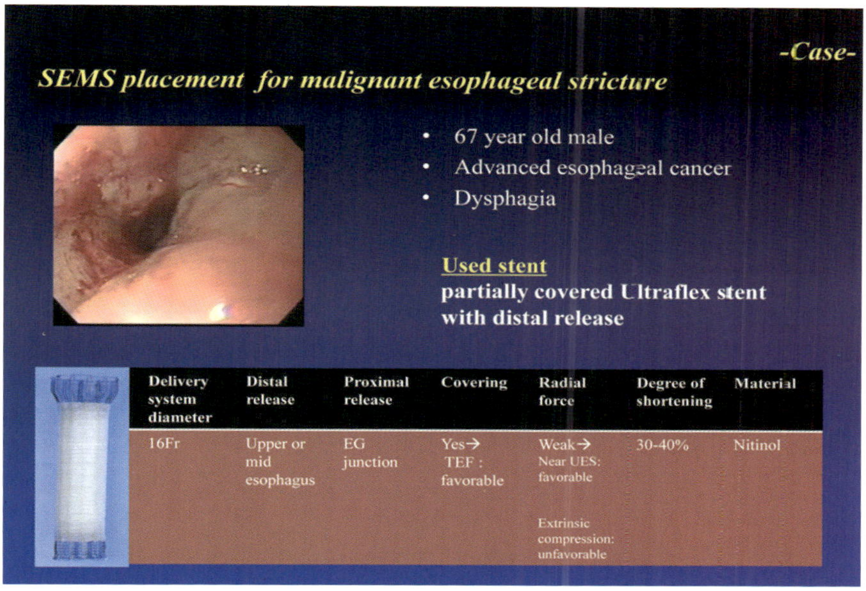

This is a 67-year-old male with advanced esophageal cancer of the mid esophagus. We used a partially covered Ultraflex stent with distal release. The stent is constructed of a single strand of nitinol that exerts a constant gentle radial pressure while minimizing traumatic tissue compression. The low radial force of the stent seems to be useful for patients with malignant strictures that are close to the upper esophageal sphincter. Stents are available in either of two different release systems. The distal release stents are used for stent placement in mid and upper esophagus while proximal release stents are used for gastro-esophageal junction lesions

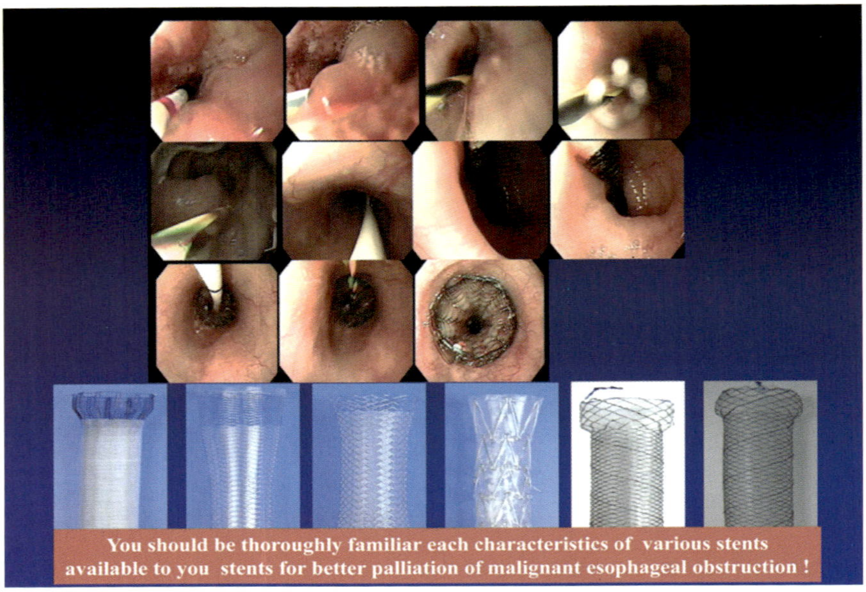

Although we used an Ultraflex stent, other stents can also be used in this patient. Prior to procedure the endoscopist should be familiar with the characteristics of each available stent.

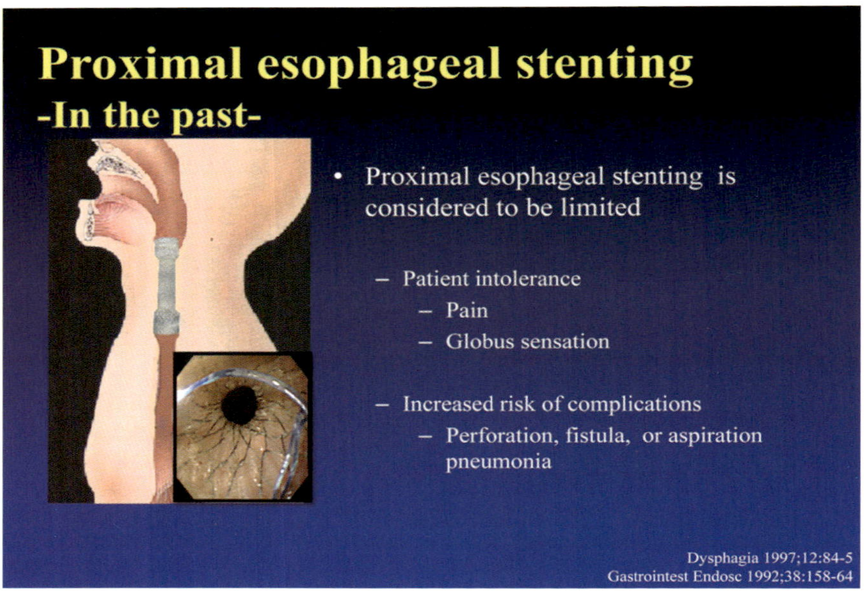

The use of stents in the proximal esophagus has traditionally been considered to be limited because of an increased risk of complications and patient intolerance.

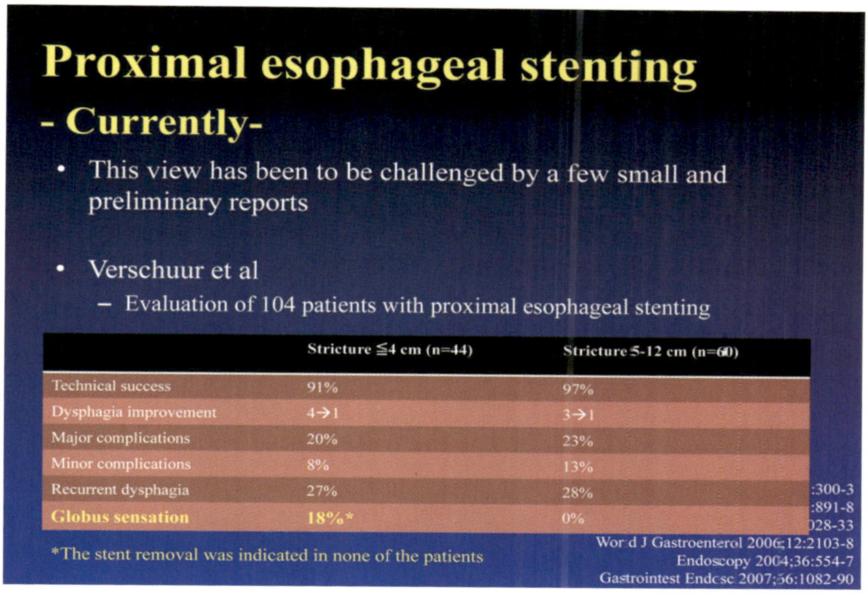

Recently this view has been challenged by a few small and preliminary reports. In a evaluation of 104 patients with proximal esophageal stenting technical success, dysphagia improvement, major complications, minor complications and recurrent dysphagia was not significantly different between patients with strictures within 4cm or between 5 to 12 cm of the UES. A foreign body sensation was significantly higher in patients with strictures within 4 cm of the UES; however, stent removal was indicated in none of the patients compared with series of stents placed in the mid or distal esophagus or gastric cardia, the complication rate in the proximal esophageal stenting is also comparable, with reported frequencies varying between 24% and 36%.

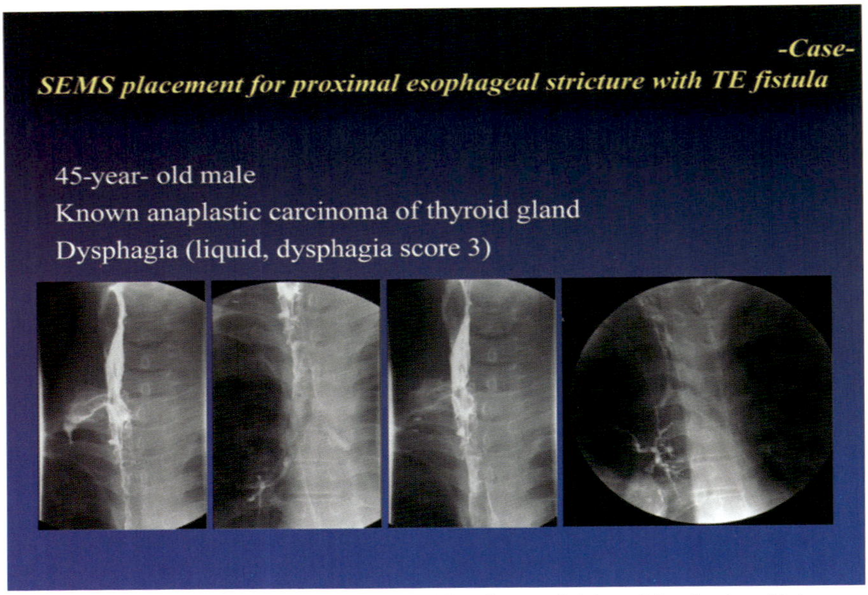

This is a barium esophagogram of a 45 year old male complaining of dysphagia, with known anaplastic cancer of the thyroid gland. On the left, Barium can be seen leaking through the tracheostomy site. The distal esophagus below the tracheostomy site cannot be seen and collections can be seen filling the bronchial tree.

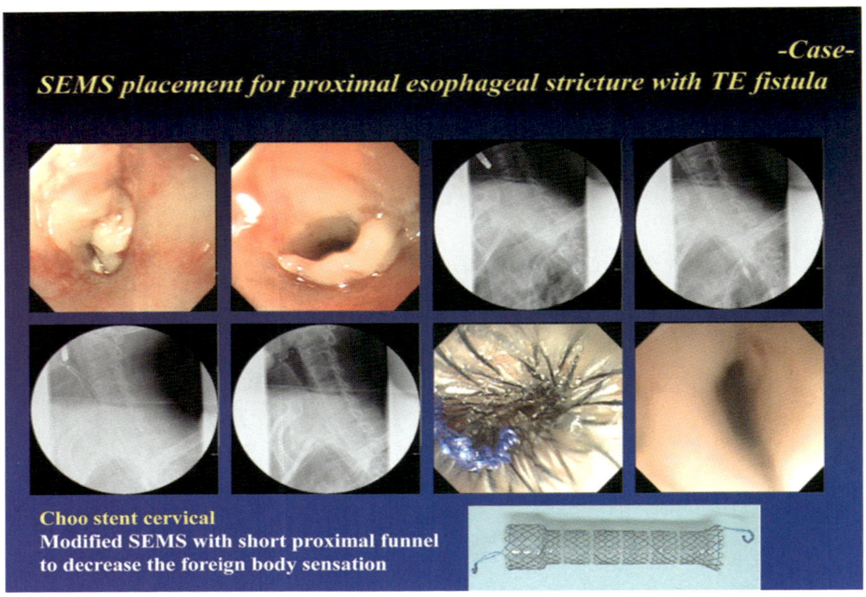

Endoscopy shows a stricture with a fistula 2cm below the UES. We decided to deploy a cervical CHOOSTENT for palliation of symptoms and sealage of the fistula. The cervical CHOOSTENT is a covered stent with a proximal funnel to minimize foreign body sensation. After successful stent deployment the patient' s dysphagia improved and no further leakage was observed on follow up exams.

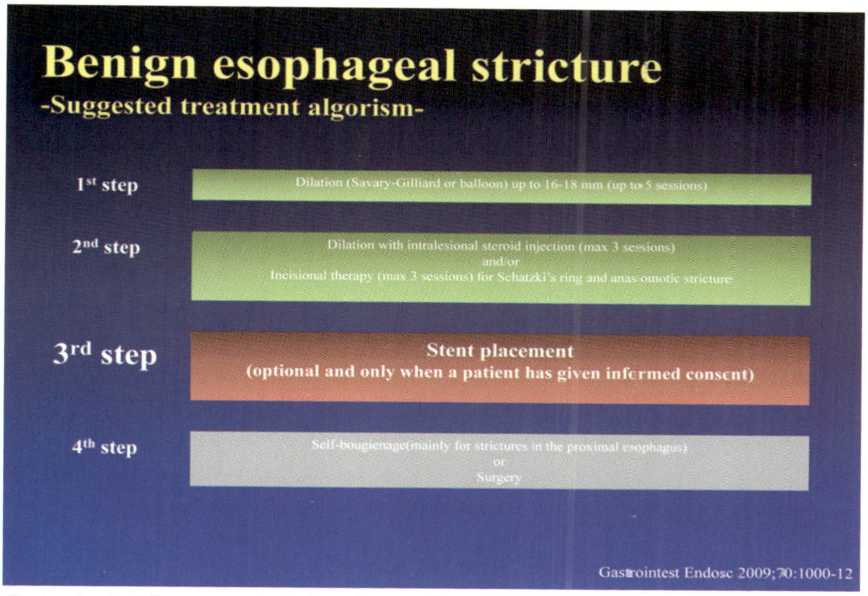

During the last few years, stents have become increasingly used for dilating refractory benign esophageal strictures. The idea is that dilation for a prolonged period of time will ultimately reduce the risk of recurrent stricture formation.

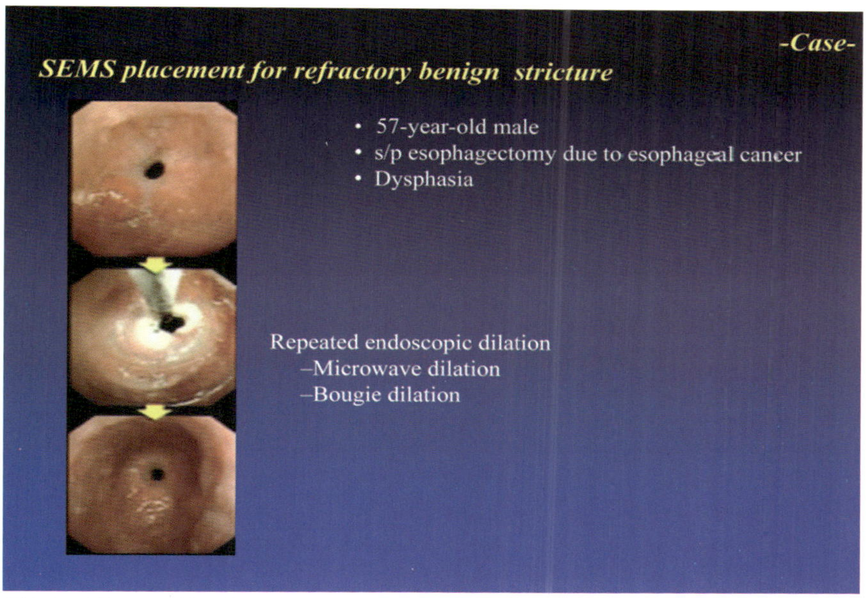

This is a 57-year-old male with an anastomotic site stricture following surgery for esophageal cancer. The stricture was refractory despite several sessions of bougie dilation and microwave therapy.

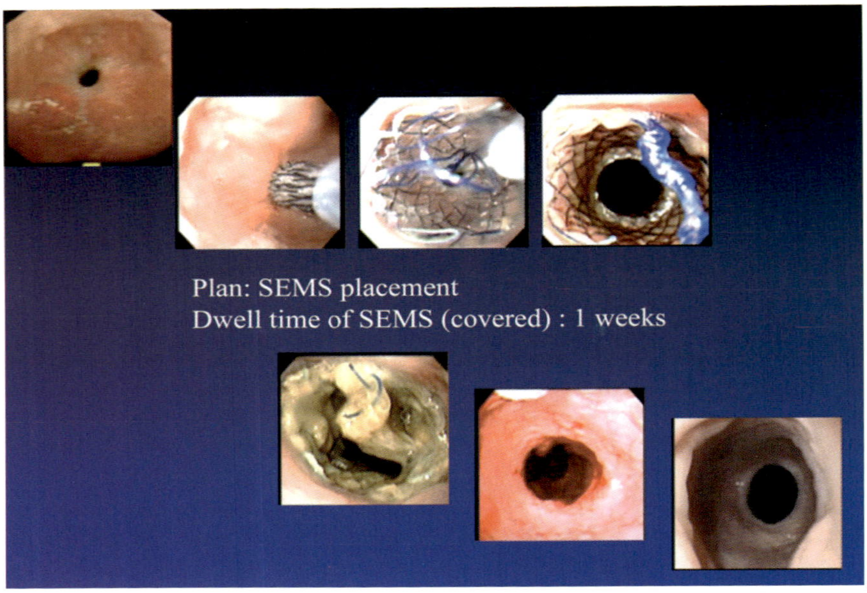

We inserted a covered SEMS for 1 week. Following removal dramatic improvement can be seen.

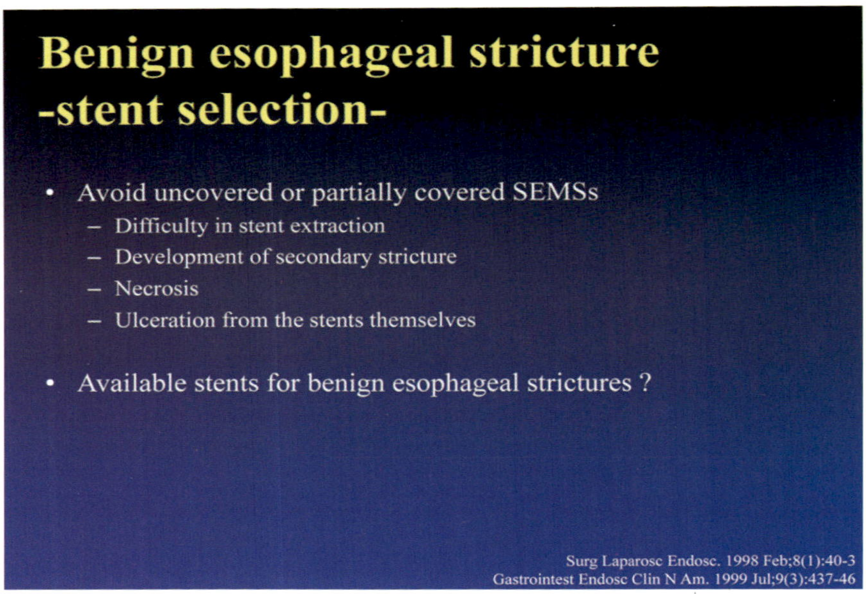

SEMSs have been used with variable success in the treatment of benign strictures. However, complications of uncovered or partially covered SEMSs include difficulty in stent extraction, development of secondary strictures, necrosis, and ulceration from the stents themselves; therefore it is best to avoid uncovered or partially covered SEMSs.

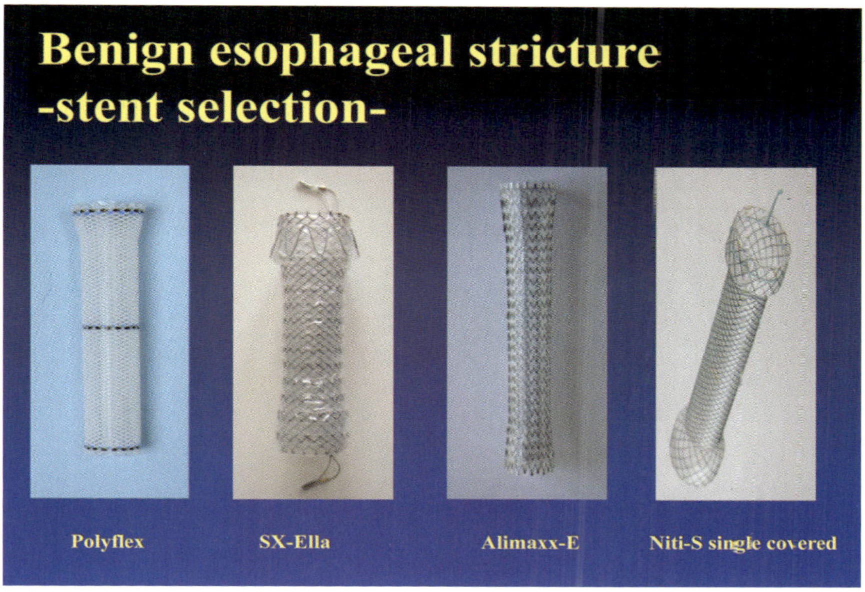

Currently available stents for benign esophageal strictures. These stents all have the common feature of easy retrieval after deployment.

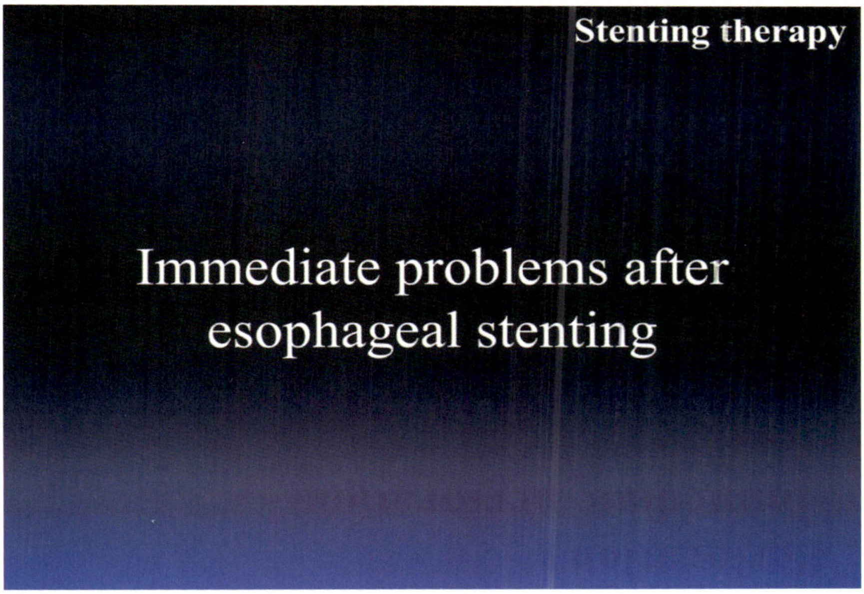

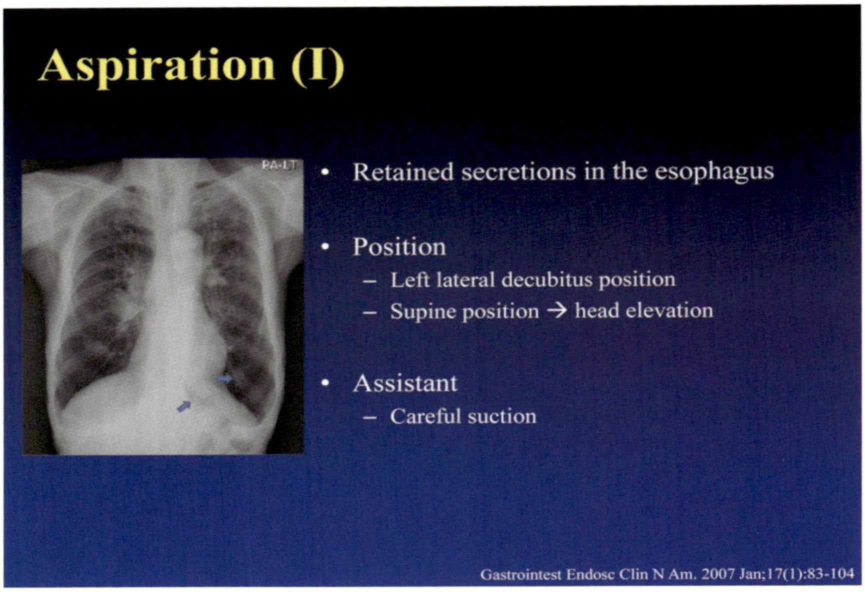

Patients who have advanced esophageal obstruction frequently have retained secretions in the esophagus. These patients are at risk for pulmonary aspiration. Placing the patient in the left lateral decubitus position and having the assistant closely monitor and suction secretions will help prevent aspiration.

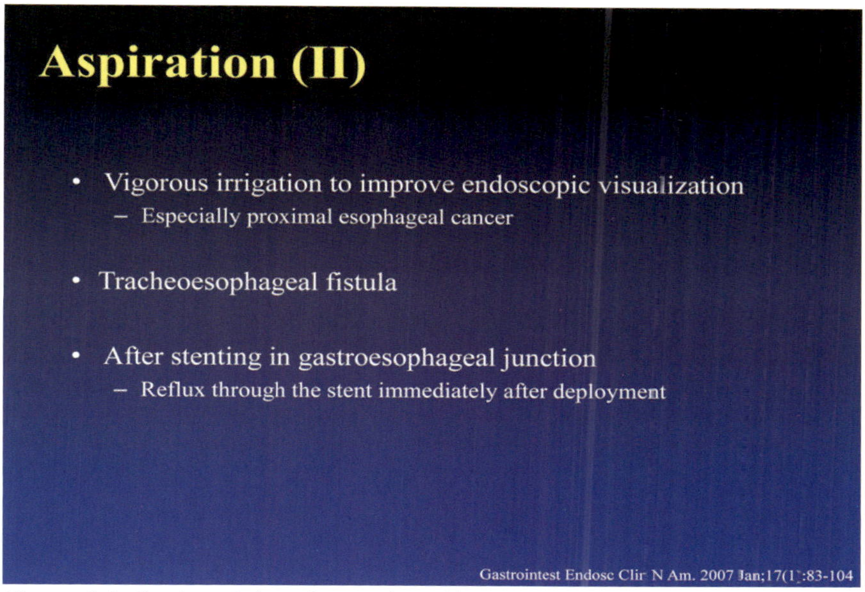

Vigorous irrigation through the endoscope channel in an attempt to clear secretions and improve endoscopic visualization may also cause aspiration. Unfortunately, fluids tend to reflux proximally from the obstruction leading to aspiration. This is more likely to occur with proximal lesions. Irrigation should be avoided in patients with tracheo esophageal fistulas when the endoscope is positioned near the fistula, since fluid is likely to pass directly into the trachea. Finally, in those patients who have gastroesophageal junction (GEJ) tumors, gastric contents can reflux through the stent immediately after deployment. Thus, while in the recovery area, patients in whom a stent has been placed across the GEJ should be kept in the left lateral decubitus position or have their head elevated if placed in the supine position to prevent aspiration during this period.

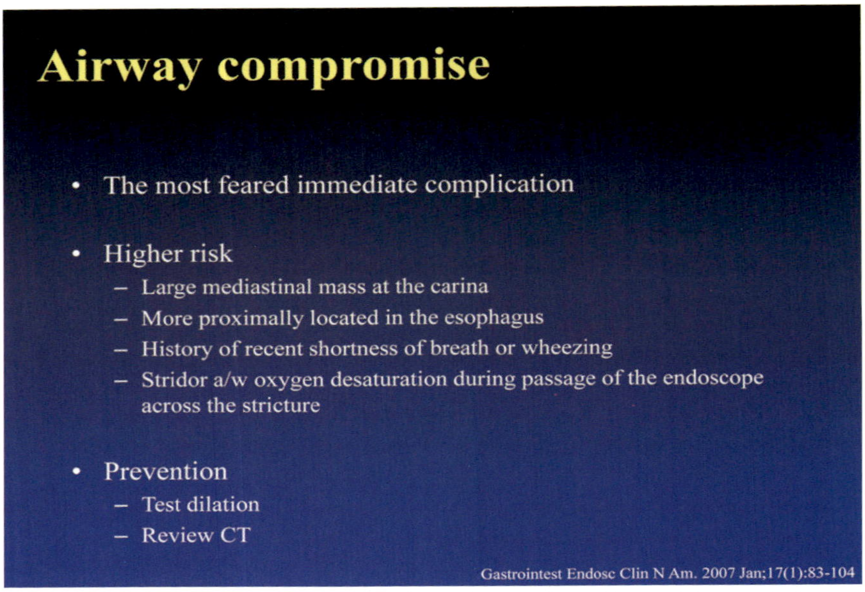

Airway compromise from tracheal obstruction is the most feared immediate complication of esophageal stent placement, It almost always occurs in the setting of large mediastinal masses that are in the area of the carina or more proximally located in the esophagus Any history of recent shortness of breath or wheezing should alert the endoscopist that there may be airway compromise In addition; the development of stridor associated with oxygen desaturation during passage of the endoscope across the stricture is a red flag. Because most patients will have had a recent chest CT, a preprocedural review with attention to the relationship of the esophagus to the mass usually will suggest some form of tracheal narrowing in those patients at risk. Some endoscopists advocate the passage of a moderate-sized rigid dilator (15 mm Savary) or inflation of a dilating balloon within the stricture as a test to see if the patient develops stridor. There is no data, however, to support this practice.

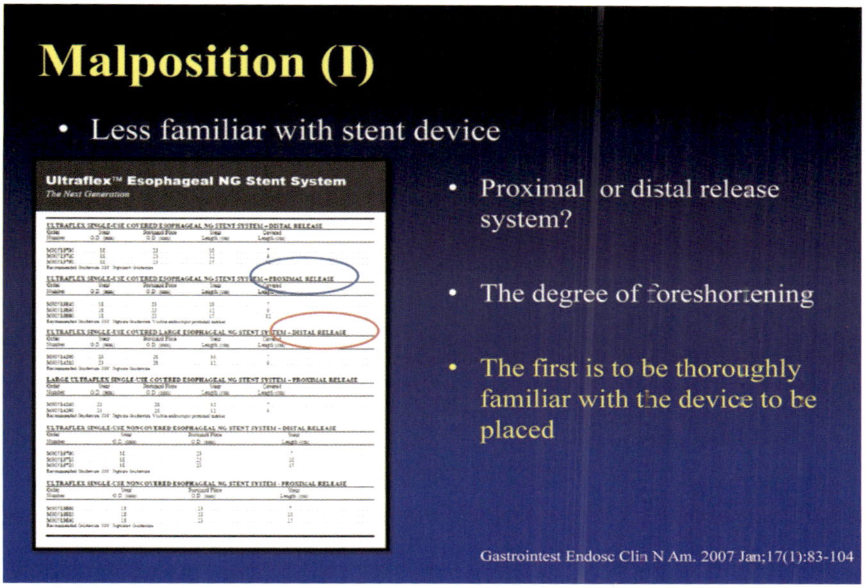

To prevent stent malposition the endoscopist must first be familiar with the stent that is to be used. Thorough knowledge of the characteristics of each stent, including the release system, and degree of foreshortening should be taken into account before deployment.

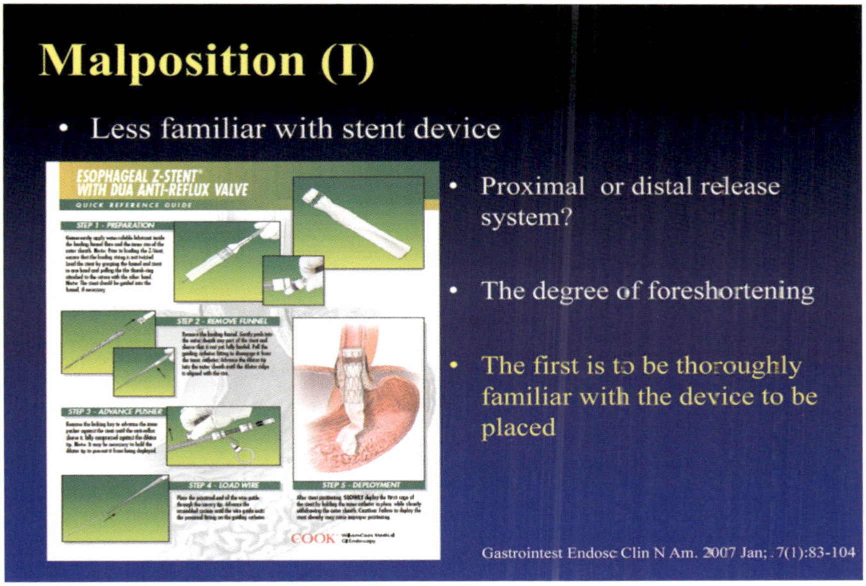

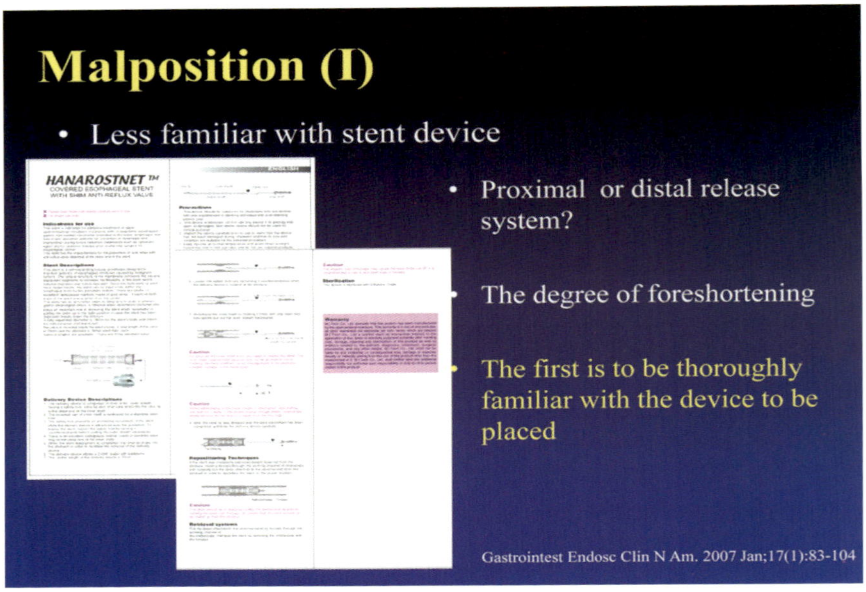

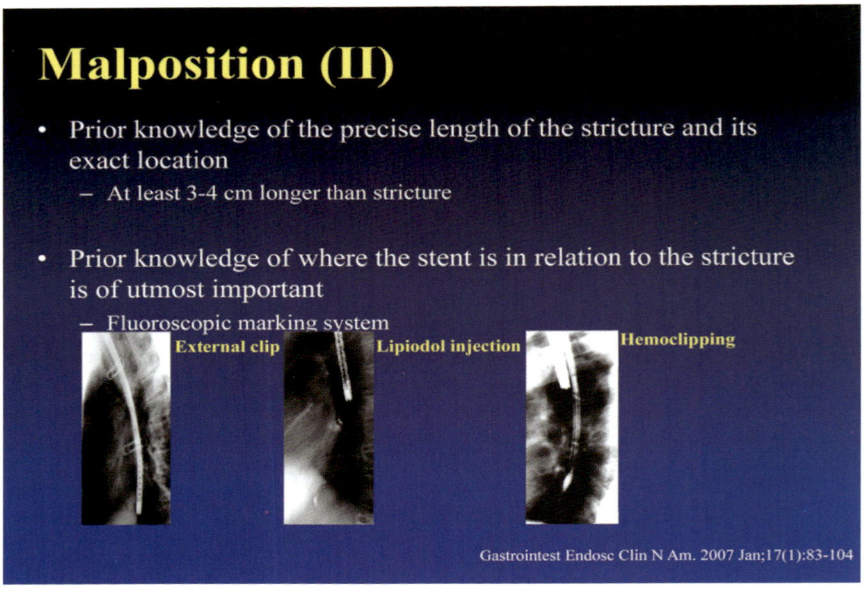

Precise knowledge of the length of the stricture and its exact location will help prevent stent malposition. Ideally, stents should be at least 3 to 4 cm longer than the stricture so as to provide room for error. Knowing where the stent is in relation to the stricture is of utmost importance. Thus, some form of fluoroscopic marking is frequently is used.

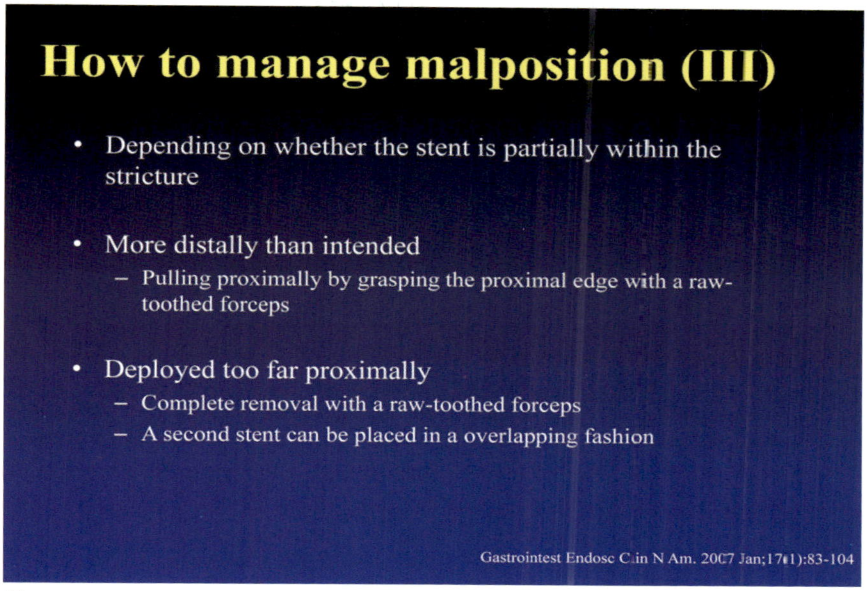

There are several options to manage stent malposition, should it occur, depending on whether the stent is partially within the stricture. If it has been deployed more distally than intended, it usually can be pulled proximally by grasping the proximal edge with a raw-toothed forceps and withdrawing the endoscope. If deployed too far proximally, it is usually not possible to push the stent forward, especially if the stent is distal release. In this situation, either the stent can be removed completely with a rat toothed forceps, or a second stent can be placed in overlapping fashion to cover the distal end of the stricture.

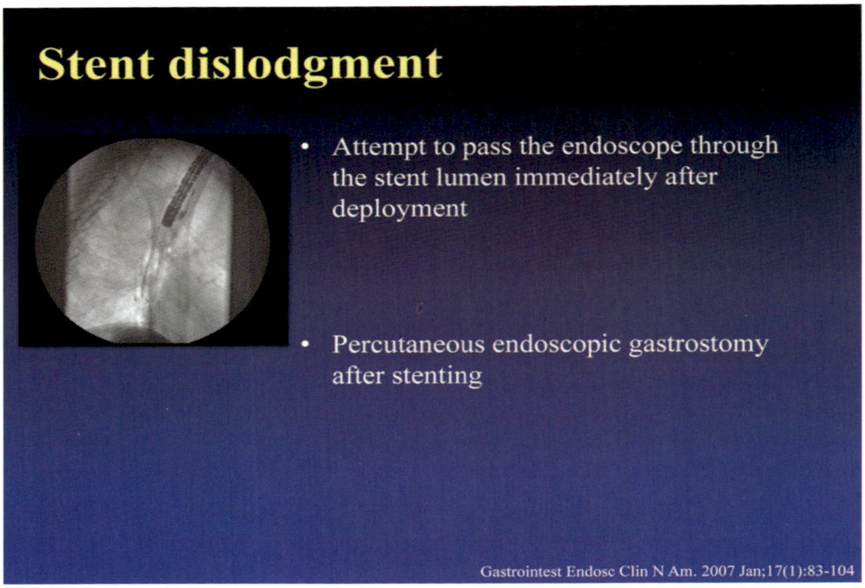

Stent dislodgment usually occurs when an attempt is made to pass the endoscope through the stent lumen immediately after deployment. This step is usually unnecessary. Another cause of stent dislodgement is placement of a percutaneous endoscopic gastrostomy tube after SEMS placement.

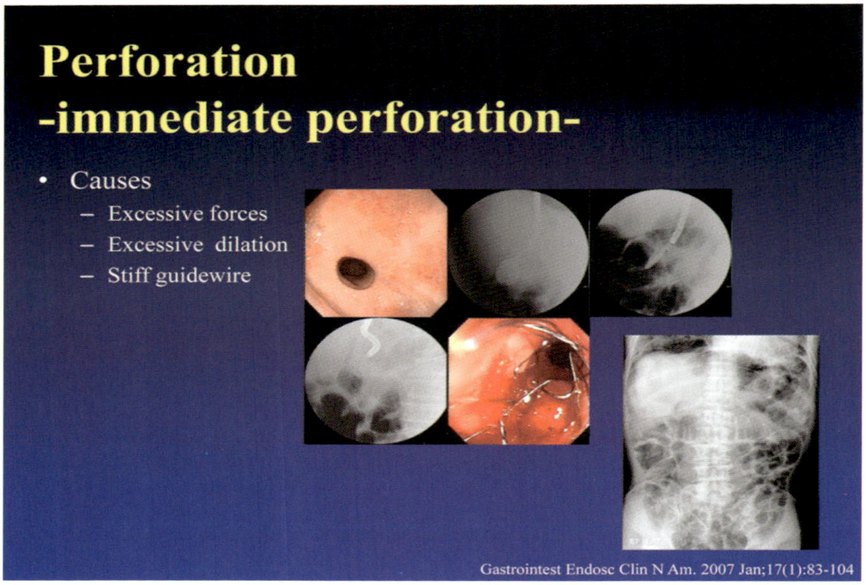

Perforation during deployment can be caused by the guide wire itself, application of excessive force to the endoscope during attempts to pass the stricture, or excessive dilation of the stricture. A stent should never be deployed unless the endoscopist is absolutely certain that the guidewire is intraluminally placed.

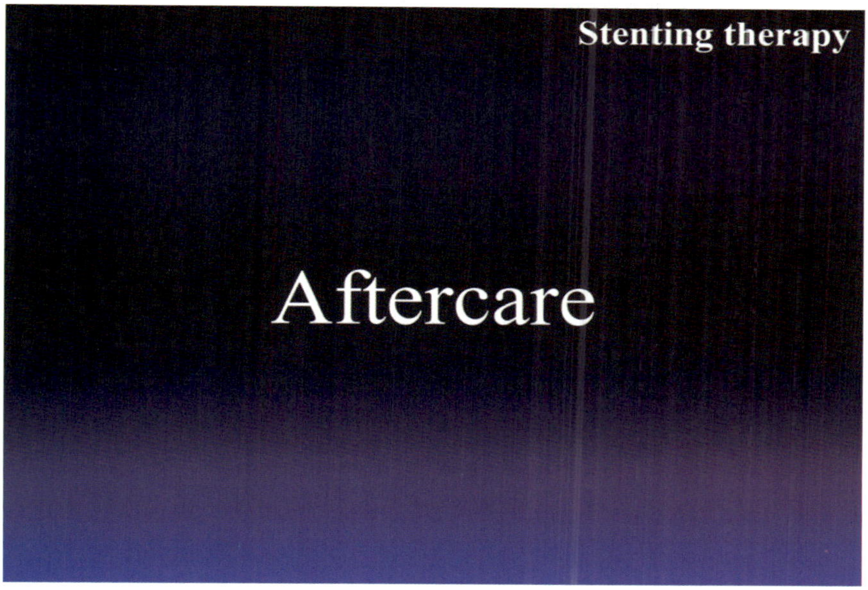

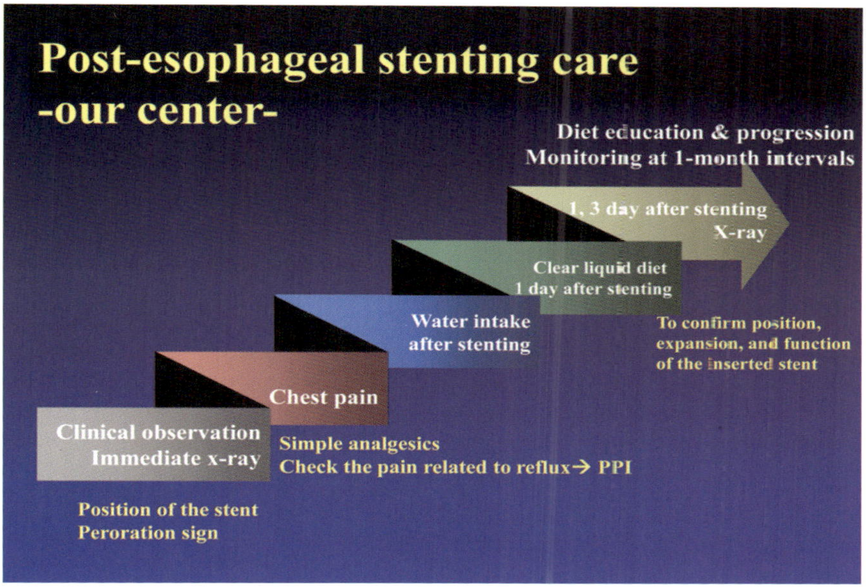

Following stent insertion, chest radiography should be carried out to verify the position of the stent and to check for signs of perforation. Following stent placement, patients can experience varying degrees of chest pain and discomfort. This is usually controlled with simple analgesia, and occasionally opiates. It is important to ascertain whether or not the chest pain is related to acid reflux. X-ray should be performed to confirm position, expansion, and function of the inserted stent 1, 3 day after stenting.

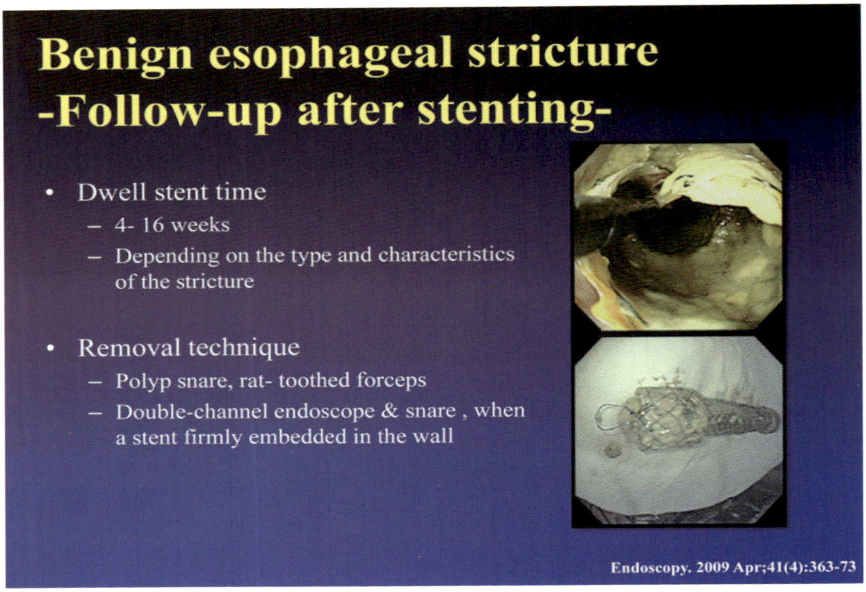

In contrast to malignant esophageal strictures, stents are removed after a period of time for benign strictures of the esophagus. Although there are no available guidelines most reports recommend a stent dwell time of 4 to 16 weeks depending on the type and characteristics of the stricture.

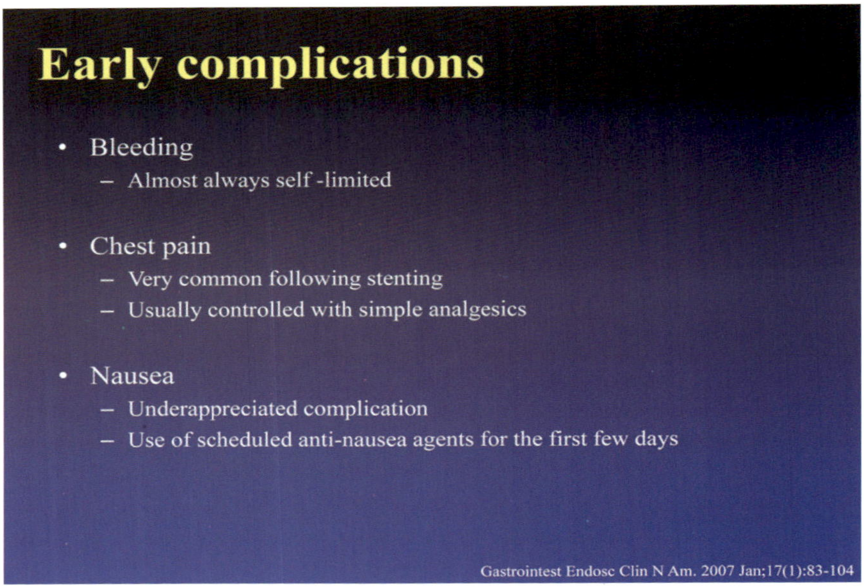

The most commonly anticipated early complications following esophageal stenting are bleeding, chest pain and nausea. Bleeding is almost always self-limited. Chest pain occurs very commonly and is usually controlled with simple analgesics. Nausea is an underappreciated complication. There is no way to avoid this, although the use of scheduled anti-nausea agents for the first few days should be considered in those patients who experience more than minimal nausea in the recovery area.

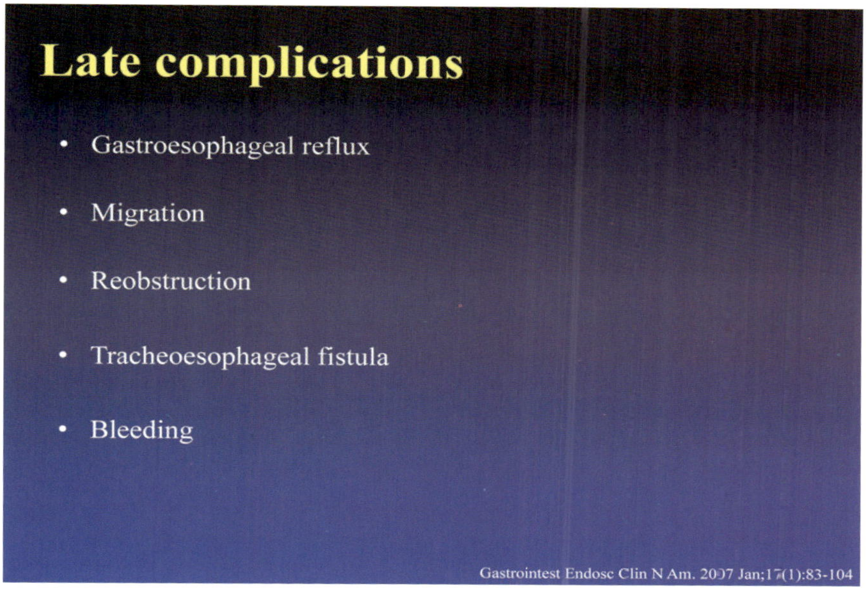

The most common late complications are gastroesophageal reflux, migration, reobstruction, tracheoesophageal fistulas, and delayed bleeding.

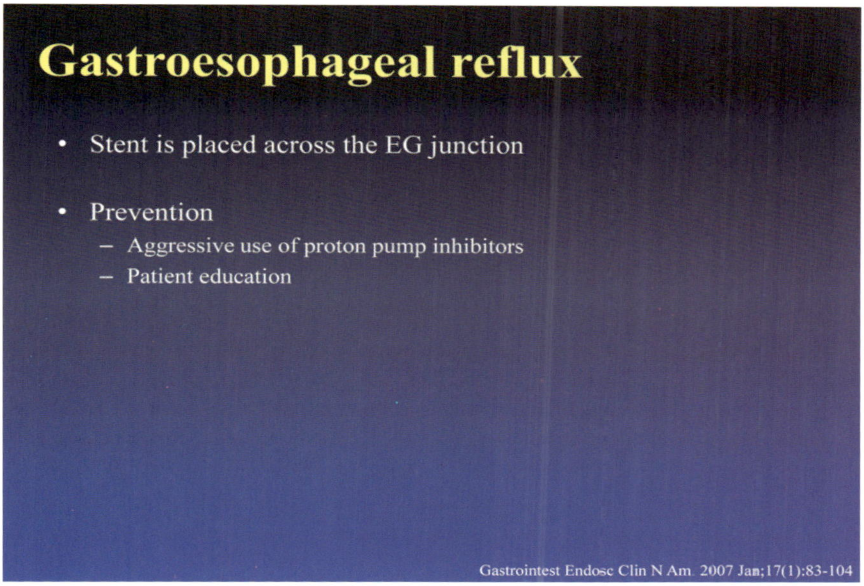

Gastroesophageal reflux disease (GERD) with or without aspiration can occur when a SEMS is placed across the GEJ. GERD and aspiration can be avoided by the aggressive use of proton pump inhibitors and patient education.

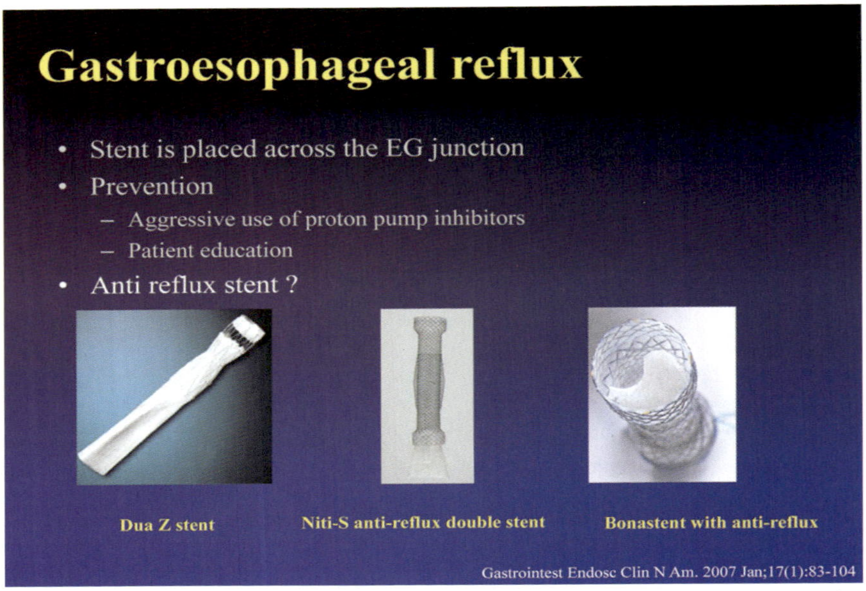

Various stents with antireflux mechanisms have been developed just for the purpose of placement across the GEJ.

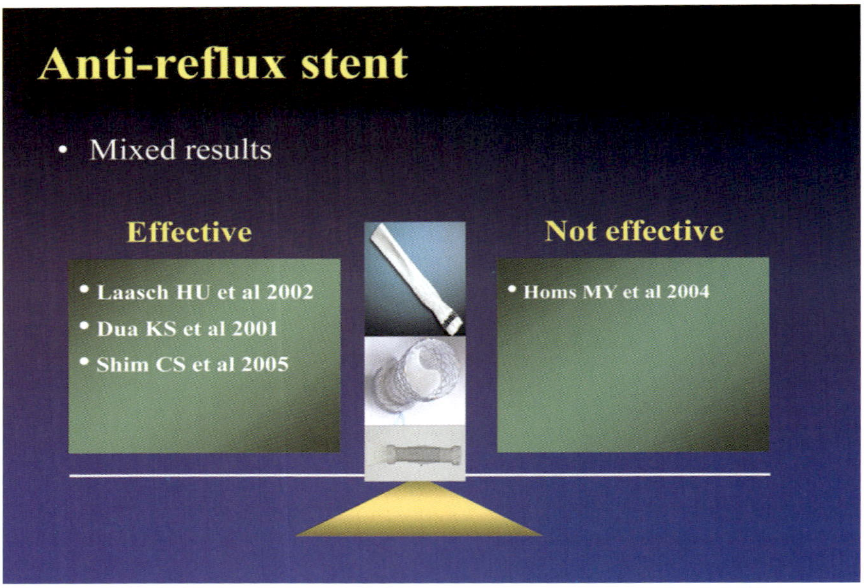

Although the available data is limited, the use of antireflux stents has yielded mixed results.

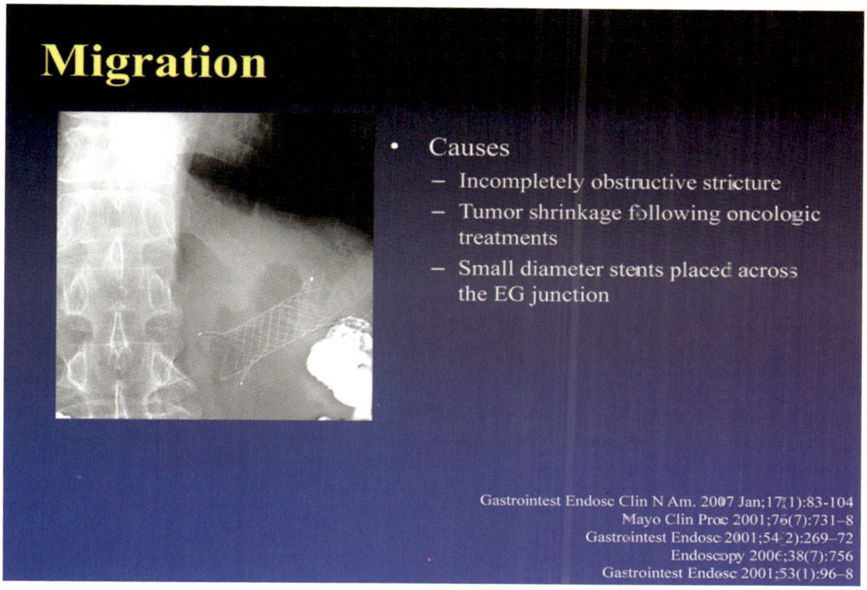

Migration of a successfully deployed stent is a relatively common complication. Migration may occur in the case of incomplete obstruction where the stent may not hold within the stricture. Tumor shrinkage following oncologic treatment also may lead to stent migration. Stents placed across very soft, polypoid tumors and smaller diameter stents placed across the GEJ are more prone to migration.

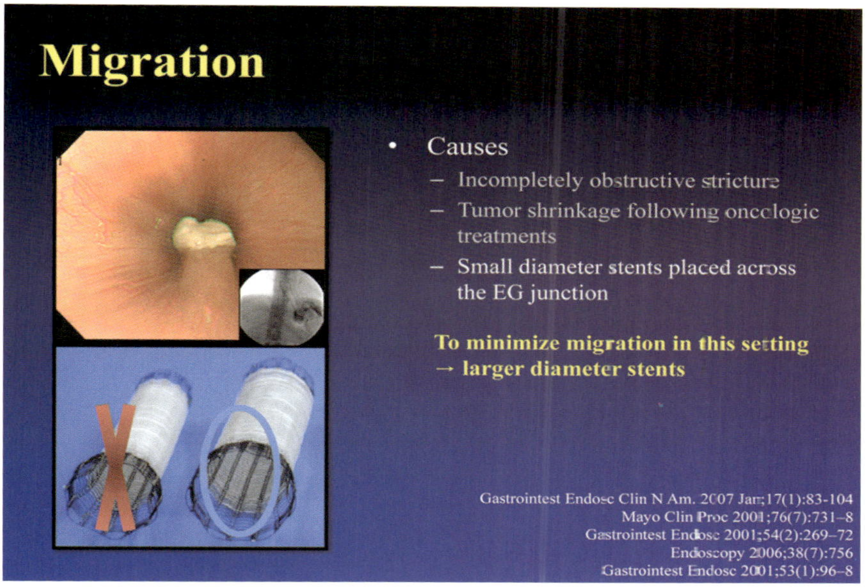

Thus to minimize migration in this setting, it is recommended that larger diameter stents be used.

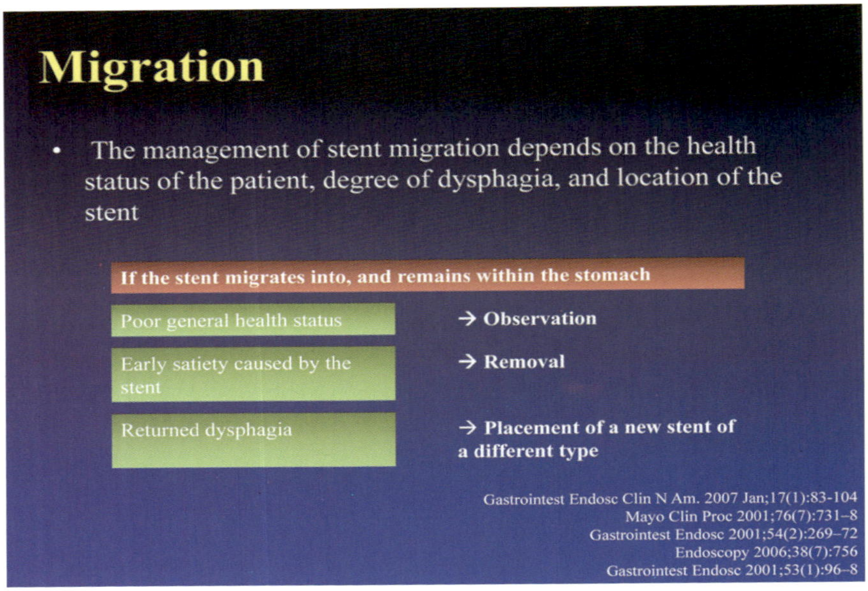

The management of stent migration depends on the health status of the patient, degree of dysphagia, and location of the stent. Most commonly, the stent migrates into, and remains within, the stomach. If the patient' s performance status is poor, it is probably best to leave the stent in place. Patients who are symptomatic because of early satiety caused by the stent should be offered stent removal. If the patient experiences recurrent dysphagia stent removal and placement of a new stent can be tried.

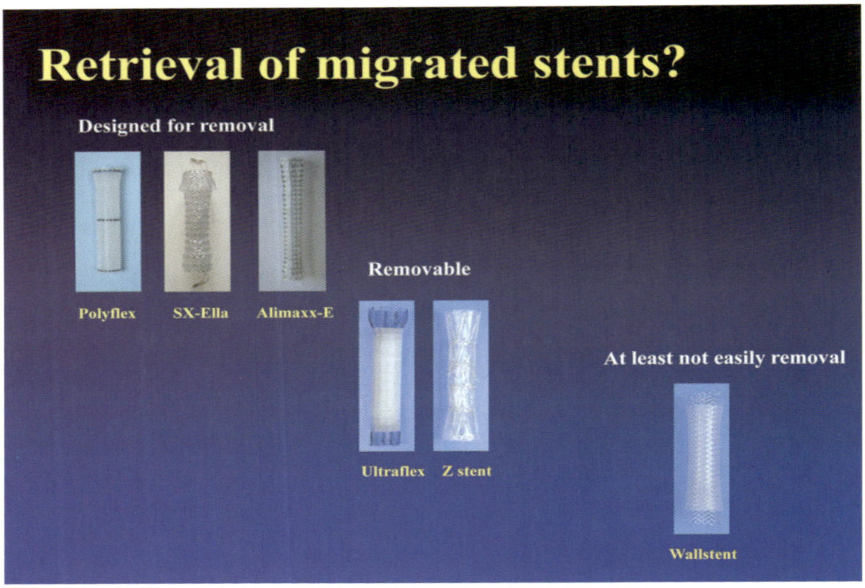

Before attempting to retrieve a migrated stent, one should first consider the design of the stent.

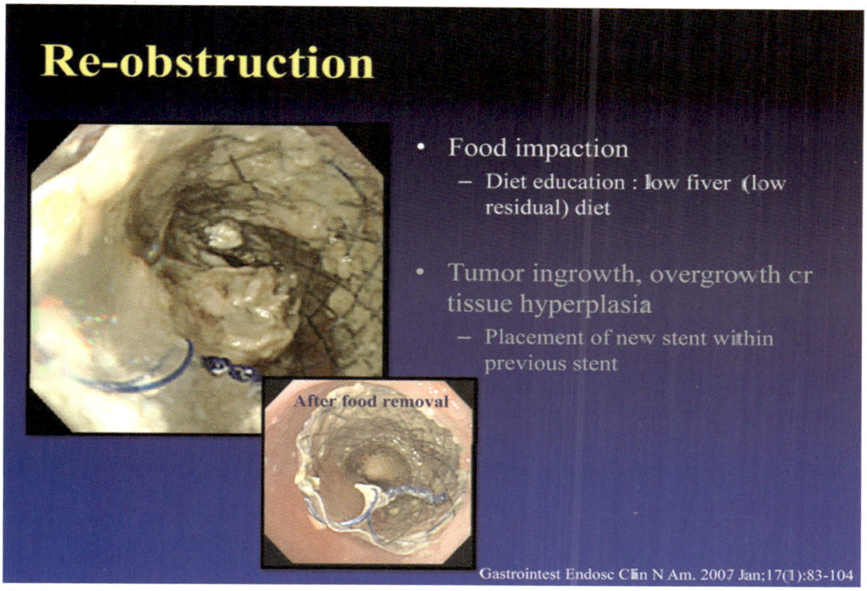

Reobstruction can occur from several mechanisms, including food impaction, tumor overgrowth, tumor ingrowth, and tissue hyperplasia. Diet education is very important for prevention of stent reobstruction due to food impaction.

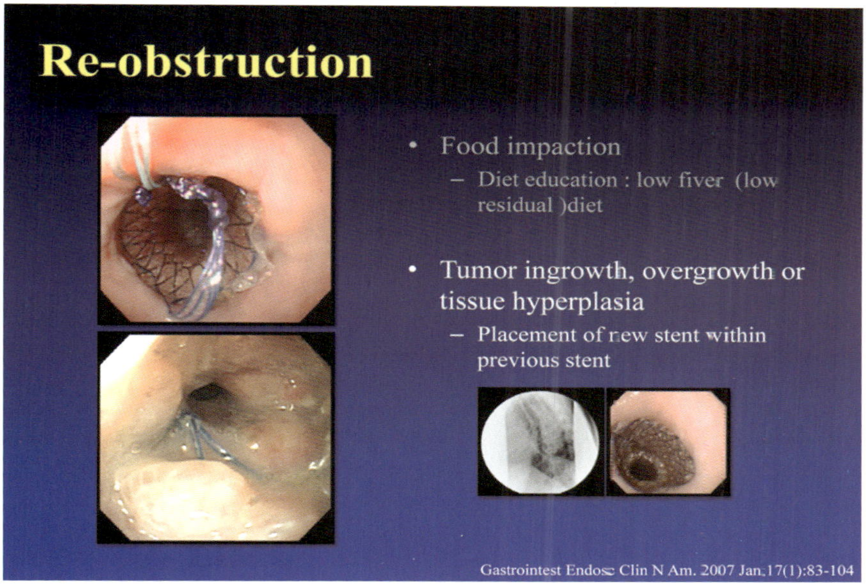

Reobstruction by tumor ingrowth, overgrowth, or tissue hyperplasia is managed best with placement of a new stent within the previous stent.

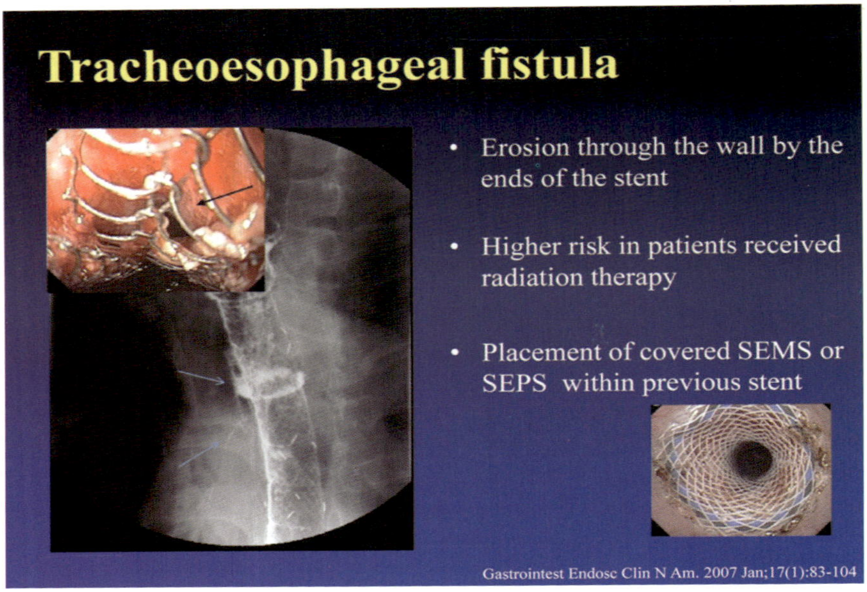

TEF as a result of the ends of the stent eroding through the wall is beyond the control of the endoscopist. This complication can be managed by placing another covered SEMS or a self-expandable plastic stent within the initial stent. The risk of SEMS-related TEF may be greater in patients who have received radiation therapy.

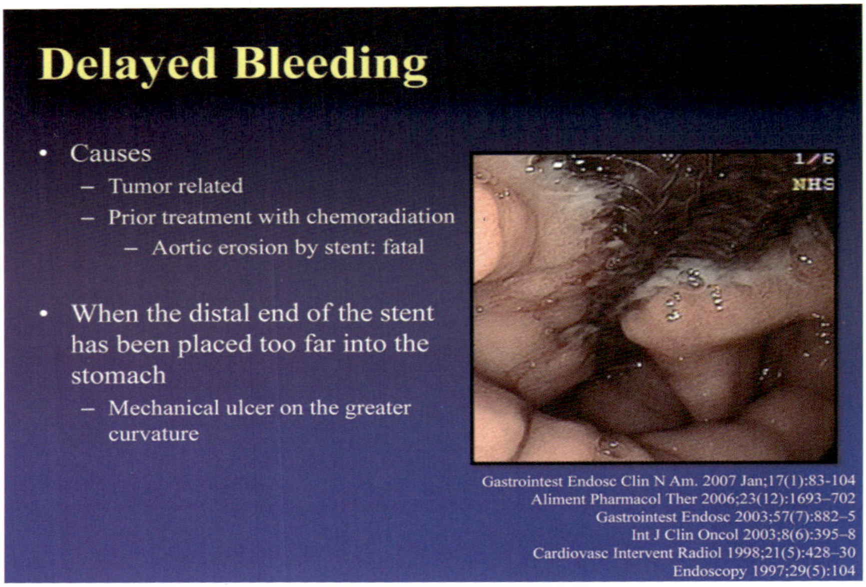

Delayed bleeding can be fatal and is largely beyond the control of the endoscopist, because it is usually tumor-related and/or caused by prior treatment with chemoradiation. Another notable cause of bleeding occurs when the distal end of the stent has been placed too far into the stomach such that it impacts the greater curvature forming a mechanical ulcer.

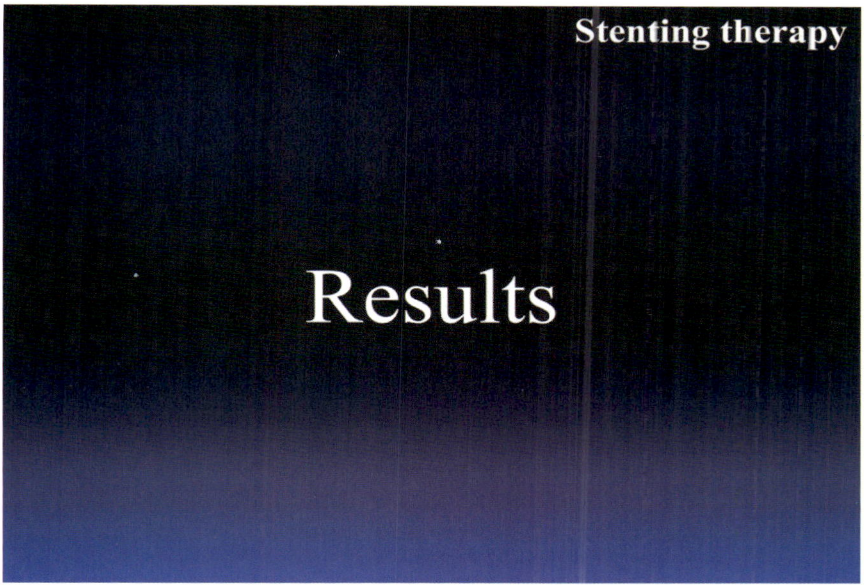

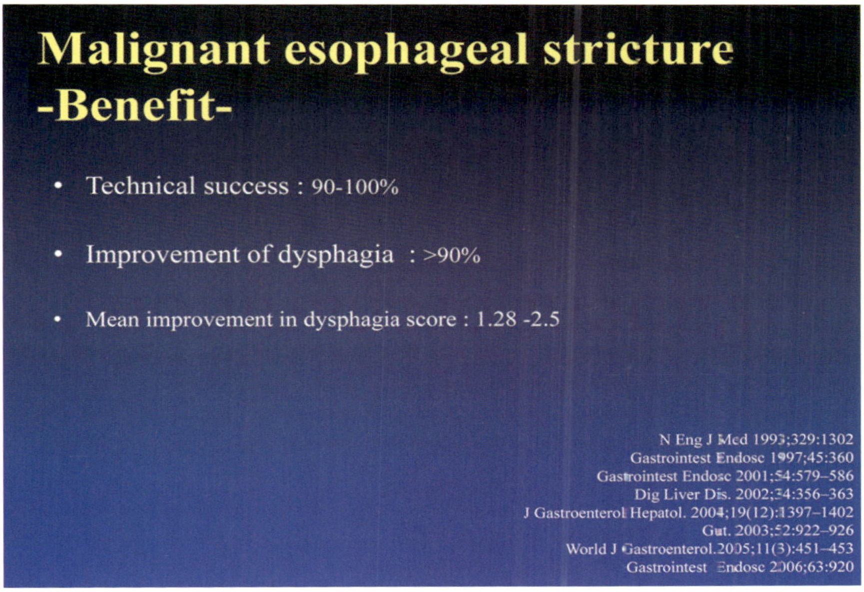

Overall the benefits of stenting is malignant esophageal strictures is well established. The technical success rate is 90-100%. Esophageal stenting improved dysphagia in over 90% patients. Mean improvement in dysphagia score is 1.28 -2.5.

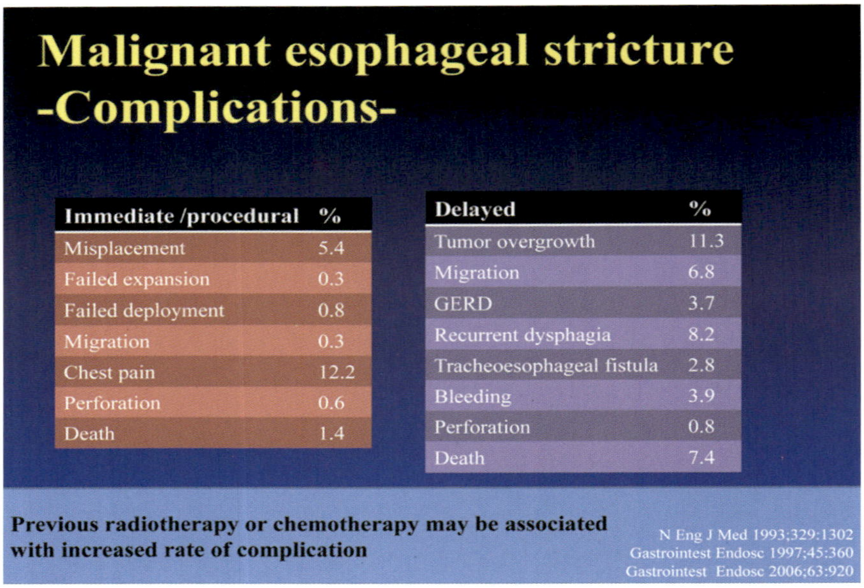

Although there are various complications that occur in varying frequency, chest pain is the most common immediate complication and tumor overgrowth is the most common delayed complication. Previous radiotherapy or chemotherapy may be associated with increased risk of developing complications.

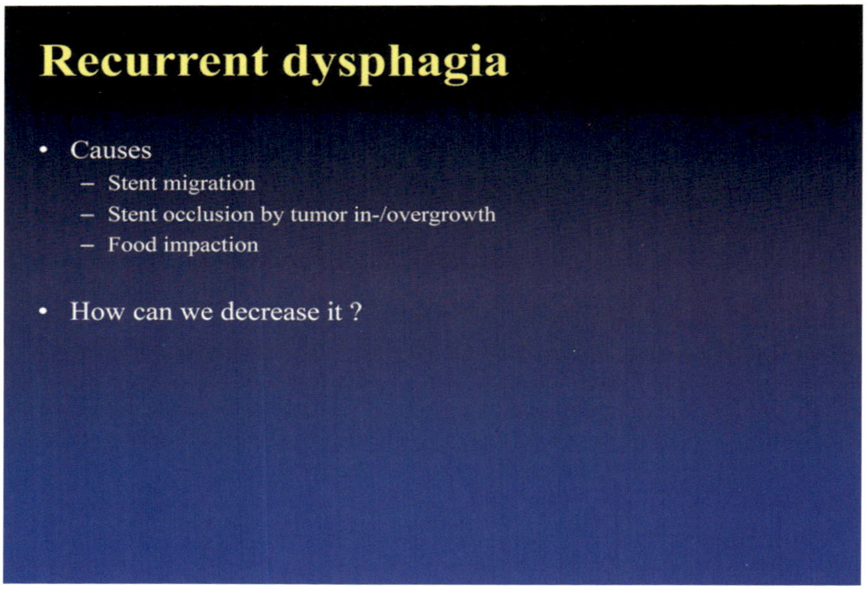

Causes of recurrent dysphagia include Stent migration, Stent occlusion by tumor in-/overgrowth, or food impaction.

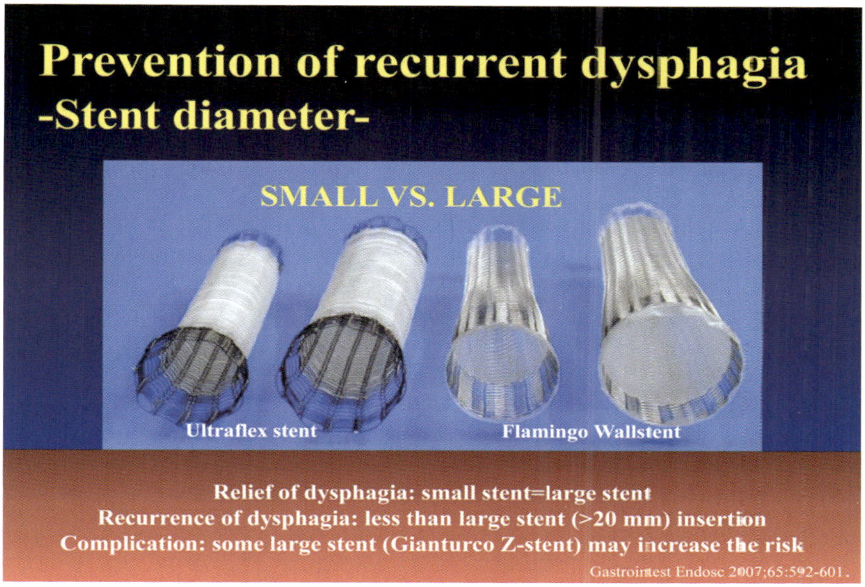

In a outcome analysis of 338 patients with esophageal or gastric cardia cancer who were treated with either small or large diameter stents(Ultraflex, Flamingo Wallstent, Gianturco Z-stent) Relief of dysphagia was equal regardless of the stent diameter, however, there was a significant increase of recurrent dysphagia in patient who inserted small stent compared to large stents. The study provides us some insights regarding the choice of stents in the management of malignant dysphagia.

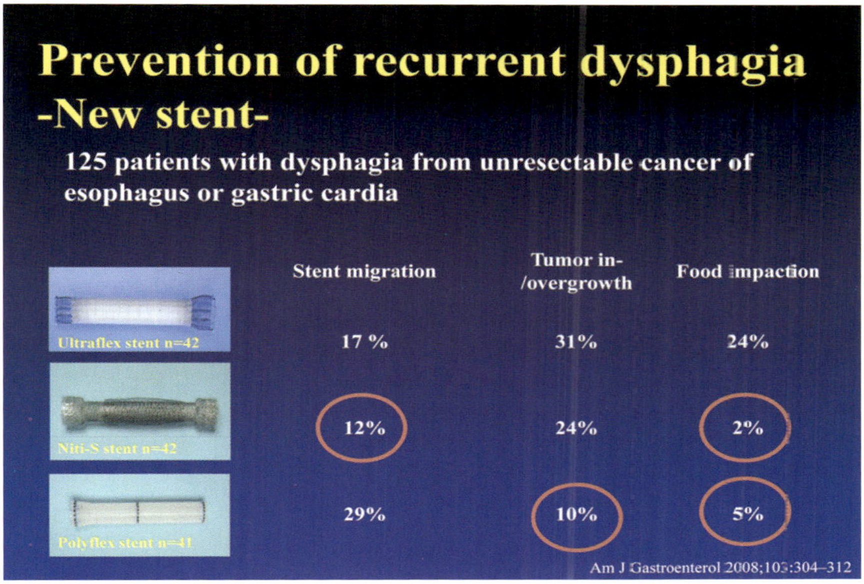

The Ultraflex stent is the most commonly used stent for palliation of malignant esophageal cancer. However in a recent study, the Niti-S stent showed a significant improvement in the rate of stent migration and food impaction. The self expandable plastic Polyflex stent showed a significant lower rate of tumor in growth and food impaction

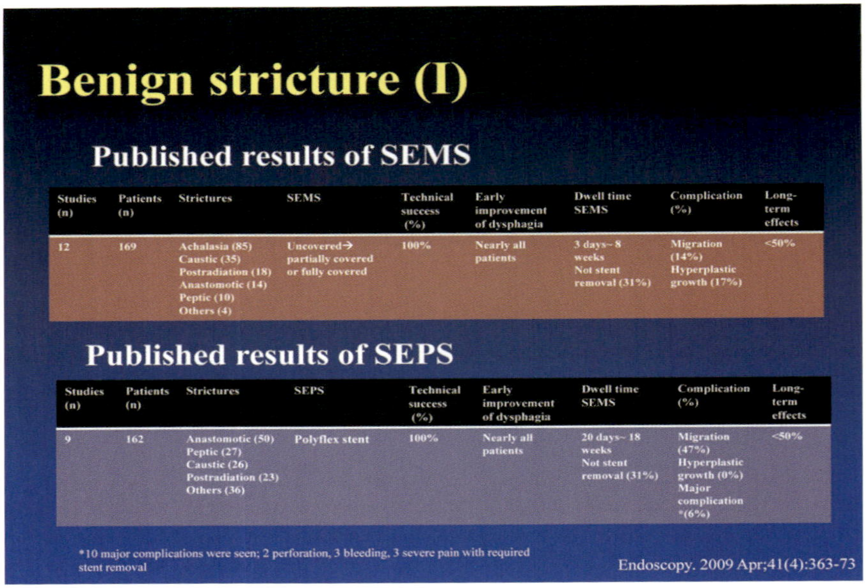

These are the published results of SEMS and SEPS for benign strictures. For SEMS the most common indication was achalasia followed by caustic and postradiation strictures. Early on uncovered stents were used, however, recently partially or fully covered stents are used more frequently. The stent dwell time varies, and in some studies the stent was not removed during the study period. Migration and hyperplastic growth were the most common complications and long term effects were seen in less than 50% of patients. The most common indication for SEPS was anastomotic strictures followed by peptic and caustic strictures. All published studies used the Polyflex stent. In contrast to SEMS hyperplastic growth rarely occurred, however the migration rate was 47% and less than 50% of patient showed long term effects.

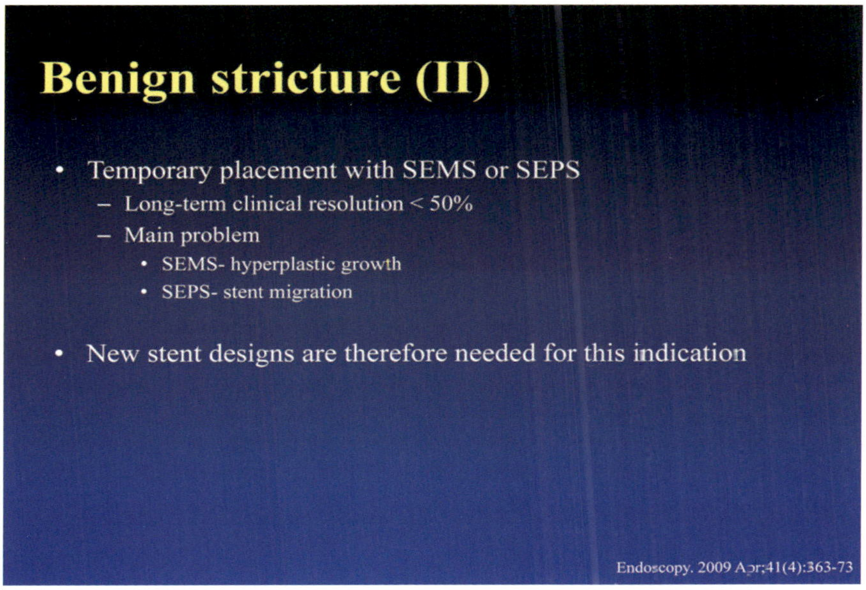

The results of stenting for benign stricture are disappointing so far, with long-term clinical resolution of the stricture achieved in less than 50% of patients. This is mainly due to hyperplastic tissue ingrowth or overgrowth (experienced with SEMS) and stent migration (SEPS) New stent designs are therefore needed for this indication.

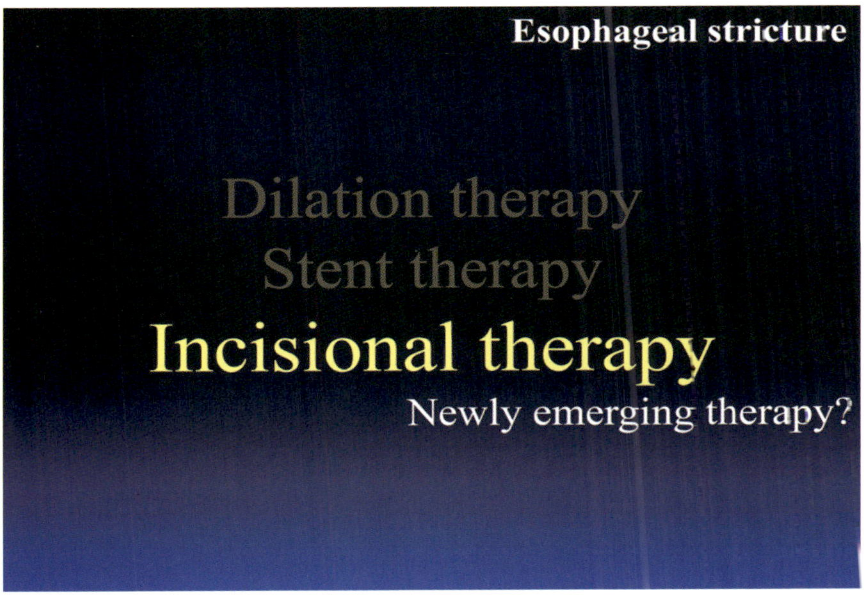

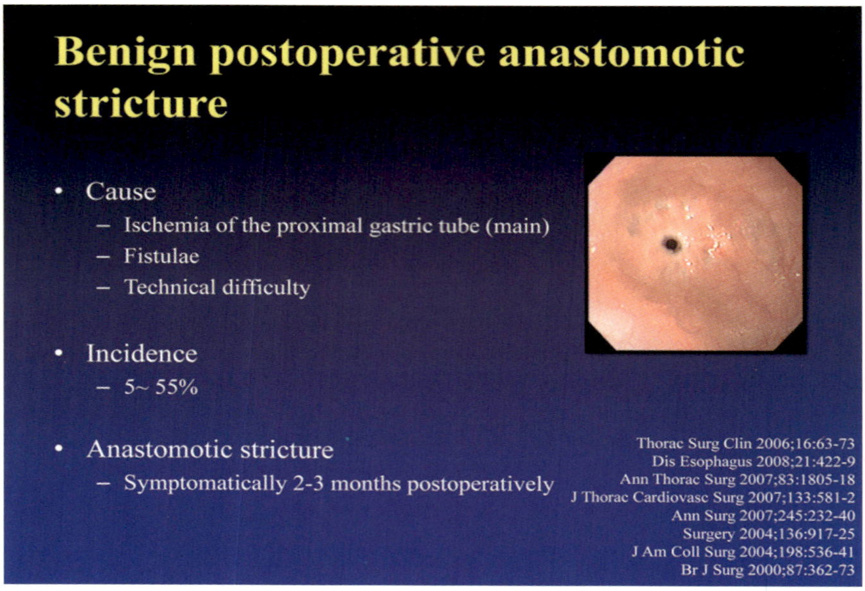

Most strictures after esophagectomy are thought to result from ischemia of the proximal gastric tube, with a smaller proportion related to fistulas or technical difficulties in the creation of the anastomosis. The reported incidence of benign postoperative gastroesophageal anastomotic strictures varies widely, from 5% to 55%. Anastomotic strictures generally present symptomatically 2 to 3 months postoperatively.

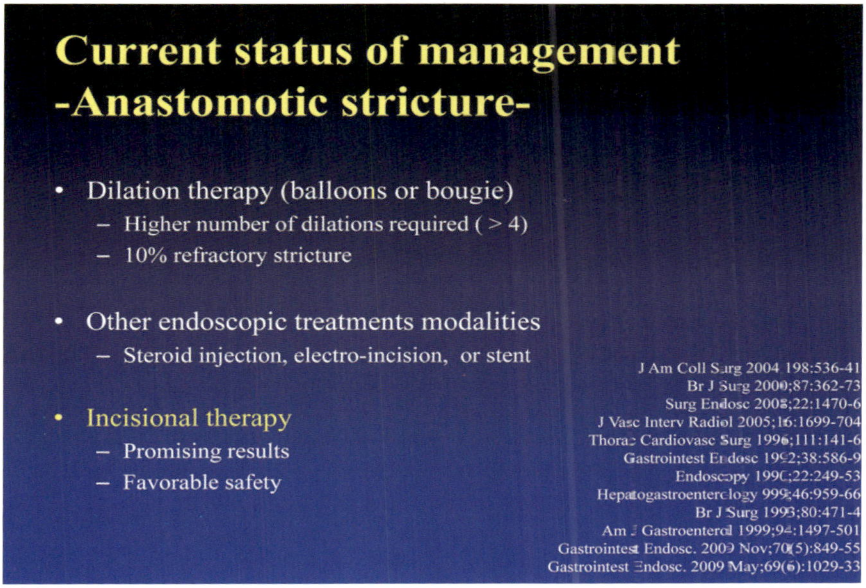

Anastomotic strictures are generally difficult to treat. Some reports indicated a higher median number of dilations required (>4), and many series recognized a subset of 10% of patients who required repeated treatment sessions due to refractory strictures. Although bougie or balloon dilations have been used most commonly, other endoscopic treatment modalities have been described, including steroid injection, electro-incision (EI), and temporary placement of a polyester-silicone self-expanding stent. Of these modalities, EI has seen the most attention of late and has shown promising results.

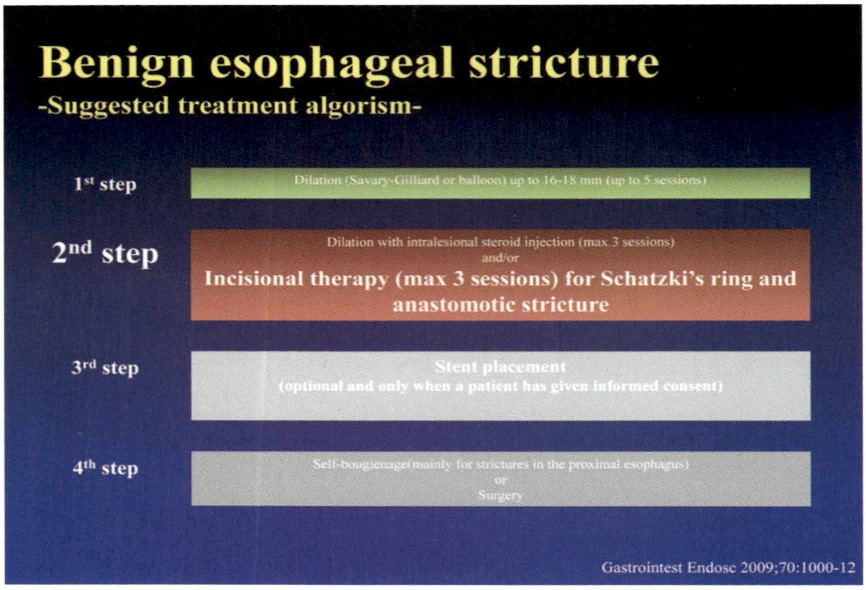

If the stricture is non-responsive to dilation therapy incisional therapy should be considered for Schatzki' s ring and anastomotic strictures.

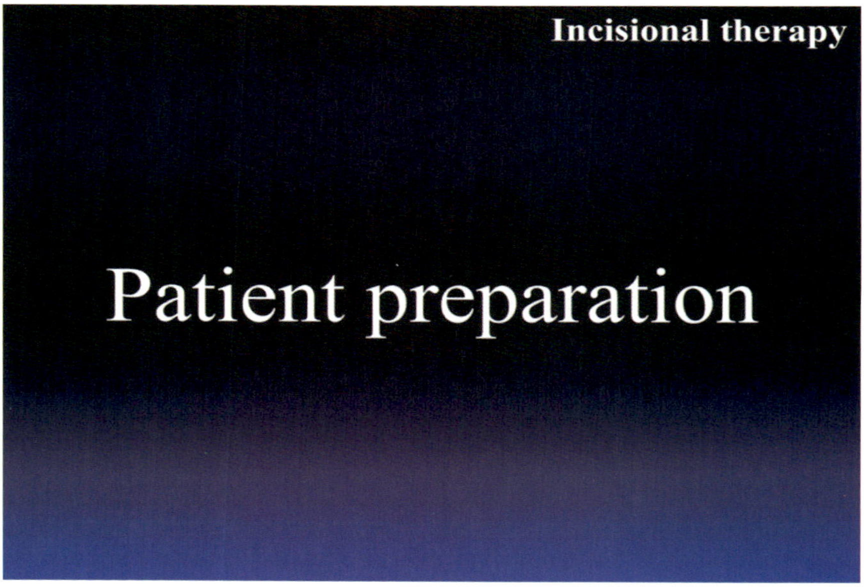

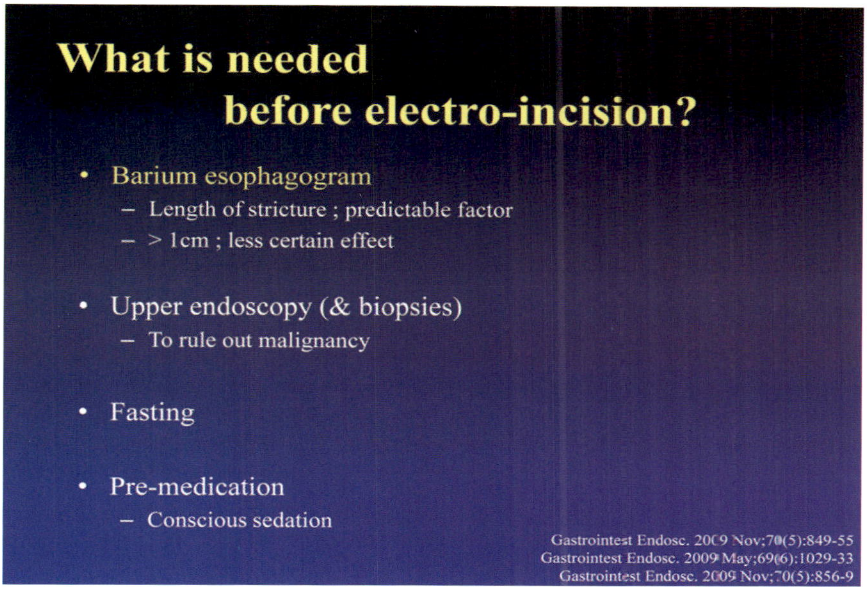

Prior to electro incision, a barium esophagogram should be obtained. The length of the stricture is an important predictor of treatment outcome. Strictures longer than 1cm have a less certain treatment effect. Endoscopy and biopsies should also be performed to rule out malignancy.

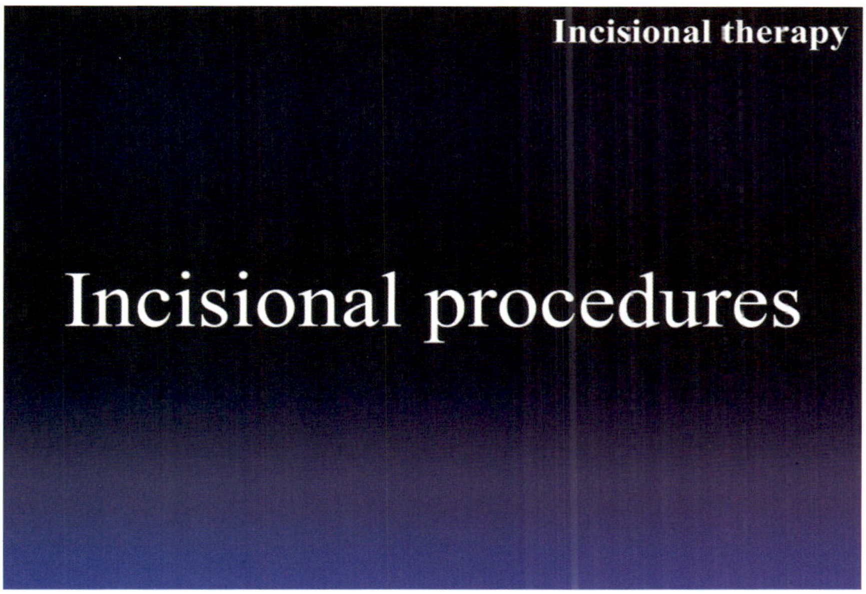

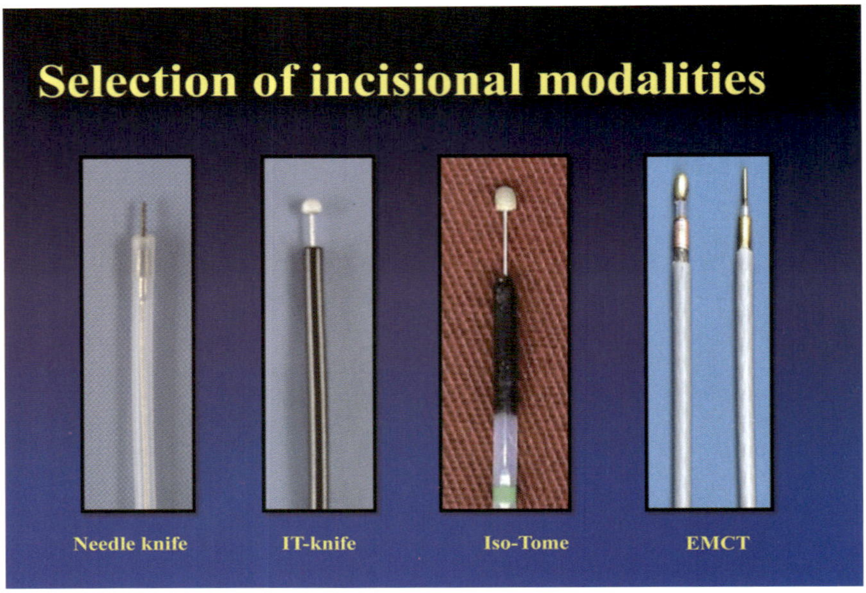

There are several modalities available for electro-incision.

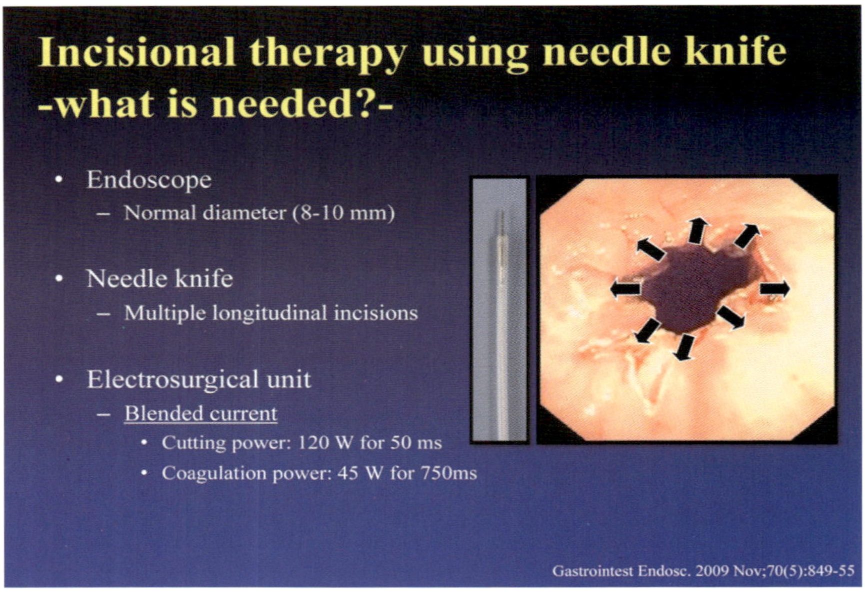

For incisional therapy with a Needle knife multiple longitudinal incisions around the circumference of the stricture are performed. The electrosurgical unit uses a blended current with a cutting power of 120W.

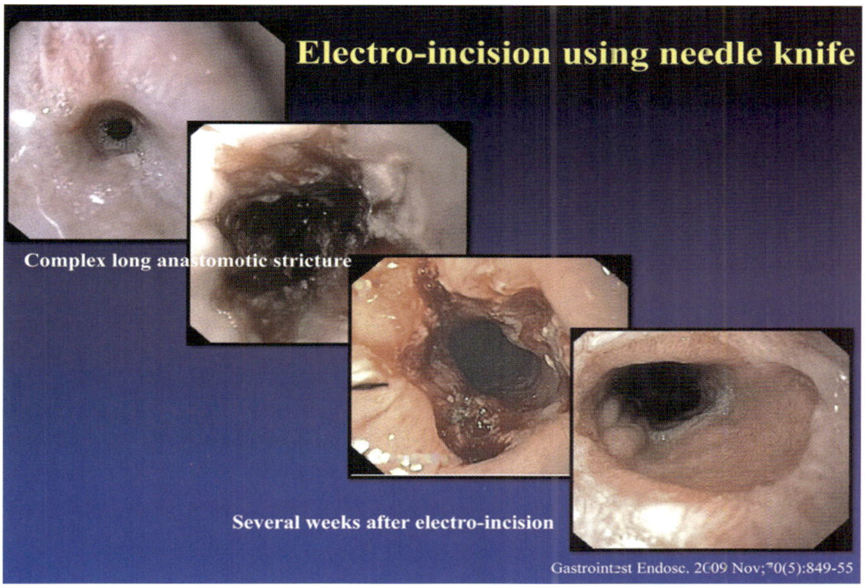

This is a patient with previous esophagectomy for esophageal cancer. A long complex anastomotic stricture in observed on endoscopy. Radial incisions are made around the stenotic ring using the needle knife. The number and radial position of the incisions were chosen to completely open the rim of the stricture. Weeks after electro-incision, dramatically improvement of the stricture can be seen.

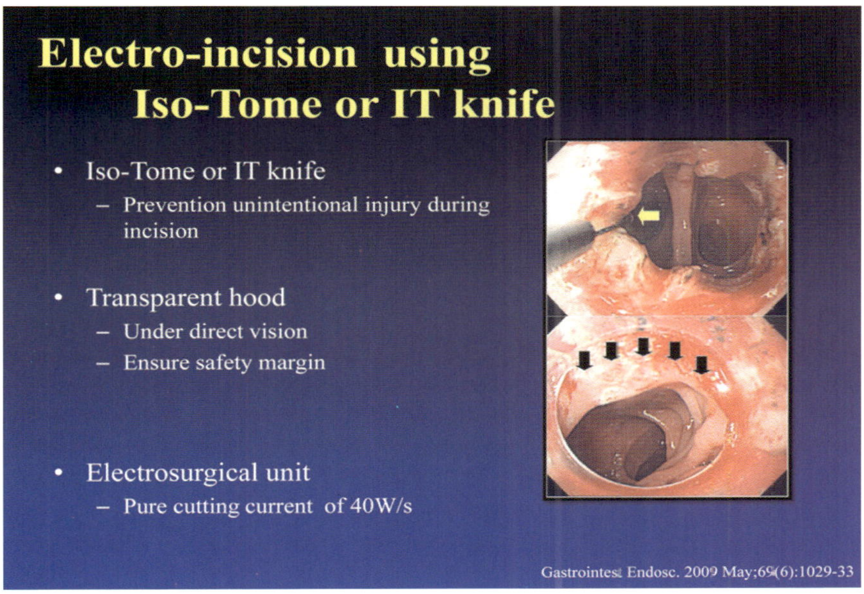

The Iso-Tome or IT knife are also used for electro incision. The Iso-Tome which has a semi-oval-shaped tip of epoxide adhesive, or an insulated-tip knife (IT-knife) can prevent unintent onal injury during incision. A transparent hood allow direct visualization while ensuring the safely margin. An electrosurgical unit was used, with a pure-cutting current at a power output setting of 40 W/S.

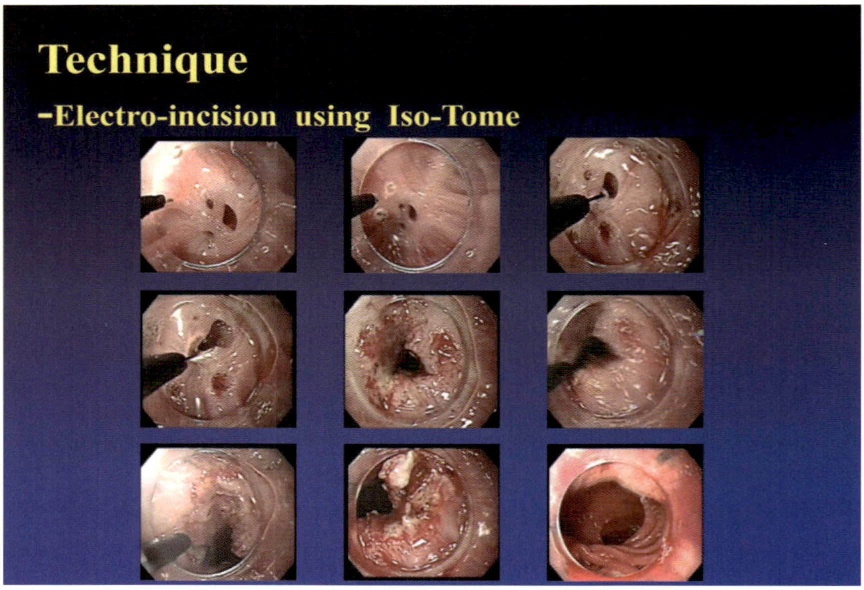

This pictures show electro-incision using the Iso-tome for an anastomotic stricture of the esophagus. The tip of a transparent hood is positioned just proximal to the stricture. Under direct vision through a transparent hood to ensure the safety margin, radial incisions parallel to the longitudinal axis of the esophagus were carefully performed by pulling up the Iso-Tome. The procedure was terminated when the endoscope could easily pass the stricture without resistance.

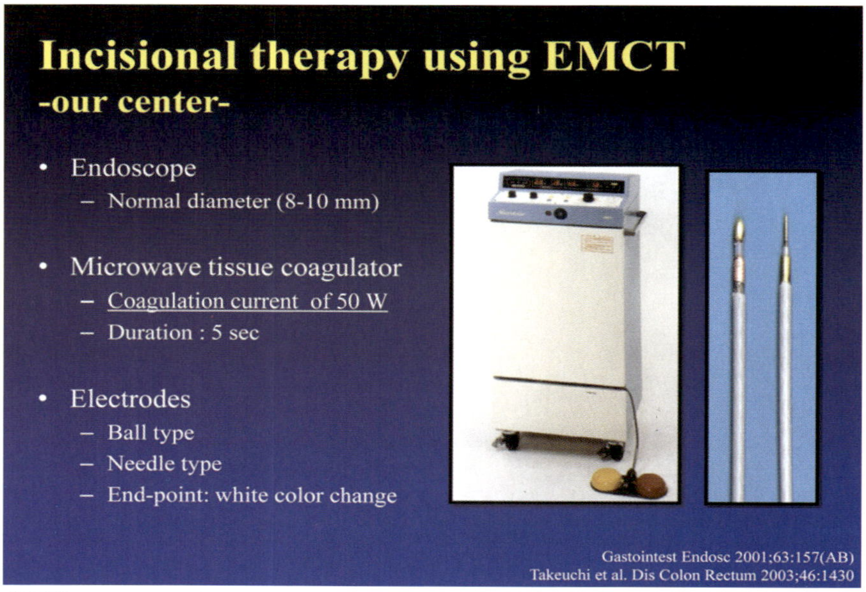

EMCT is not a commonly used modality. However it has been used for incisional therapy for anastomotic strictures refractory to dilation treatment. The microwave tissue coagulator is set at a coagulation current of 50W for duration of 5 seconds. Ball or needle type electrodes are contacted with the stricture in a radial direction.

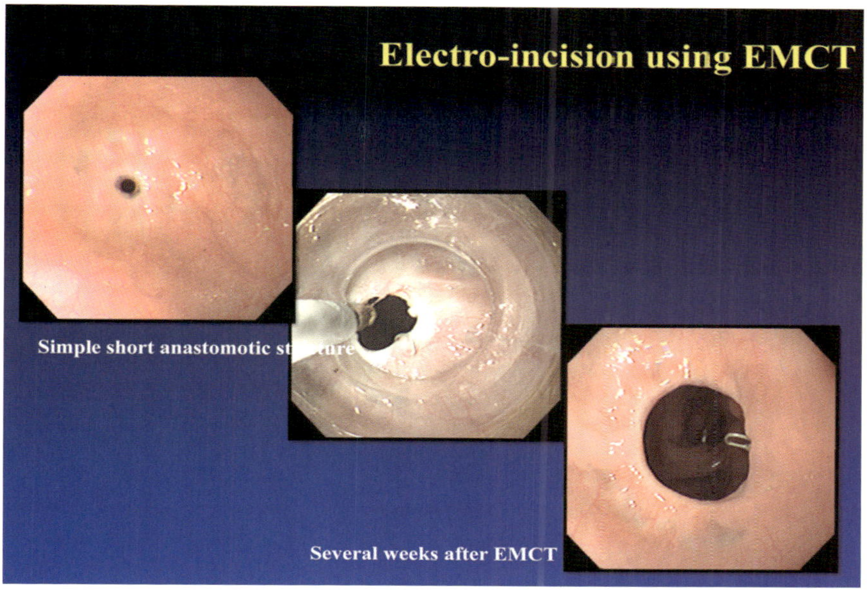

A simple short anastomotic stricture is seen in patient who underwent esophagectomy for esophageal cancer. Electro-incision using EMCT was performed. Tissue coagulation is performed in a radial direction until the tissue comprising the stenotic ring shows a white color.

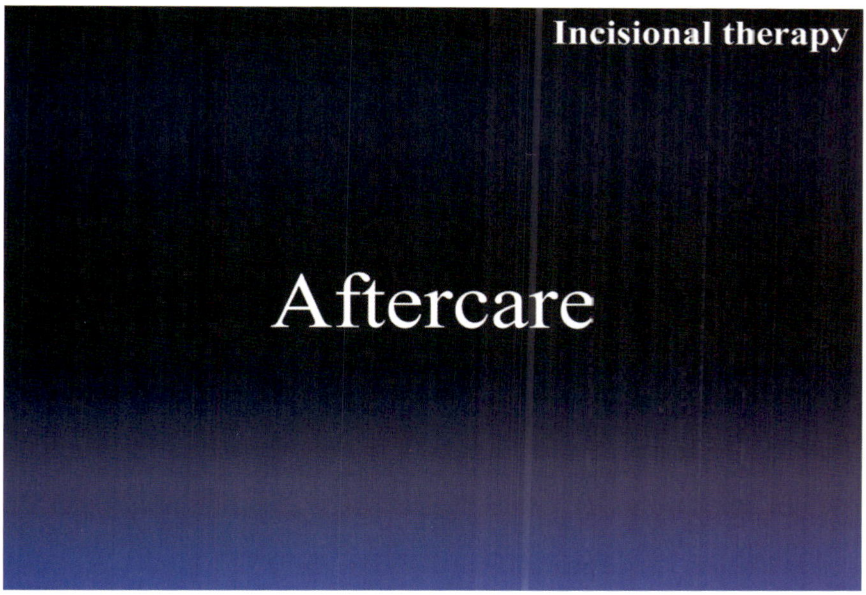

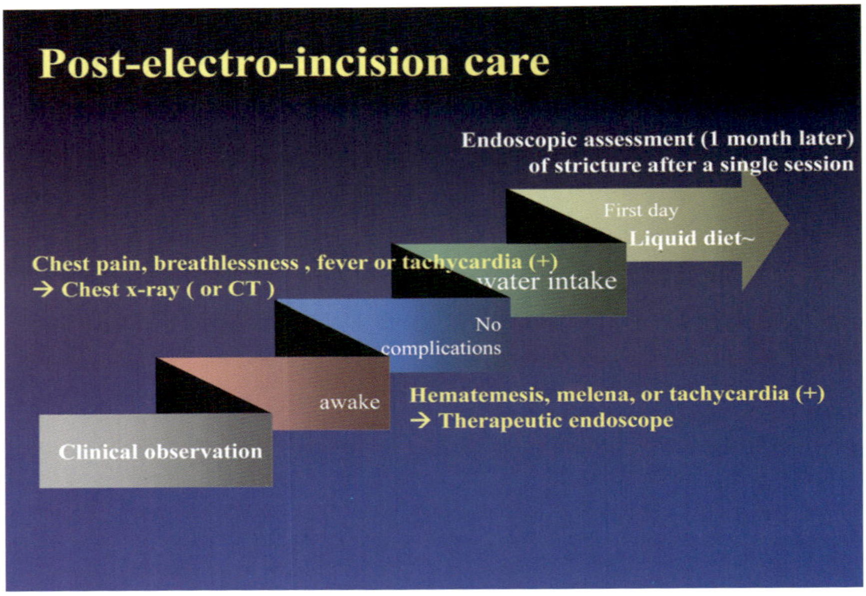

Patients should be closely observed after electroincision. Chest X-ray is not essential but should be performed urgently in patients who develop pain, breathlessness, fever, or tachycardia. Therapeutic endoscopy should be considered urgently in patients who develop hematemesis, melena or tachycardia. We recommended the patient drink water when awake and alert and without evident complications. Clinical evaluation and follow up endoscopy should be performed at least 1 month after the procedure.

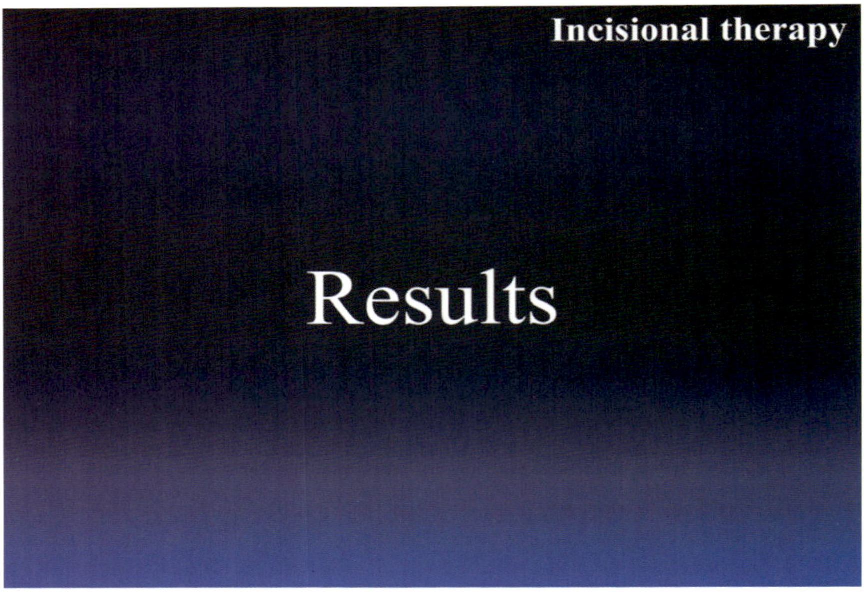

Published results of incisional treatment for benign anastomotic stricture

Author	Year	Patients (n)	Modality	F/U	Efficacy*	Complication
Ko BM	2001	20	EMCT	NA	100%	0%
Hordijk	2006	12	Needle	12 month	85%	0%
Hordijk*	2009	60*	Needle	6 month	80.6%	0%
Lee TH	2009	24	Iso-Tome/IT	24 month	87.5%	0%

*Comparison study between savary and needle knife; Savary =Needle knife

Gastointest Endosc 2001;63:157(AB)
Gastrointest Endosc. 2006 Jan;63(1):157-63
Gastrointest Endosc. 2009 Nov;70(5):849-5
Gastrointest Endosc. 2009 May;69(6):1029-33

The cumulative safety experience with electro-incision of anastomotic strictures has been favorable

The overall safety experience with electro-incision of anastomotic strictures has been favorable, but data is still limited.

Restricture after incisional treatment

The rate of restricture

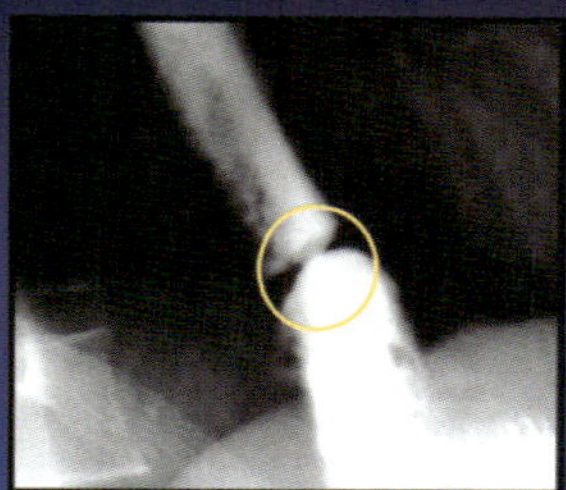

VS.

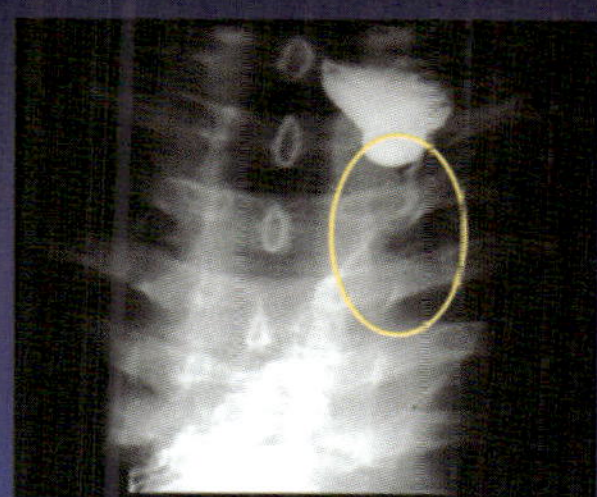

short-segment(< 1 cm) 4%

long-segment(>1 cm) 66.7%

A long-segment stricture was the only risk factor for restricture

Gastrointest Endosc. 2009 Nov;70(5):849-5
Gastrointest Endosc. 2009 May;69(6):1029-33

Restricture may occur after incisional treatment, usually in long segment strictures. In a recent report, the restricture rate for strictures less than 1cm was 4% in contrast to 66.7% for long segment strictures.

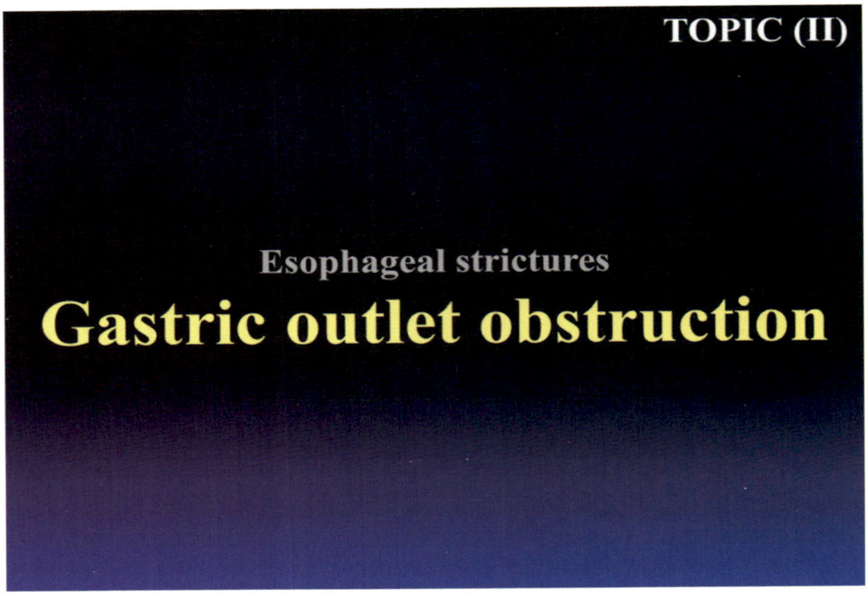

This topic will review various endoscopic treatments for gastric outlet obstruction.

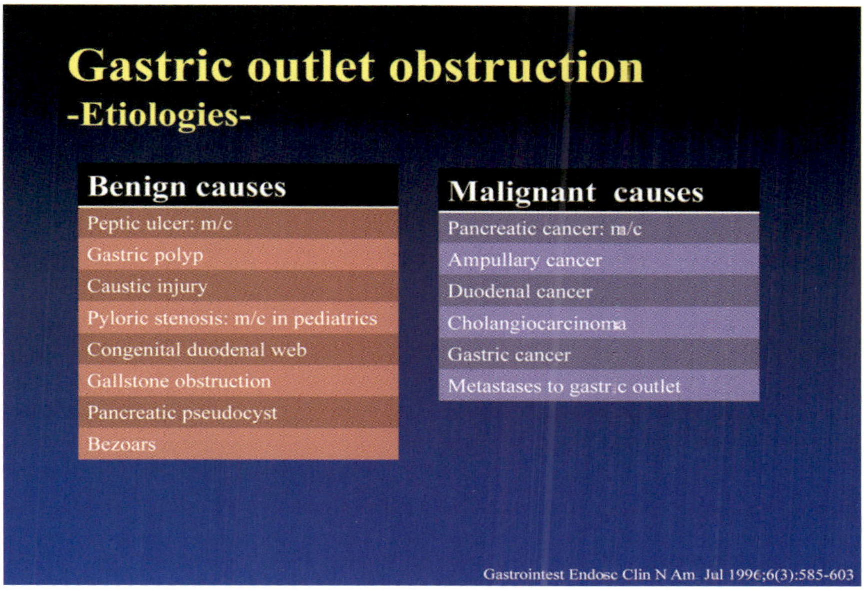

Clinical entities that can result in GOO generally are categorized into 2 groups-benign and malignant. The major benign causes of gastric outlet obstruction are PUD, gastric polyps, ingestion of caustics, pyloric stenosis, congenital duodenal webs, gallstone obstruction, pancreatic pseudocysts, and bezoars. Pancreatic cancer is the most common malignancy causing GOO. Outlet obstruction may occur in 10-20% of patients with pancreatic carcinoma. Other tumors that may obstruct the gastric outlet include ampullary cancer, duodenal cancer, cholangiocarcinoma, and gastric cancer. Metastases to the gastric outlet also may be caused by other primary tumors.

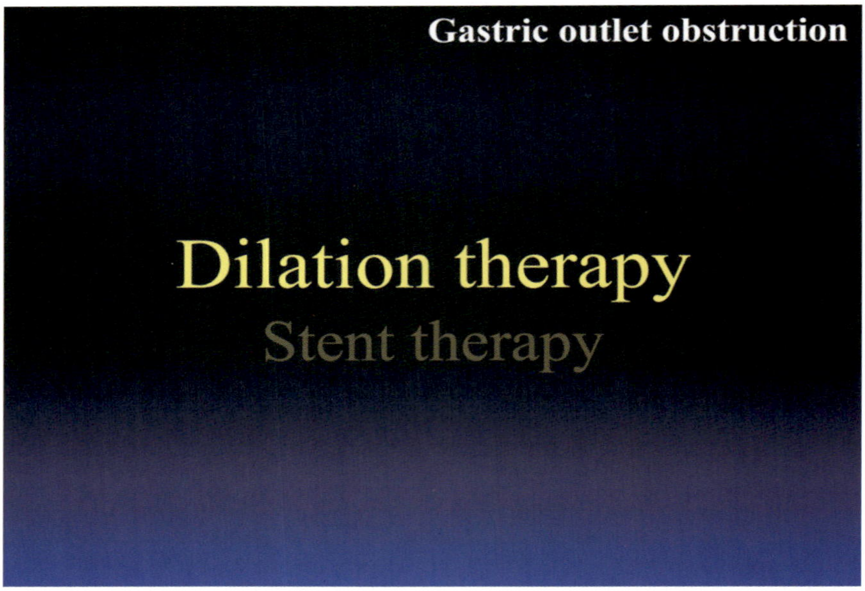
Gastric outlet obstruction
Dilation therapy
Stent therapy

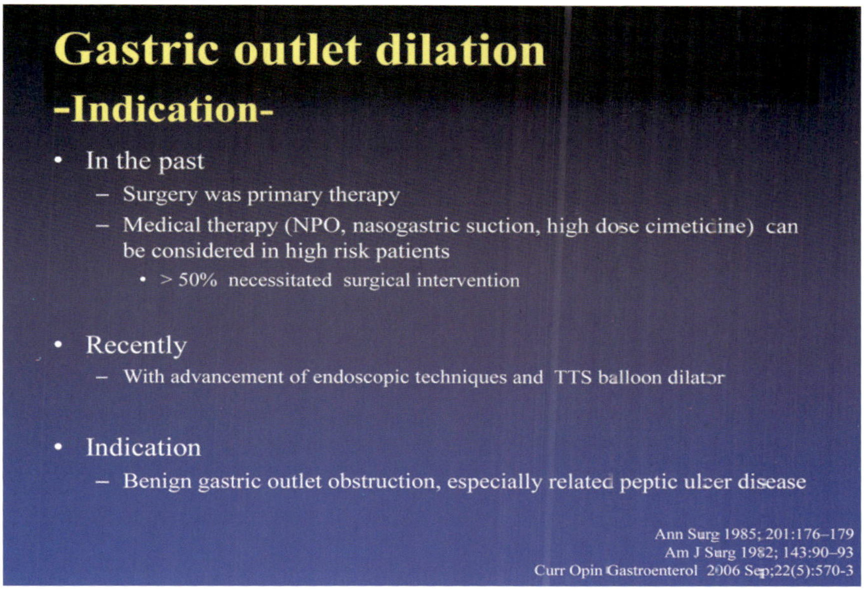

Traditionally, treatment of benign gastric outlet obstruction has been surgical. In high risk patients medical therapy was considered, however obstruction persisted in more than 50% and necessitated surgical intervention. With advances in endoscopic techniques and the advent of 'through-the-scope' (TTS) balloon dilating catheters, Endoscopic balloon dilation has emerged as the most effective first-line therapy in most patients and in those who are at high risk for surgery.
Balloon dilation for benign gastric outlet obstruction is especially useful in their treatment of obstruction related to peptic ulcer disease.

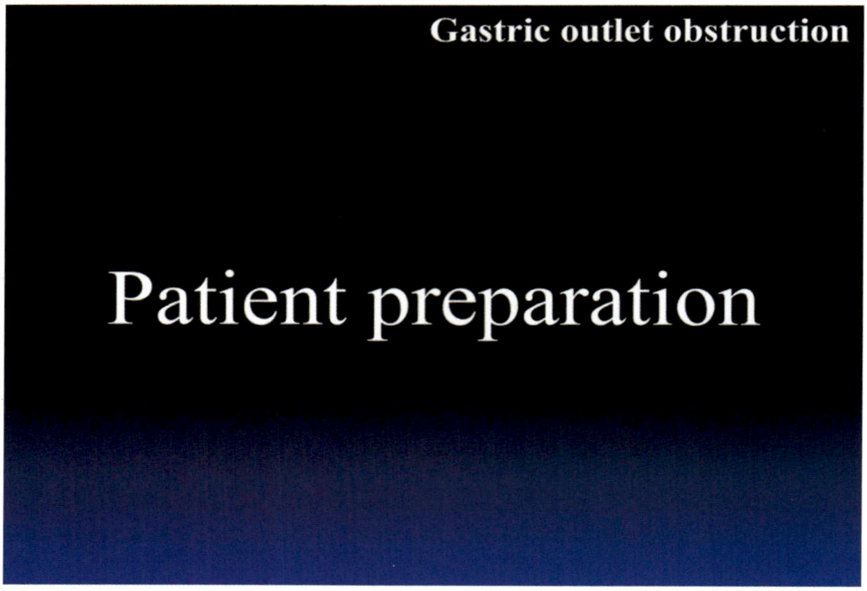
Gastric outlet obstruction
Patient preparation

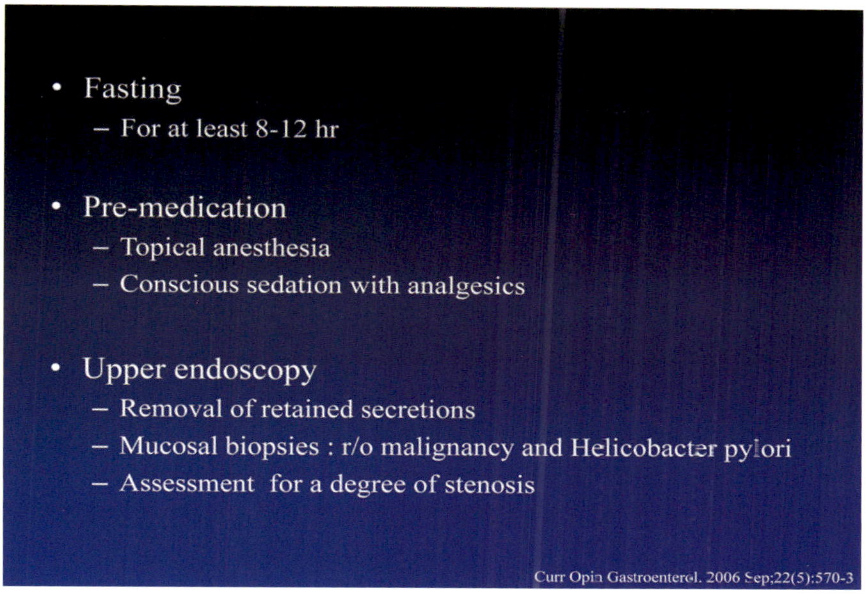

Prior to endoscopy, the patient should be fasted for at least 8-12 h. During standard upper endoscopy, the stomach and pyloric channel are carefully examined for the presence of active or chronic ulcer disease. A large channel gastroscope will allow for suction and removal of retained secretions. Multiple biopsies should be taken from the ulcer edges and gastric mucosa to exclude malignancy and Helicobacter pylori, respectively. The pyloric or duodenal stricture is assessed for the degree of stenosis by measuring its luminal diameter in reference to the outer diameter of the endoscope and by the ability to advance the endoscope through the stricture into the distal duodenum.

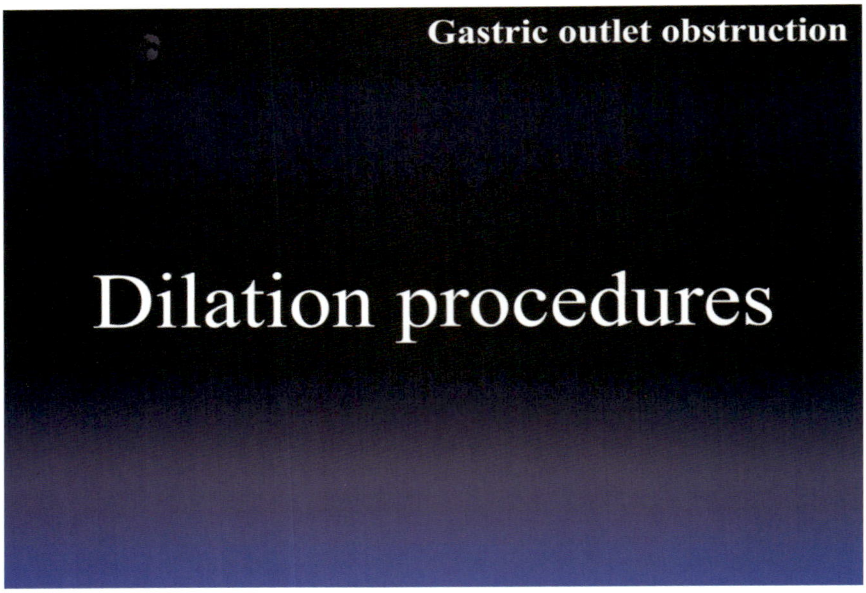

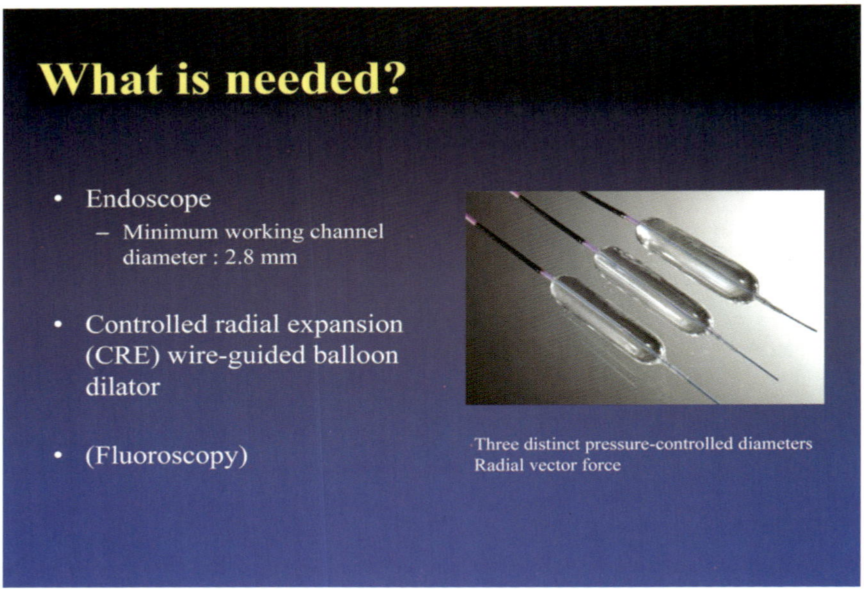

Currently, there are a number of commercially available balloon dilators of different sizes and lengths. The most commonly used are the controlled radial expansion (CRE) wire-guided balloon dilators. These balloons are designed to deliver three distinct pressure-controlled diameters with a high degree of radial vector force at any given pressure. The tip is flexible and minimizes the risk of perforation. When fluoroscopy is not utilized, dilation is performed under direct endoscopic guidance.

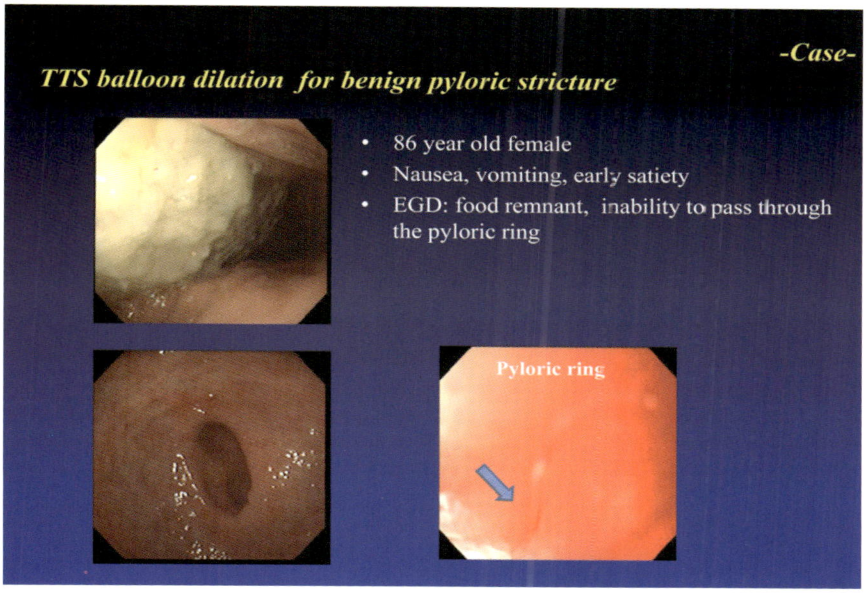

This is an 86-year-old female, complaining of nausea and early satiety Endoscopy showed a large amount of remnant food and a pyloric stricture. The endoscope was inability to pass through the pyloric ring.

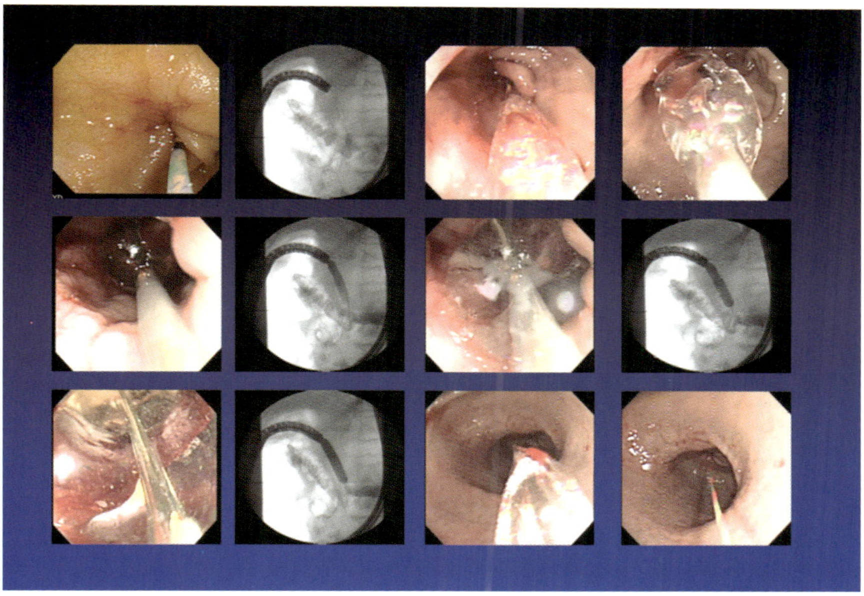

Under direct endoscopic guidance the CRE balloon catheter is passed through the stricture. The 8-9-10 mm CRE balloon is advanced through the channel of endoscope. The floppy tip is positioned across the stricture. Once in place, the CRE balloon is advanced over the guidewire, leaving one third of the balloon beyond the stricture. The CRE balloon is then inflated 8, 9, and then 10 mm for 3 min at each diameter.

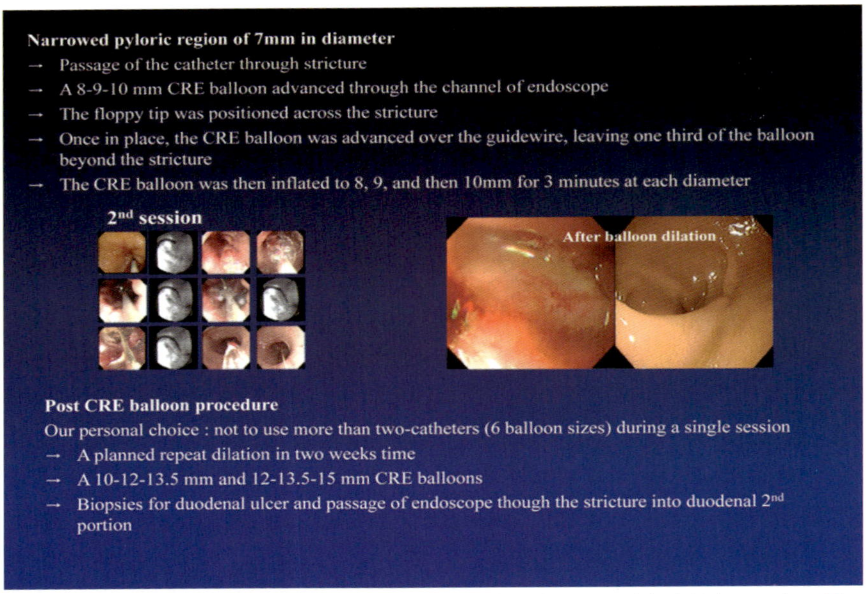

When to repeat dilation depends on the degree of stenosis and success of the initial procedure. The procedure should be repeated within two weeks for high-grade strictures. A planned repeat dilation was performed in two weeks time. We decided not to use more than two-catheters during a single session, 10-12-13.5 mm and 12-13.5-15 mm CRE balloons were used for the second dilation. Balloon dilation allowed passage of the endoscope into the duodenum and for biopsies of a duodenal ulcer.

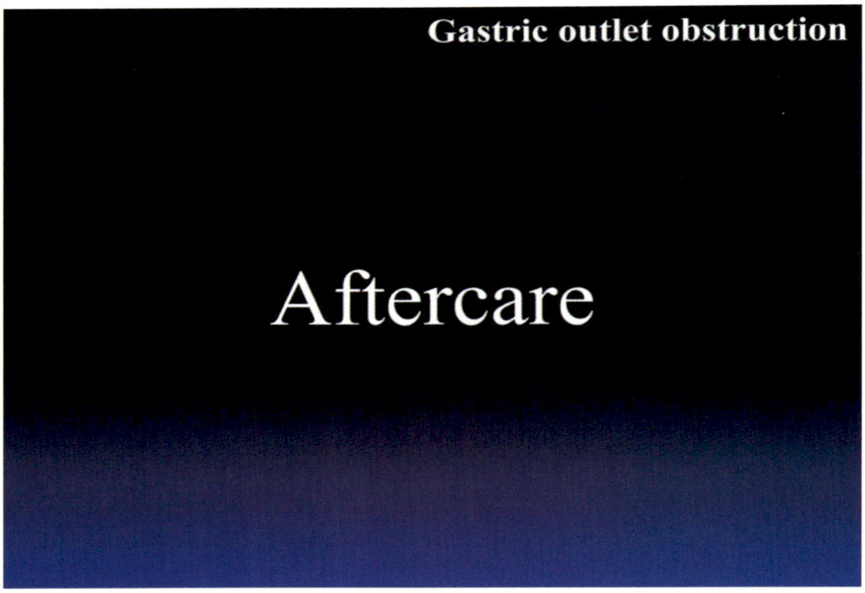

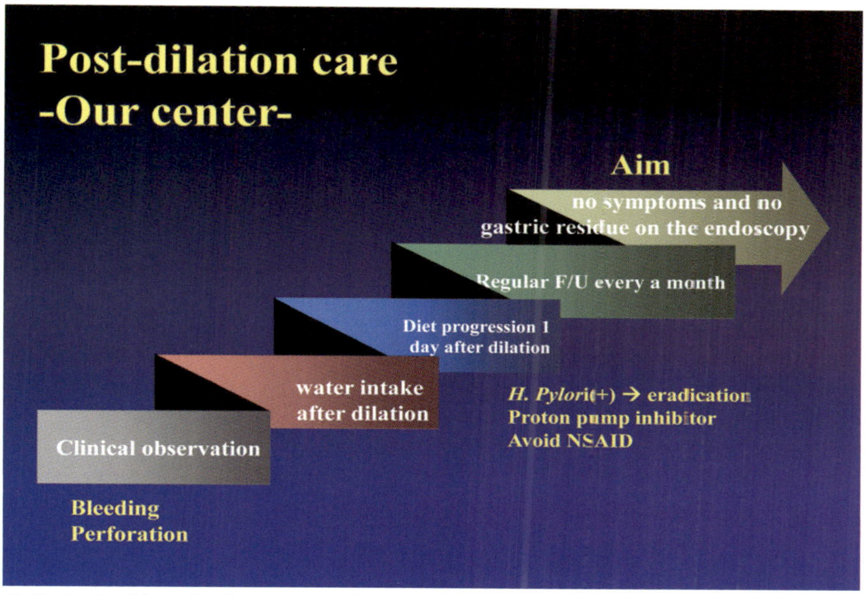

Patients should be closely observed after gastric outlet dilation. We recommended the patient initially drink water if the patient was awake and had no complications such as bleeding or perforation. We started a liquid diet 1 day after dilation and then advanced diet carefully in a stepwise pattern. The procedure is repeated in 1-2 weeks until obstructive symptoms improve. Helicobacter pylori should be eradicated if present, and ulcer disease should be aggressively treated to prevent recurrence.

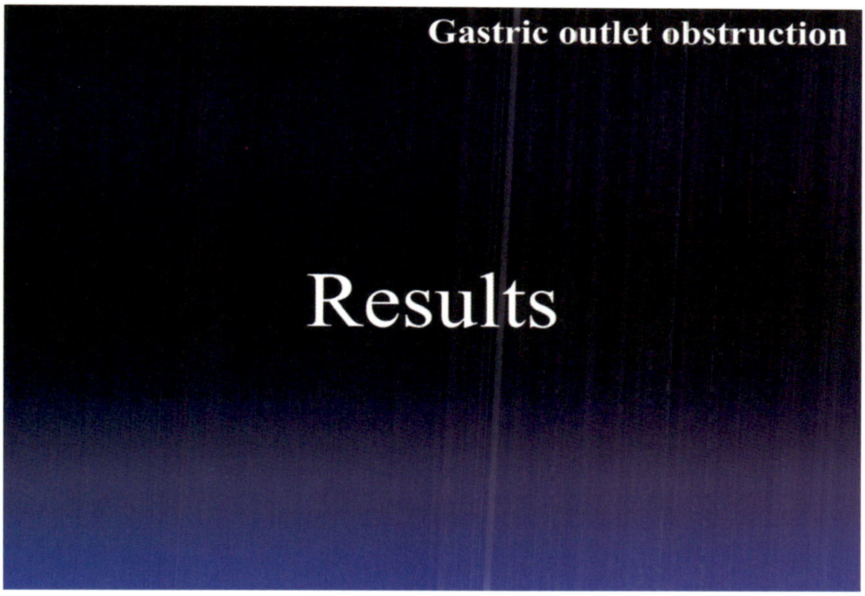

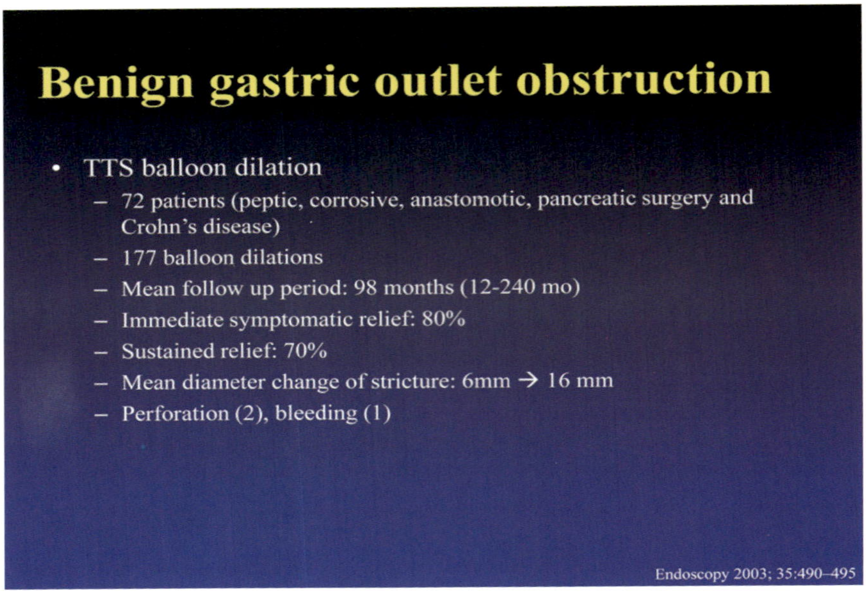

A recent study evaluated the outcome of TTS balloon dilation in 72 patients with gastric outlet obstruction secondary to various causes (peptic, corrosive, anastomotic, pancreatic surgery, and Crohn' s disease). Immediate symptomatic relief was achieved in 80% of patients and sustained relief was seen in 70% of patients. The mean diameter of the stricture increased from 6mm before dilation to 16mm after dilation. Perforation occurred in two patients and arterial bleeding occurred in one patient.

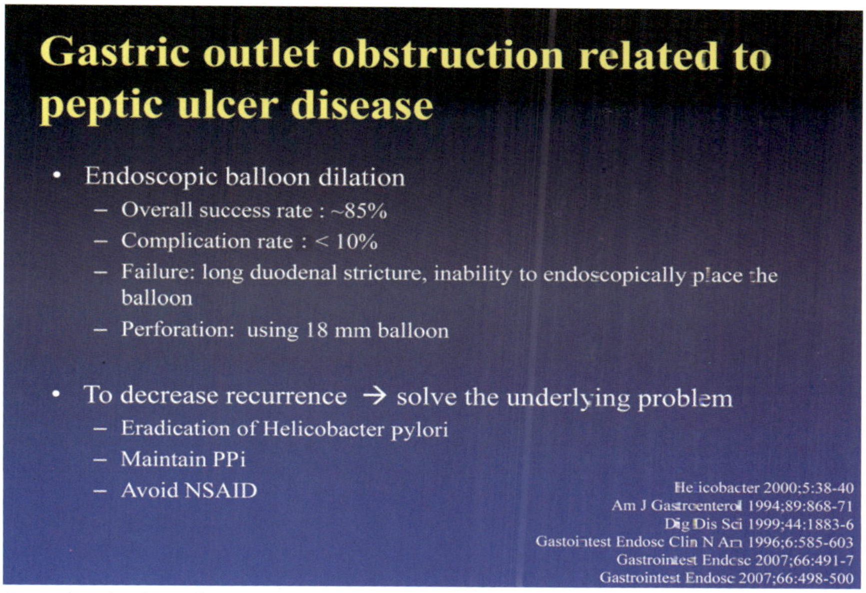

In gastric outlet obstruction related to peptic ulcer, overall success rates for endoscopic dilation(s) were up to 85%, with complications of perforation and bleeding occurring in fewer than 10% of cases. Failures were primarily associated with long duodenal strictures or inability to endoscopically place the balloons. Perforations were most often seen when using balloons reaching 18 mm in diameter. Endoscopic balloon dilation is now widely accepted as the first line therapy for benign GOO. Unfortunately, recurrence of stricture may develop, especially if the endoscopist only focuses on fixing the stenosis without resolving the underlying problems, such as Helicobacter pylori infection, nonsteroidal anti-inflammatory drug (NSAID) and aspirin use, and acid hypersecretion.

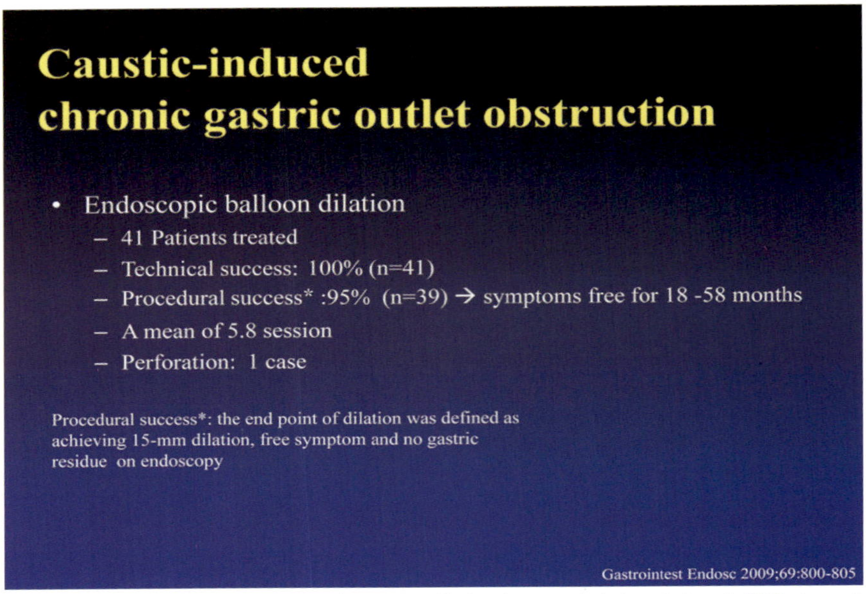

A retrospective analysis, of endoscopic balloon dilation for caustic induced chronic GOO showed promising results. After a mean of 5.8 sessions 39 of 41 patients remained symptom free for 18 to 58 months. These results suggest that endoscopic balloon dilation may be a safe, effective, and long-lasting alternative to surgery for caustic-induced gastric outlet obstruction.

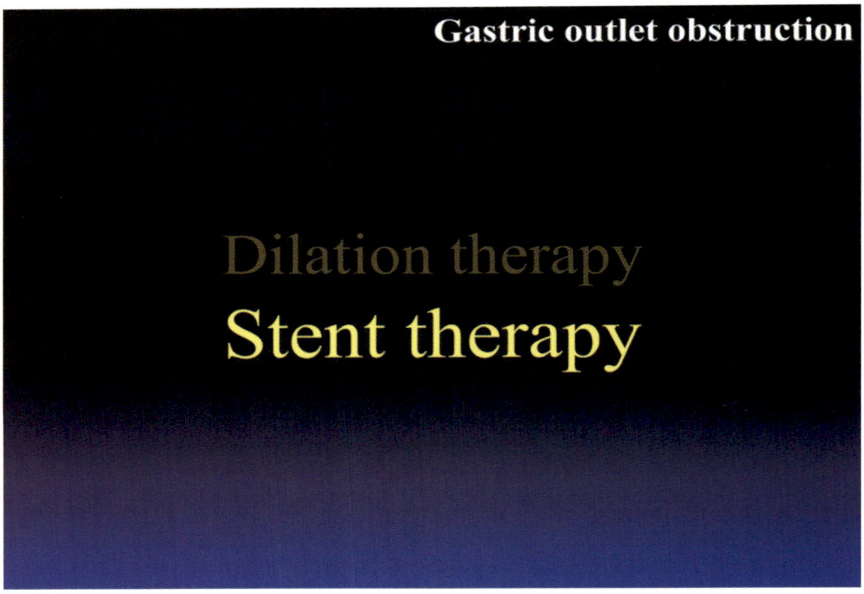

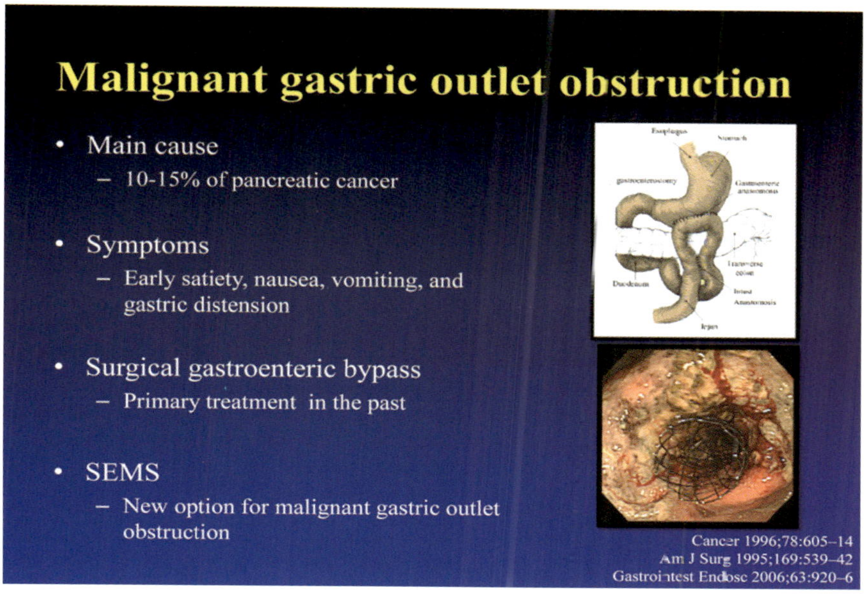

Malignant gastric outlet obstruction is a common complication of advanced pancreatic cancer. It occurs in 10% to 15% of patients with pancreatic cancer and manifests as a stricture of the proximal duodenum. Clinical presentations include early satiety, nausea, vomiting, and gastric distension. Until recently, the management of this complication consisted of surgical gastroenteric bypass with or without associated biliary bypass. Over the past decade, the endoscopic deployment of self-expanding metal stents (SEMS) has emerged as a new option for restoration of enteric patency.

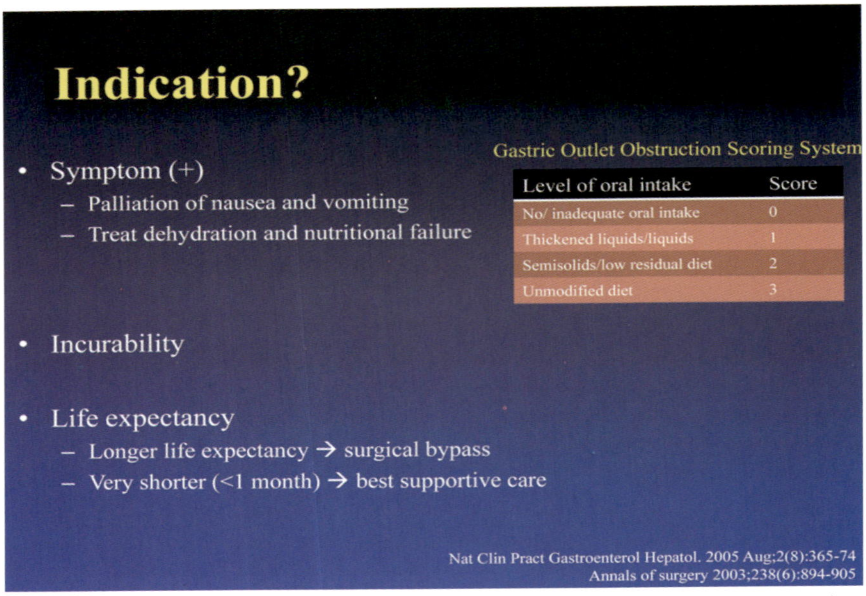

Gastroduodenal stents can be considered in symptomatic patients with malignant gastric outlet obstruction. Stent treatment should be indicated in patients with incurable cancer. The life expectancy of the patient should be considered first. When life expectancy is long surgical bypass is preferred. In patients with a very short life expectancy, best supportive care is the optimal choice.

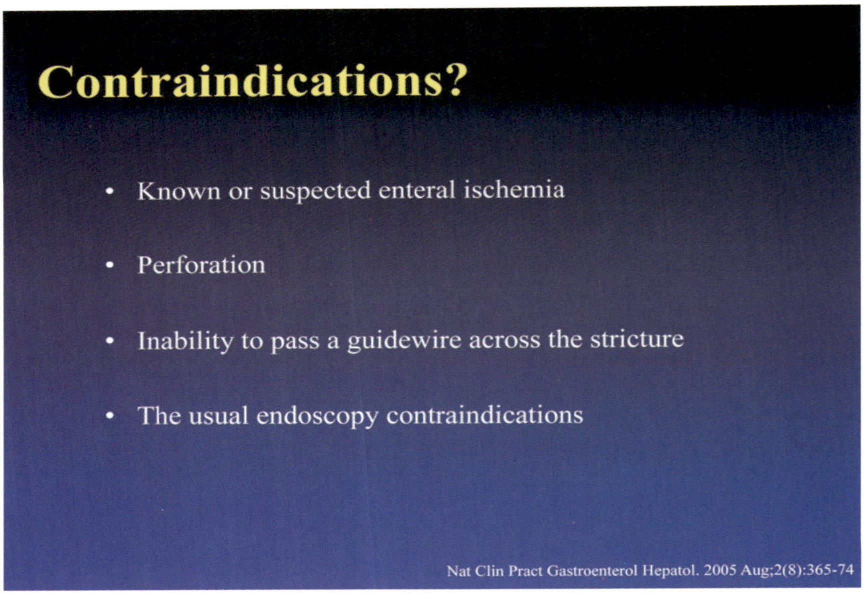

Contraindications to gastroduodenal stent placement include known or suspected enteral ischemia or perforation, inability to pass a guidewire across the stricture, and the usual endoscopy contraindications.

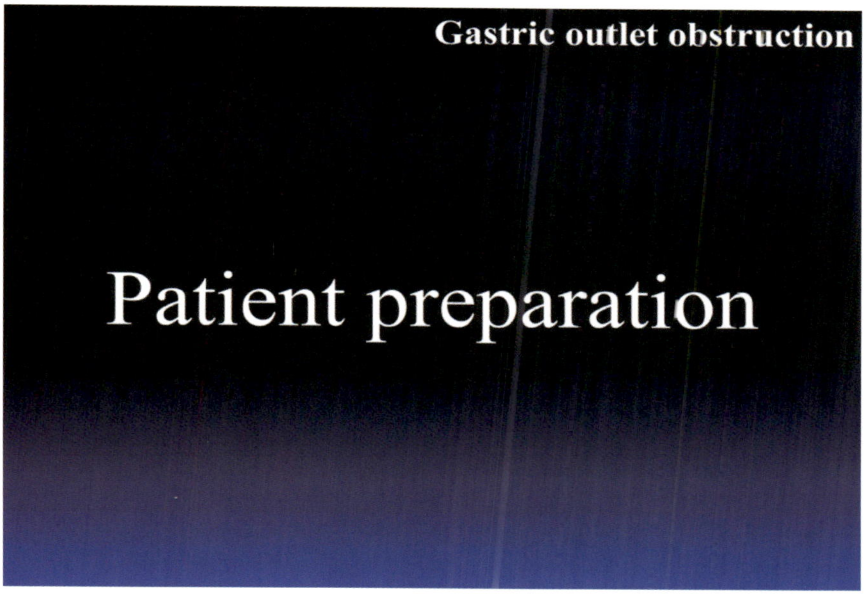
Gastric outlet obstruction
Patient preparation

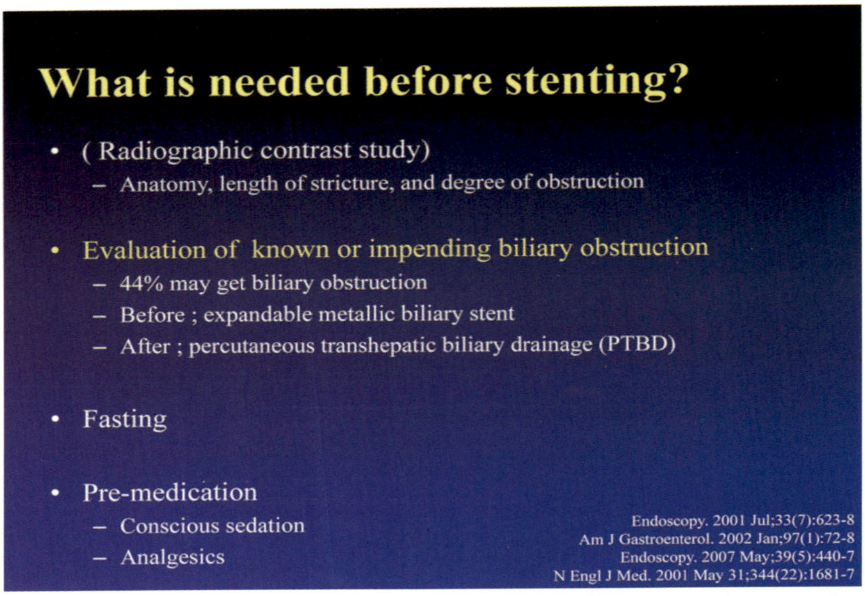

Although not absolutely necessary, it is helpful to obtain a radiographic contrast study to assess the anatomy, length of the stricture, and degree of obstruction, especially in cases where it is unclear if the obstruction is functional. Coexistent biliary obstruction is commonly present since it typically develops earlier than gastric outlet obstruction (at least in patients with pancreatic cancer). If there is known or impending biliary obstruction, an expandable metal biliary stent should be placed before the duodenal stent because it is difficult to obtain biliary tree access once a duodenal stent has been placed across the papilla. A percutaneous transhepatic approach may be required to treat a biliary obstruction that develops after duodenal stent placement.

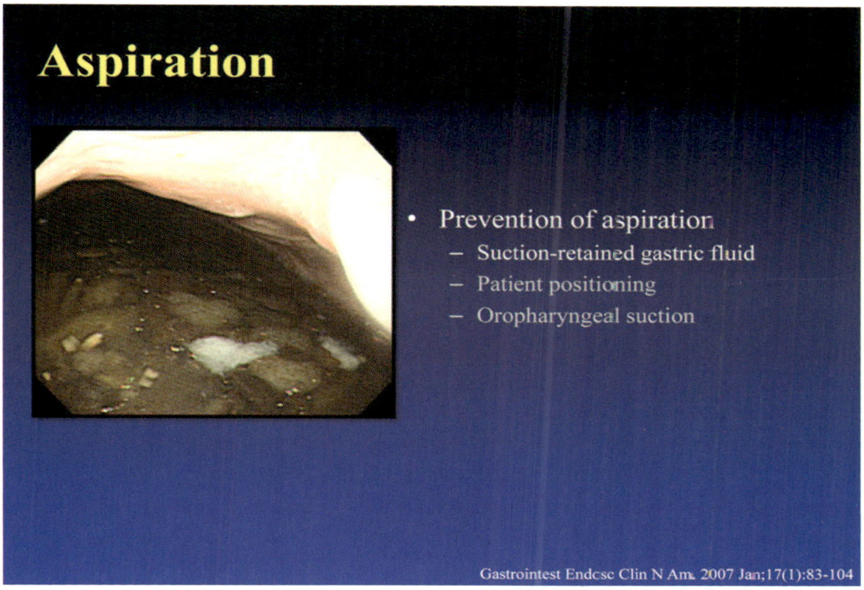

To prevent the aspiration of gastric content during procedure, endoscopic suction and removal of retained gastric content prior to stent insertion is essential.

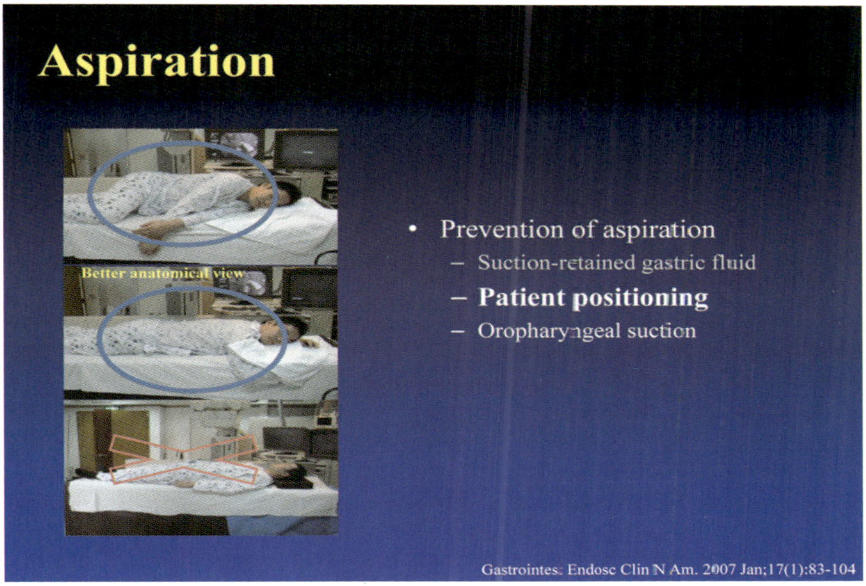

The patient should be placed in the left lateral decubitus or prone position. Prone position allows for a better anatomic view under fluoroscopy. Supine position should be avoided because of the high risk of aspirating retained gastric contents.

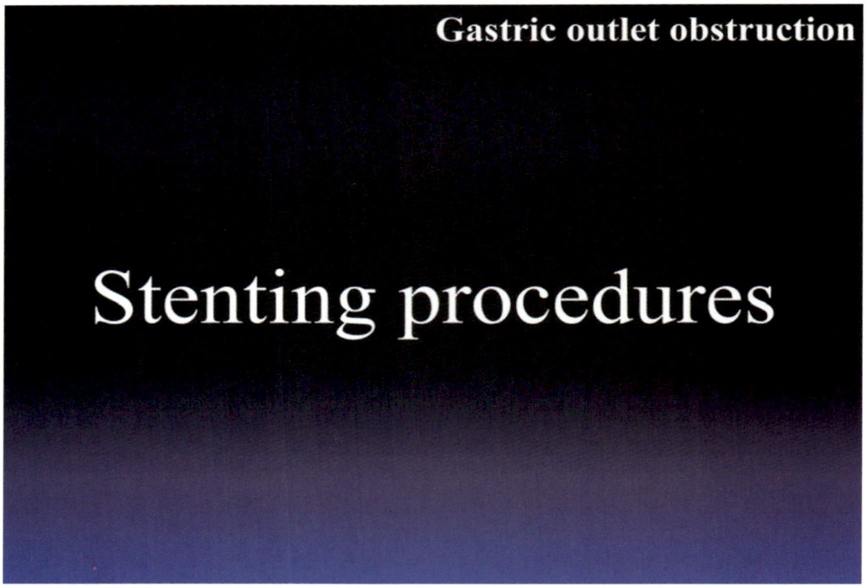

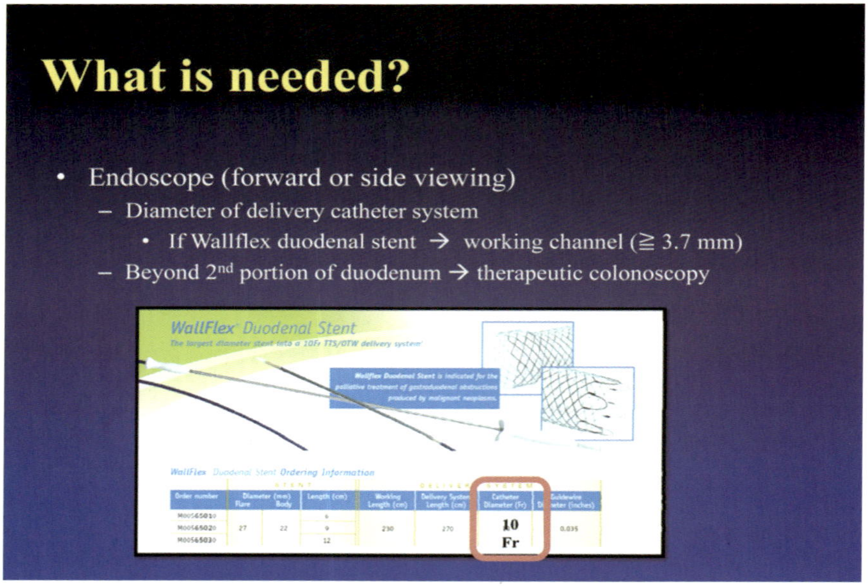

Prior to procedure, an adequate endoscope should be chosen with consideration of the delivery catheter system and location of the obstruction. If the Wallflex is planned to be used, an endoscope with a therapeutic working channel ($\geq$ 3.7 mm) is required to allowing passage of the 10Fr delivery system. When stents are placed beyond the proximal and second duodenum, a therapeutic channel adult colonoscope is usually required.

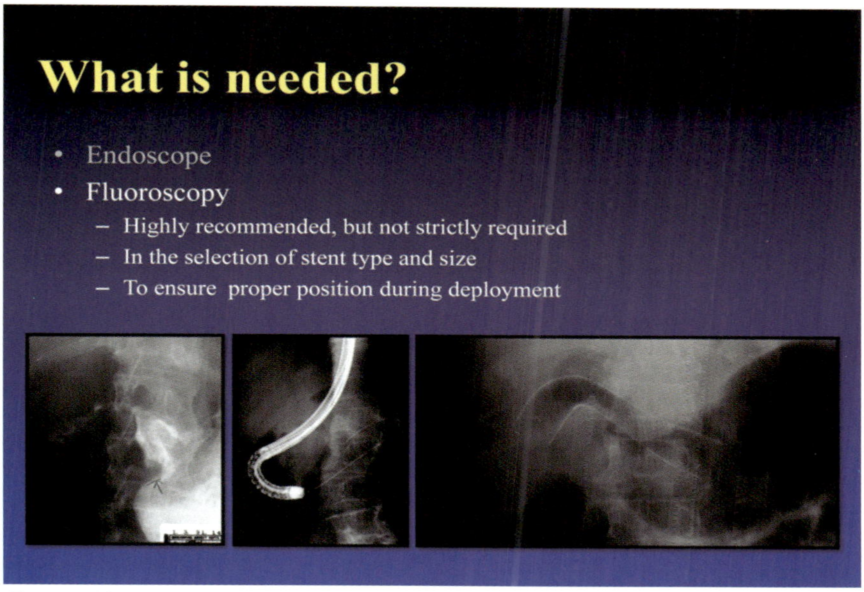

The use of fluoroscopy is highly recommended, but not strictly required for proper stent placement. Fluoroscopy allows identification of contrast dye to delineate the stricture, defining its length and geometry, both of which greatly aid in the selection of stent type and size. Use of fluoroscopy during deployment helps to ensure proper position and may minimize misdeployments or other complications.

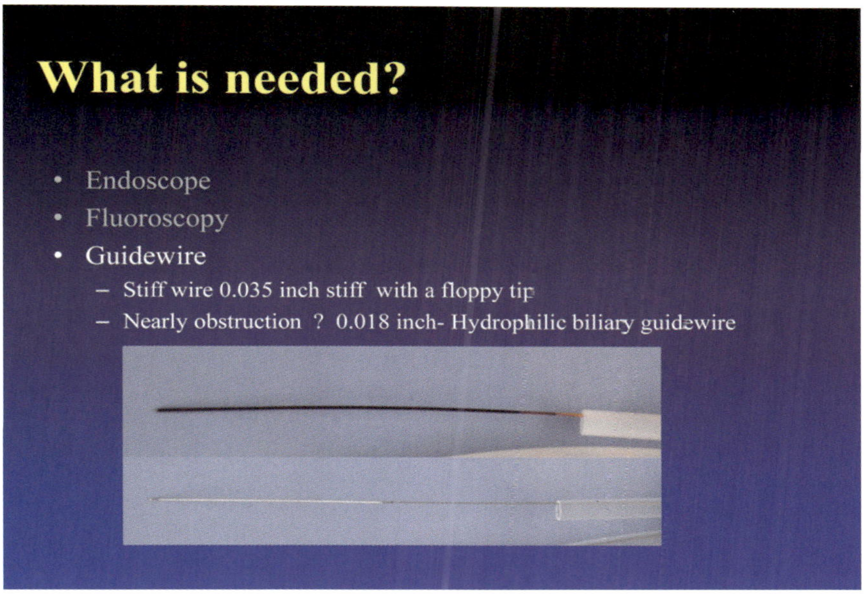

If the endoscope passes easily through the lesion, a 0.035 inch guidewire with a floppy tip is placed through the endoscope channel. If the endoscope cannot be passed easily through the lesion, a hydrophilic biliary guidewire preloaded through standard biliary accessories can be used to traverse the stricture.

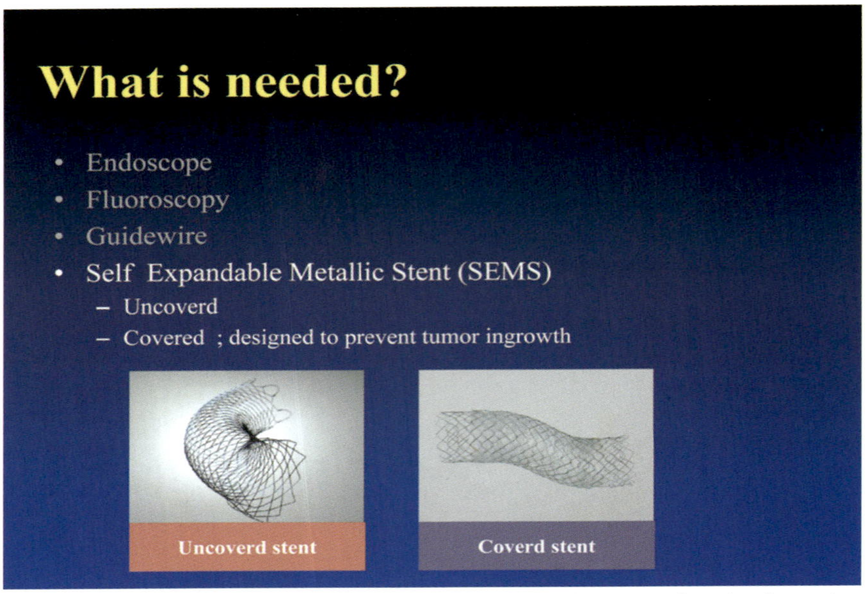

Uncovered SEMSs are now widely used for the palliation of malignant gastric outlet obstruction Nevertheless, a number of complications have also been observed with SEMSs, most frequently, stent obstruction caused by tumor ingrowth, mucosal hyperplasia, tumor overgrowth, or food impaction. Covered stents were designed to prevent the former 2 problems, which are caused by the inward growth of tumorous or hyperplastic tissue across the interstices of the stent mesh.

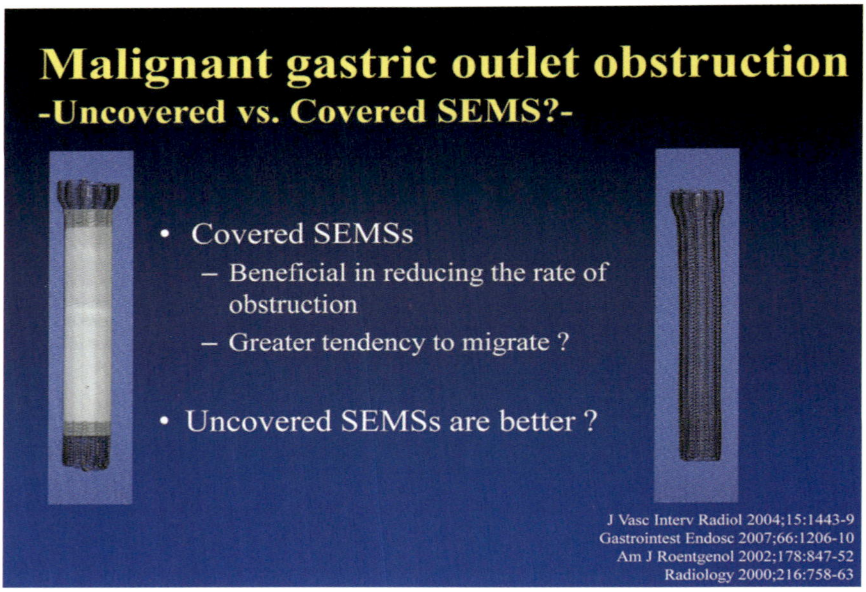

Previous studies indicated that although covered SEMSs are beneficial in reducing the rate of obstruction, they may have a greater tendency to migrate. However, supporting evidence for the efficacy of covered SEMS is lacking.

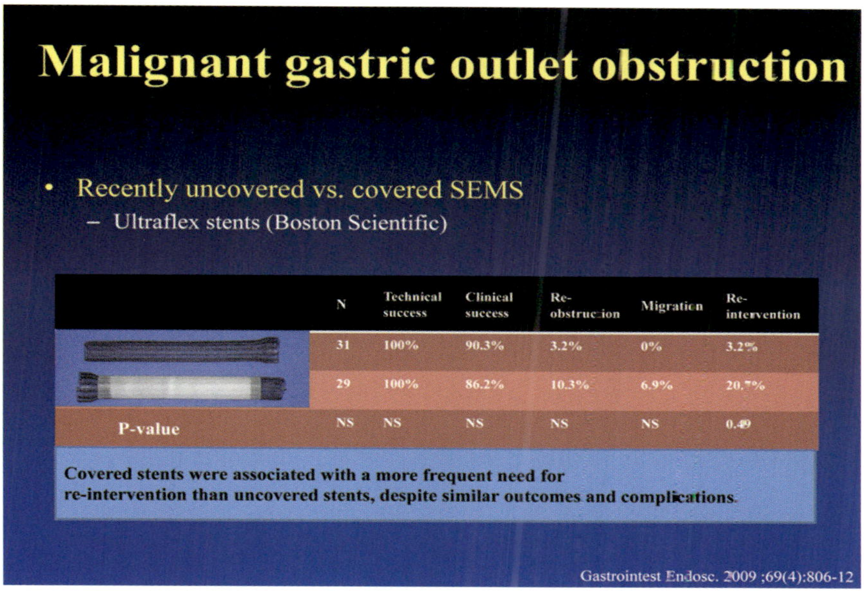

In a retrospective comparison of uncovered and covered SEMSs in 60 patients with malignant gastric outlet obstruction, covered stents were comparable with the uncovered ones in terms of feasibility and complications but were associated with an increased need for repeated interventions.

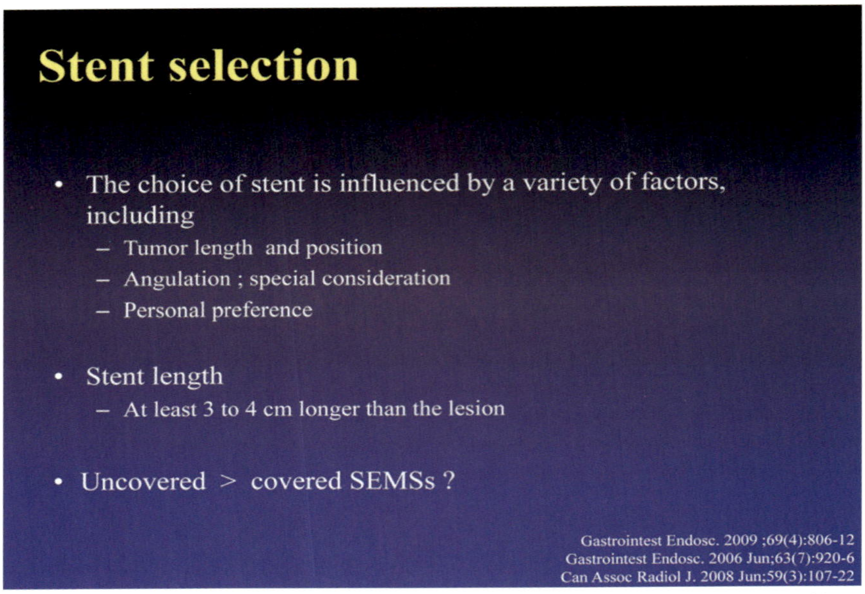

The choice of stents is influenced by a variety factors including tumor length and position, angulation, and personal preference. In malignant gastric outlet obstruction, angulation should be specially considered because the proximal and distal aspects of the stent should conform to the natural curves of the stomach and duodenum. Stent should be 3-4 centimeters longer than underlying stricture. At present, uncovered stents appear to be better in palliation of gastric outlet obstruction because uncovered stents are less prone to re-intervention; however these results require confirmation in larger randomized trials.

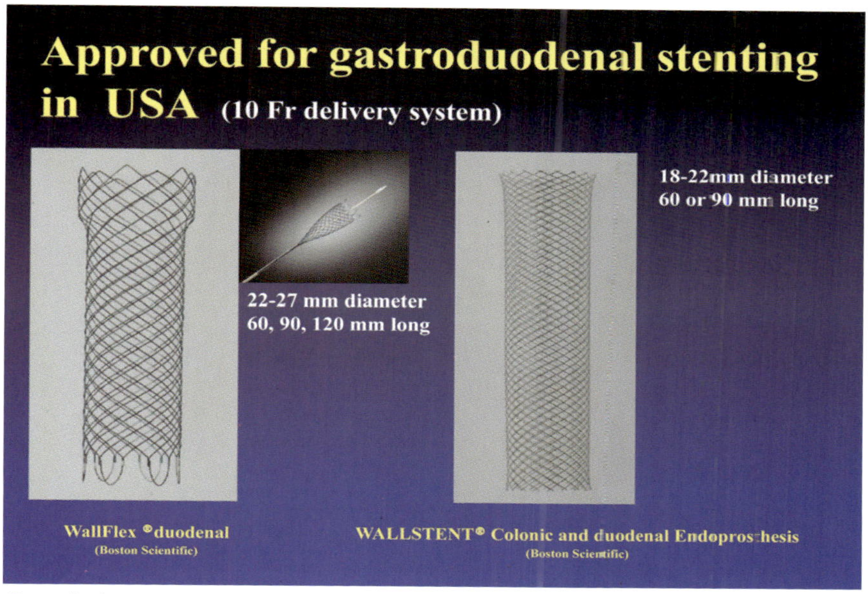

Currently, there are two stents approved by the Food and Drug Administration for palliation of malignant gastroduodenal obstruction, the duodenal Wallflex and colonic/duodenal WALLSTENT.

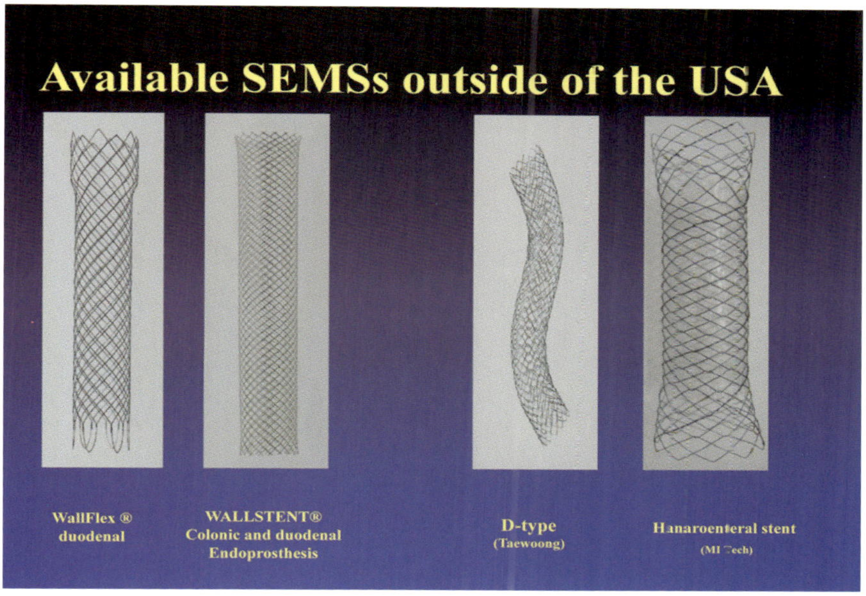

Outside of the U.S., a variety of SEMS designed for gastroduodenal use are available. These include the D-type stent, and Hanaroenteral stents.

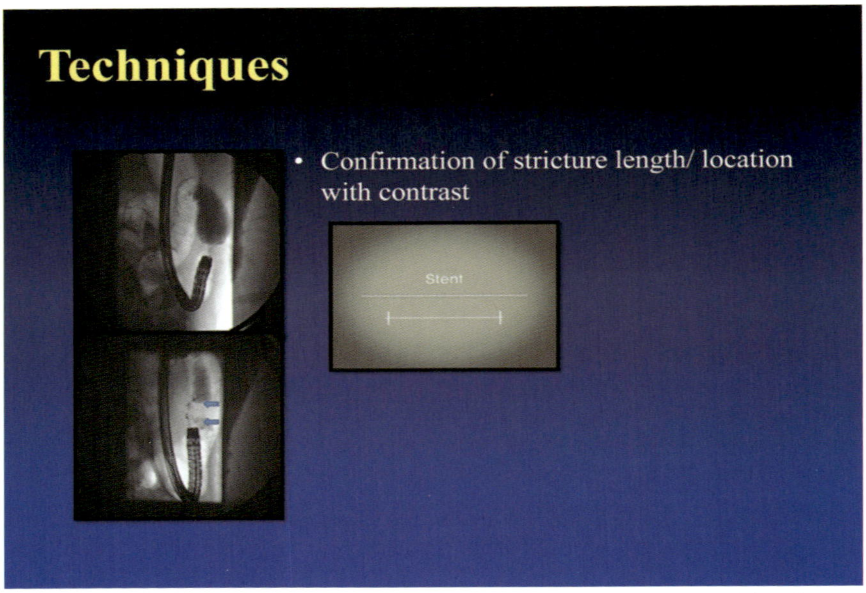

Fluoroscopy is used to Confirm the length and location of the of stricture. The Stent should be 3-4 centimeters longer than underlying stricture.

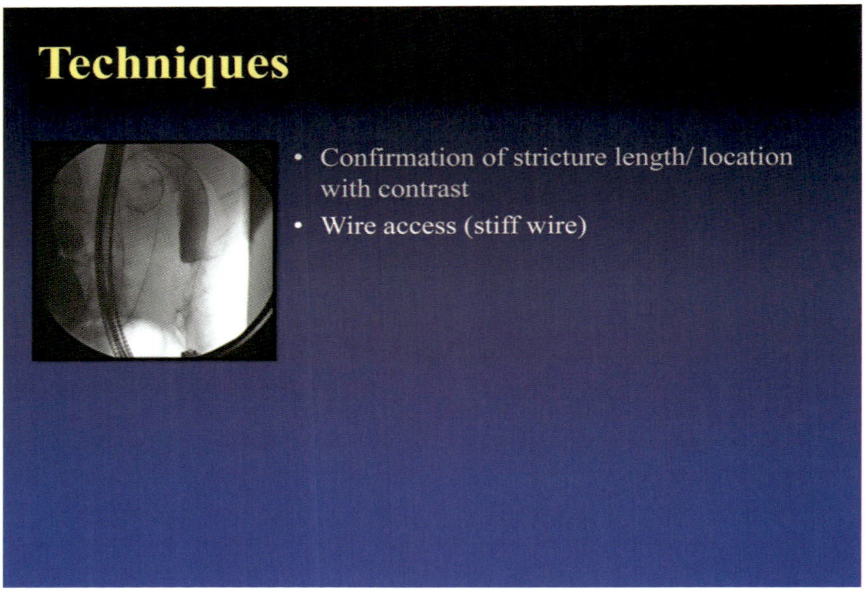

For guidewire access a 0.035-inch stiff guidewire is commonly used under fluoroscopic guidance. In difficult situations where the lumen is hard to locate or pass through, a round tip cannula with contrast injection helps with guidewire insertion.

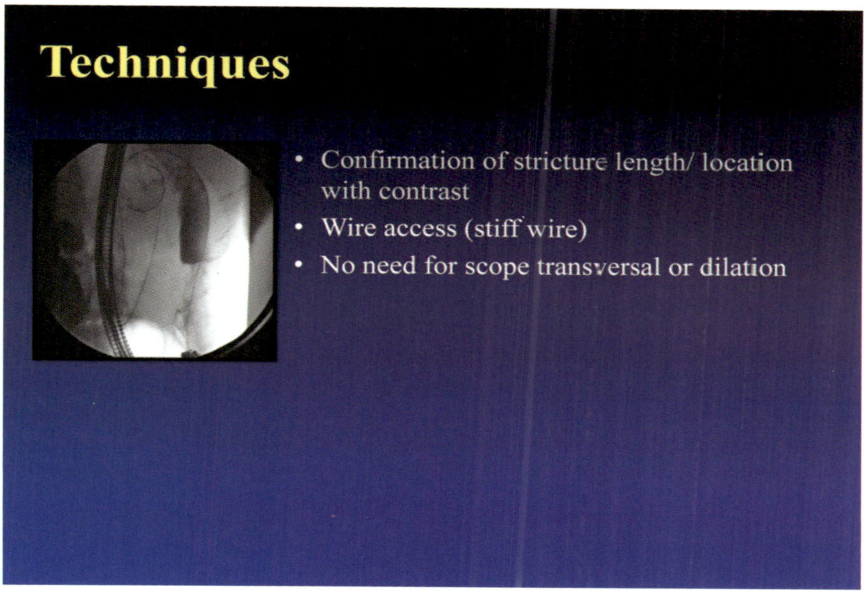

There is no need to traverse or pre-dilate the stricture prior to procedure.

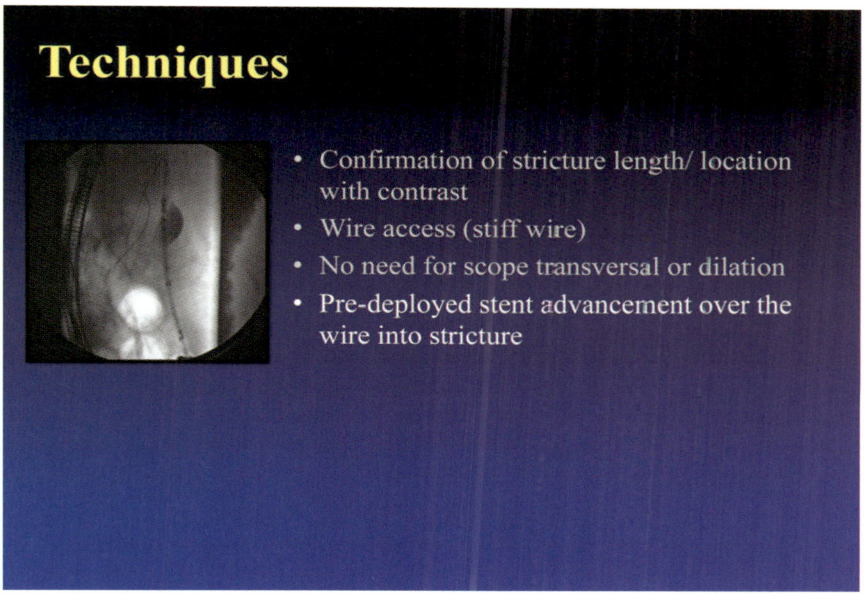

Before advancing the pre-deployed stent over the guidewire, the extension tube of the delivery system should be primed with abundant saline for a smooth delivery. The endoscope should be reduced to a relatively straight position to allow the distal portion of the stent to pass through the stricture.

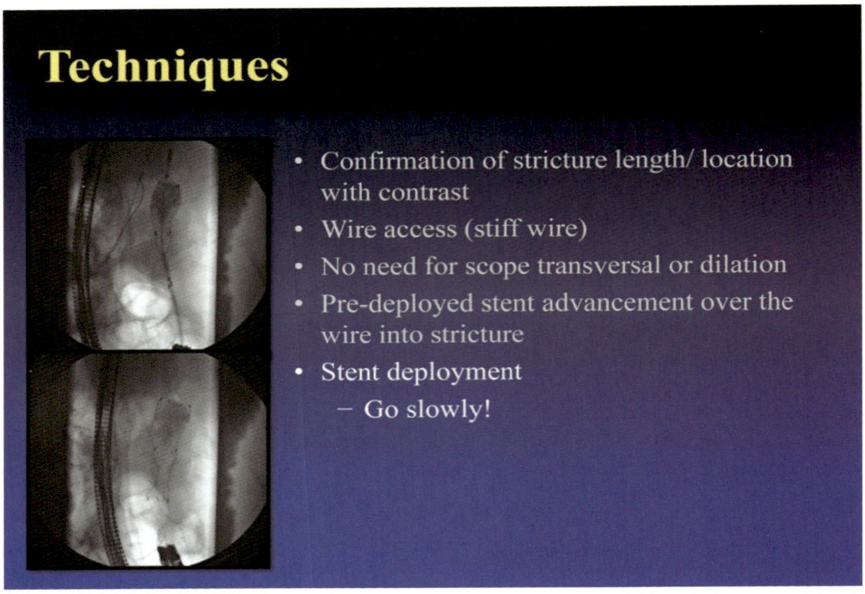

Once the position of the stent is confirmed. Deployment is performed slowly. While deploying, the position of the stent frequently needs adjustment as it has a tendency to slip distally from the expected delivery site.

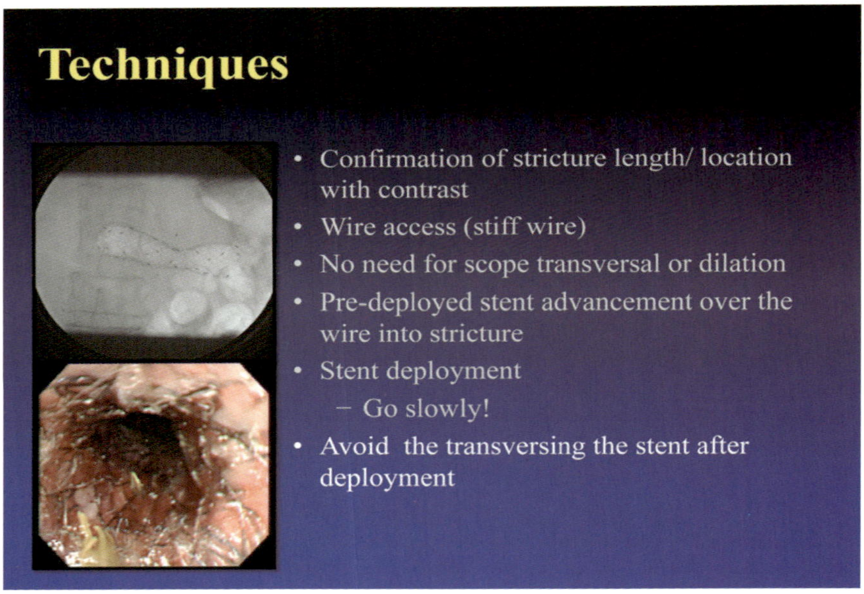

The endoscope should not routinely be passed through the stent lumen to check for patency as the stent could take some time to achieve full deployment.

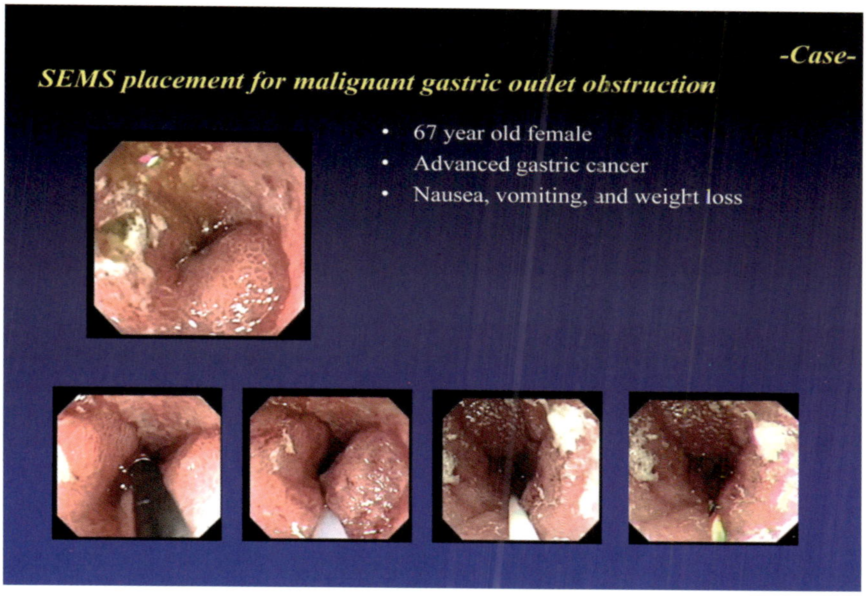

This is a 67-year-old female with advanced gastric cancer. We used a duodenal Wallstent for palliation of gastric outlet obstruction. A 0.035-inch stiff guidewire was inserted across the obstruction site using fluoroscopy and the stent was advanced over the guidewire into the stricture.

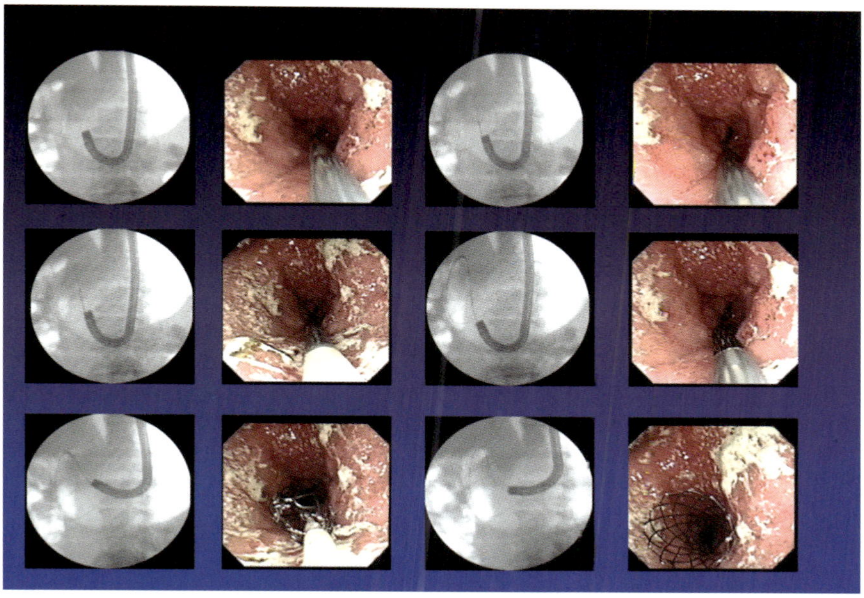

Looping of the endoscope makes it difficult to pass the stent through the operating channel, it easier to deploy and adjust the stent when endoscope is straightened and as close to the stricture as possible. When deploying, the endoscopist should adjust the stent position as it frequently slips distally from the delivery.

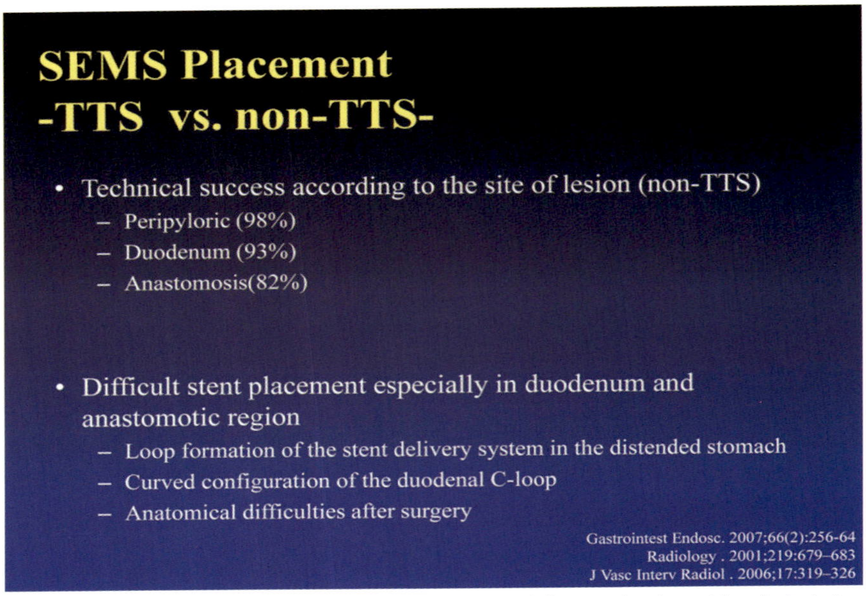

Looping of the endoscope makes it difficult to pass the stent through the operating channel, it easier to deploy and adjust the stent when endoscope is straightened and as close to the stricture as possible. When deploying, the endoscopist should adjust the stent position as it frequently slips distally from the delivery.

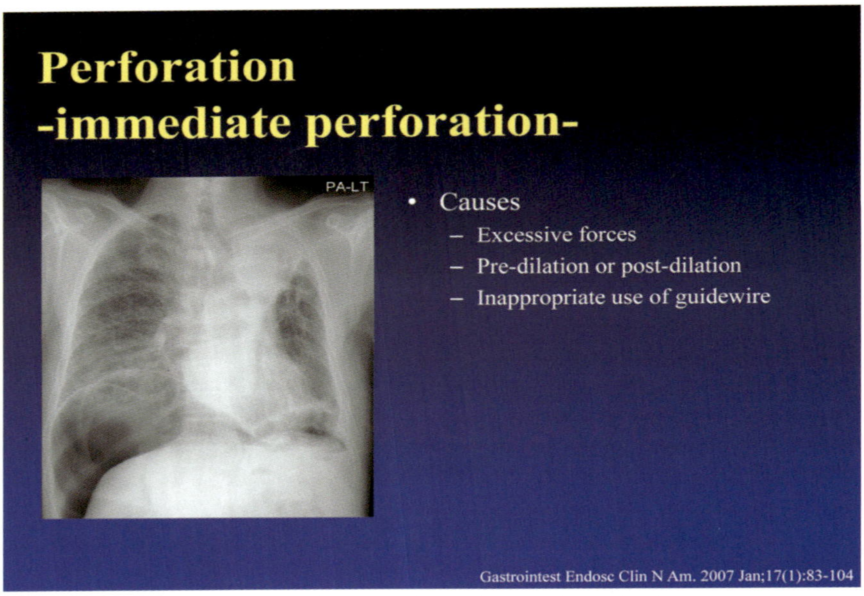

Perforation during deployment can be caused by application of excessive force to the endoscope during attempts to pass the stricture, pre-or post-dilation of the stricture, or inappropriate use of the guidewire.

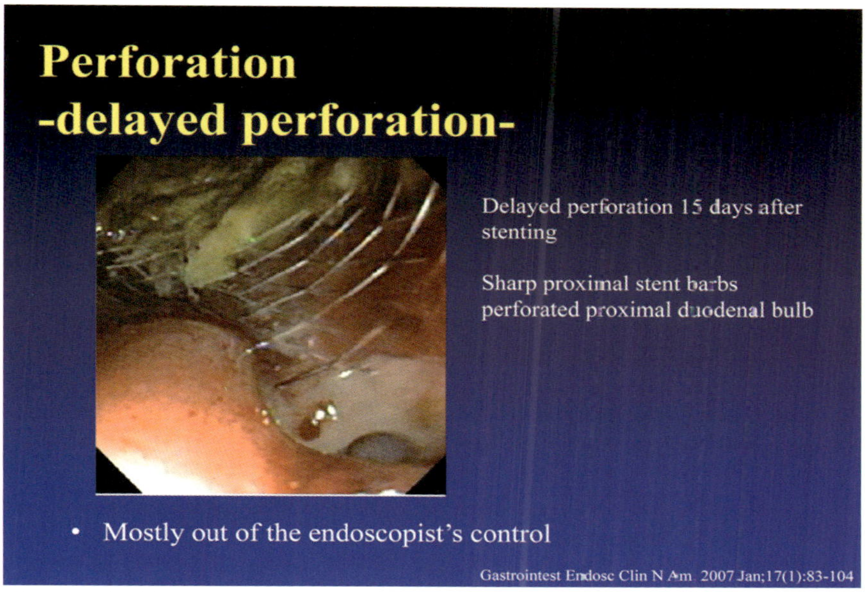

This picture is a delayed perforation 15 days after duodenal stenting. Delayed perforation is mostly out of the endoscopist's control.

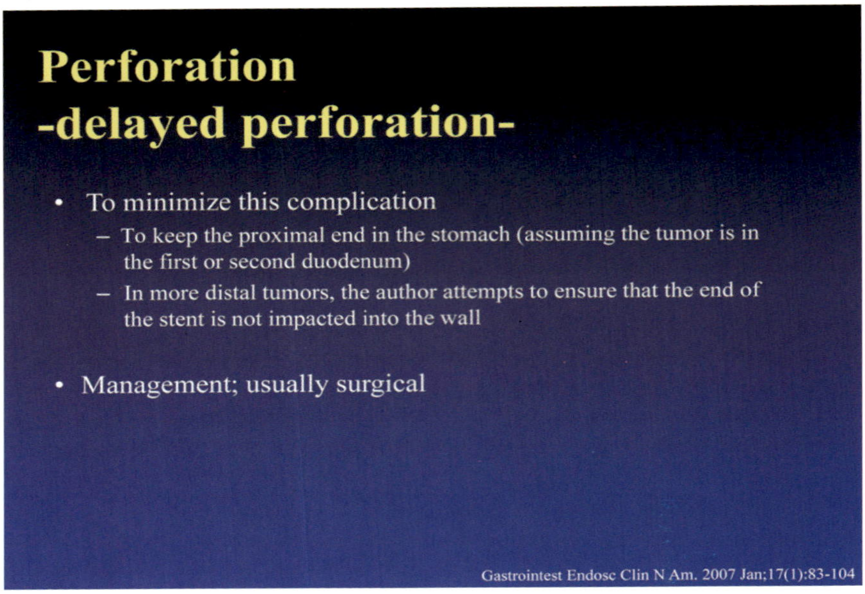

Although mostly out of the endoscopist' s control, it may be minimized two ways. The first is to keep the proximal end in the stomach (assuming the tumor is in the first or second duodenum). The stent is unlikely to perforate the gastric antrum. In more distal tumors, the author attempts to ensure that the end of the stent is not impacted into the wall. This can be achieved by placing the stent around a bend with the end into a straight segment, although it may not be possible in all situations. Management of delayed perforation, should it occur, is usually surgical.

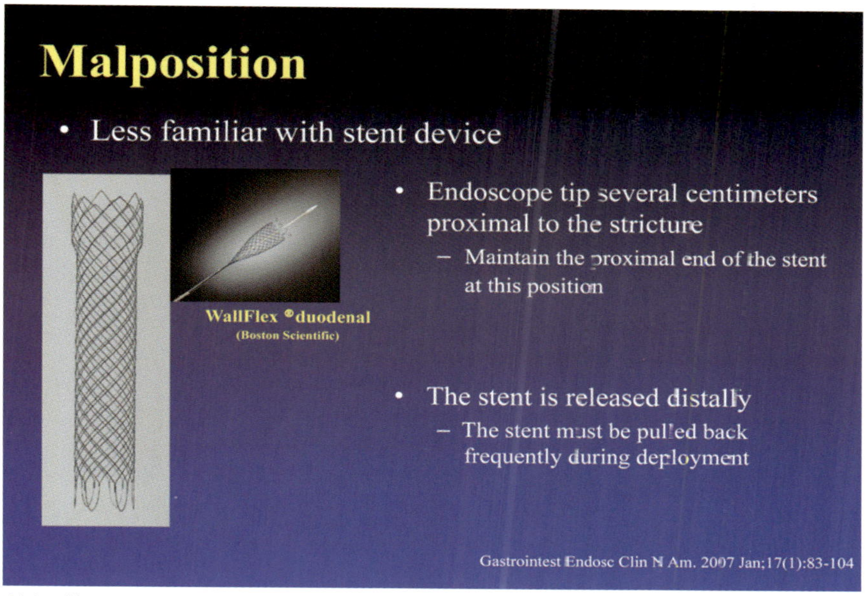

Malposition may be more likely to occur during deployment, because it may be underappreciated how much the Enteral Wallstent foreshortens. The endoscopist should keep the endoscope tip several centimeters proximal to the stricture and maintain the proximal end of the stent at this position. Because this stent is released distally (distal in terms of the endoscopist), the stent must be pulled back frequently during deployment, as is moves away from the endoscopist (distally) as it shortens.

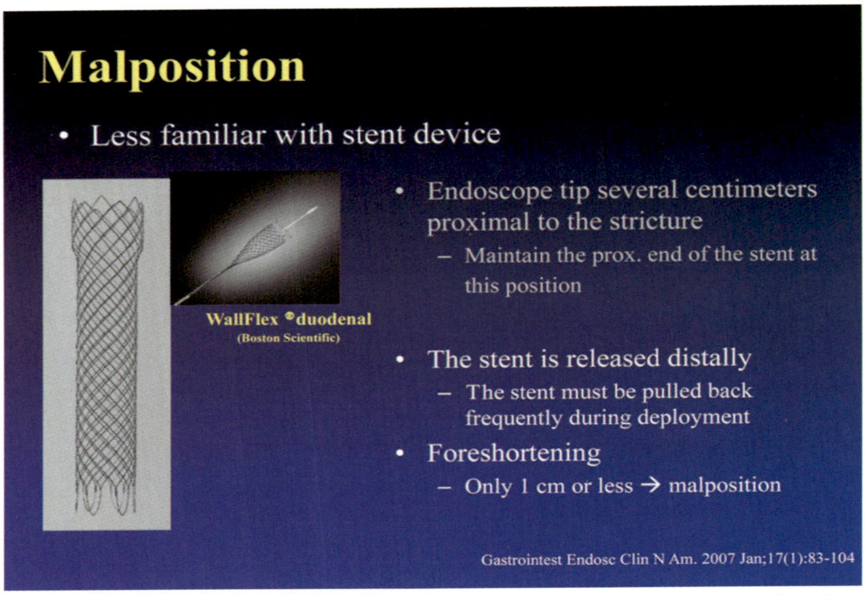

The endoscopist also should be aware that the bare metal wires are not endoscopically visible through the delivery sheath until the stent has deployed partially. At this point, the stent may be positioned too far distally than desired. Thus, the endoscopist needs to communicate with the assistant during deployment, and the stent deployment should proceed slowly. It is also worth noting that the stent will continue to shorten after the procedure until it fully expands. Thus, if only 1 cm or less is beyond one or both margins of the tumor at the time complete deployment, the stent is likely to be too short when fully expanded several days later.

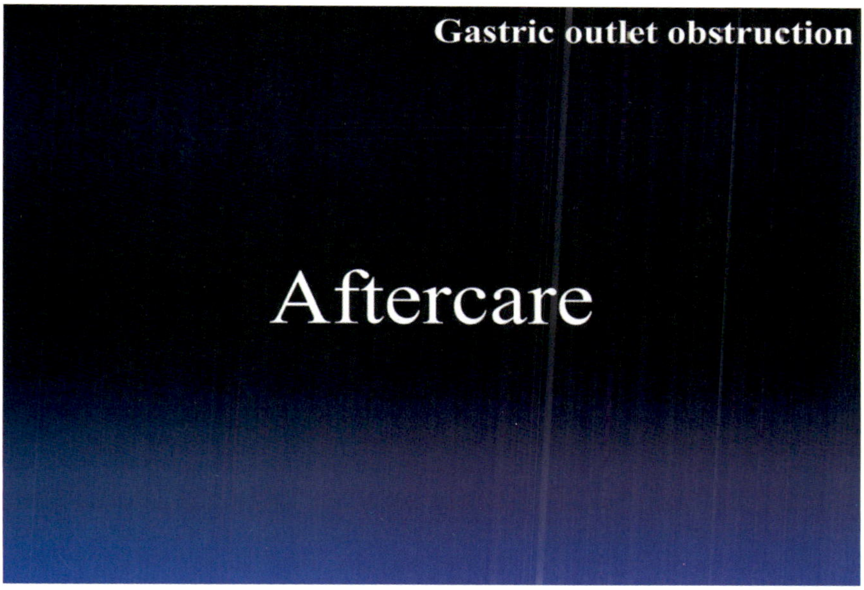

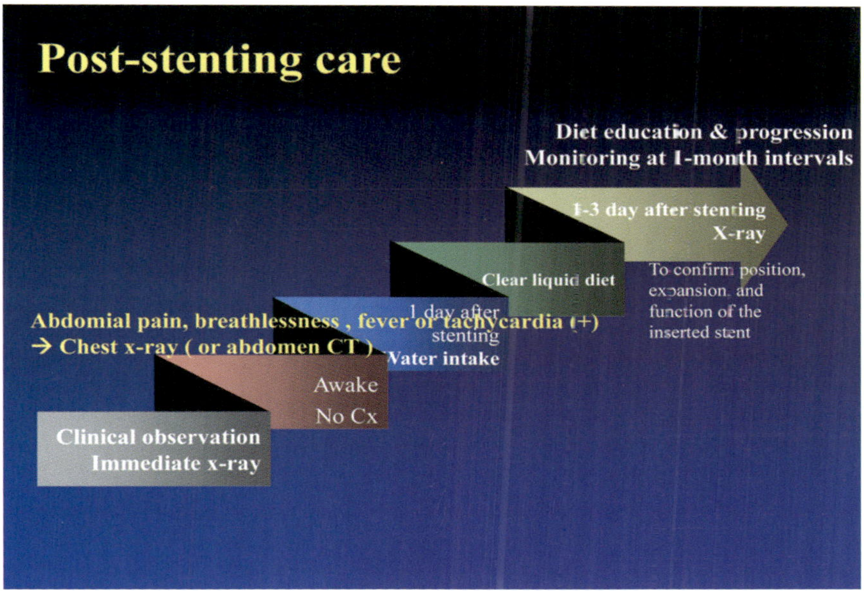

Following stent insertion, X-ray should be carried out to verify the position of the stent and to check for signs of perforation. Following stent placement, patients can experience varying mild abdominal pain or discomfort while the stent is still in the process of expanding. This is usually controlled with simple analgesia. X-ray should be performed to confirm position, expansion, and function of the inserted stent 1, 3 day after stenting.

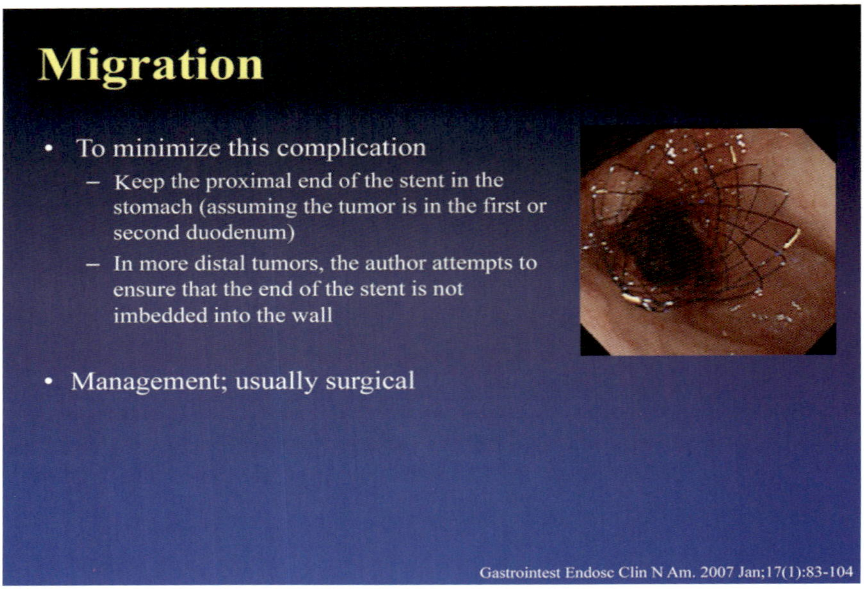

Migration is a rare event following placement of the Enteral Wallstent, because the stent is uncovered completely. Thus, if stent migration occurs, it is likely that there was not a significant stricture. Finding minimal to no stricture or finding that a therapeutic channel endoscope easily passes through the stricture suggests that mechanical obstruction may not be the cause of the clinical finding of a dilated and fluid-filled stomach. Gastroparesis or peritoneal seeding may be the cause for the patient' s symptoms.

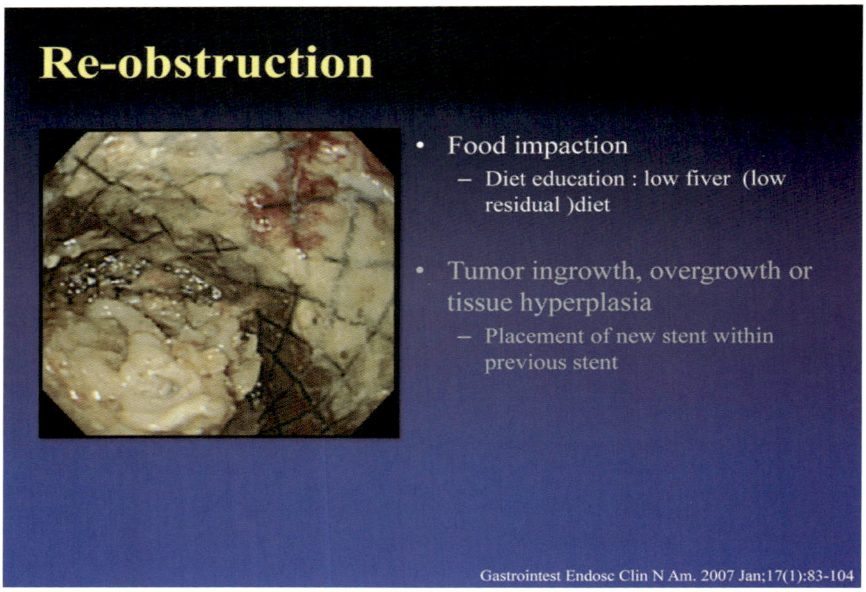

Obstruction by food is less likely to occur than with esophageal stents. Nonetheless, patients should be instructed to consume a low-fiber (low-residue) diet to reduce the risk of food impaction within the stent.

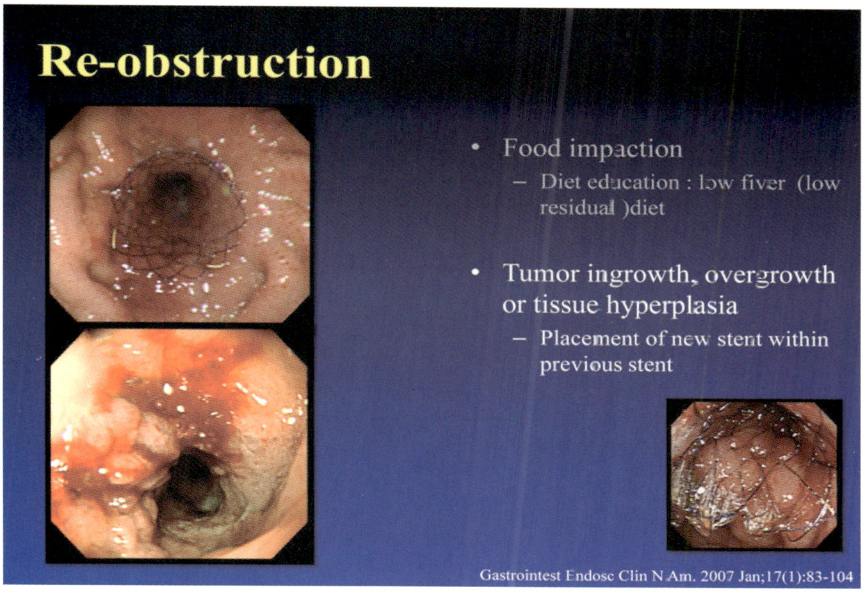

Reobstruction by tumor ingrowth, overgrowth, or tissue hyperplasia is managed best with placement of a new stent within the previous stent.

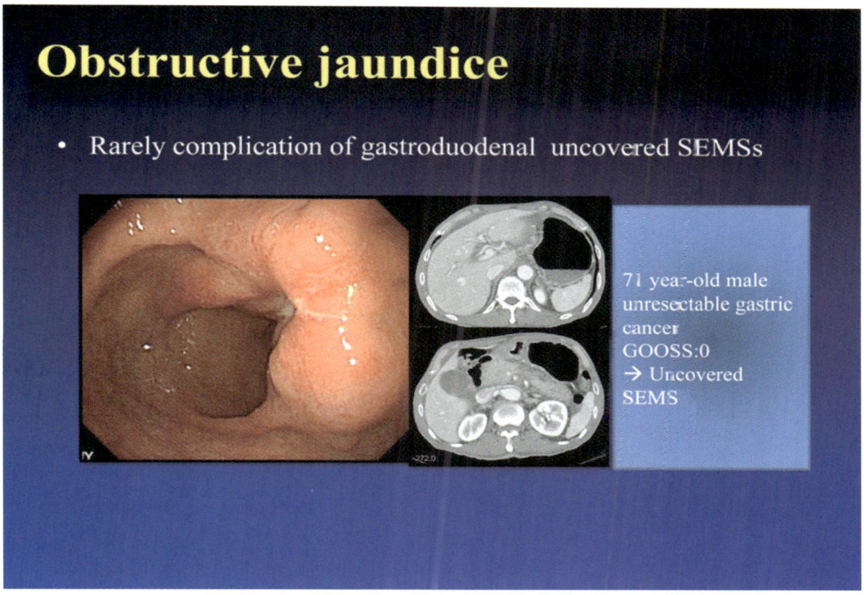

If pre-evaluation of coexistent biliary obstruction precedes stent insertion, obstructive jaundice rarely occurs following placement of gastroduodenal uncovered stents. This 71 year old male with inoperable advanced gastric cancer underwent stenting with a uncovered SEMS for gastric outlet obstruction. The initial abdominal CT scan showed mild intrahepatic duct dilation.

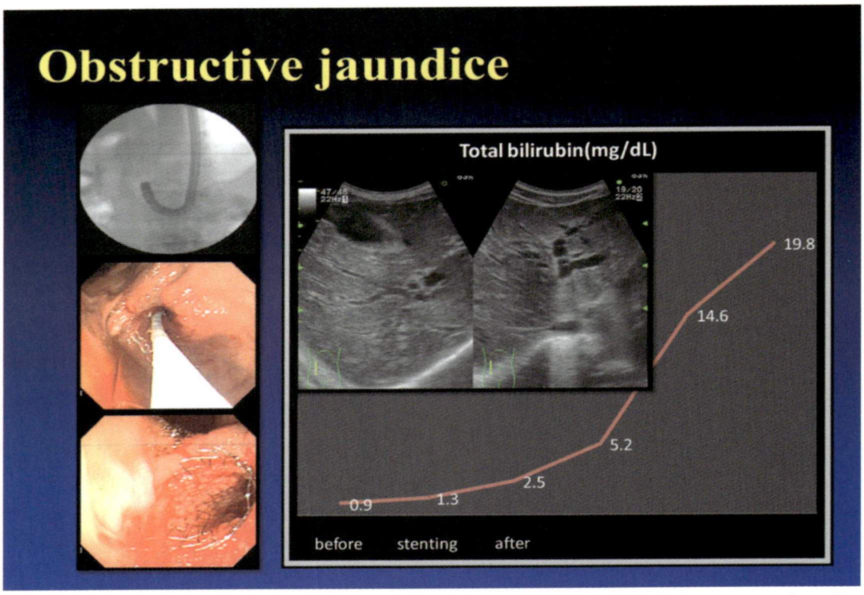

After deployment of the uncovered stent the patients obstructive symptoms improved, however 2 weeks later he developed jaundice and ultrasonography showed severe intrahepatic duct dilatation. The patient eventually underwent percutaneous transhepatic biliary drainage.

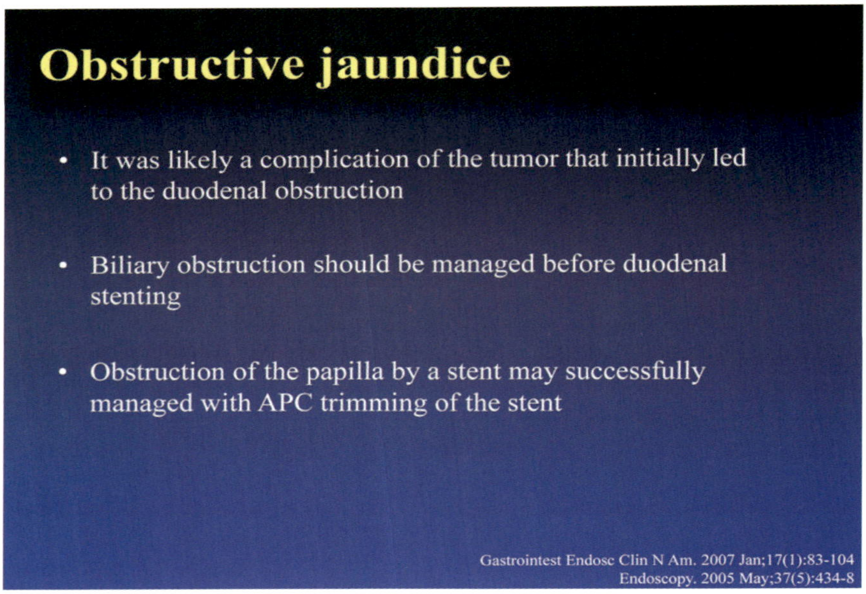

As in this case obstructive jaundice following an uncovered stent for gastric outlet obstruction is mainly due to overlooked coexisting biliary obstruction, rather than the stent itself. Obstruction of the papilla by the stent itself has been reported and managed with APC trimming of the stent.

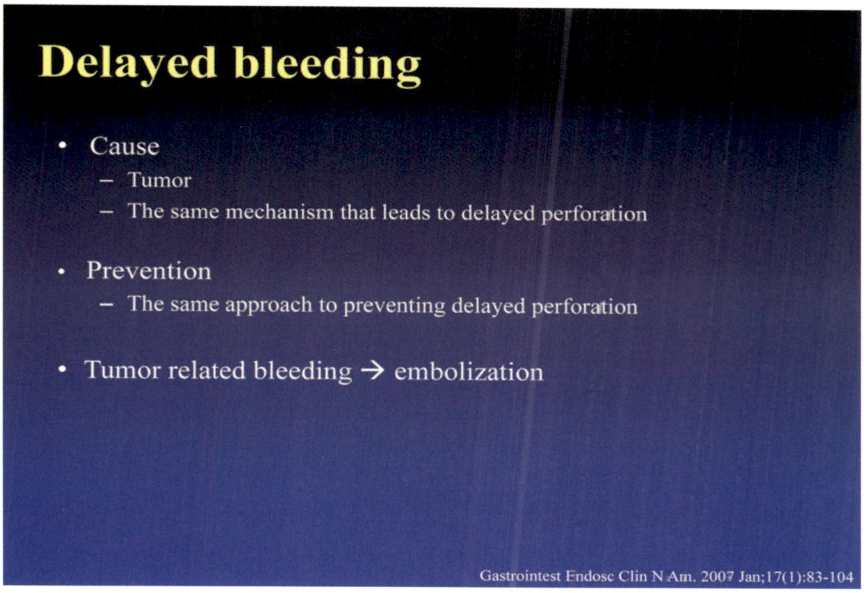

Delayed bleeding is likely to be caused by the tumor, although the same mechanism that leads to delayed perforation may lead to ulcer formation and bleeding. Thus, the same approach to preventing that complication also may prevent bleeding. Tumor-related bleeding may be managed by embolization.

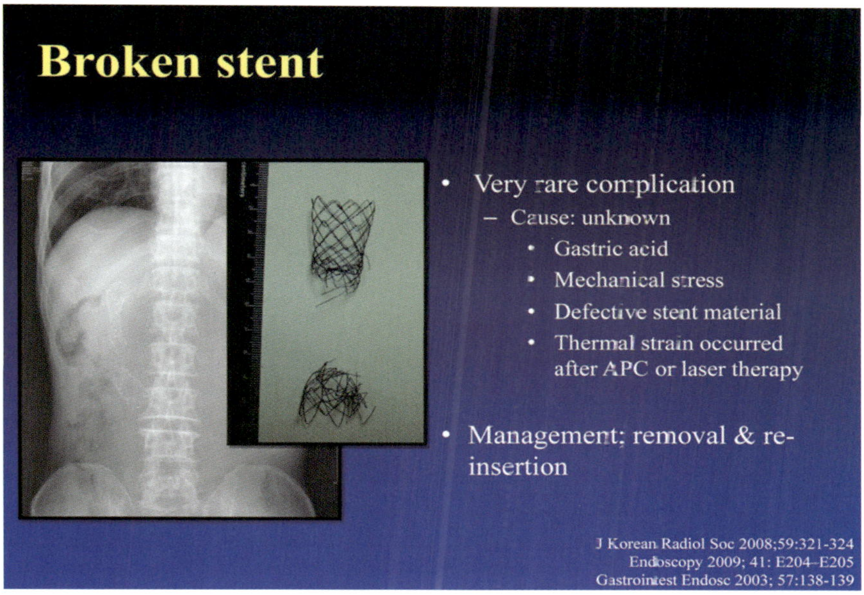

Broken stents are a very rare complication. The cause of the complication is unknown, however it may be related to gastric acid, mechanical stress, defective stent material, or thermal strain occurring after APC or laser therapy. The management of a broken stent is removal and reinsertion of new stent.

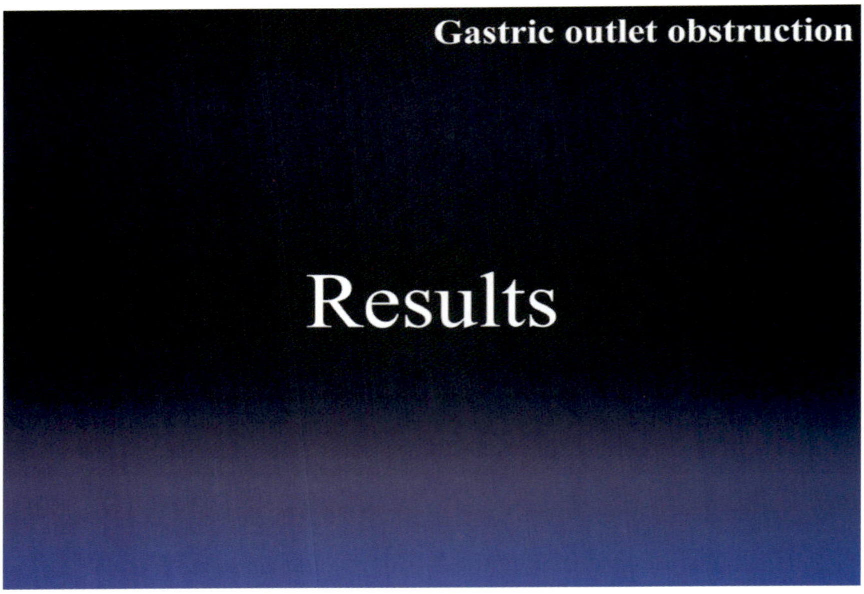

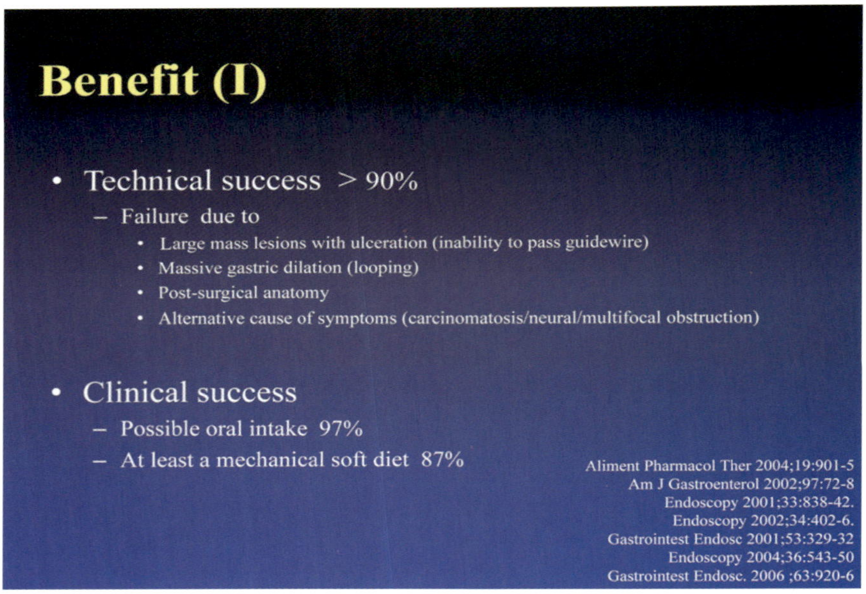

Technical success rates for SEMS in malignant GOO are generally over 90%. Technical failure results from large mass lesions with ulceration, massive gastric dilation, post-surgical anatomy or alternative symptoms. A comprehensive review of 32 case series including 606 patients unable to take oral intake reported successful stent deployment in 97% of patients, and oral intake was possible in all successful cases, with 87% of patients capable of eating at least a mechanical soft diet.

Benefit (II)

-A systematic review of 44 studies-

	Stent	Gastrojejunostomy
Technical success(%)	972/1012 (96)	203/204 (99)
Clinical success(%)	**890/1000 (89)**	**79/110 (72)**
Complication(%)		
Early major complications	43/609 (7)	6/159 (4)
Late major complications	171/950 (18)	34/201 (33)
Minor complications	66/732 (9)	66/201 (33)
Persistent obstructive symptoms	43/535 (8)	10/106 (9)
Reintervention	147/814 (18)	1/38 (1)
Mean hospital stay(day, [range])	7 (2-18)	13 (7-30)
Mean survival (day, [range])	105(23-210)	164(64-348)

Stent > Gastrojejunostomy : initial clinical success
Stent = Gastrojejunostomy : technical success, complication, and persistent symptoms

BMC Gastroenterol 2007;7:18

No differences between stent placement and gastrojejunostomy were found in technical success, early and late major complications and persisting symptoms. Initial clinical success was higher after stent placement. Recurrent obstructive symptoms were more common after stent placement. Hospital stay was prolonged after GJJ compared to stent placement. SEMS placement seems to be associated with an improved quality of life and decreased length of hospital stay making it a superior treatment option.

Complications

-A systematic review of 32 studies-

Complication		%
Procedural mortality		0
Severe complication		1.2
	Perforation	0.7
	Bleeding	0.5
Nonsevere complications		26.7
	Stent occlusion	17.2
	Stent migration	5.1
	Pain	2.5
	Biliary	1.3
	Other	0.7

Endoscopy 2004;36:543-50

According to a systematic review of 32 case series regarding gastroduodenal stenting. There were no procedure-related mortalities. Severe complications such as bleeding and perforation were observed in seven patients (1.2%). Stent migration was reported in 5%, and stent obstruction occurred in 18% mainly due to tumor infiltration.

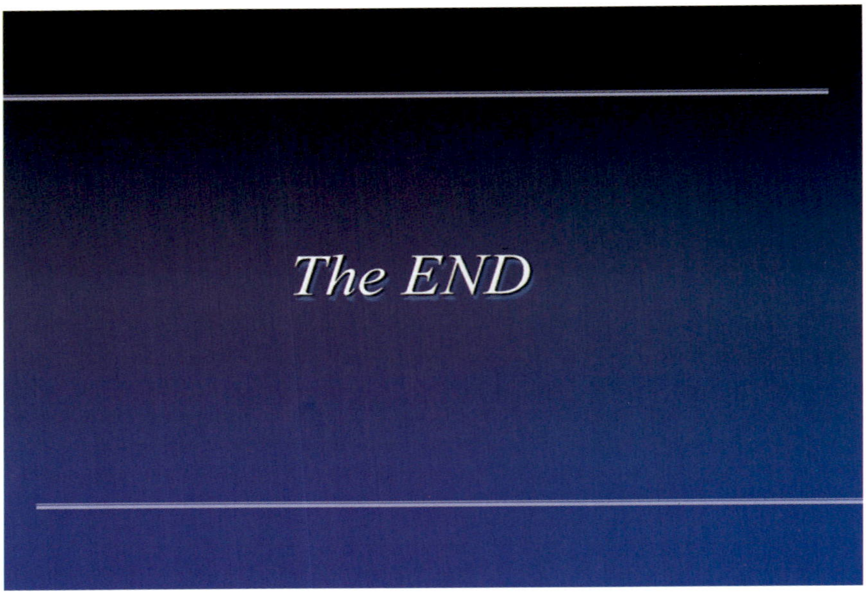

Strictures of the upper GI tract are not uncommonly encountered in the clinical practice and can pose a challenge to the gastroenterologist. It is important to know what techniques and instruments are indicated for different situations. Endoscopic treatment is a reliable and safe procedure in skilled, expert hands with a high success rate and low morbidity and mortality.

Chapter 8

Guideline for Infection Control and Antibiotics Prophylaxis During GI Endoscopy

Educational Video Nominated for a 2009 ASGE Audiovisual Award

Won Young Cho, M.D. Ph D.
Joo Young Cho, M.D. Ph D.

Chapter 8 Guideline for Infection Control and Antibiotics Prophylaxis During GI Endoscopy

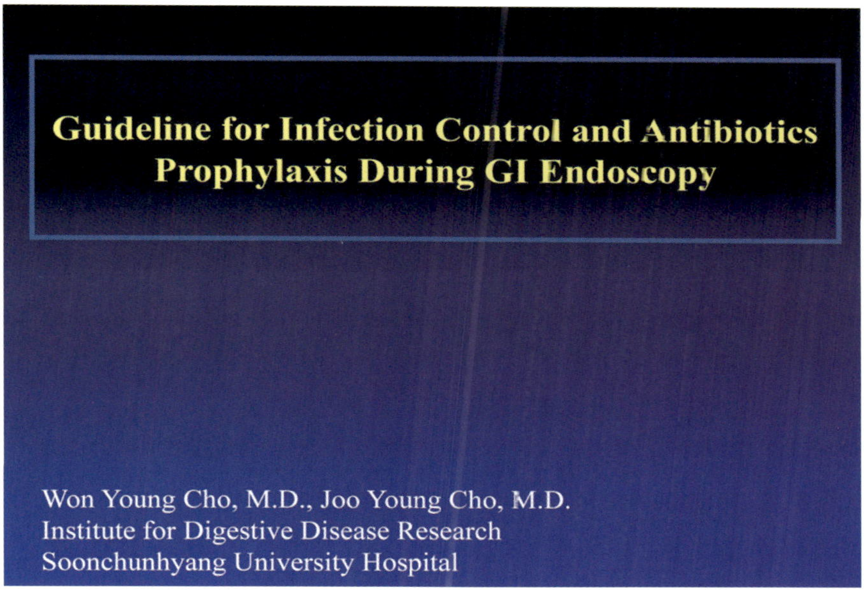

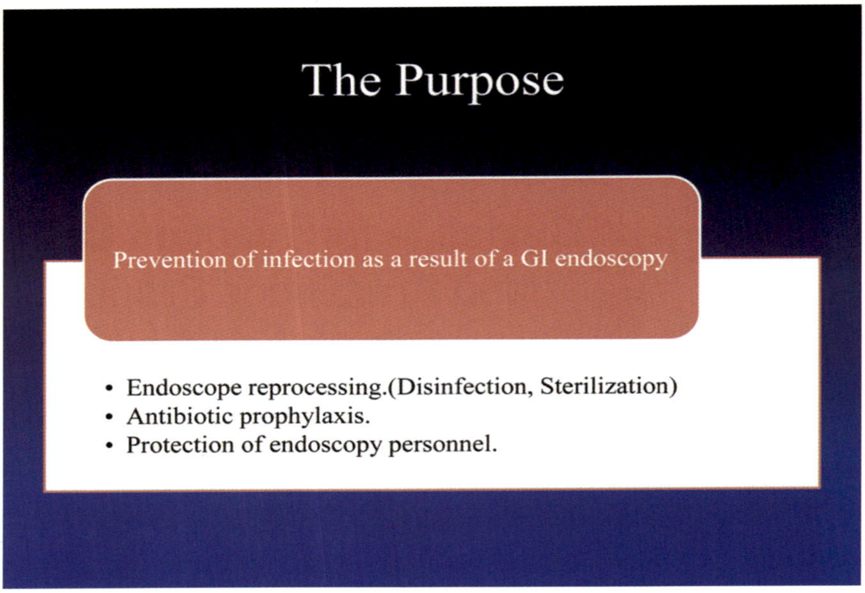

The purpose of this chapter is to provide information and promote understanding, which leads to the prevention of infection as a result of a GI endoscopy.
We will discuss measures to prevent infection, including endoscope reprocessing, antibiotic prophylaxis, and protection of endoscopy personnel.

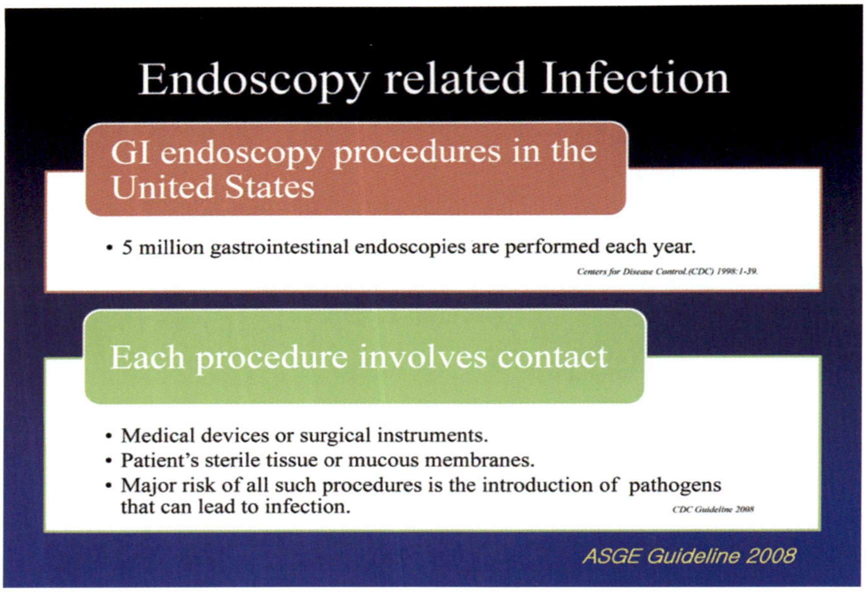

Over 5 million gastrointestinal endoscopies are performed each year. Each procedure involves contact of medical devices or surgical instruments with the patient' s sterile tissue or mucous membranes. The major risk of all such procedures is the introduction of pathogens that can lead to infection.

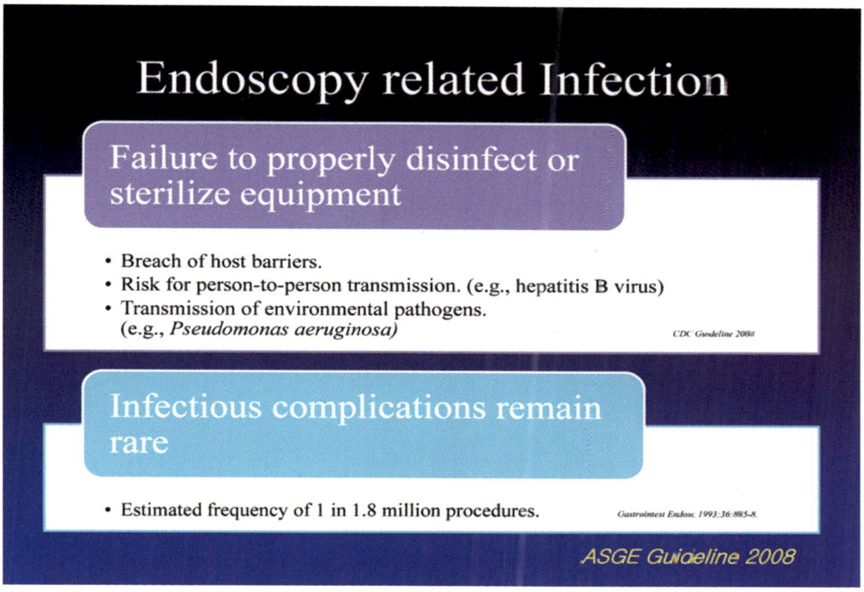

Failure to properly disinfect or sterilize endoscopy equipment, when there is a breach of host barriers. Increases the risk for person-to-person transmission, (e.g., hepatitis B virus) and transmission of environmental pathogens.
Infectious complications remain rare with an estimated frequency of 1 in 1.8 million procedures.

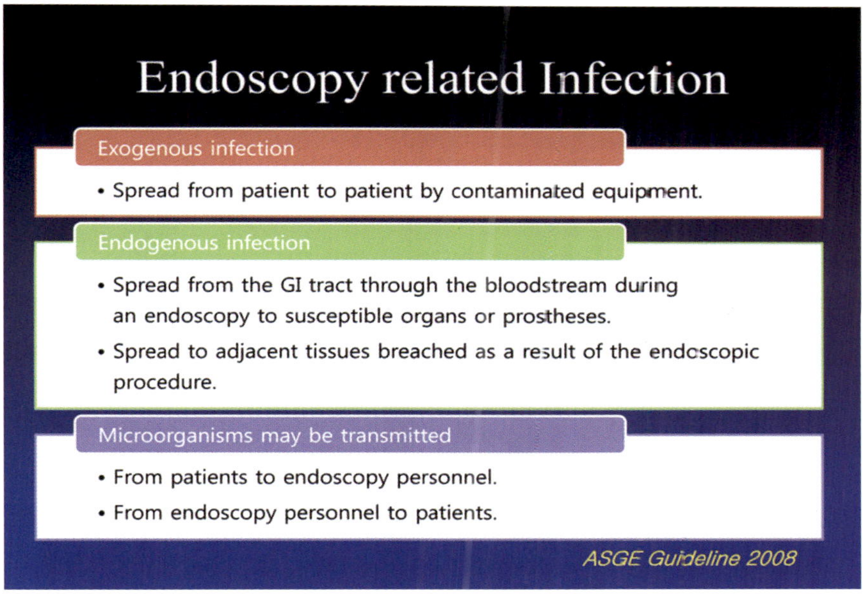

Exogenous infections spread from patient to patient by contaminated equipment.
Endogenous infection spread from the GI tract through the bloodstream during an endoscopy to susceptible organs or adjacent tissues breached as a result of the endoscopic procedure.
Microorganisms may be transmitted from patients to endoscopy personnel, or from endoscopy personnel to patients.

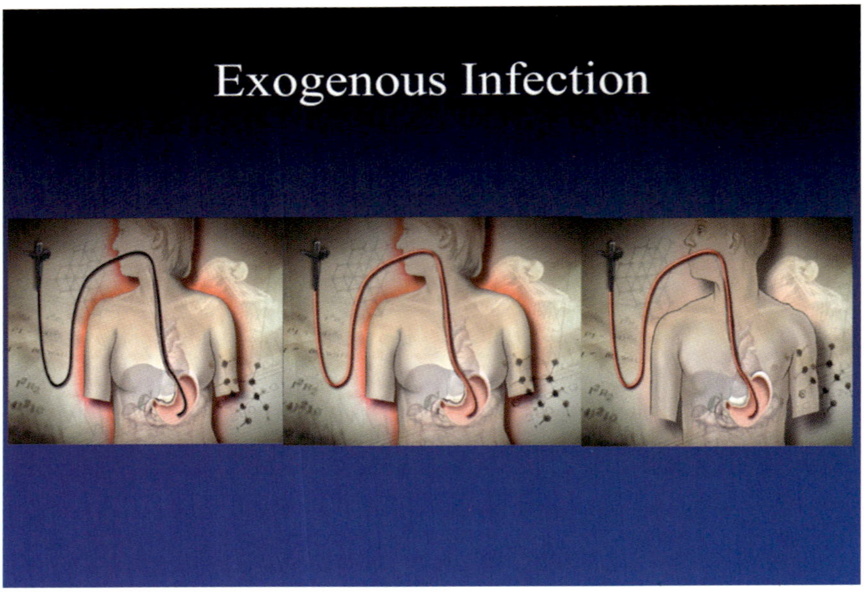

These pictures demonstrate exogenous infection. If the endoscope is not properly reprocessed following endoscopy of an infected patient pathogens can be transmitted to another patient during endoscopy.

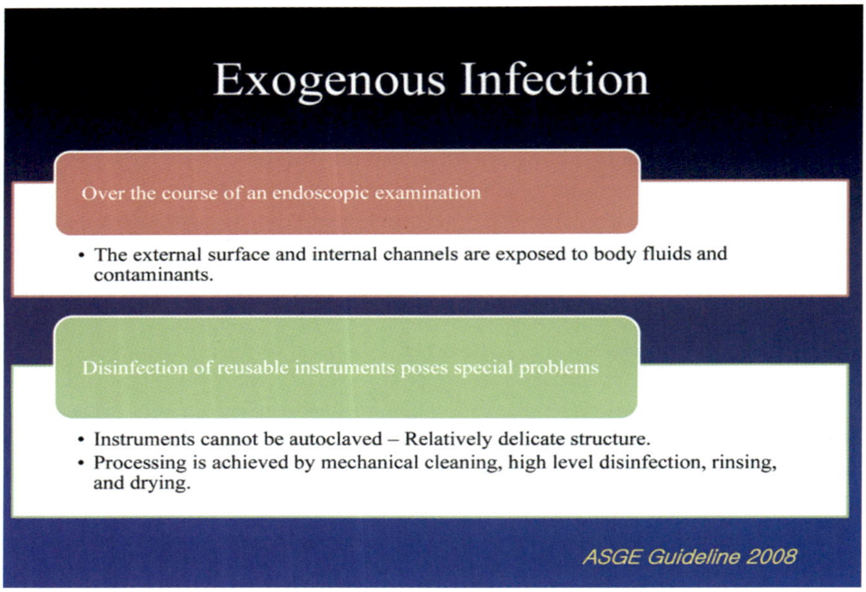

Over the course of an endoscopic examination, the external surface and internal channels are exposed to body fluids and contaminants.
Due to their relatively delicate structure, disinfection of reusable endoscopic instruments poses special problems as they cannot be autoclaved. Therefore, processing is achieved by mechanical cleaning, high level disinfection, rinsing, and drying.

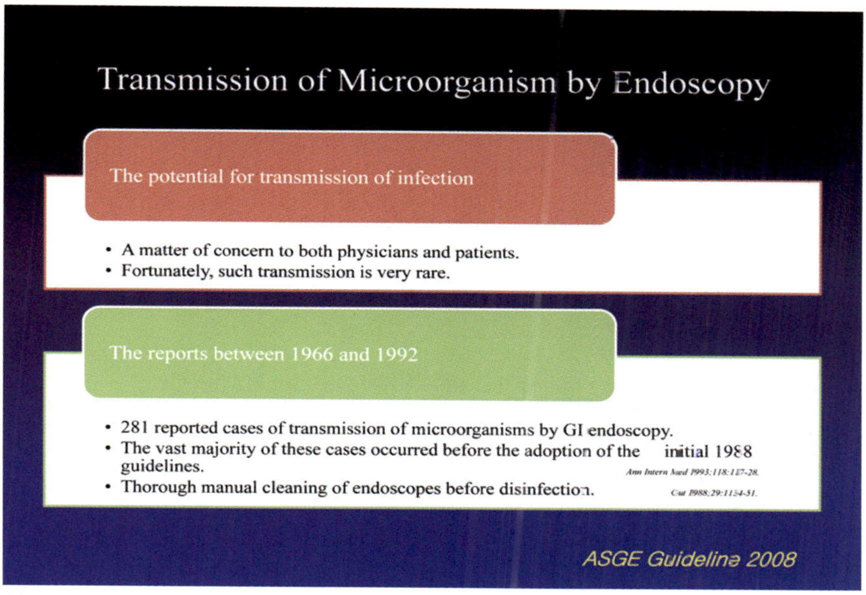

The potential for transmission of infection is a matter of concern to both physicians and patients. Fortunately, such transmission is very rare.

281 cases of transmission of microorganisms by GI endoscopy were reported between 1966 and 1992. The vast majority of these cases occurred before the adoption of the initial 1988 guidelines.

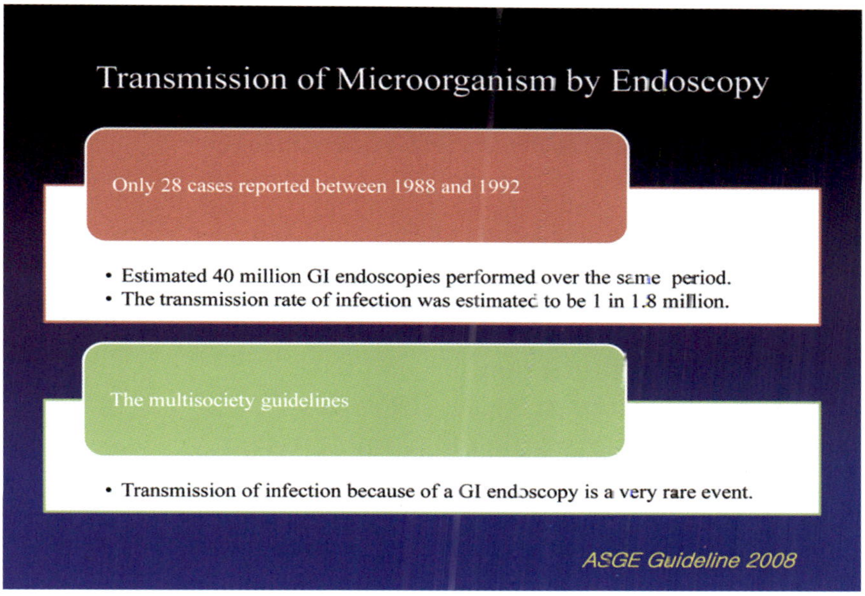

During an estimated 40 million GI endoscopies performed through 1988 to 1992 Only 28 cases of infection were reported.

Although there argue that this estimation is underestimated, it is evident that transmission of infection because of a GI endoscopy is a very rare event.

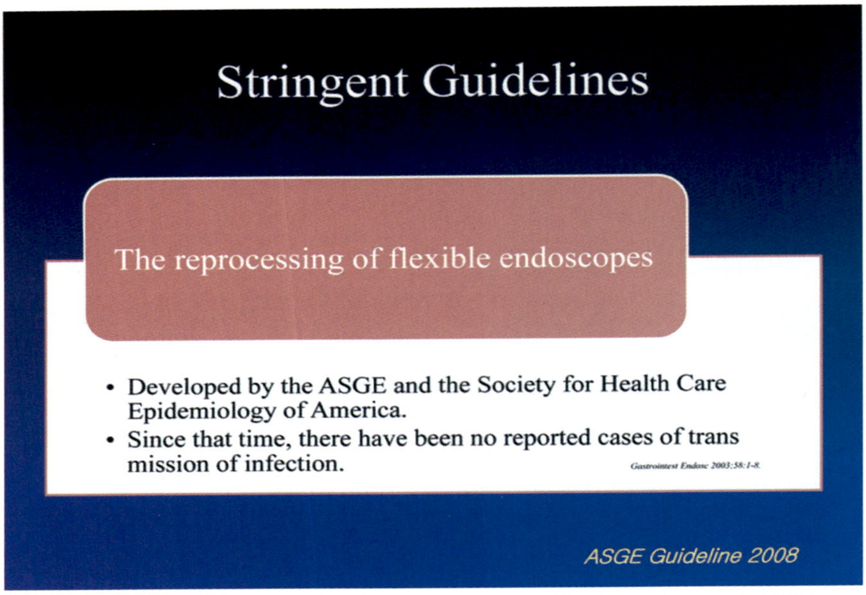

With the adoption of stringent guidelines for the reprocessing of flexible endoscopes in 2003, there have been no reported cases of transmission of infection.

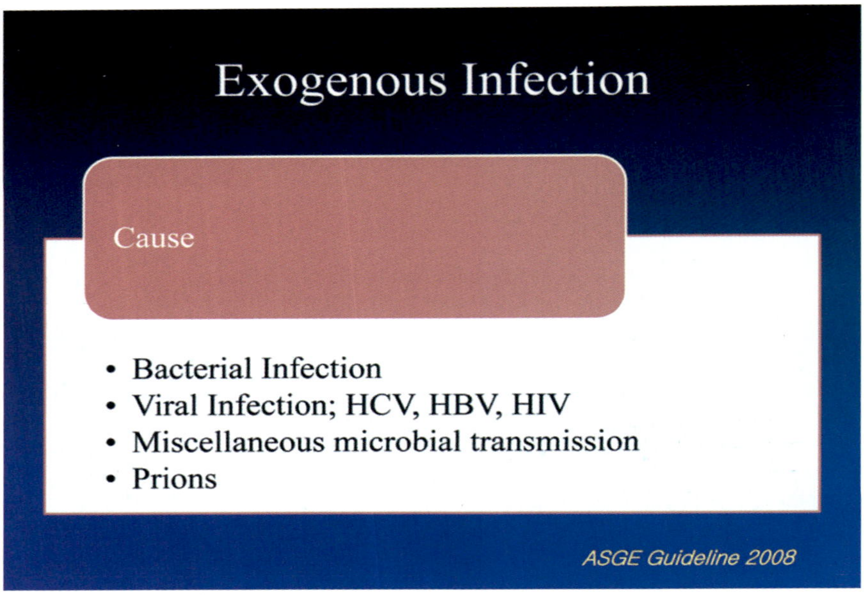

Causes of exogenous Infection are, bacterial Infection, Viral Infections(HCV, HBV, HIV), Miscellaneous microbial transmission and prions.

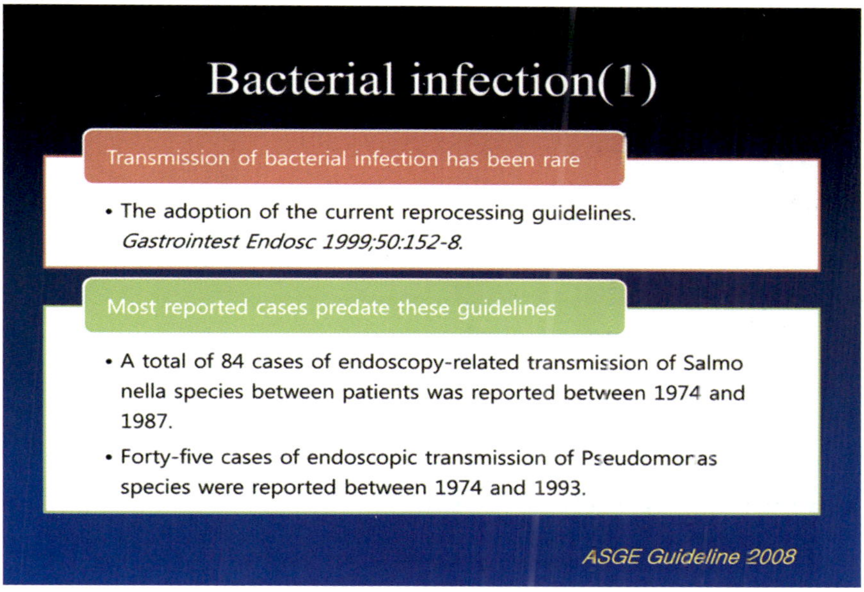

Transmission of bacterial infection has been rare after the adoption of the current reprocessing guidelines and most reported cases predate these guidelines.

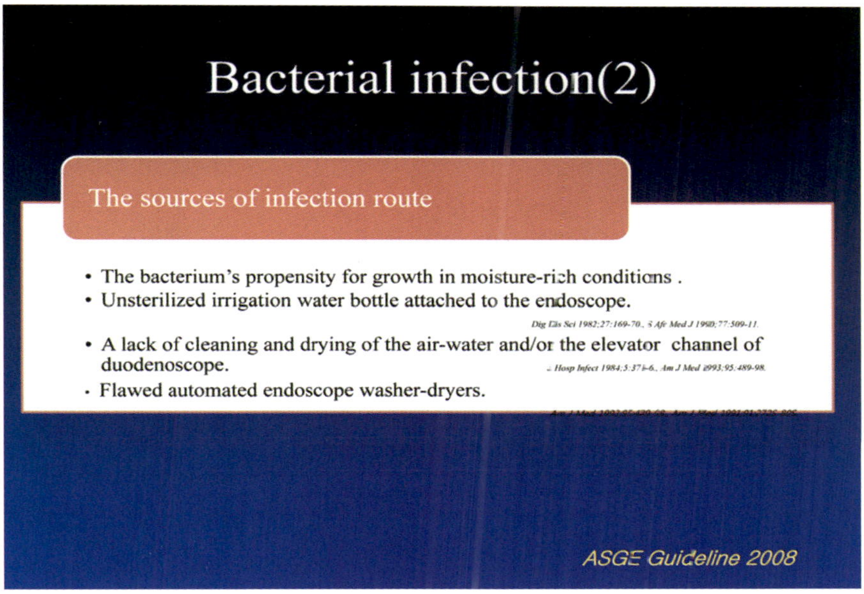

The sources of infection route are the bacterium' s propensity for growth in moisture-rich condition.

Unsterilized irrigation water bottle attached to the endoscope.

A lack of cleaning and drying of the air, water or the elevator channel of the duodenoscope.

And flawed automated endoscope washer-dryers.

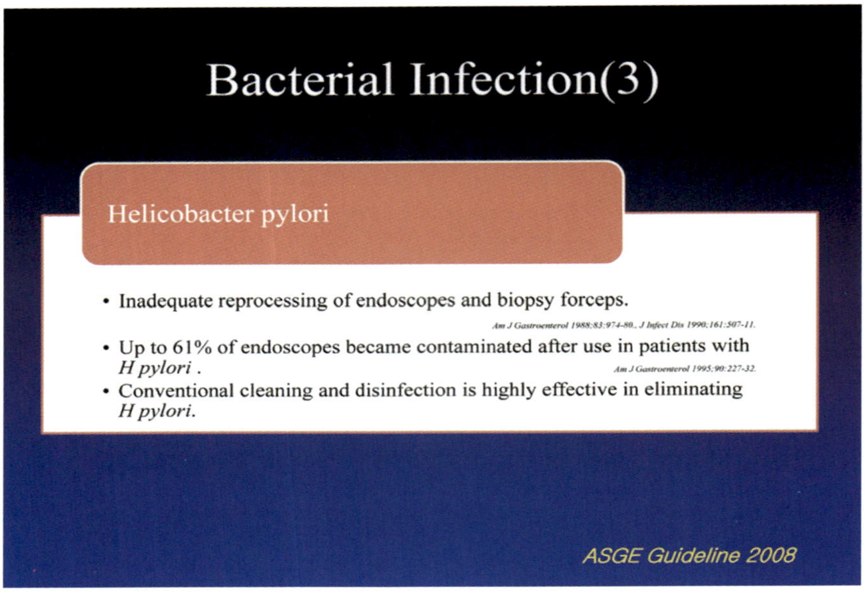

Helicobacter pylori infection can be caused by Inadequate reprocessing of endoscopes and biopsy forceps. Up to 61% of endoscopes become contaminated after use in patients with H pylori. Conventional cleaning and disinfection is highly effective in eliminating H pylori.

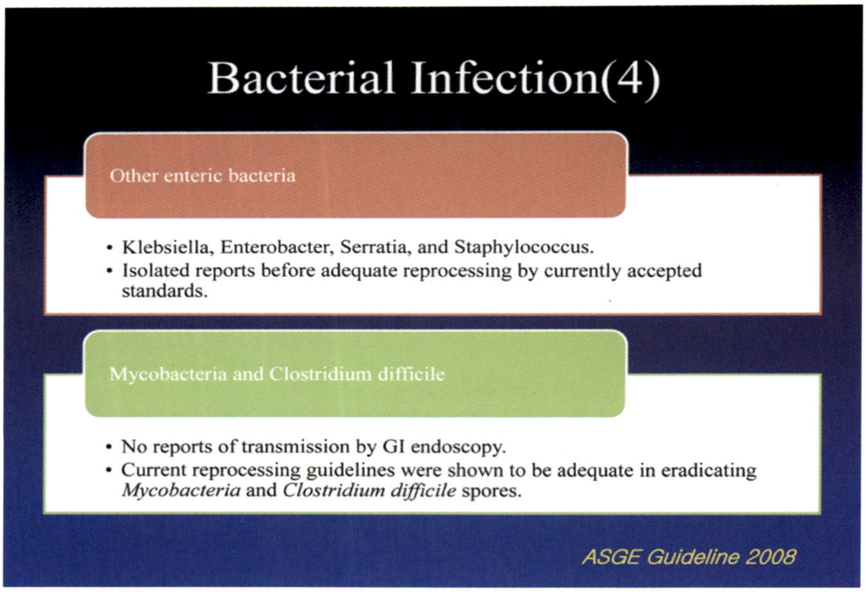

Endoscopic infection of other enteric bacteria, are rare and there are only isolated reports. There are no reports of Mycobacteria and Clostridium infection and current reprocessing guidelines were shown to be adequate in eradicating these pathogens.

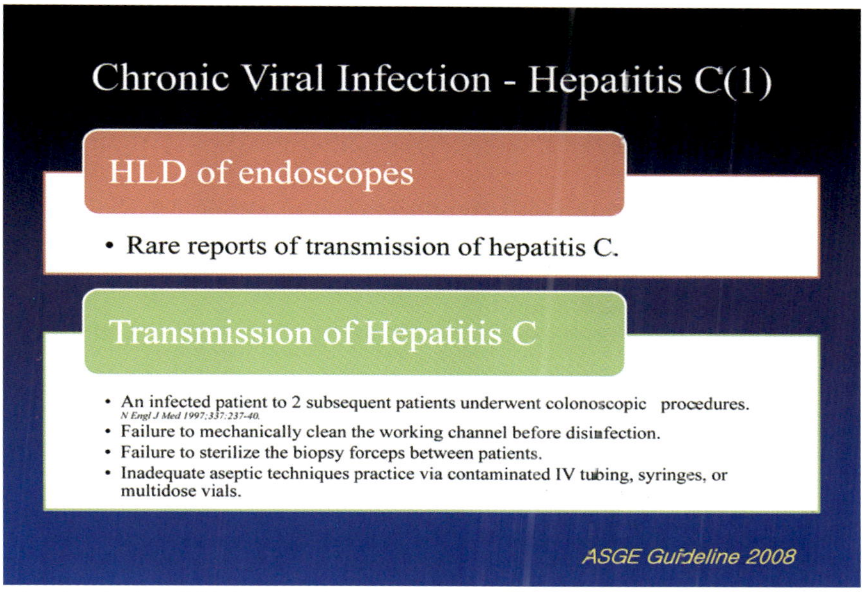

After the adoption of HLD there have been rare reports of transmission of hepatitis C. Transmission of Hepatitis C may occur with inadequate disinfection of the endoscope or accessories.

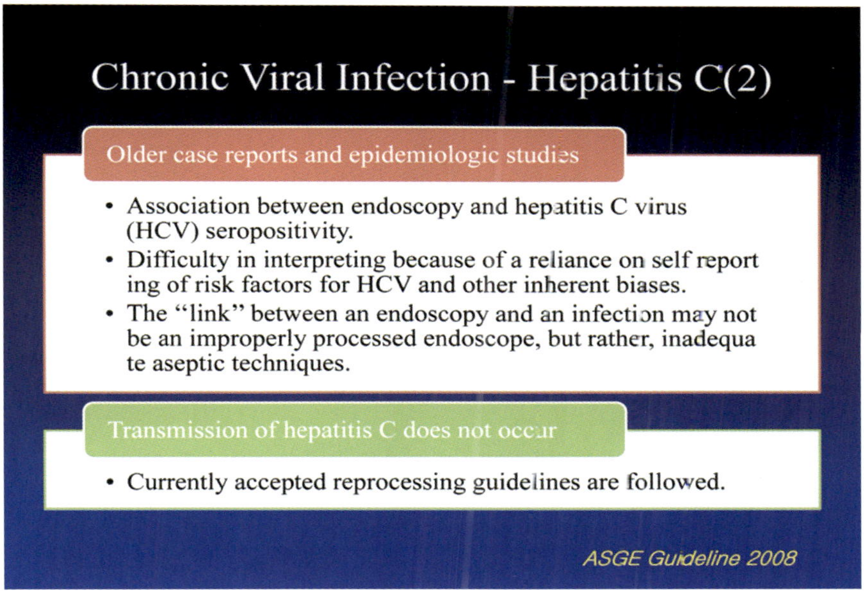

There have been older case reports of hepatitis C transmission. However, transmission of hepatitis C does not occur when currently accepted reprocessing guidelines are followed.

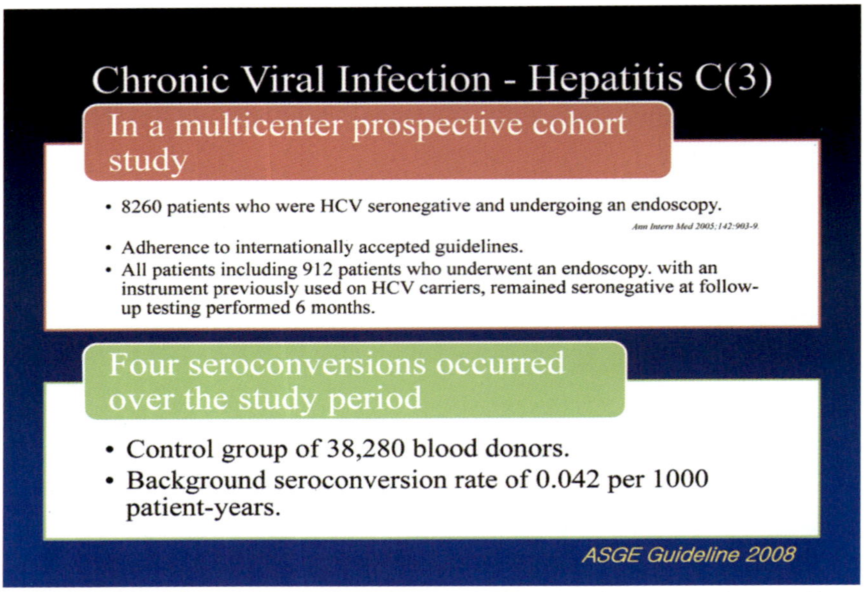

In a multicenter prospective cohort study, all of 8260 patients who underwent an endoscopy with an instrument previously used on HCV carriers remained sero negative at follow-up testing performed 6 months.

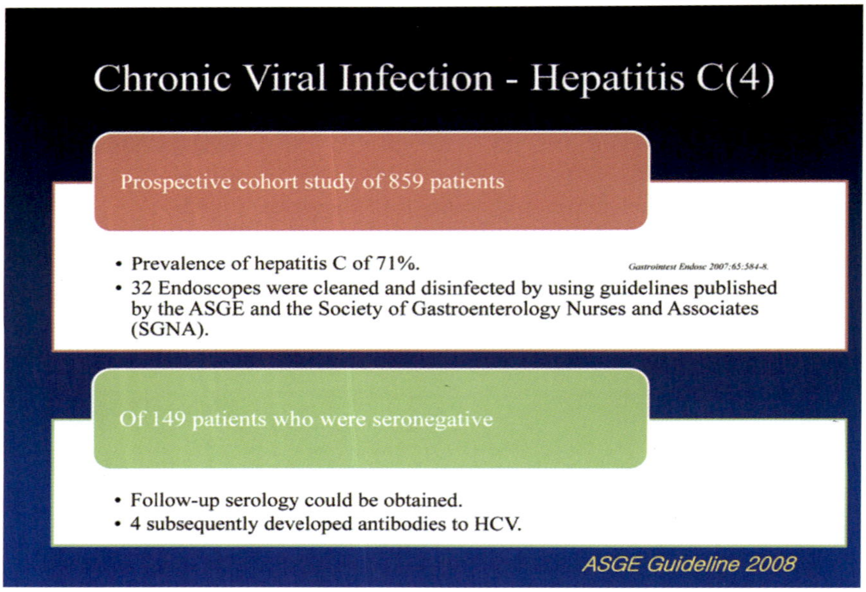

In another prospective cohort study of 859 patients with a 71% prevalence of hepatitis C, Of the 149 patients who were seronegative, 4 developed antibodies to HCV.

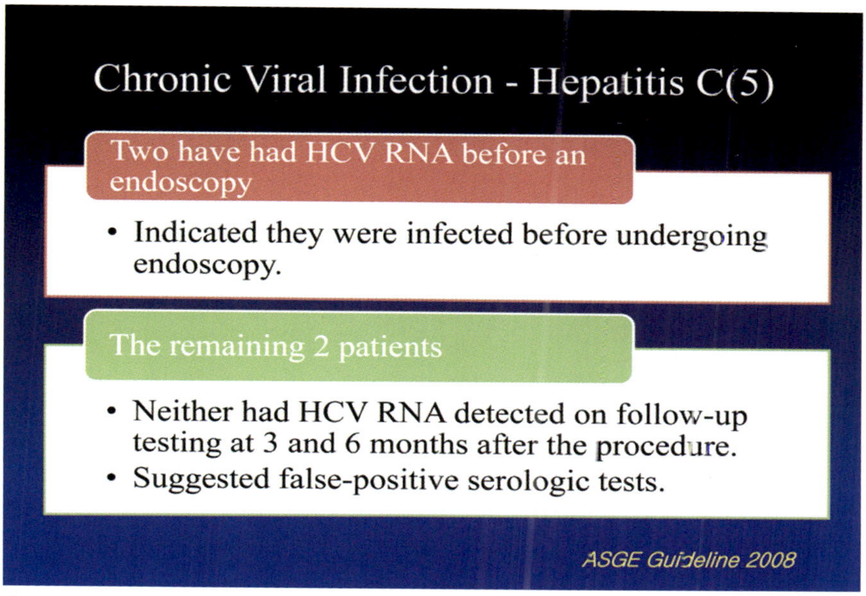

Two have had HCV RNA before an endoscopy indicated they were infected before undergoing endoscopy. The remaining 2 patients neither had HCV RNA detected on follow-up testing at 3 and 6 months after the procedure. Suggesting false-positive serologic tests.

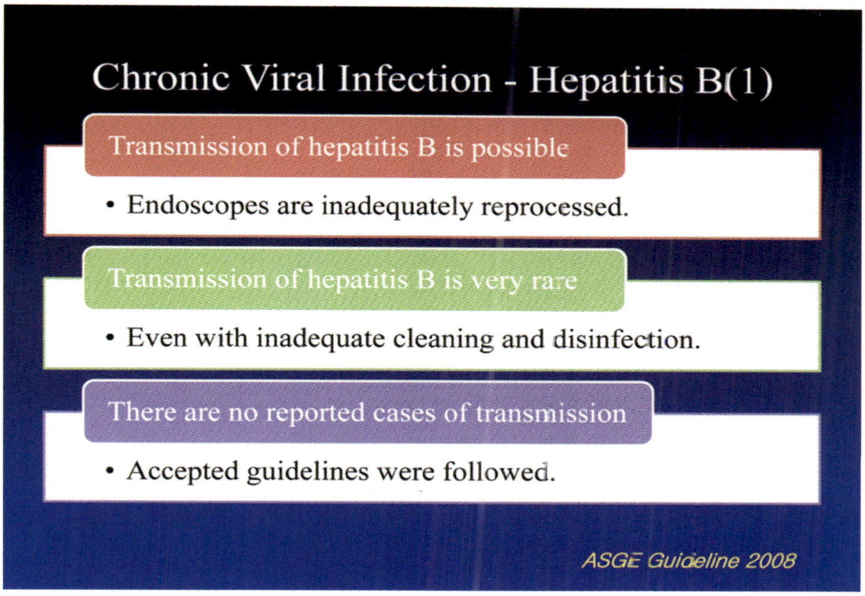

Although extremely rare, transmission of hepatitis B is possible if endoscopes are inadequately reprocess. There are no reported cases of transmission.

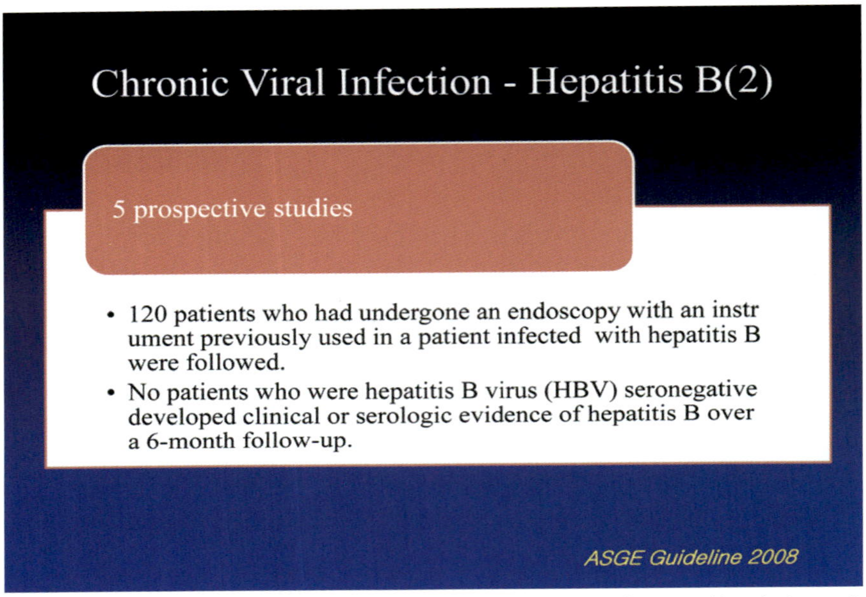

In 5 prospective studies, none of 120 patients who had undergone an endoscopy with an instrument previously used in a patient infected with hepatitis B developed clinical or serologic evidence of hepatitis B over a 6-month follow-up.

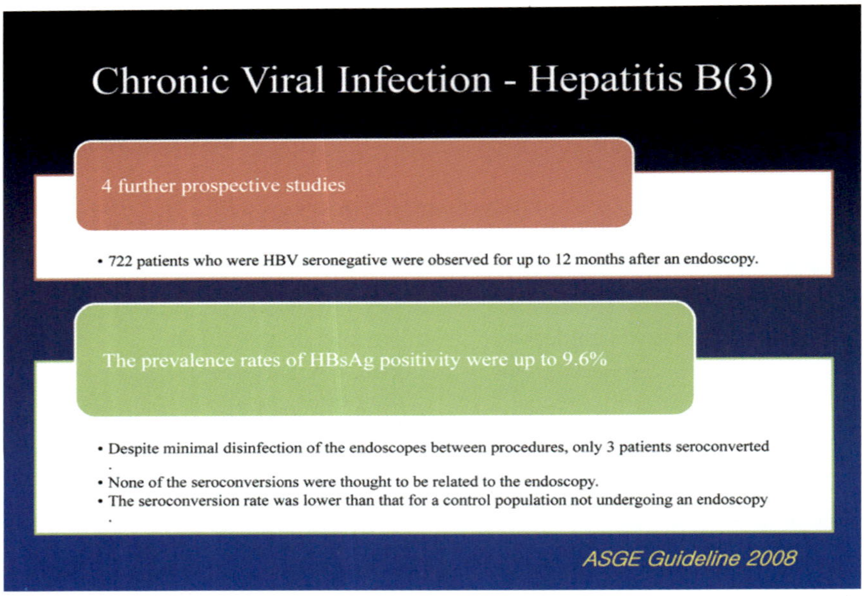

In 4 further prospective studies, only 3 of 722 patients who were HBV seronegative seroconverted. The seroconversion rate was lower than that for a control population not undergoing an endoscopy. None of the seroconversions were thought to be related to the endoscopy.

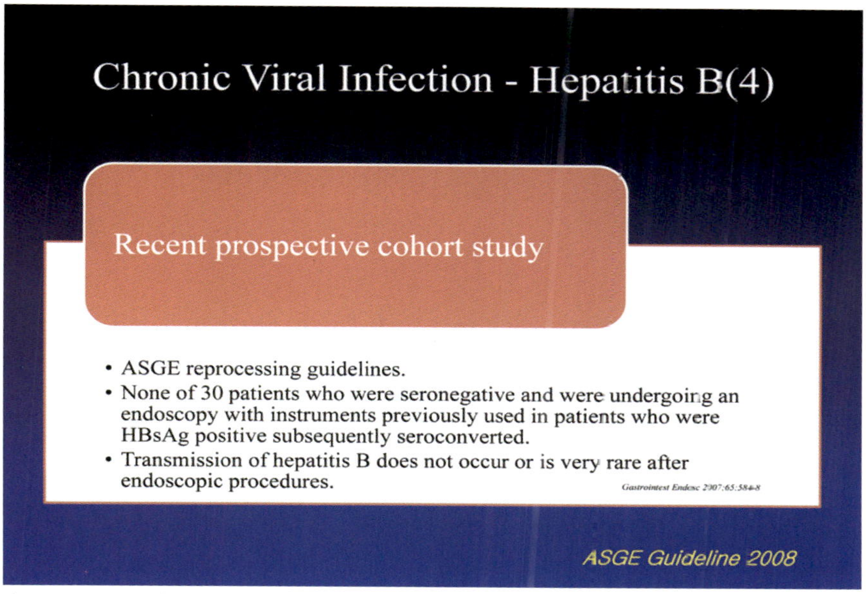

A recent prospective cohort study also showed that transmission of hepatitis B does not occur or is very rare after endoscopic procedures when adhering to ASGE reprocessing guidelines.

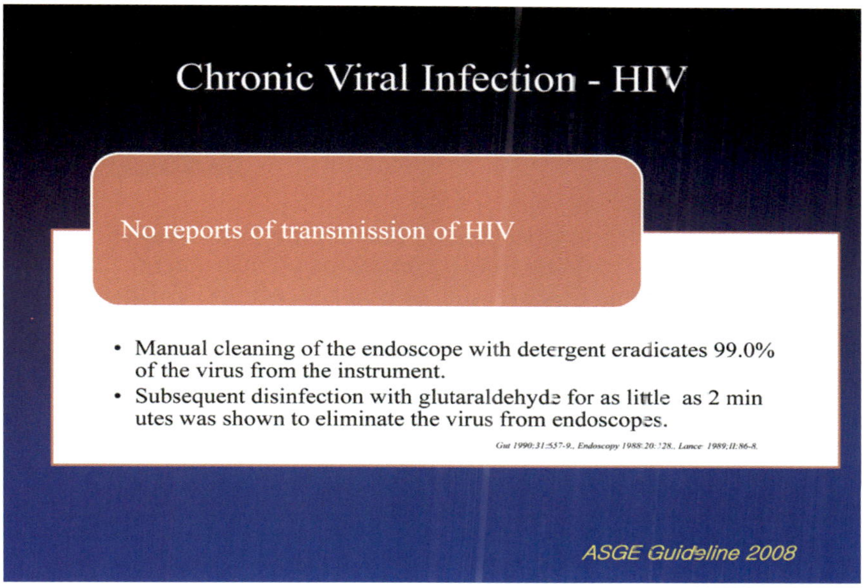

There are no reports of transmission of HIV following endoscopy. Manual cleaning and subsequent disinfection was shown to eliminate the virus from endoscopes.

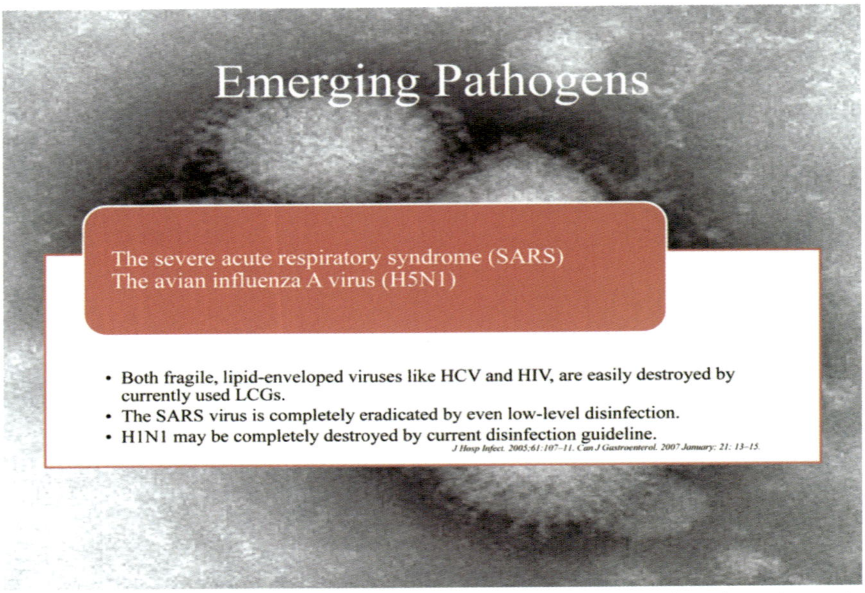

Both the severe acute respiratory syndrome (SARS) and avian influenza A virus (H5N1) are completely eradicated by even low-level disinfection. Though there are no reports, H1N1 may also be completely destroyed by the current disinfection guideline.

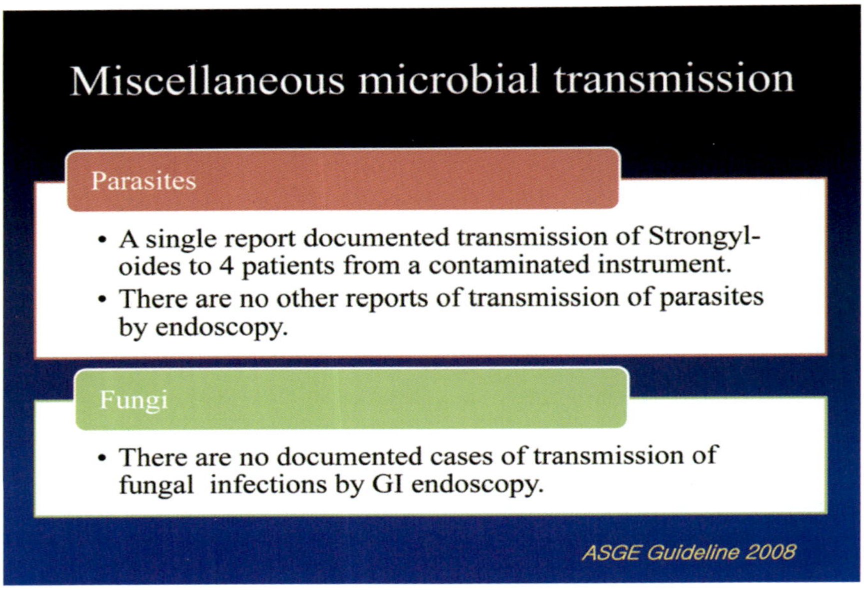

There is only 1 documentaion of parasitic transmission from a contaminated instrument and there are no documented cases of transmission of fungal infections by GI endoscopy.

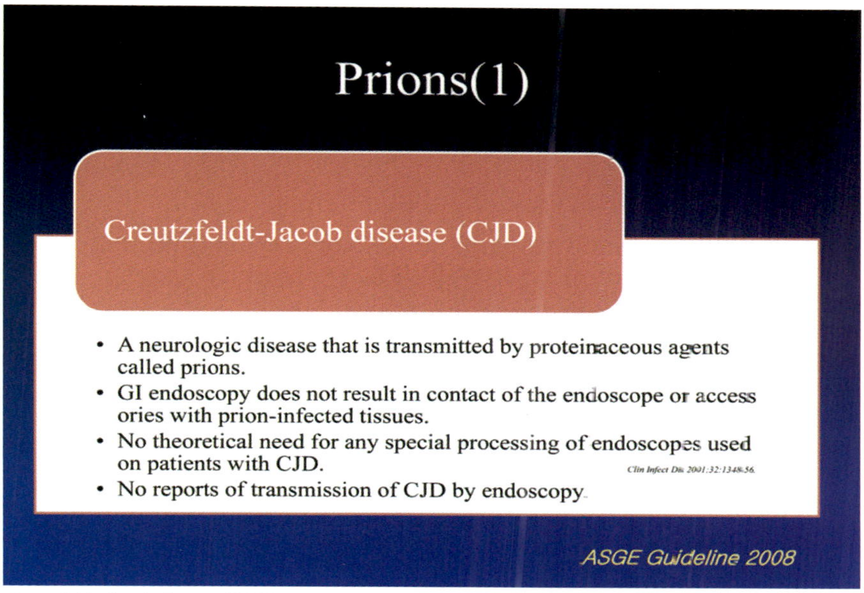

Creutzfeldt-Jacob disease (CJD) is a neurologic disease that is transmitted by mutated prion proteins. GI endoscopy does not result in contact of the endoscope or accessories with prion-infected tissues. And there have been no reports of transmission of CJD by endoscopy.

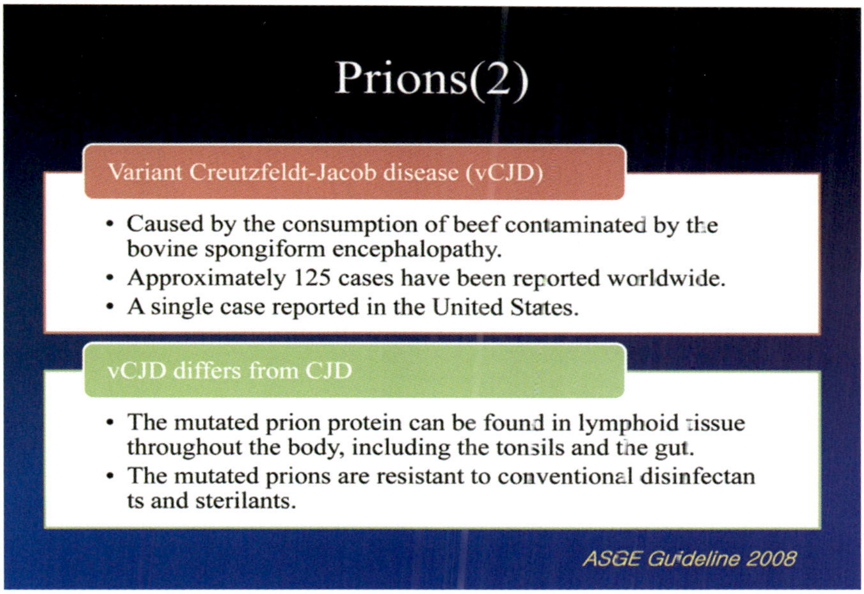

Variant Creutzfeldt-Jacob disease (vCJD) is caused by the consumption of beef contaminated by the bovine spongiform encephalopathy. Approximately 125 cases have been reported worldwide. vCJD differs from CJD in that the mutated prion protein can be found in lymphoid tissue throughout the body, including the tonsils and the gut. The mutated prions are resistant to conventional disinfectants and sterilants.

Prions(3)

The European Society of Gastrointestinal Endoscopy (ESGE)

- Recommends that an endoscopy be avoided in patients with known vCJD.
- When an endoscopy is unavoidable, use of an instrument dedicated for patients with vCJD.
- Use of an endoscope that is approaching the end of its useful life.
- Can be destroyed after use or quarantined until needed for other patients with vCJD.

ASGE Guideline 2008

The European Society of Gastrointestinal Endoscopy (ESGE) Recommends that an endoscopy be avoided in patients with known vCJD. And when an endoscopy is unavoidable, the endoscope should be destroyed after use or quarantined until needed for other patients with vCJD.

Resistance and Level of Disinfection or Sterilization

Resistant	Pathogen	Level
↓	Prions(Creutzfeldt-Jakob Disease)	Prion reprocessing
	Bacterial spores (*Bacillus atrophaeus*)	Sterilization
	Coccidia (*Cryptosporidium*)	
	Mycobacteria (*M. tuberculosis, M. terrae*)	High
	Nonlipid or small viruses (polio, coxackie)	Intermediate
	Fungi (*Aspergillus, Candida*)	
	Vegetative bacteria (*S.aureus, P. aeruginosa*)	Low
	Lipid or medium sized viruses (HIV, herpes, hepatitis B)	
Susceptible		

CDC Guideline 2008
Russell AD. J. Hosp. Infect. 1998:43:S57-68 .
Favero MS. Disinfection, sterilization, and preservation. 2001:881-917.

This table showed the relationship between the resistance of the orgasm and the level of disinfection or sterilization.

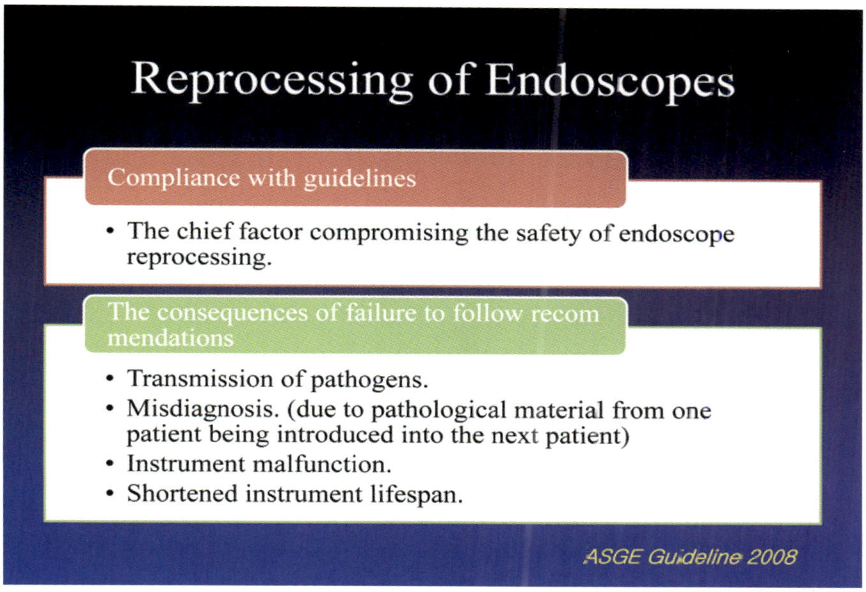

Stringent adherence to multisociety guidelines is the single best protection against patient-to-patient transmission of microorganisms by endoscopy.

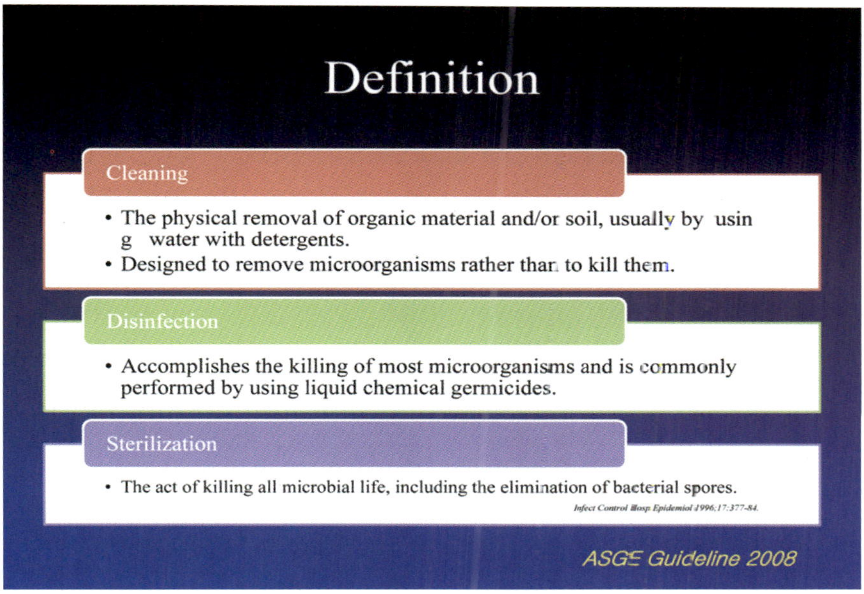

Cleaning is the physical removal of organic material usually by using water with detergents and is designed to remove microorganisms rather than to kill them. Disinfection accomplishes the killing of most microorganisms and is commonly performed by using liquid chemical germicides. Sterilization is the act of killing all microbial life, including the elimination of bacterial spores.

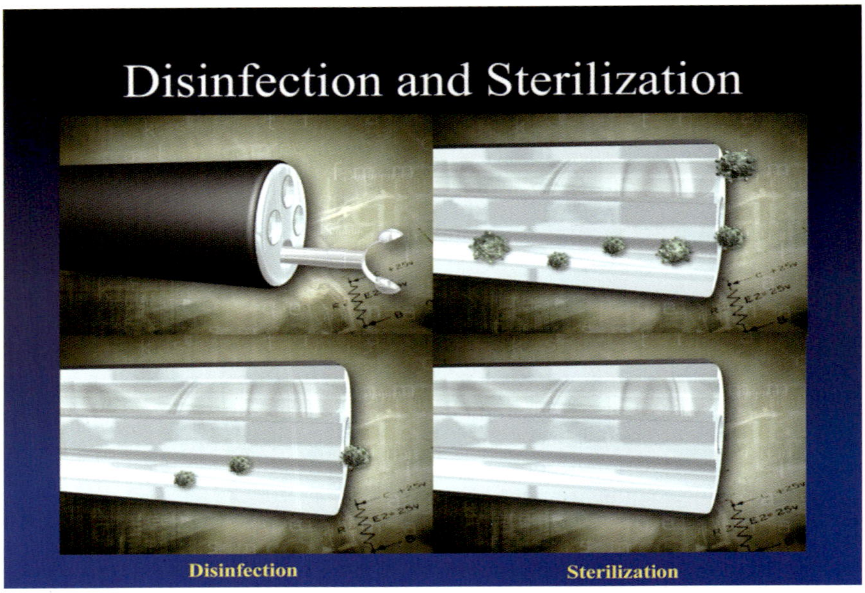

These pictures demonstrate disinfection and sterilization. Disinfection kills most of the organisms contaminating the endoscope. Sterilization destroys or eliminates all forms of microbial life including bacterial spores.

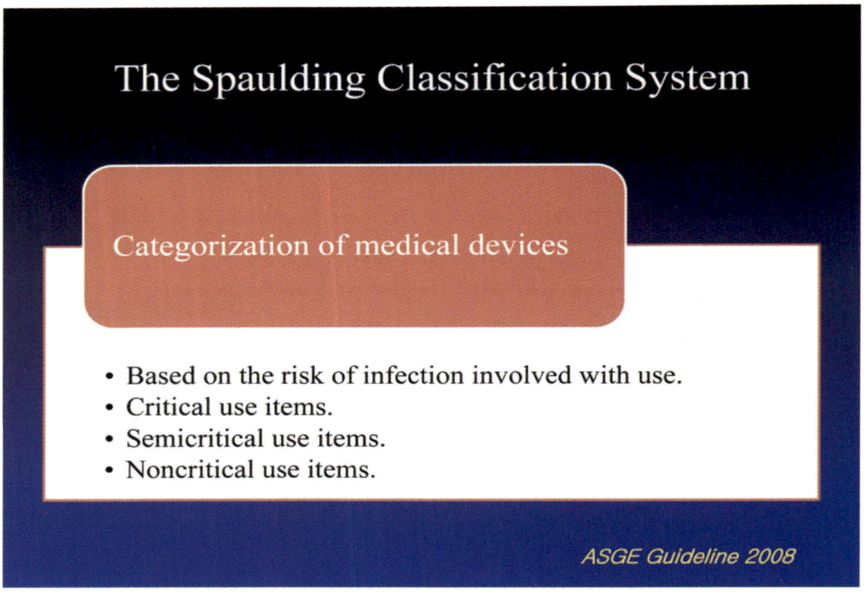

The Spaulding Classification System categorizes medical devices based on the risk of infection involved with use.

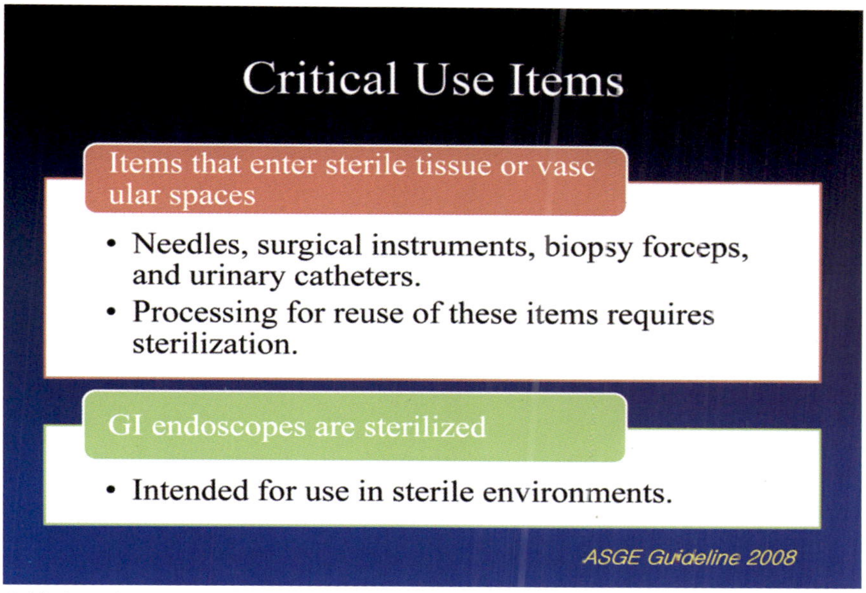

Critical use items are items that enter sterile tissue or vascular spaces, such as needles, biopsy forceps, surgical equipment and catheters. Processing for reuse of these items requires sterilization.

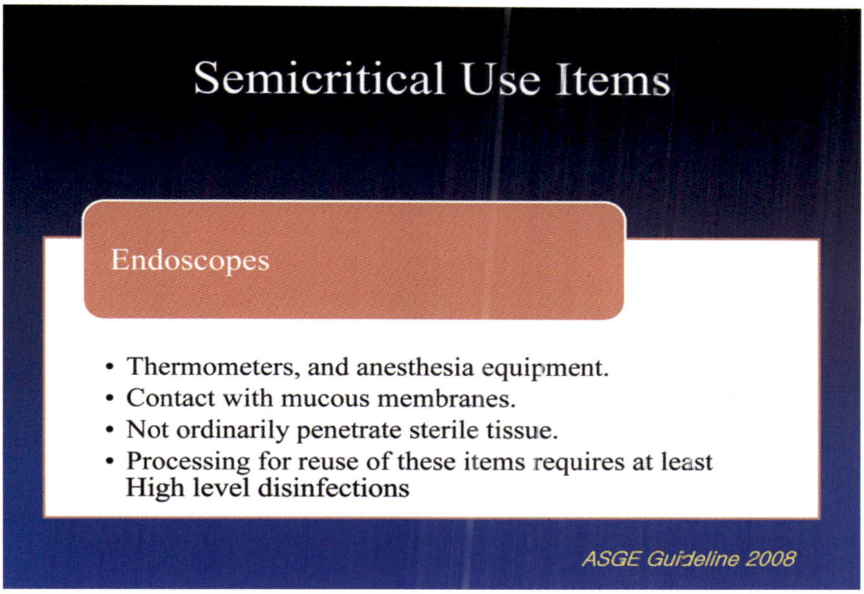

Semicritical use items such as endoscopes are contacted with the mucous membranes. Processing for reuse of these items requires at least High level disinfections.

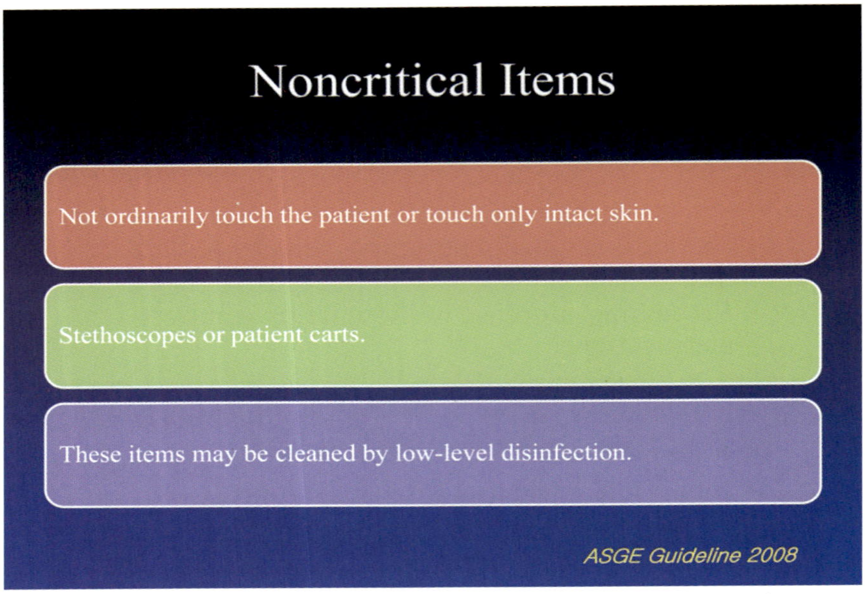

Noncritical use items normally do not touch the patient or touch only intact skin. These items may be cleaned by low-level disinfection.

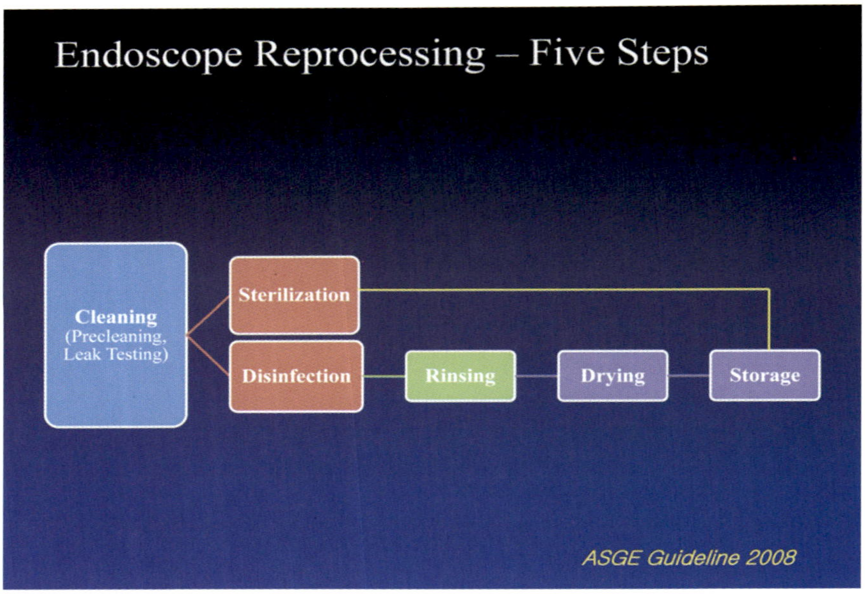

Endoscope Reprocessing can be arranged into five Steps, Cleaning, Sterilization or Disinfection, Rinsing, Drying and Stroage.

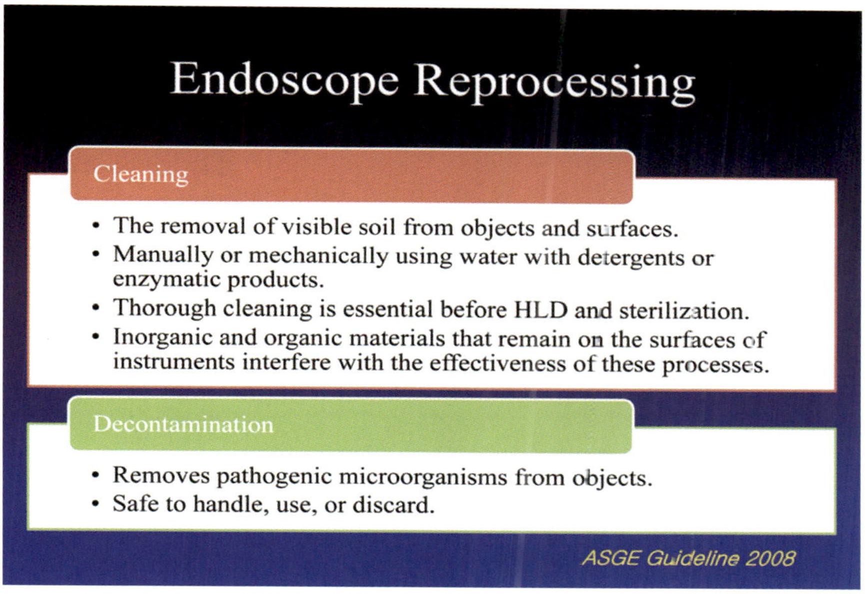

Thorough cleaning is essential before HLD and sterilization.

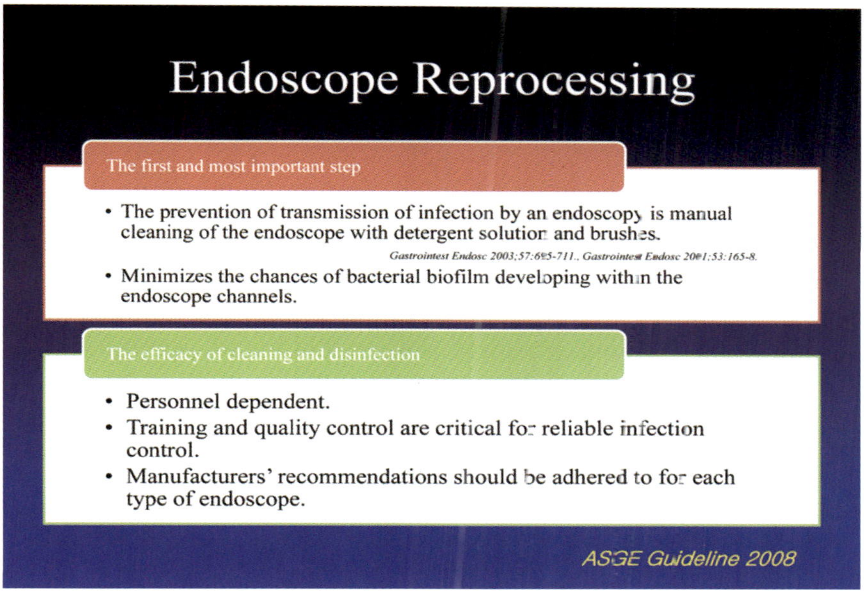

The first and most important step of endoscopic processing is manual cleaning of the endoscope with detergent solution and brushes. Manual cleaning minimizes the chances of bacterial biofilm developing within the endoscope channels.

The efficacy of cleaning and disinfection is personnel dependent. Training and quality control are critical for reliable infection control. The manufacturers' recommendations should be adhered to for each type of endoscope.

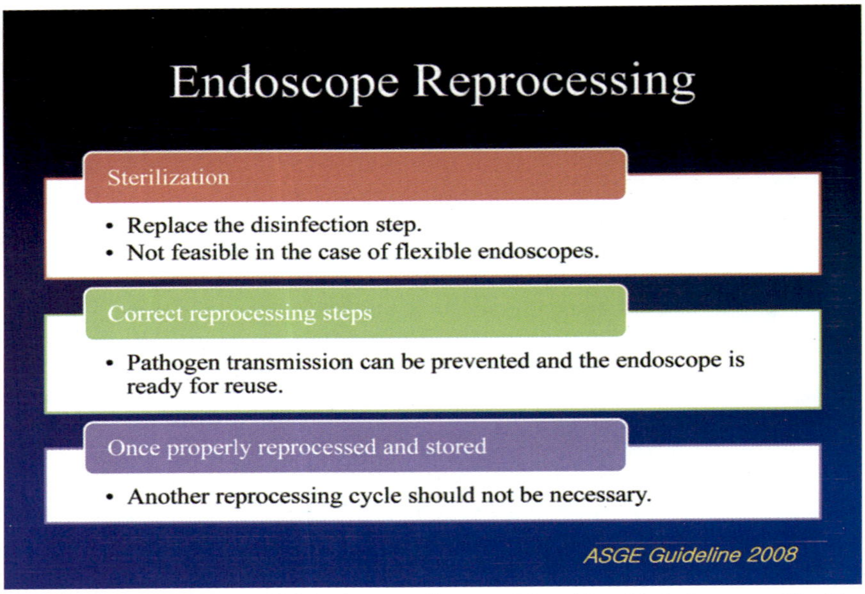

Sterilization can replace the disinfection step. However it is not feasible in the case of flexible endoscopes. Through the correct reprocessing steps pathogen transmission can be prevented and once properly reprocessed and stored another reprocessing cycle should not be necessary.

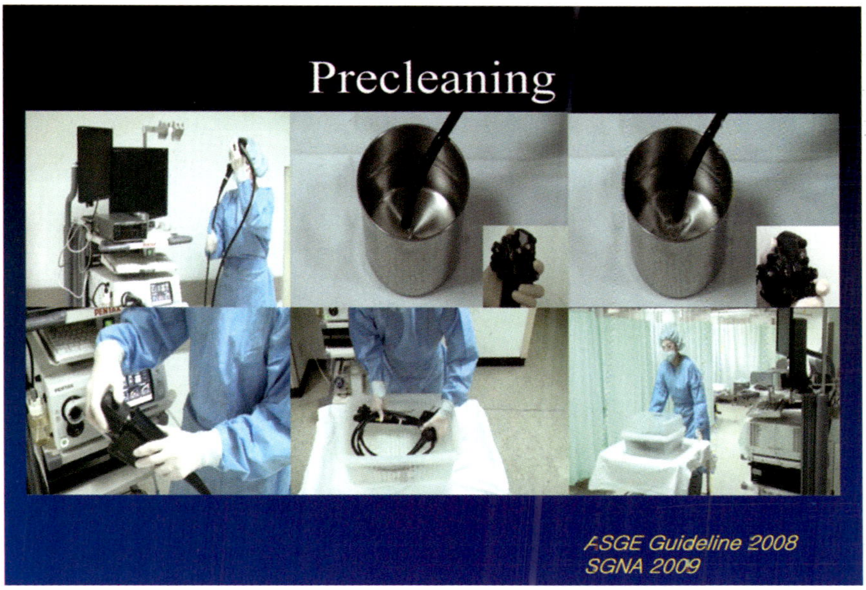

These pictures demonstrate precleaning of the endoscope following endoscopy.

1. The insertion tube is wiped with a disposable, lint-free wet cloth soaked in freshly prepared detergent solution.
2. The distal end of the endoscope is placed into detergent solution
3. Alternate suction of detergent solution and air is performed several times through the biopsy/suction channel until the solution is visibly clean.
4. This process is finished by suctioning air and releasing air bubbles in the detergent.
5. The endoscope is detached from the light source and suction pump.
6. The protective video cap is attached.
7. The endoscope is coiled and placed in a container with detergent solution. The container should be large enough that the endoscope will not be damaged by being coiled too tightly.
8. Finally, transport the endoscope is transported to the reprocessing area in an enclosed container.

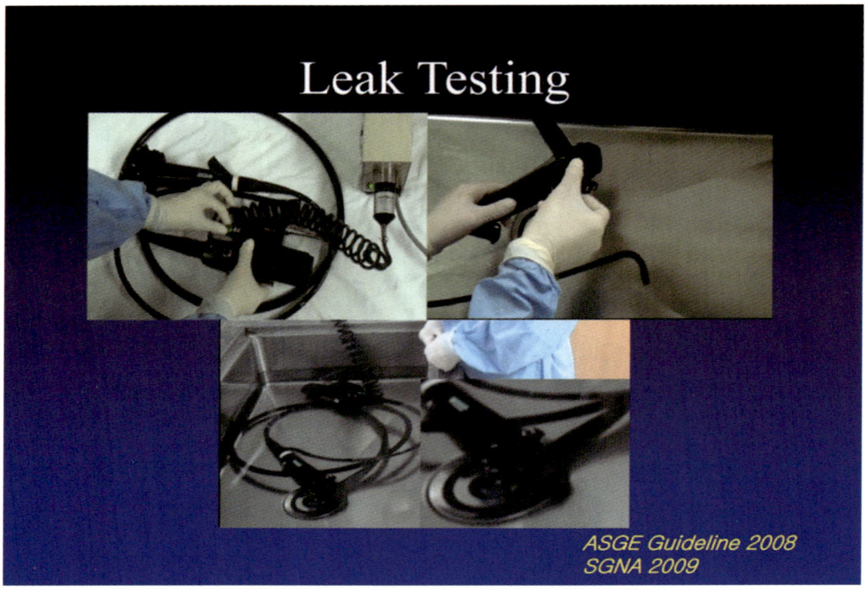

Leak testing detects damage to the interior or exterior of the endoscope.

1. Suction valves, air water valves, biopsy valves and all parts that are designated disposable are removed.
2. The leak tester is attached to the endoscope and the endoscope is pressurized before submerging in water.
3. With the pressurized insertion tube completely submerged, the distal portion of the scope is flexed in all directions, observing for bubbles.
4. The entire endoscope is submerged. The control head, freeze and release buttons, as well as the insertion tube, and distal bending should be checked for bubbles coming from the interior of the scope.

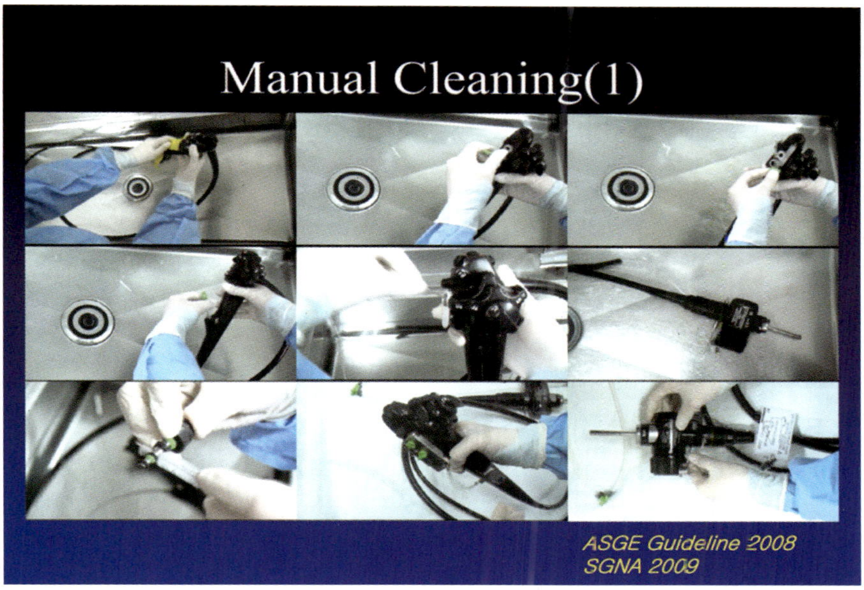

1. After removal of all disposable parts, the endoscope in immersed in a sink with a freshly-made solution of water and detergent formulated for endoscopes.
2. All debris from the exterior of the endoscope is washed and the instrument is wiped with a lint free cloth while submerged in the detergent solution.
3. Whenever practical, leave the endoscope submerged in the detergent solution when performing all subsequent cleaning steps to prevent splashing of contaminated fluid and aerosolization of bioburden.
4. All accessible endoscope channels including the body, insertion tube and the umbilicus of the endoscope are brushed. Use a brush size compatible with each channels used.
5. After each passage, the brush should be rinsed in the detergent solution, removing any visible debris before retracting and reinserting it.
6. Brushing is continued until there is no debris visible on the brush.
7. A small, soft brush is used to clean all removable parts, including inside and under the suction valve, air/water valve, and biopsy port cover and openings.
8. Finally, the endoscope manufacturer' s cleaning adapters for suction, biopsy, air, and water channels are attached

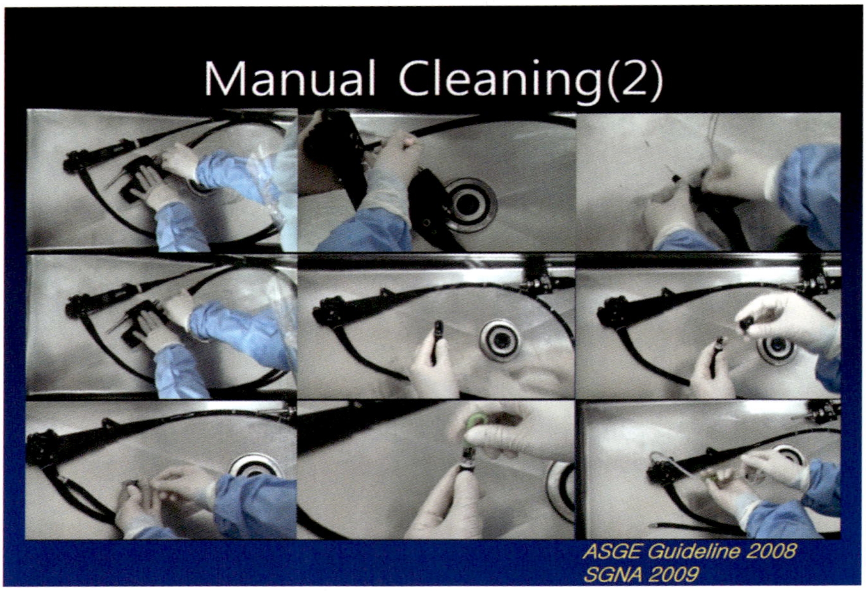

The processing of manual cleaning is different for each device and manufacturer.

1. However the process of brushing all accessible endoscope channels of the endoscope with a compatible brush, rinsing the brush in detergent solution, and removing any visible debris before retracting and reinserting it is same.
2. The elevator channel of a duodenoscope has a small and complex lumen this channel requires manual reprocessing.
3. Brushing is performed with a manufacturers specific brush.
4. Flushing of the channel is performed using a 2- to 5milliliter syringe.

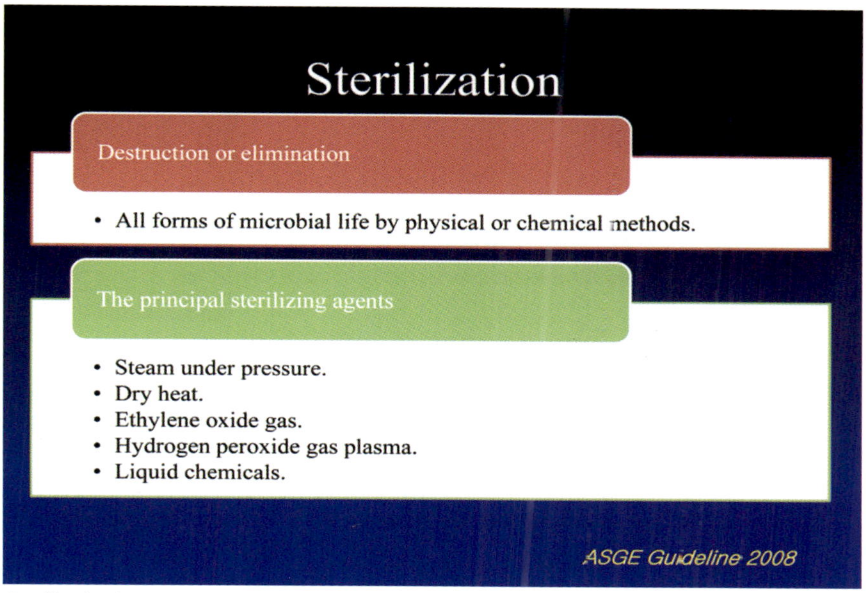

Sterilization is the destruction or elimination of all forms of microbial life by physical or chemical methods. The principal sterilizing agents are steam under pressure. Dry heat. Ethylene oxide gas. Hydrogen peroxide gas plasma, and Liquid chemicals.

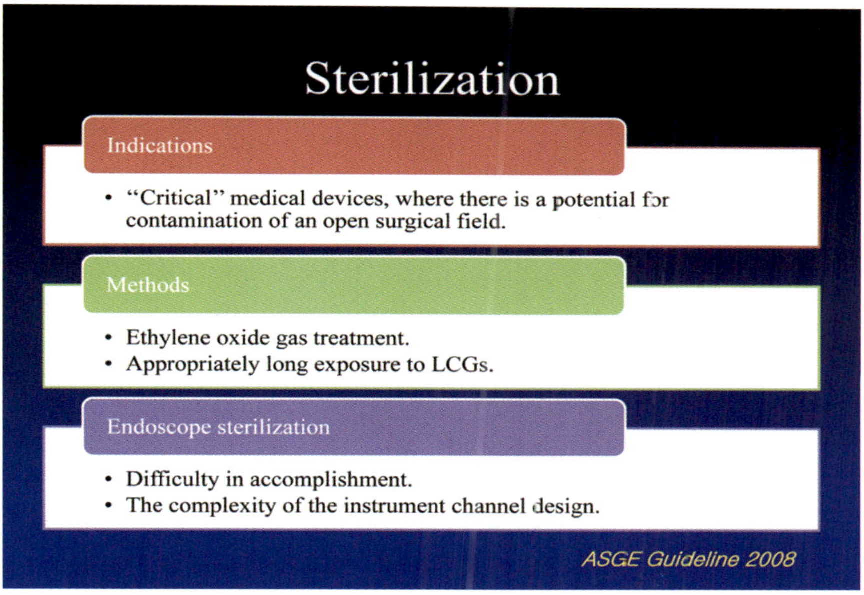

Sterilization is critical for medical devices, where there is a potential for contamination of an open surgical field. Due to the complexity of the instrument channel design, endoscope sterilization difficult to accomplish.

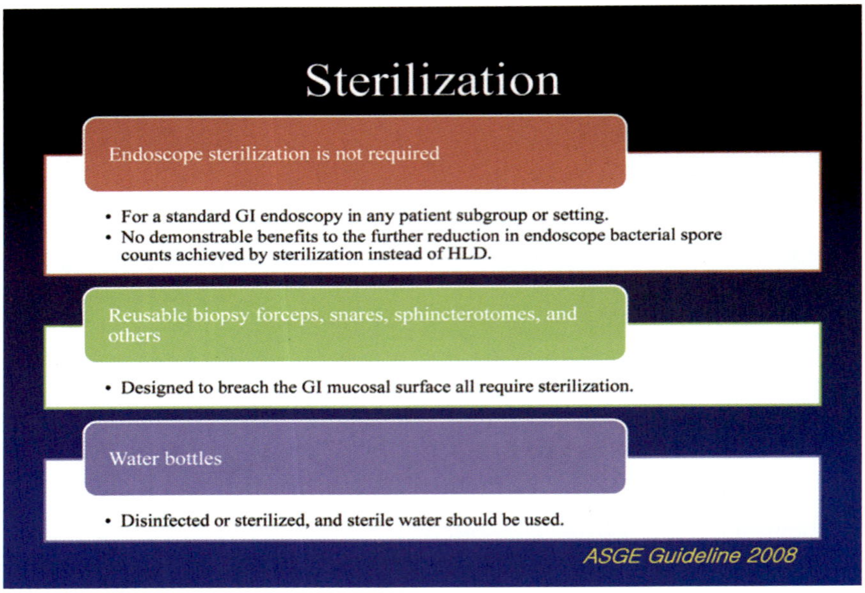

Endoscope sterilization is not required for a standard GI endoscopy. Reusable biopsy forceps, snares, sphincterotomes, and others designed to breach the GI mucosal surface all require sterilization. Water bottles should be disinfected or sterilized, and sterile water should be used.

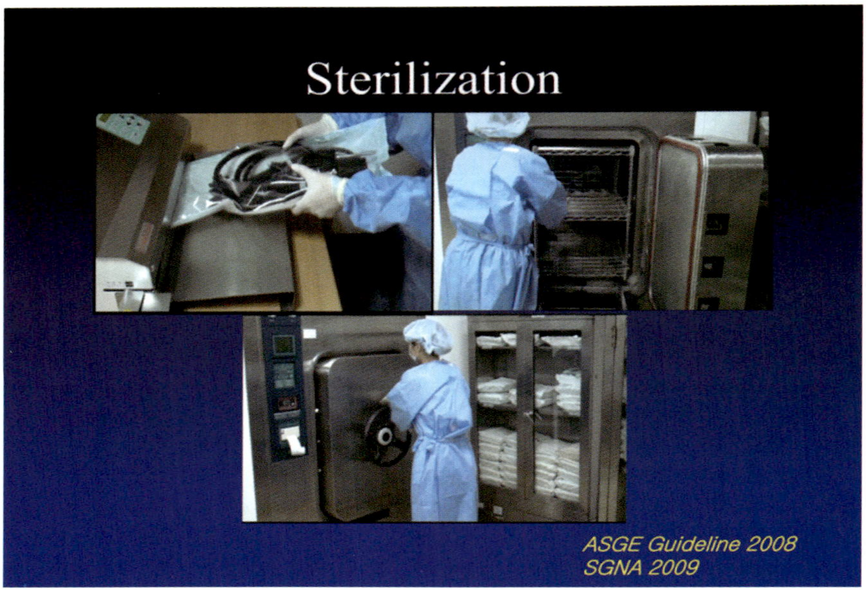

These pictures demonstrate sterilization of the endoscope. The endoscope is sealed in a package appropriate for ethylene oxide(ETO) gas sterilization. Following sterilization, the endoscope must be aerated to remove toxic ETO gas residuals.

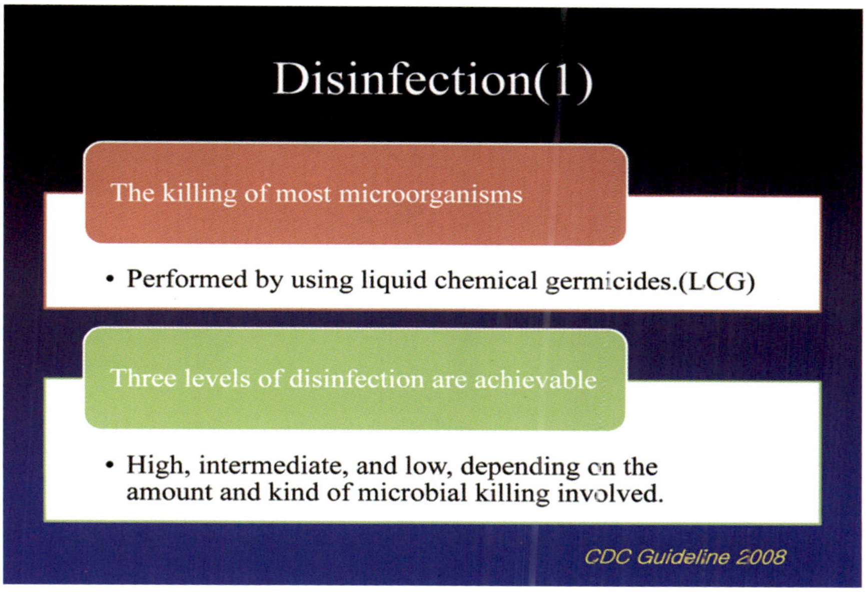

Disinfection kills most microorganisms by using liquid chemical germicides.(LCG)
There are three levels of disinfection High, intermediate, and low, depending on the amount and kind of microbial killing involved.

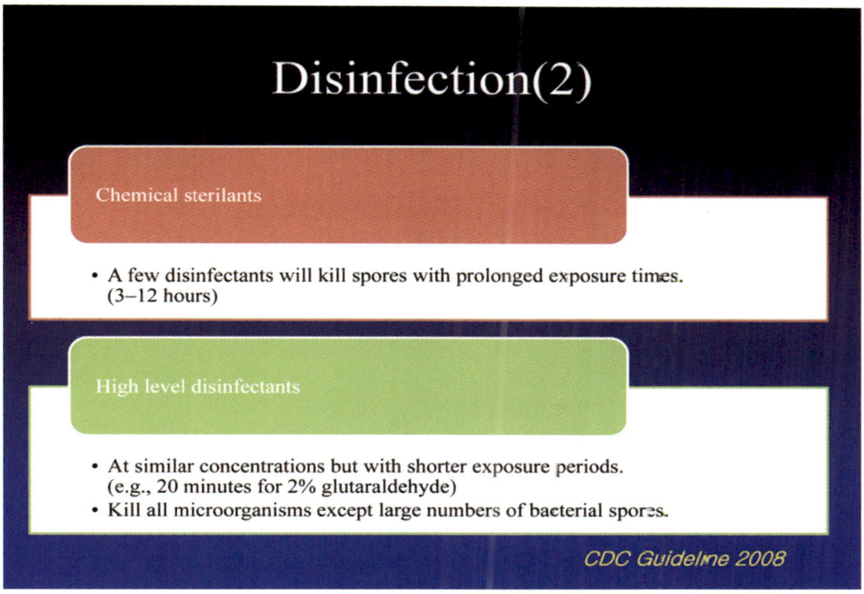

Chemical sterilants will kill spores with prolonged exposure times. (3-12 hours)
High level disinfectants well kill all microorganisms except large numbers of bacterial spores, at similar concentrations but with shorter exposure periods.

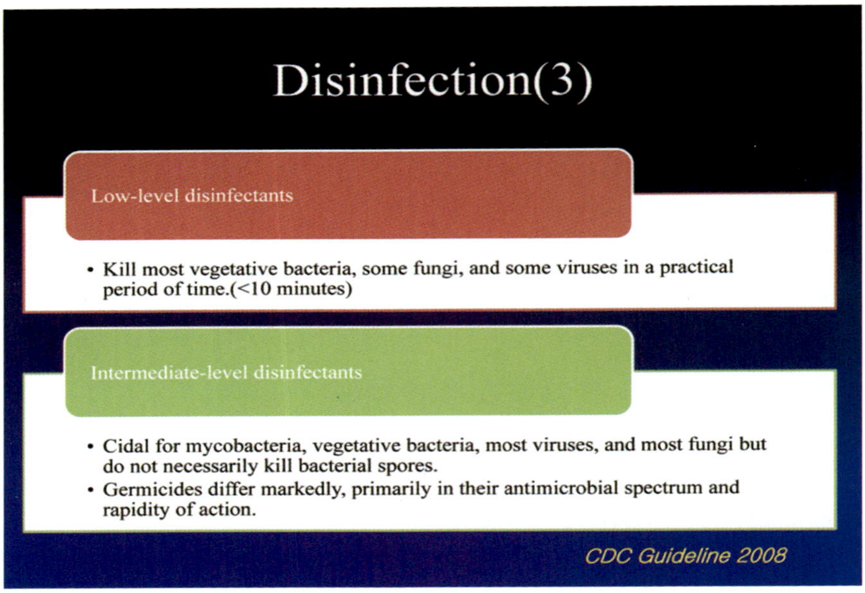

Low-level disinfectants kill most vegetative bacteria, some fungi, and some viruses in a practical period of time.(<10 minutes). Intermediate-level disinfectants kill mycobacteria, vegetative bacteria, most viruses, and most fungi but do not necessarily kill bacterial spores. Germicides differ markedly, primarily in their antimicrobial spectrum and rapidity of action.

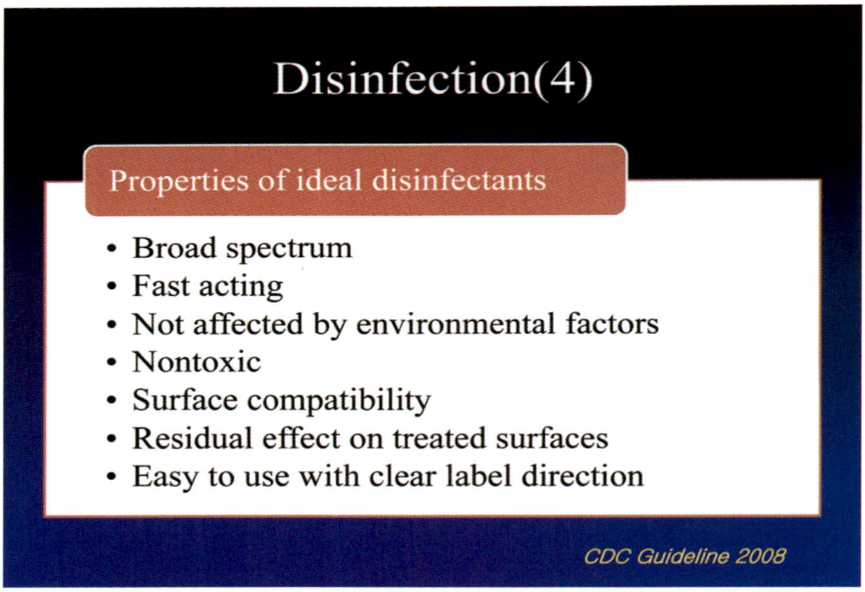

Properties of ideal disinfectants are broad spectrum, fast acting, not affected by environmental factors, nontoxic, surface compatibility, residual effect on treated surfaces and easy to use with clear label direction.

Disinfection(5)

Properties of ideal disinfectants

- Odorless
- Economical
- Solubility
- Stability
- Cleaner
- Environmentally friendly

CDC Guideline 2008

Properties of ideal disinfectants are odorless, economical, solubility, stability, cleaner and environmentally friendly.

Disinfection(6)

	HydrogenPeroxide (HP) (7.5%)	Paracetic acid(PA)(0.2%)	Glutaraldehyde (2.0%)	Orthophthalaldehyde(0.05%)	HP/EA(7.35%/0.23%)
HLD	30min/20℃	NA	20-90min/20-25℃	12min/20℃, 5min/25℃ in AER	15min/20℃
Sterilization	6h/20℃	12min/50-55℃	10h/20-25℃	None	3h/20℃
Activation	No	No	Yes(alkaline glut)	No	No
Reuse Life	21D	Single use	14-30D	12D	14D
Shelf Life Stability	2yr	6mo	2yr	2yr	2yr
Disposable Restrictions	None	None	Local	Local	None
Materials-compatibility	Good	Good	Excellent	Excellent	No data
Monitor minimum effective concentrration	Yes(6%)	No	Yes(1.5% or higher)	Yes(0.3% OPA)	No
Safety	Serious eye damage(safety glass)	Serious eye and skin damage(concentrated)	Respiratory	Eye irritant, stains skin	Eye damage
Processing	Manual or automated	Automated	Manual or automated	Manual or automated	Manual
Organic material resistance	Yes	Yes	Yes	Yes	Yes
OSHA exposure limit (time-weighted average for a 8-hour workday)	1ppm TWA	None	None	None	HP-1ppm TWA
Cost profile(per cycle)	+(manual), ++(automatic)	++++(automatic)	+(manual), ++(automatic)	++(manual)	++(manual)

Rutala WA. Infect Control Hosp. Epidemiol. 1999;20:69-76.

This table showed the summary of the various disinfectants commercially available.

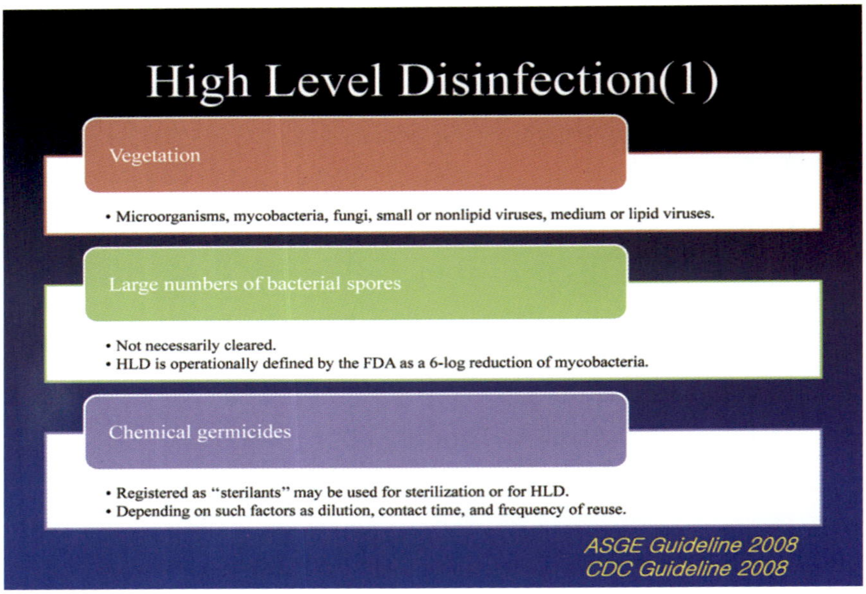

High Level Disinfection will kill all vegetative bacteria and all other microorganisms. However large number of bacterial spores are not necessarily cleard.
HLD is operationally defined by the FDA as a 6-log reduction of mycobacteria.
Chemical germicides registered as ''sterilants'' may be used for HLD.

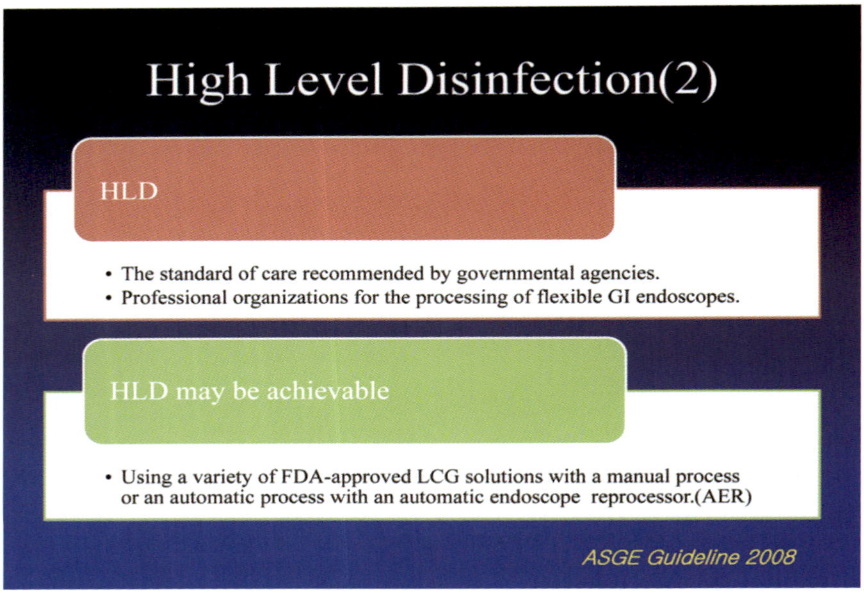

High Level Disinfection is the standard of care recommended by governmental agencies. And professional organizations for the processing of flexible GI endoscopes. HLD may be achievable using a variety of FDA-approved liquid chemical germicide solutions with manual or automatic systems.

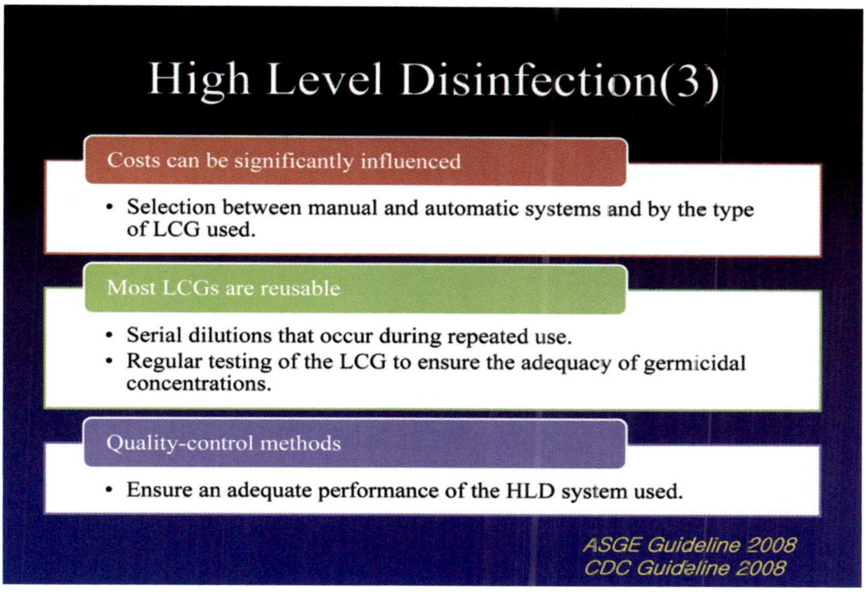

The cost of HLD can be significantly influenced by the selection between manual and automatic systems and by the type of LCG used.
Most LCGs are reusable and regular testing of the LCG to ensure the adequacy of germicidal concentrations should be performed.
Quality-control methods ensure an adequate performance of the HLD system used.

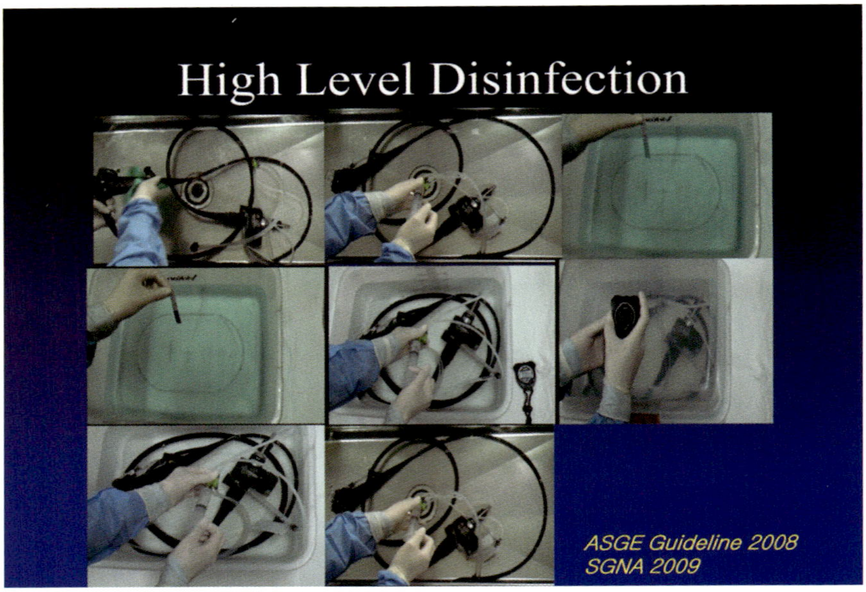

These pictures demonstrate high level disinfection of the endoscope

1. The endoscope and all removable parts are thoroughly washed with clean water to remove residual debris and detergent.
2. Water is purged from all channels using forced air. the exterior of the endoscope is dried with a soft, lint-free cloth to prevent dilution of the liquid chemical germicide used in subsequent steps.
3. The product should be tested for the MEC according to the label on the test strip container. It is essential that the level of active ingredient be at or above that required to kill and/or inactivate the desired microorganisms.
4. The disinfectant is injected into all channels of the endoscope until it can be seen exiting the opposite end of each channel. Care should be taken so that all channels are filled with the chemical for complete microbial destruction, and that no air pockets remain within the channels.
5. The soaking basin should be covered with a tight-fitting lid to minimize the hazard from chemical vapor.
6. The endoscope should be soaked in the high-level disinfectant/sterilant for the time/temperature required to achieve high level disinfection. A timer should be used to verify soaking time.
7. All channels should be purged completely with air before removing the endoscope from the high-level disinfectant.
8. The endoscope and its removable part are thoroughly rinsed and the channels of the endoscope are flushed with clean water.

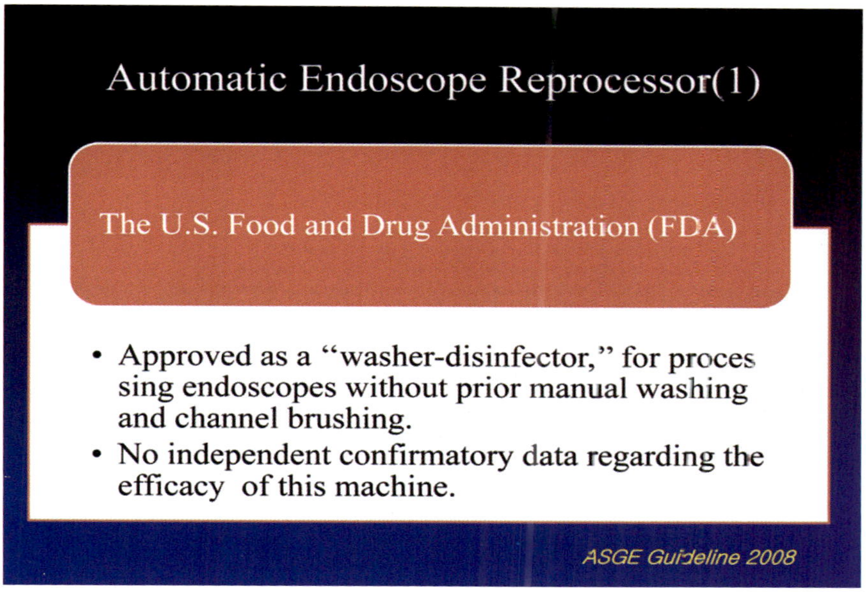

The Automatic Endoscope Reprocessor is a FDA approved "washer-disinfector," for processing endoscopes without prior manual washing and channel brushing.
However there is no independent confirmatory data regarding the efficacy of this machine.

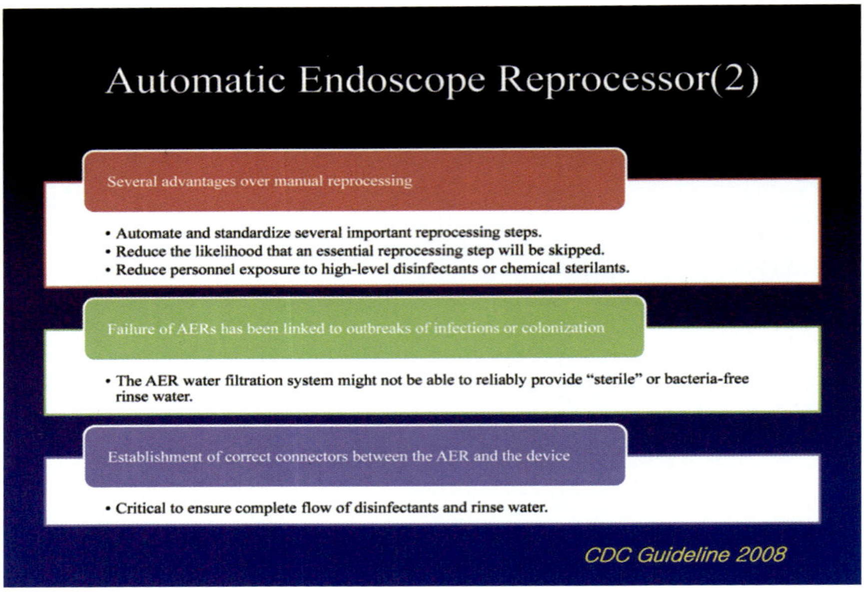

The Automatic Endoscope Reprocessor has several advantages over manual reprocessing.
It can automate and standardize several important reprocessing steps therefore reducing the likelihood that an essential step will be skipped. It can also reduce personnel exposure to high-level disinfectants or chemical sterilants.
Failure of AERs has been linked to outbreaks of infections or colonization.
Establishment of correct connectors between the AER and the device is critical to ensure complete flow of disinfectants and rinse water.

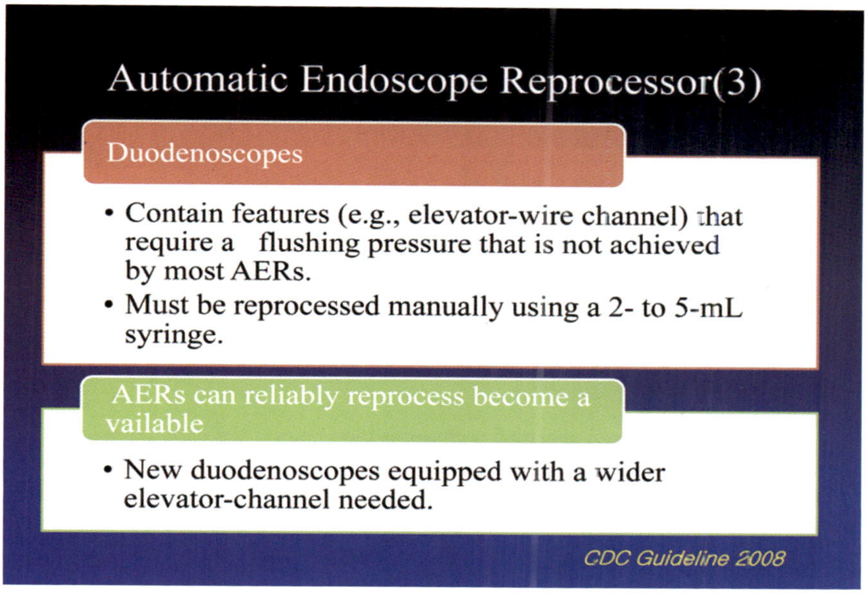

In most cases duodenoscopes should be reprocessed cmanually because they have elevator-wire channels that require a flushing pressure that is not achieved by most AERs.
For AER reprocess to become available new duodenoscopes equipped with a wider elevator-channel are needed.

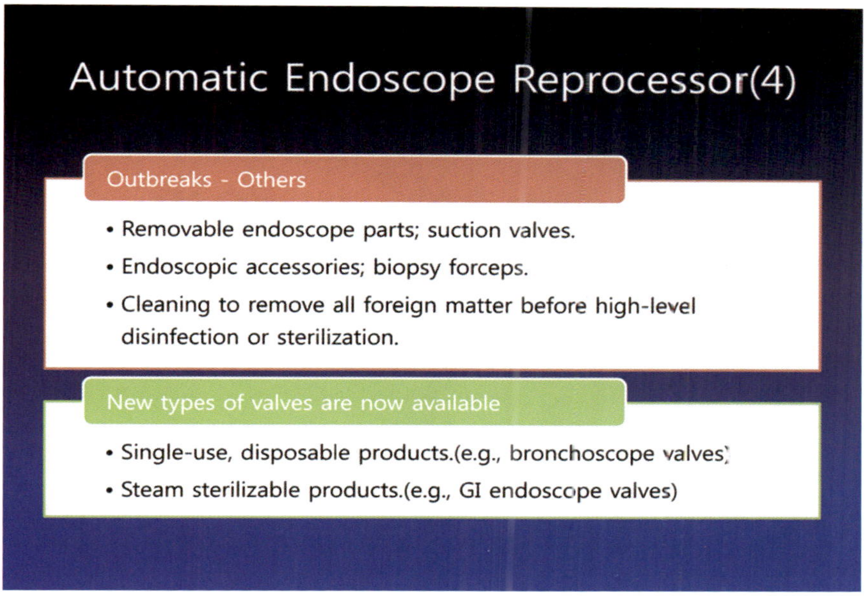

Removable endoscope parts such as suction valves and endoscopic accessories; biopsy forceps should be manually cleaned to remove all foreign matter before high-level disinfection or sterilization.
New types of valves such as single-use, disposable valves or steam sterilizable products are now available.

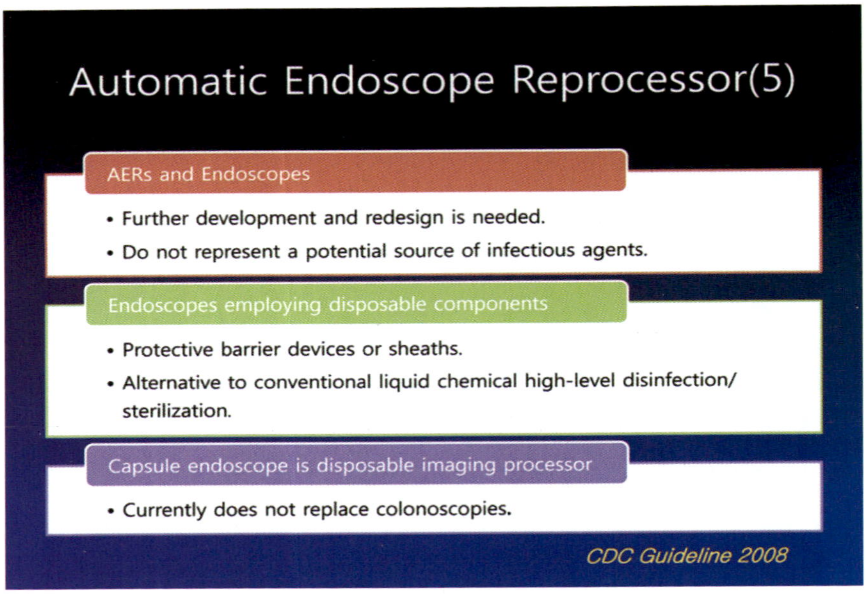

For a fully automated endoscope reprocessor system, further development and redesign of AERs and endoscopes is needed.
Endoscopes employing disposable components such as protective barrier devices or sheaths, maybe an alternative to conventional liquid chemical high-level disinfection/sterilization.
Capsule endoscope is also an alternative, however it currently cannot replace colonoscopies.

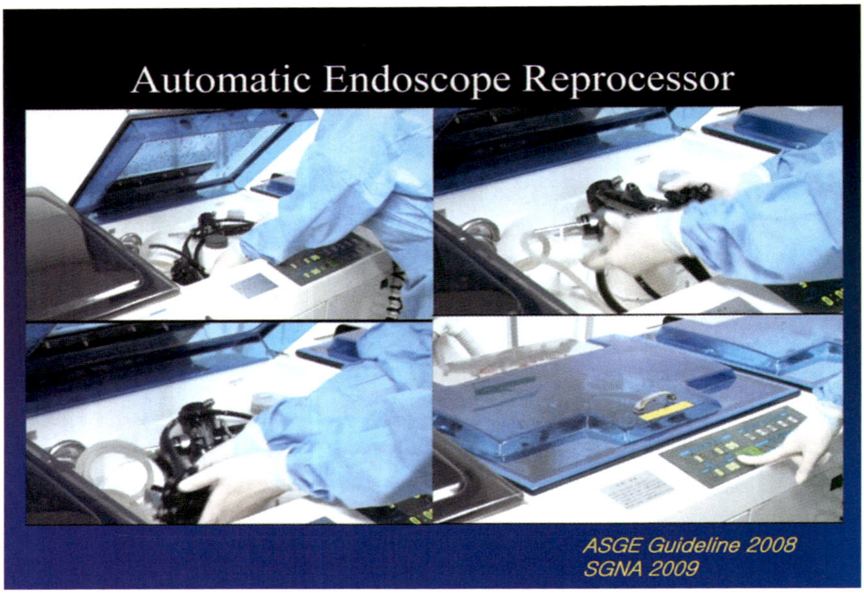

If automatic endoscope reprocessor is available, it is necessary to follow all steps for the manual cleaning of the endoscope prior to using an automatic endoscope reprocessor.

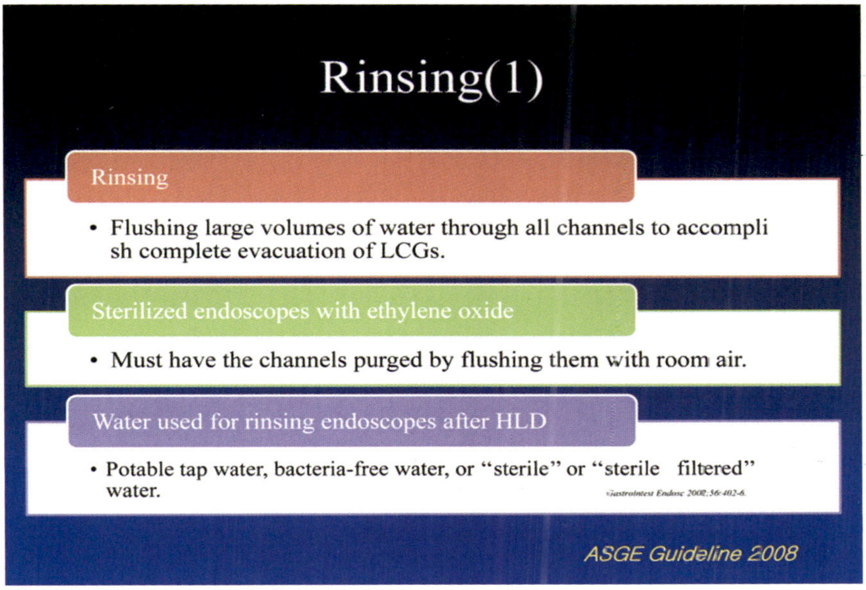

Rinsing utilizes flushing large volumes of water through all channels to accomplish complete evacuation of LCGs.
Sterilized endoscopes are rinsed with ethylene oxide, and water is used for rinsing endoscopes after HLD.

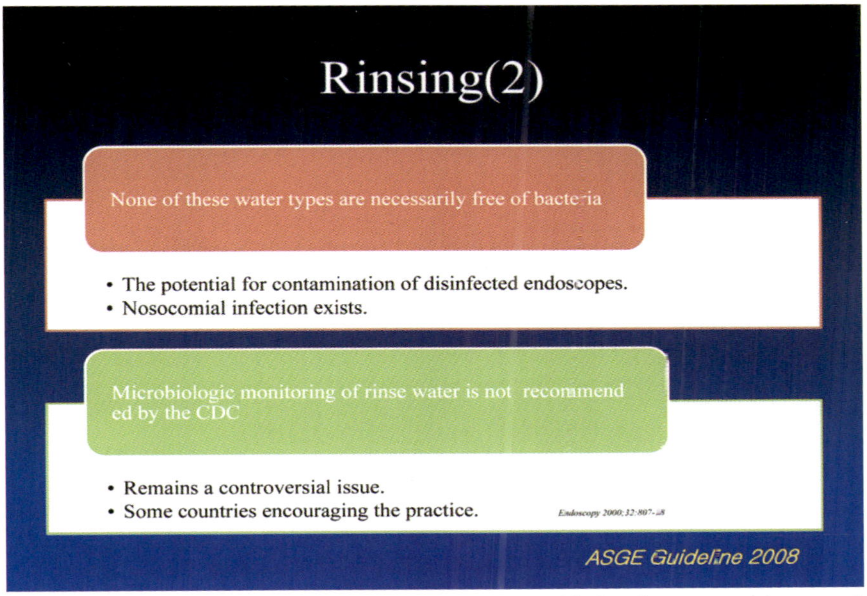

The water used in rinsing is not necessarily free of bacteria and is therefore a potential source of contamination of disinfected endoscopes.
Currently microbiologic monitoring of rinse water is not recommended by the CDC.
However, this remains a controversial issue.

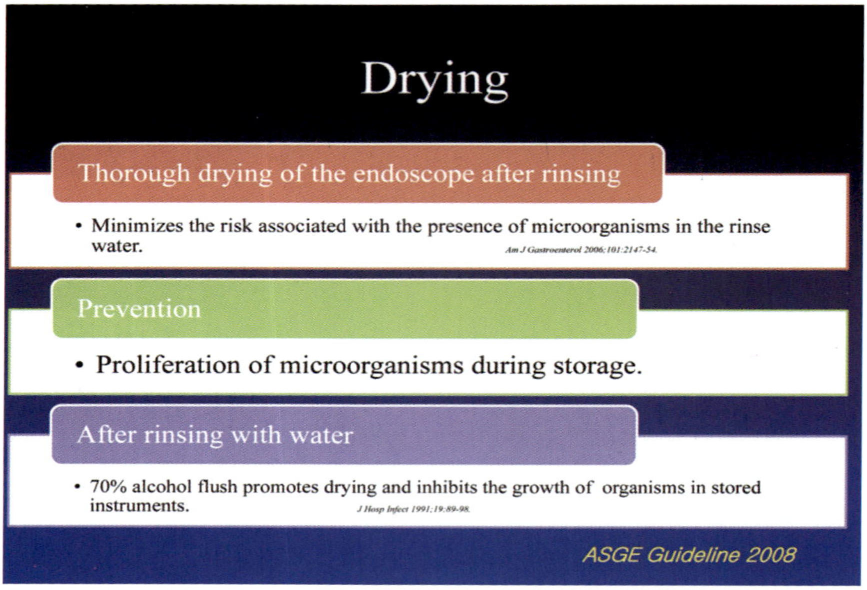

Thorough drying of the endoscope after rinsing minimizes the risk associated with the presence of microorganisms in the rinse water.
Drying prevents the proliferation of microorganisms during storage.
After rinsing with water 70% alcohol flush promotes drying and inhibits the growth of organisms in stored instruments.

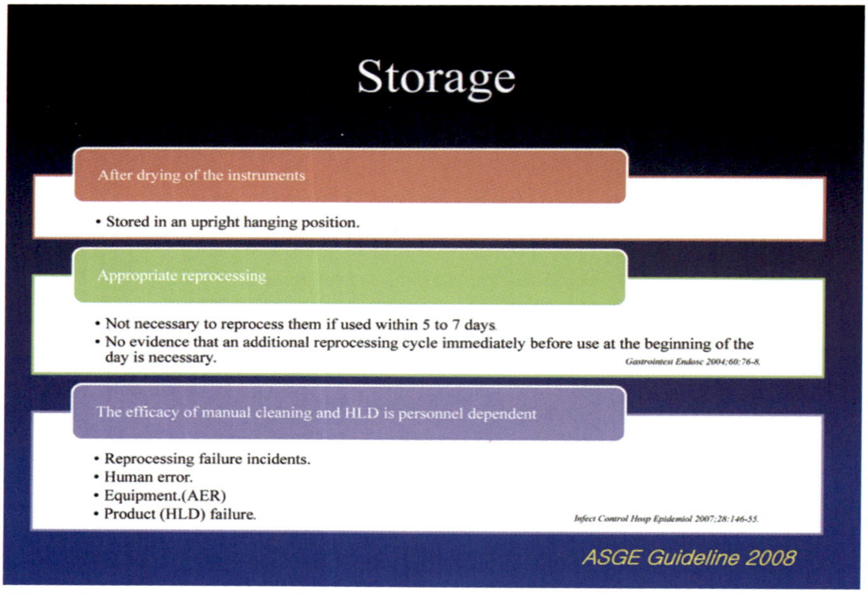

After drying the instruments should be stored in an upright hanging position.
Reprocessing is not needed if instruments are used within 5 to 7 days.
There is no evidence that an additional reprocessing cycle immediately before use at the beginning of the day is necessary.

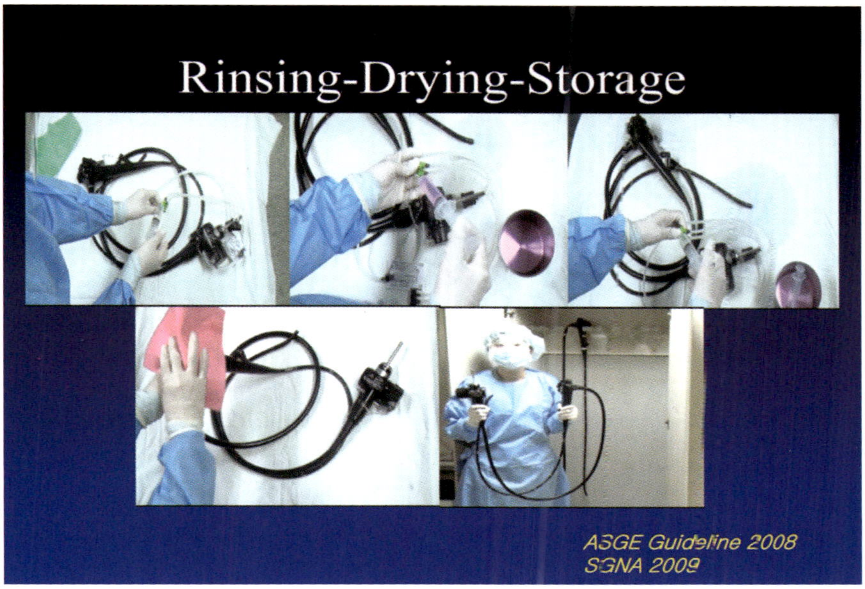

These pictures demonstrate rinsing, drying and storage of the endoscope.

1. All channels are purge with air until dry.
2. All channels including accessory channels are flushed all channels, with 70% isopropyl alcohol until the alcohol can be seen exiting the opposite end of each channel.
3. All channels are purged with air. Note that alcohol mixes with the remaining water on the channel surfaces and acts to encourage evaporation of the residual water as air flows through the channel.
4. All channels of the adapters are removed.
5. The exterior of the endoscope is dried with a soft, clean lint-free towel.
6. The endoscope is hung vertically with the distal tip hanging freely in a clean, well-ventilated, dust-free area.

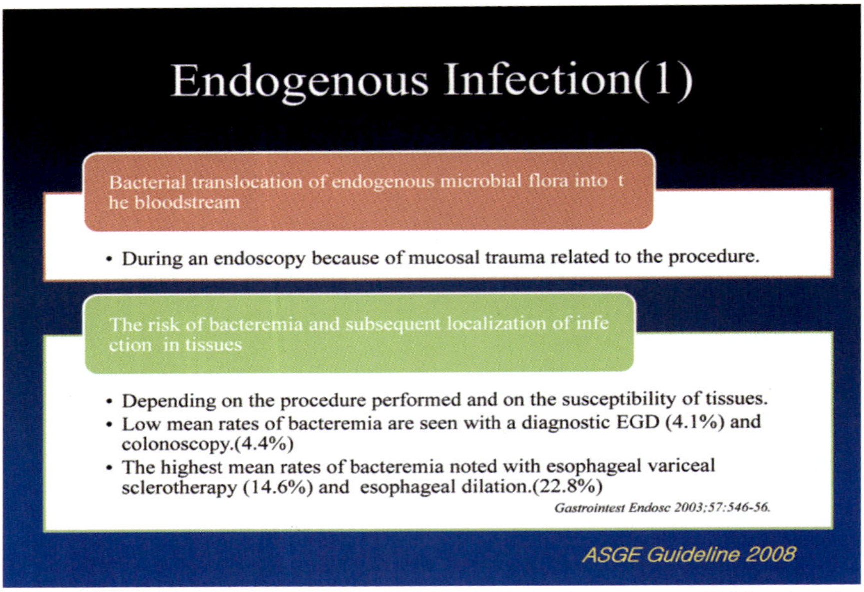

Endogenous Infection is caused by bacterial translocation of endogenous microbial flora into the bloodstream during an endoscopy because of mucosal trauma related to the procedure.
The risk of bacteremia and subsequent localization of infection in tissues depends on the procedure performed and on the susceptibility of tissues.

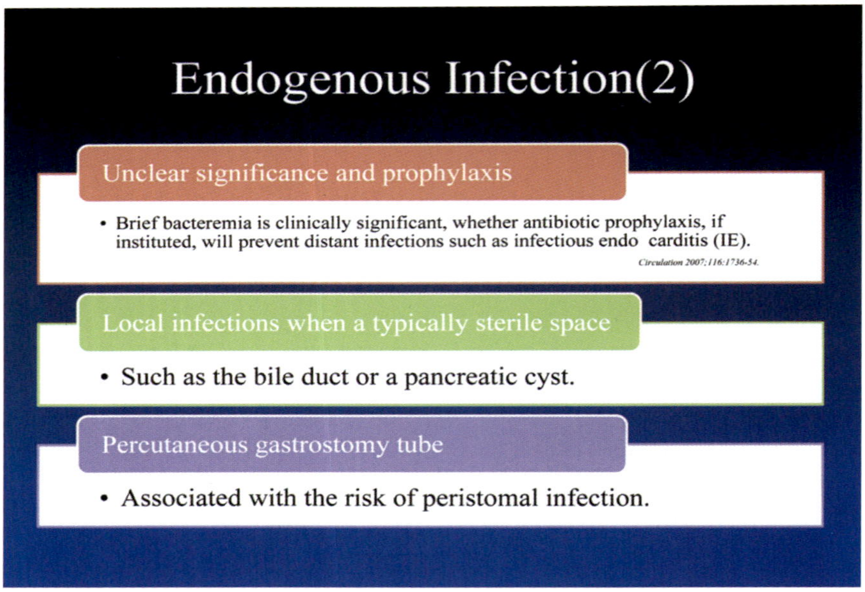

The significance and need for antibiotic prophylaxis for endogenous infection is still unclear.
Local infections may occur when a typically sterile space such as the bile duct or a pancreatic cyst are exposed.
Percutaneous gastrostomy tube is associated with the risk of peristomal infection.

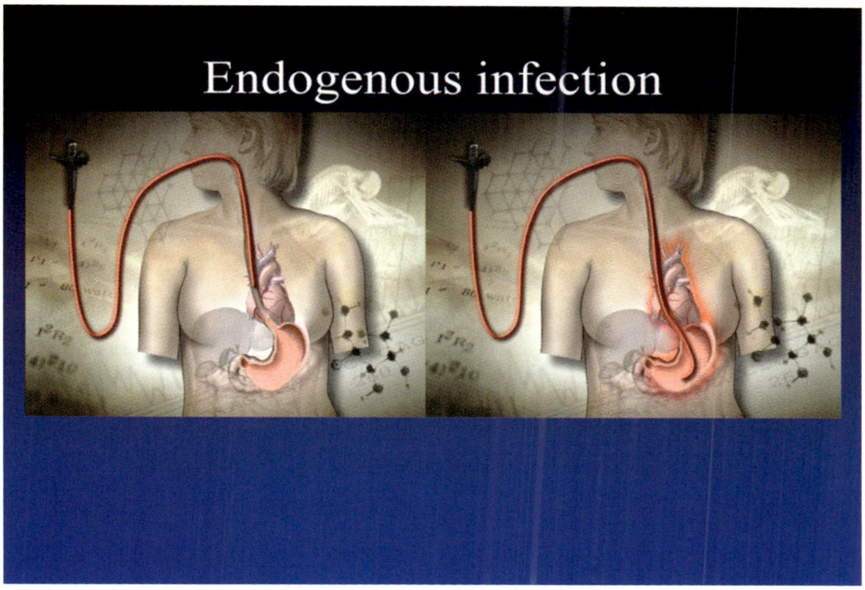

These pictures demonstrate endogenous infection. The endoscopic can be infection by bacteremia that occurs during the endoscopic procedure.

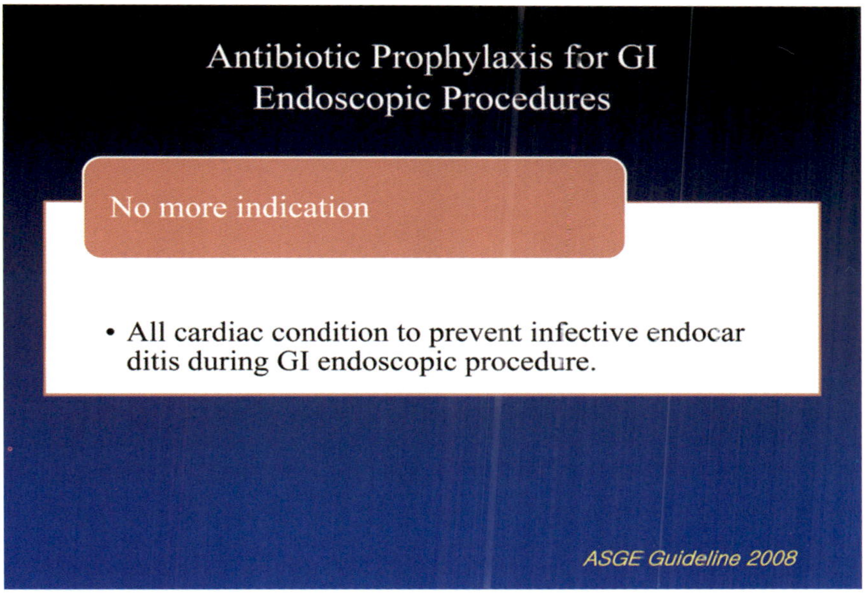

Antibiotic Prophylaxis for the prevention infective endocarditis is no longer recommended.

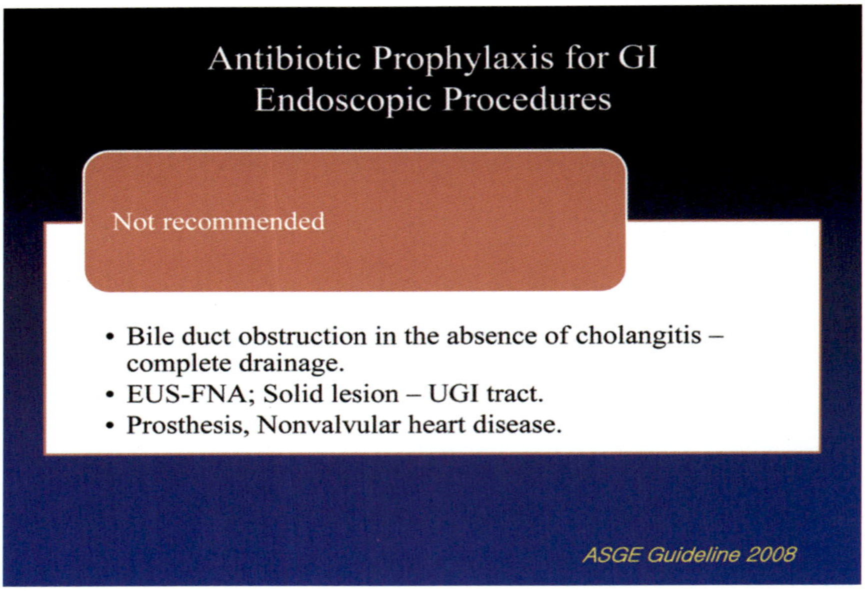

Antibiotic prophylaxis for GI endoscopic procedures are not recommended for complete bile duct obstruction in the absence of cholangitis. EUS-FNA of solid lesions in the UGI tract and patient with prosthesis, or nonvalvular heart disease.

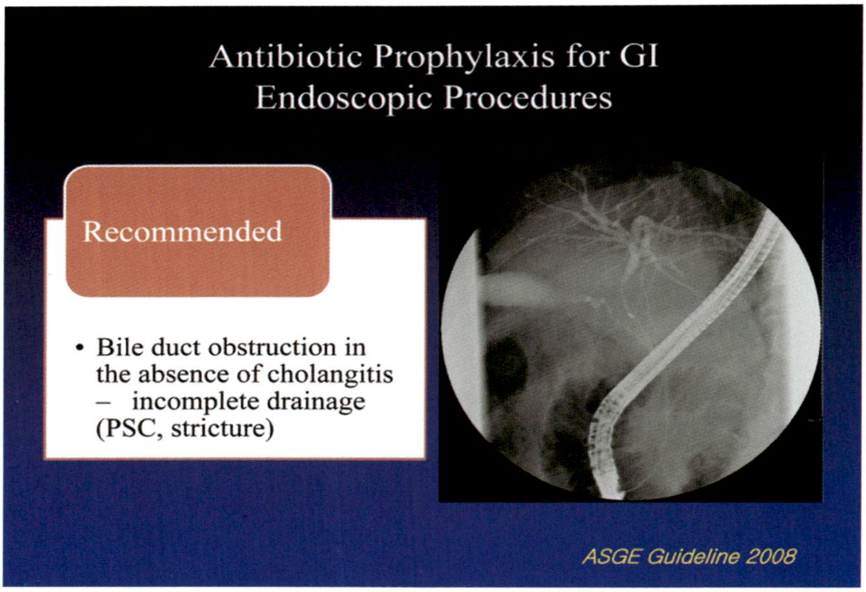

Antibiotic prophylaxis for GI endoscopic procedures is recommended for incomplete bile duct obstruction in the absence of cholangitis.

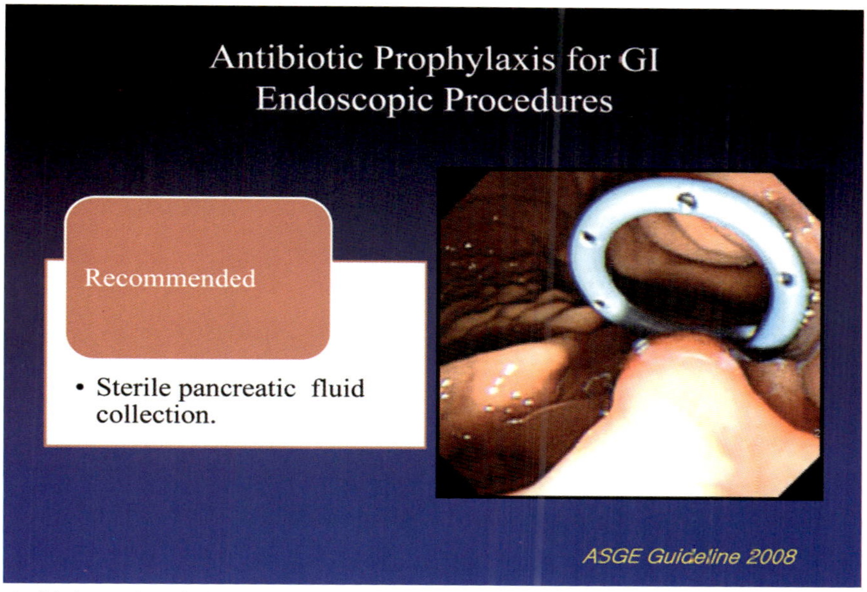

Antibiotic prophylaxis for GI endoscopic procedures is recommended for sterile pancreatic fluid collection.

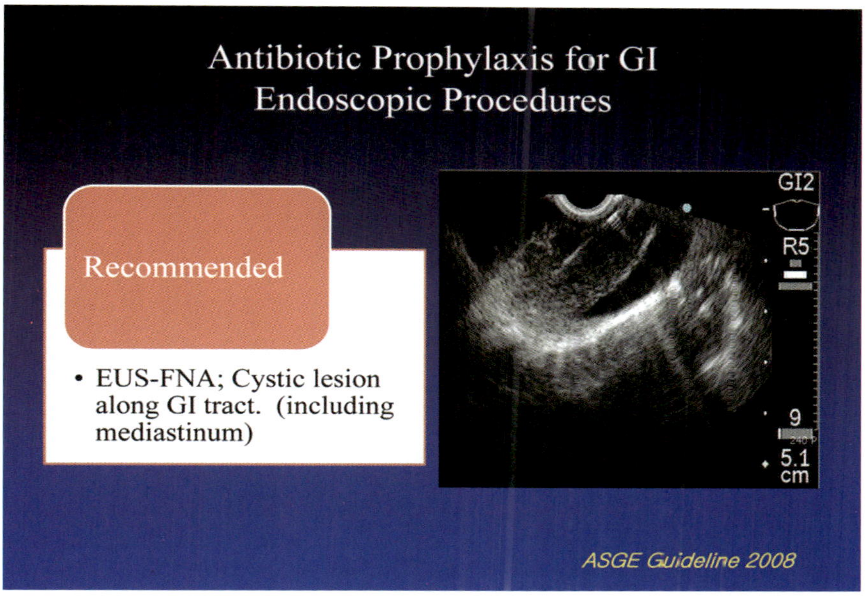

Antibiotic prophylaxis for GI endoscopic procedures is recommended for EUS-FNA of cystic lesions of the GI tract. (including the mediastinum)

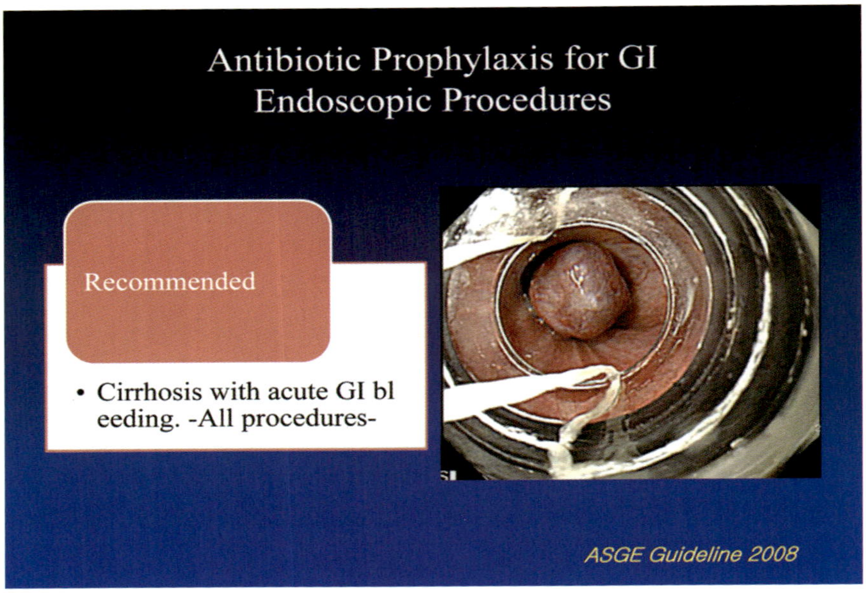

Antibiotic prophylaxis for GI endoscopic procedures is recommended for all GI prodedure in cirrhotic patients with acute GI bleeding.

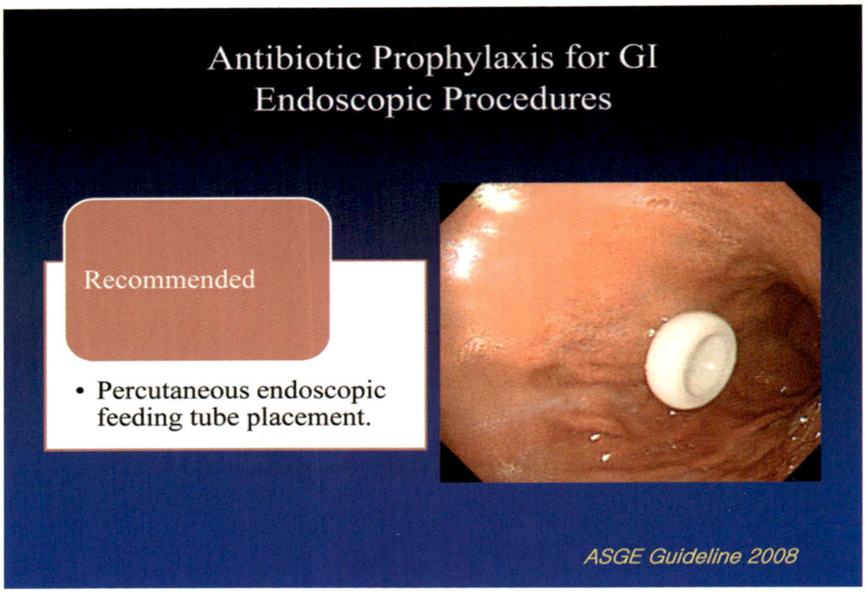

Antibiotic prophylaxis for GI endoscopic procedures is recommended for percutaneous endoscopic feeding tube placement.

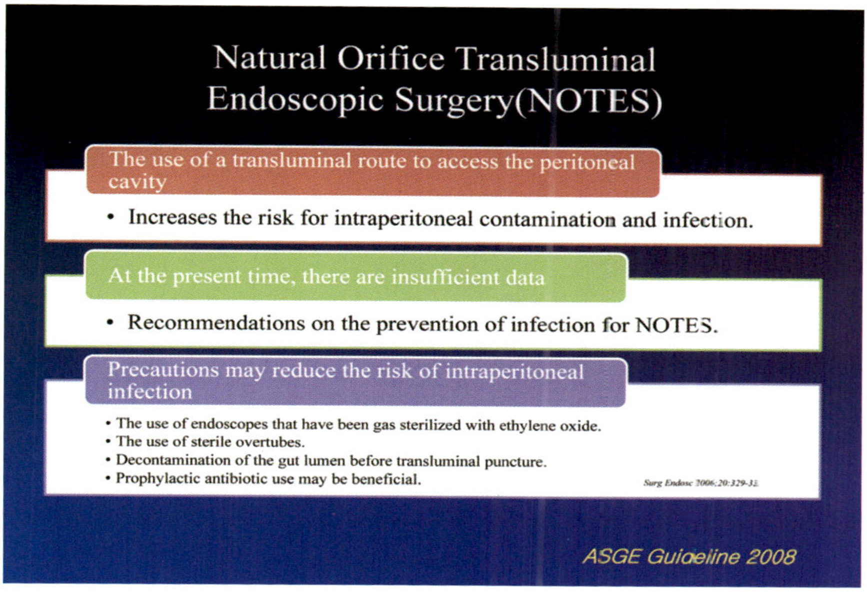

NOTES uses a transluminal route to access the peritoneal cavity which increases the risk for intraperitoneal contamination and infection. However at the present time, there is insufficient data to recommend a specific method for the prevention of infection.
The use of endoscopes that have been gas sterilized with ethylene oxide.
The use of sterile overtubes.
Decontamination of the gut lumen before transluminal puncture.
And the use of prophylactic antibiotic use may be beneficial.

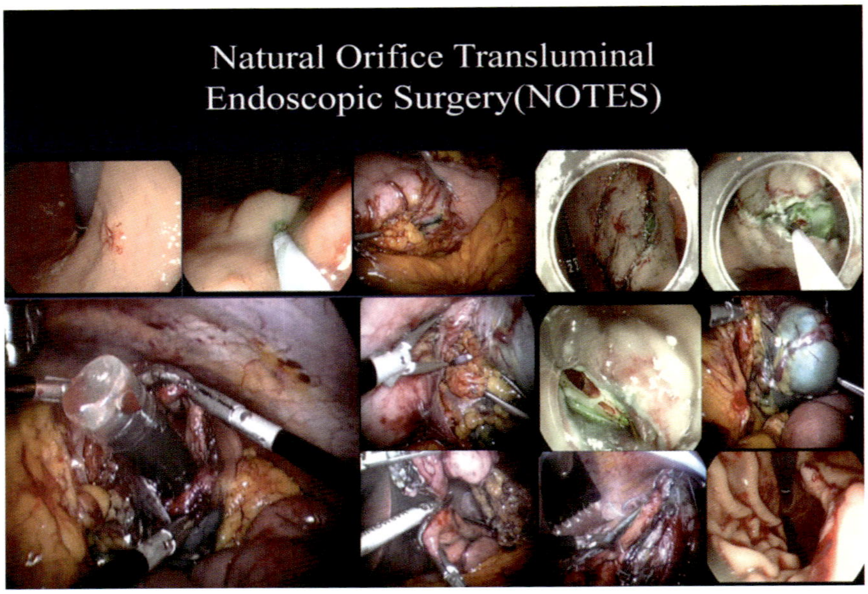

NOTES uses a transluminal route to access the peritoneal cavity which increases the risk for intraperitoneal contamination and infection. However at the present time, there is insufficient data to recommend a specific method for the prevention of infection.
The use of endoscopes that have been gas sterilized with ethylene oxide, The use of sterile overtubes. Decontamination of the gut lumen before transluminal puncture, And the use of prophylactic antibiotic use may be beneficial.

Transmission of Infection from Endoscopy Personnel to Patients

Small and task dependent

- Considered a low-risk task for such transmission.
- The lack of direct contact between the endoscopist and patients' tissues.
- No documented cases.

ASGE Guideline 2008

Transmission of Infection from patients to endoscopy personnel is small and task dependent
This is due to the lack of direct contact between the endoscopist and patients' tissues.

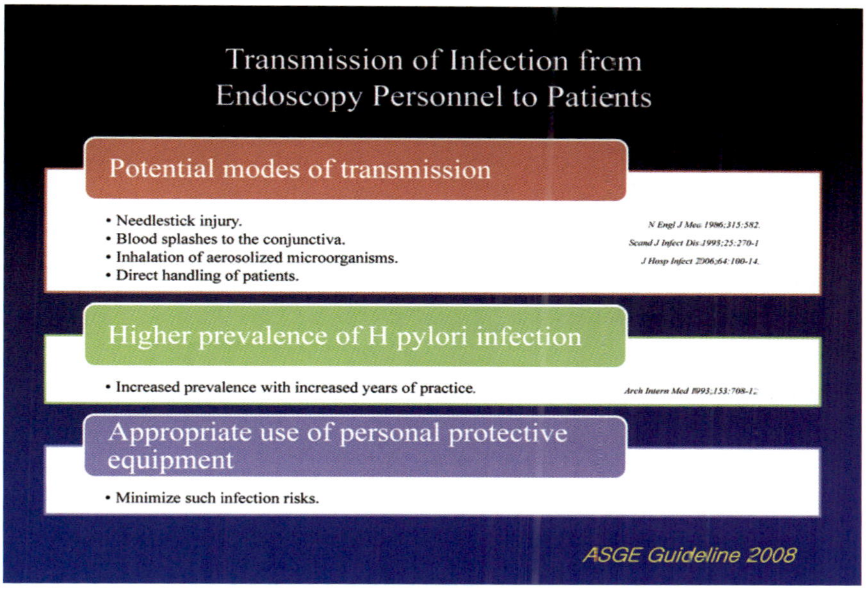

Potential modes of transmission are needle stick injury, blood splashed to the conjunctive, inhalation of aerosolized microorganisms and direct handling of patients.
Appropriate use of personal protective equipment minimizes infection risks.

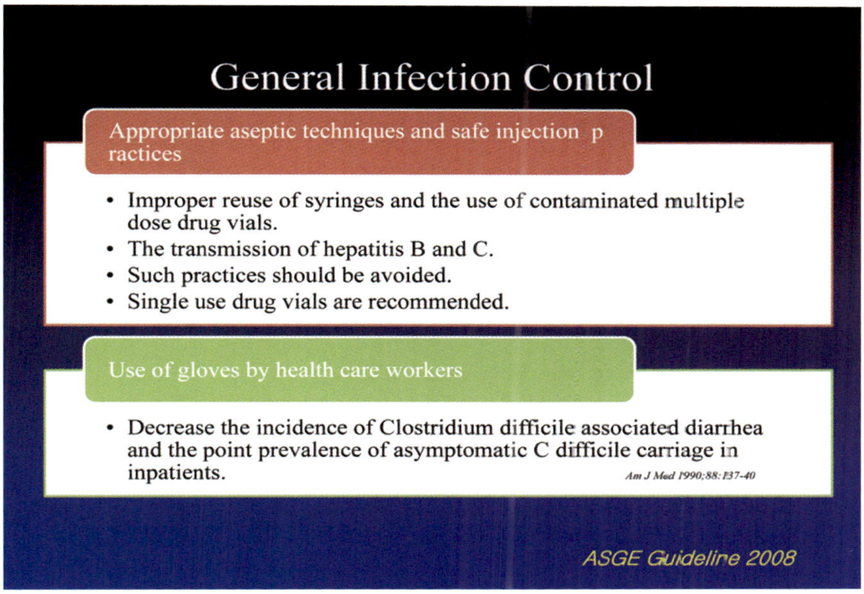

General infection control starts with appropriate aseptic techniques and safe injection practices
Use of gloves by health care workers is also important.

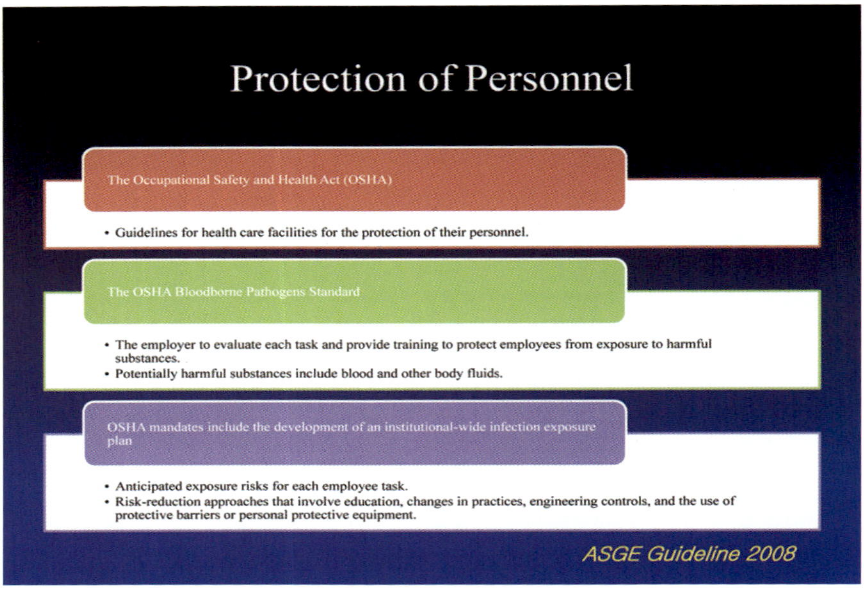

The Occupational Safety and Health Act (OSHA) Provides guidelines for health care facilities for the protection of their personnel. The employer is to evaluate each task and provide training to protect employees from exposure to harmful substances. OSHA mandates include the development of an institutional-wide infection exposure plan.

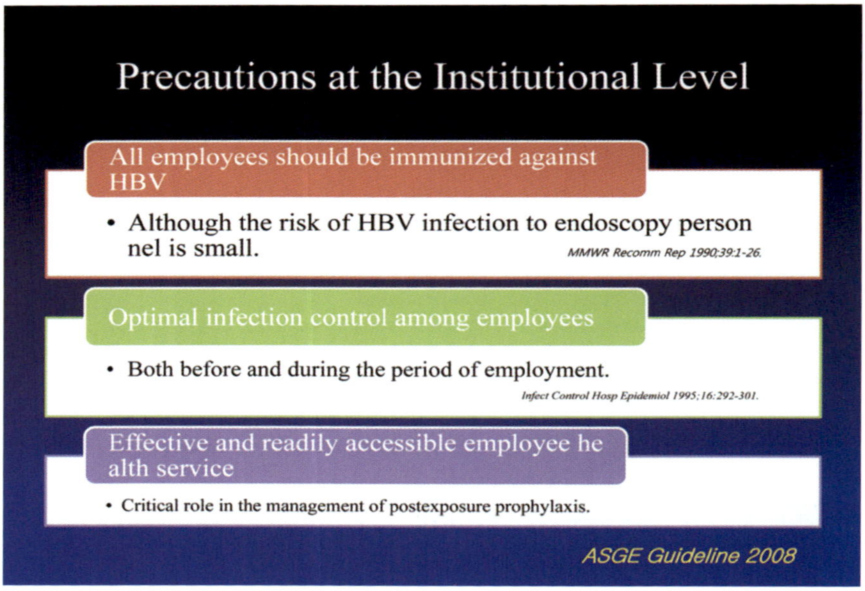

For institutions, all employees should be immunized against HBV. Optimal infection control among employees both before and during the period of employment and effective and readily accessible employee health service should be provided.

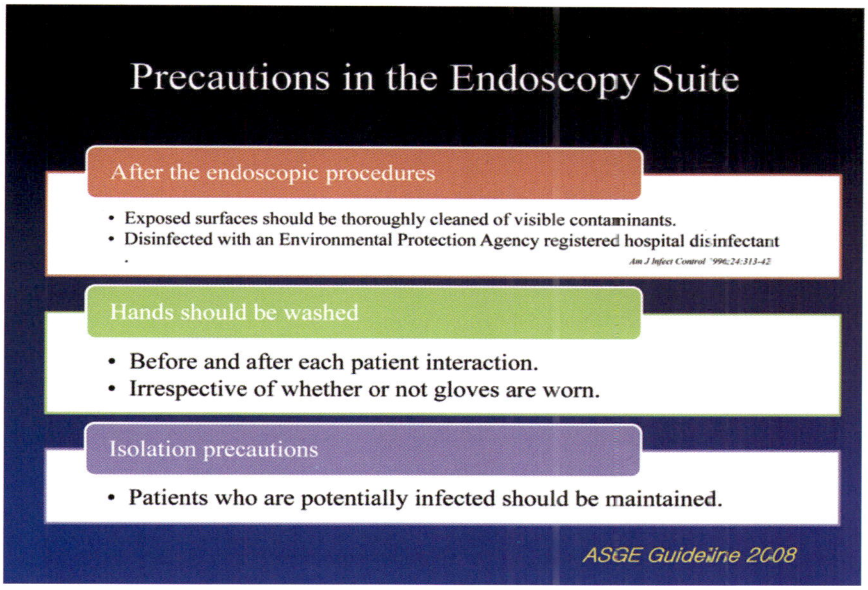

In the endoscopy suite following endoscopy exposed surfaces should be thoroughly cleaned of visible contaminants. hands should be frequently washed and isolation precaution should be taken.

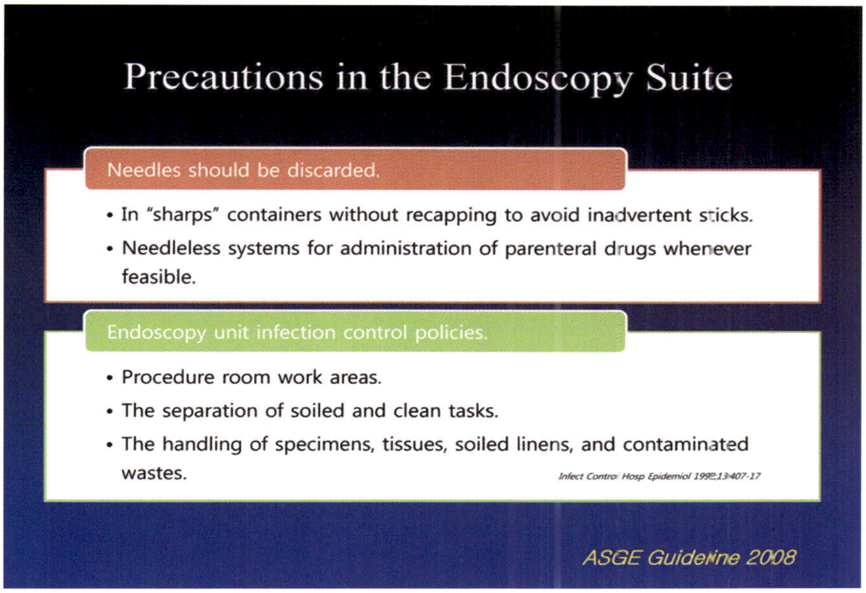

Following endoscopy, needles should be properly discarded and endoscopy unit infection control policies maintained.

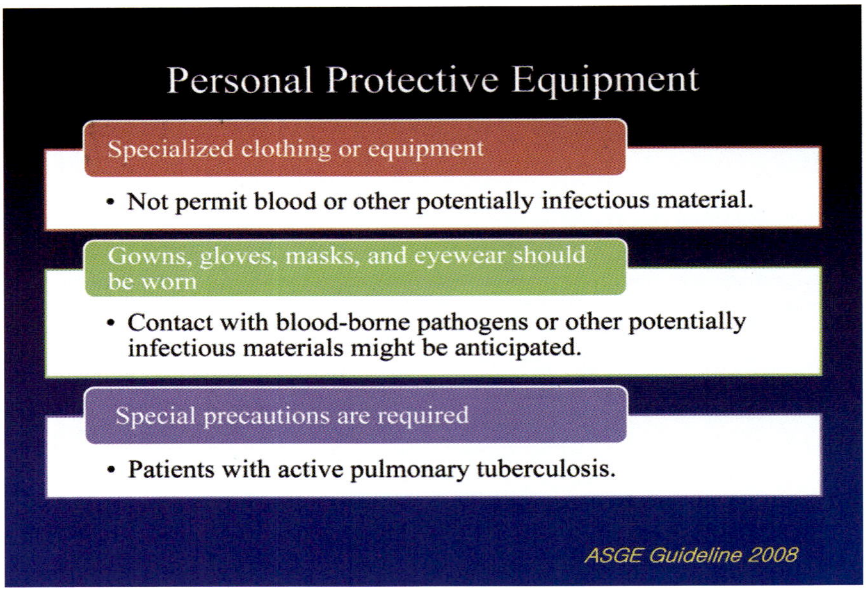

Personal Protective Equipment, including Gowns, gloves, masks, and eyewear should be worn Special precautions are required for patients with active pulmonary tuberculosis.

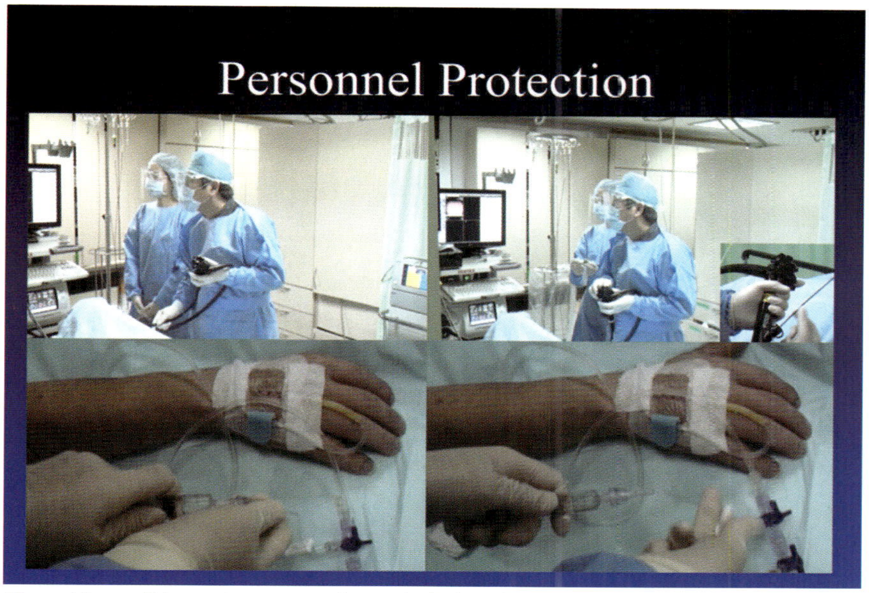

These pictures will demonstrate personnel protection in the endoscopy suite.
During the procedure, all accessories are hung on a hanger and covered with a protective sheath to minimize contamination.
The endoscopist and assistant are equipped with protective masks, facial shields and gowns to minimize contact of aerosolized and other contaminants.
During therapeutic endoscopy with the patient sedated, frequent injections may be required. A needleless injection may help prevent infection in this case.

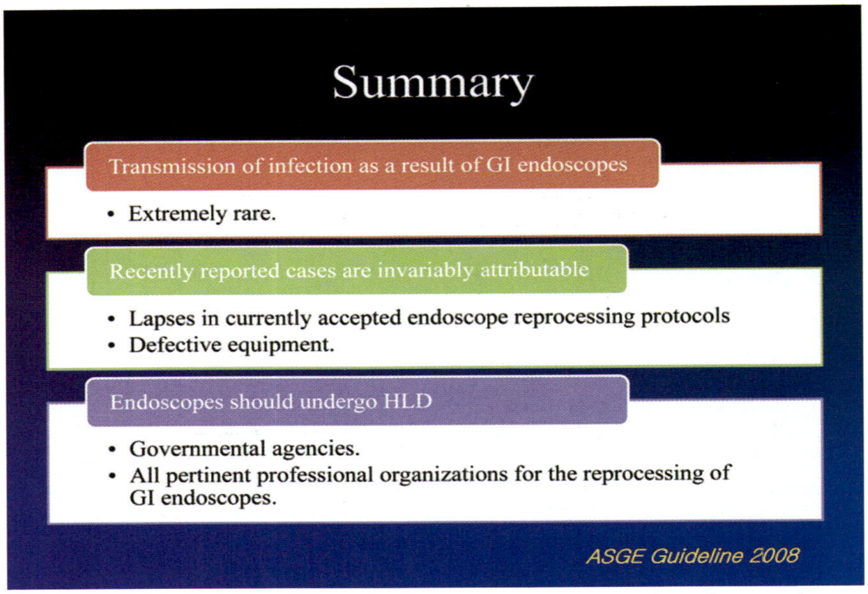

Transmission of infection as a result of GI endoscopes is extremely rare. Recently reported cases are mainly due to lapses in currently accepted endoscope reprocessing protocols and Defective equipment. Endoscopes should undergo HLD.

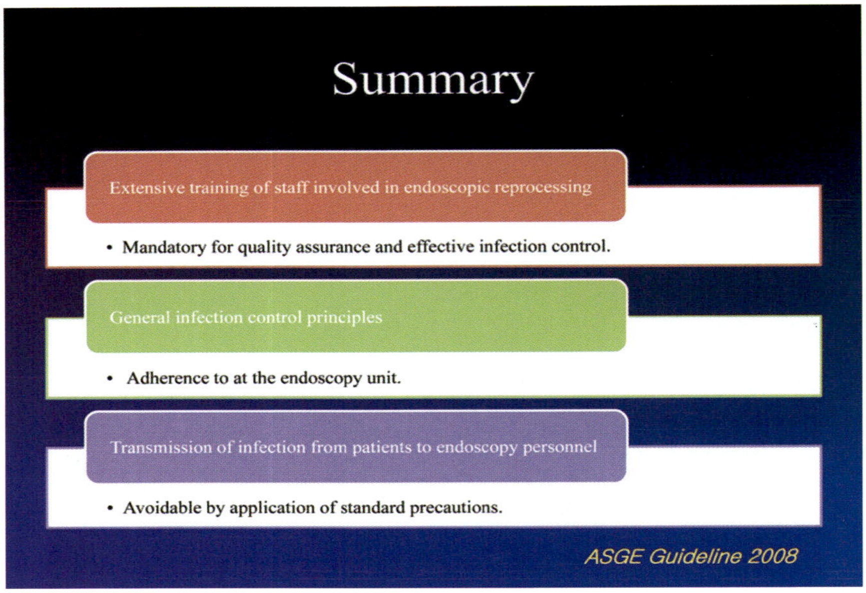

Extensive training of staff involved in endoscopic reprocessing is mandatory for quality assurance and effective infection control. General infection control principles should be adhered to at the endoscopy unit. Transmission of infection from patients to endoscopy personnel should be avoidable by application of standard precautions.

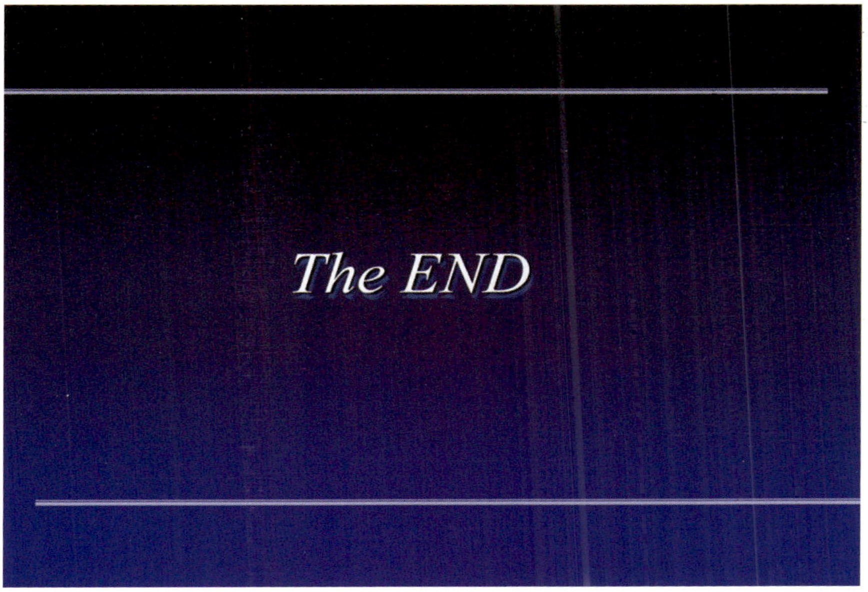
The END

Index

A

B

C

D

E

F

G

H

I

R

S

T

U

V

W

Z